Molecular Toxicology

Color figures and supplementary material for *Molecular Toxicology*, Second Edition, may be found at the companion website:

http://www.oup.com/us/MolTox2ed

Molecular Toxicology
Second Edition

P. DAVID JOSEPHY
BENGT MANNERVIK

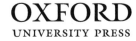

OXFORD
UNIVERSITY PRESS

2006

OXFORD
UNIVERSITY PRESS

Oxford University Press, Inc., publishes works that further
Oxford University's objective of excellence
in research, scholarship, and education.

Oxford   New York
Auckland   Cape Town   Dar es Salaam   Hong Kong   Karachi
Kuala Lumpur   Madrid   Melbourne   Mexico City   Nairobi
New Delhi   Shanghai   Taipei   Toronto

With offices in
Argentina   Austria   Brazil   Chile   Czech Republic   France   Greece
Guatemala   Hungary   Italy   Japan   Poland   Portugal   Singapore
South Korea   Switzerland   Thailand   Turkey   Ukraine   Vietnam

Copyright © 2006 by Oxford University Press, Inc.

Published by Oxford University Press, Inc.
198 Madison Avenue, New York, New York 10016

www.oup.com

Oxford is a registered trademark of Oxford University Press

Library of Congress Cataloging-in-Publication Data
Josephy, P. David.
Molecular toxicology/P. David Josephy, Bengt Mannervik—2nd ed.
    p. cm.
ISBN-13   978-0-19-517620-9
ISBN   0-19-517620-0
1. Molecular toxicology.   I. Mannervik, Bengt.   II. Title.
RA1220.3.J67   2005
615.9--dc22   2005011274

9 8 7 6 5 4 3 2 1

Printed in the United States of America
on acid-free paper

To the memory of our dear mothers:

Goldie Josephy, 1924–2002
Lisbeth Eriksson, 1917–1996

Preamble

$\triangleright$

The

Molecular

Basis

of

Toxicity

E very cell encounters toxic insults by molecules present in its environment or arising by chemical processes occurring intracellularly. In order to survive, protect its genetic material, and give rise to viable progeny, the cell relies on a wide range of biochemical processes for defense. These protective mechanisms include membrane-bound transporters, small molecules such as glutathione, enzymes for biotransformation and detoxication, and proteins effecting the repair of damaged macromolecules such as DNA. The toxic agent, X, may be exemplified by drugs, anticancer agents, environmental pollutants, and industrial chemicals. However, noxious molecules are also formed from natural cellular constituents, particularly through the chemistry of reactive oxygen species. The toxic molecule may eventually be eliminated, often in a modified form. Membrane transporters facilitate the exit of toxic agents and the products of their biotransformation. Enzymes catalyze the derivatization, oxidation, and conjugation of toxicants, and they effect the repair of damaged DNA. The cellular response to toxic insults also involves integrated biological processes, including the activation of signaling pathways, the regulation of gene expression and cell division, and programmed cell death (apoptosis). *Molecular Toxicology* unravels the key processes in this cellular drama, from the biochemical perspective. Many specific examples are given, but the cast has endless variations. The main emphasis of the book is to introduce molecular principles and the key biochemical players, and to foster a deeper understanding of the molecular basis of toxicology.

$\triangleright$

Acknowledgments, Second Edition

The authors gratefully acknowledge the contributions of the many individuals who have assisted us in preparing this second edition. Chantal Guillemette, Université Laval, Quebec, Canada, wrote the chapter on glucuronosyltransferases. Material for specific sections or "sidebars" was contributed by the following: Christine Ambrosone, Roswell Park Cancer Institute, Buffalo, New York (molecular epidemiology); Brenda L. Coomber, University of Guelph (apoptosis); Monique Cosman, Lawrence Livermore National Laboratory, Livermore, California (NMR structure determination of DNA adducts); Scott Grossman, Bristol-Myers Squibb Pharmaceutical Research Institute, Princeton, New Jersey (drug toxicity is not always due to a metabolite); Rosalie Elesperu, US Food and Drug Administration (human genetic diseases); Patrick E. Hanna, Medicinal Chemistry and Pharmacology, University of Minnesota and David Hein, Pharmacology and Toxicology, University of Louisville School of Medicine (NAT multiplicity); James Kirkland, University of Guelph (human nutrition and cancer); Larry Marnett, Vanderbilt University, Nashville, Tennessee (cyclic DNA adducts); Marcel Schlaf, University of Guelph (ligand field theory and P450 spin states); Frances Sharom, University of Guelph (MRP and Pgp proteins).

Each of the following experts helped the project greatly by reading a section or chapter and suggesting corrections and improvements: Fred Beland, National Center for Toxicological Research, Jefferson, Arkansas; Bruce Demple, Harvard University School of Public Health, Boston, Massachusetts; James S. Felton, Lawrence Livermore National Laboratory, Livermore, California; Hansruedi Glatt, Deutsches Institut für Ernährungsforschung, Potsdam, Germany; Denis M. Grant, University of Toronto, Canada; Jack A. Hinson, University of Arkansas for Medical Sciences, Little Rock, Arkansas; David J. Jollow, Medical University of South Carolina, Charleston, South Carolina; Jean McGowan-Jordan, Children's Hospital of Eastern Ontario, Ottawa, Canada; Iain Lambert, Carleton University, Ottawa, Canada; Edward L. LeCluyse, University of North Carolina, Chapel Hill, North Carolina; Ronald P. Mason, National Institute of Environmental Health Sciences, Research Triangle Park, North Carolina; David Phillips, Institute of Cancer Research, Sutton, Surrey, UK; Paul R. Ortiz de Montellano, University of California, San Francisco; Adrian Schwan, University of Guelph; Ingeborg Schmidt-Krey, Max-Planck-Institute of Biophysics, Frankfurt-am-Main, Germany. Tomas Hansson, Stockholm University, pointed out several errors in the first edition. Uwe Oehler, University of Guelph, provided expert computing assistance. Ylva Ivarsson, Carolina Orre, Sanela Kurtovic, Mikael Nilsson, and Johanna Mannervik assisted with the preparation of the figures.

We also thank the graduate students in the Josephy and Mannervik laboratories for additional proofreading and suggestions. Responsibility for the remaining errors is that of the primary authors.

Note: Protein and DNA structural figures for this edition were prepared on DS ViewerPro software from Accelrys Inc. (http://www.accelrys.com/dstudio/ds_viewer/).

$\triangleright$

Contents

Part Three Molecular Principles Applied to Specific Toxicants

Molecular Toxicology is a book devoted to the fundamental biochemical processes underlying the biotransformation and toxicity of chemical substances that cause damage to cells. The focus is mainly on mammalian cells. We consider a wide variety of toxic substances: endogenous metabolites, natural products (toxins), drugs, pesticides, persistent environmental pollutants, mutagens and carcinogens, industrial chemicals, and chemical warfare agents. The book is aimed at readers (whether students, researchers, physicians, or practicing pharmacologists/toxicologists) who are seeking a deeper understanding of the molecular basis of the discipline of toxicology.

We have deleted the preliminary discussion of elementary aspects of biochemistry and molecular biology that was given in the first edition. These topics (such as protein purification, DNA structure, and DNA sequencing) are by now sufficiently standard that any introductory textbook in biochemistry offers a satisfactory presentation, and we assume that the reader has already mastered this material.

We feel that the structure of the book has been substantially improved in this completely rewritten second edition. The first part is entitled Toxicity at the Cellular Level. We begin with a chapter on the toxicology of oxygen, describing the roles of enzyme systems in detoxifying reactive oxygen species. We examine specific biomolecular targets of toxic agents (whether endogenous or exogenous): lipids, protein, and DNA. Lipid peroxidation and the formation of covalent adducts to protein and DNA are precursors of cellular toxicity and serve as biomarkers of exposure. We discuss the chemistry of protein and DNA adduct formation and the experimental methods for detecting and identifying adducts. DNA is the indispensable macromolecule and so the repair of DNA damage is summarized. Next, the consequences of imperfect repair (or erroneous replication) of DNA are explained in chapters on the processes of mutagenesis and carcinogenesis. In presenting the science of oncogenes and tumor suppressors, our emphasis is on the analysis of these genes as molecular targets of mutagens, without attempting comprehensive coverage of the fields of signal transduction and cell-cycle control. Finally, we provide an elementary mathematical analysis of cell survival and the shape of dose–response curves, and ponder the biological implications of this "target theory" model of cellular life and death.

The second part is entitled Enzymology of Biotransformation. The cellular and organismal response to toxic agents (again, both endogenously generated, such as oxidants, and exogenous, such as drugs and pollutants) is largely determined by biotransformation. Metabolic processes mediated by families of enzymes transform the unlimited array of potentially toxic substances along more or less predictable pathways (figure I-1).

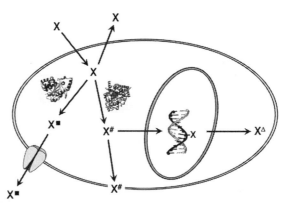

FIGURE I-1.

Overview of the cellular biotransformation of a foreign compound (xenobiotic, X). Following entry to the cell, X can either be eliminated, by passive diffusion or active transport, or be metabolized by intracellular enzymes. Conjugation reactions catalyzed by enzymes produce metabolites that are suitable for export via membrane-associated transport proteins (lower left). Other metabolic pathways generate reactive products, which facilitate their further metabolism, but may also promote reactions with DNA or other biological targets. The DNA adducts can lead to mutations, but excision of the adduct and reparative DNA synthesis counteract the genotoxicity. Many compounds of endogenous origin are metabolized in the same manner as are xenobiotics. *Note*: A full-color version of this figure appears on the website.

At the heart of the book, we concentrate on two key families of enzymes: the P450 monooxygenases, which catalyze oxidation of most drugs, pollutants, and carcinogens; and the glutathione transferases, which use the nonprotein sulfhydryl glutathione to trap reactive electrophiles. Transport proteins such as MRP and Pgp ship these glutathione adducts out of the cell. These enzyme families are examined in detail from multiple vantage points, including chemical mechanisms, substrate selectivity, protein structure, and the biology of their genetics and regulation. The receptors (such as AHR, PXR, and CAR) that mediate the transcriptional responses to xenobiotic exposure were mainly unknown at the time of the first edition, but are now presented as full members of the cast. Next, some of the enzymes that catalyze conjugation of nucleophilic sites (–OH, –COOH, $-NH_2$, etc.) on xenobiotics are considered: N-acetyltransferases, sulfotransferases, and glucuronosyltransferases. The toxicology of many classes of drugs, pollutants, and carcinogens is highlighted in this part of the book, including caffeine, nicotine, nitrosamines, aflatoxin (figure I-2), alkylating agents, and chlorinated aromatics.

In this presentation, we have broken free from the time-honored division of biotransformation reactions into "Phase 1" and "Phase 2" processes. In this classification, which dates back to the 1940s, "Phase 1" describes oxidation, reduction, and hydrolysis reactions, which can be regarded as "functionalization" processes, introducing hydroxyl groups or other functions into the substrate. "Phase 2" encompasses conjugation reactions, such as glucuronidation and sulfation, which yield water-soluble urinary metabolites. A recent textbook describes this classification as

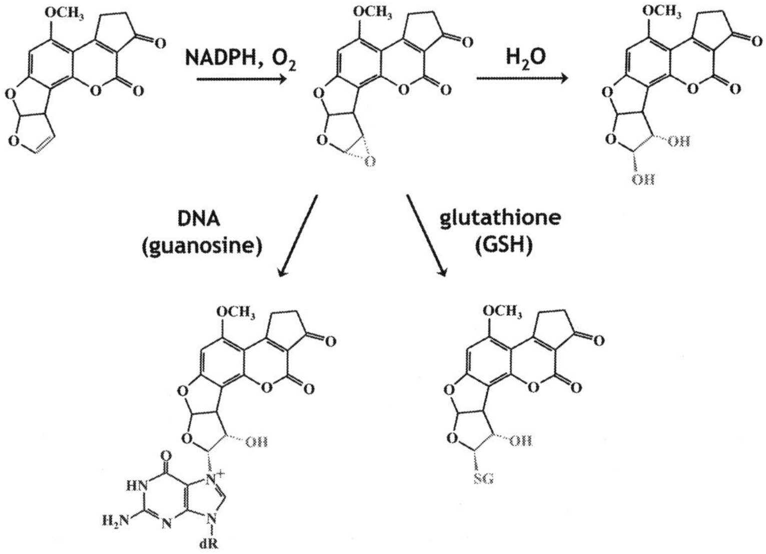

FIGURE I-2.
An example of biotransformation: aflatoxin B1 (AFB1). In humans, the mycotoxin AFB1 is a strong hepatocarcinogen, owing to a cytochrome P450-catalyzed monooxygenation leading to a reactive epoxide. The epoxide forms a promutagenic adduct with guanine in DNA, unless it is hydrolyzed to a diol (facilitated by membrane-bound epoxide hydrolase) or scavenged by glutathione (catalyzed by glutathione transferase). AFB1-exposed individuals lacking glutathione transferase M1-1 and simultaneously having high-risk genotypes of a single-strand DNA repair enzyme and epoxide hydrolase have a significantly increased risk of hepatocellular carcinoma. *Note*: A full-color version of this figure appears on the website. (*Kirk, G. D.; Turner, P. C.; Gong, Y.; Lesi, O. A.; Mendy, M.; Goedert, J. J.; Hall, A. J.; Whittle, H.; Hainaut, P.; Montesano, R.; Wild, C. P. Hepatocellular carcinoma and polymorphisms in carcinogen-metabolizing and DNA repair enzymes in a population with aflatoxin exposure and hepatitis B virus endemicity.* Cancer Epidemiol. Biomarkers Prev. **2005**, 14, *373–379*).

"simple and convenient," but we disagree. We believe that the distinction between "Phase 1" and "Phase 2" processes, which has no connection to the standard enzyme classification systems used in biochemistry, is antiquated. A useful classification system groups together things that are similar and distinguishes things that are different. Why, then, should we group oxidation and hydrolysis as "Phase 1"? Mechanistically, these reactions have nothing in common. The reaction that most resembles hydrolysis is glutathione conjugation: both processes entail the reaction of a xenobiotic electrophile with a cellular nucleophile (water or glutathione). And yet one classifies glutathione conjugation as a "Phase 2" reaction. The generalization that "Phase 1" enzymes introduce functional groups is also not valid; P450-catalyzed N-demethylation, for example, is the removal rather than the introduction of a functional group. Important processes of xenobiotic metabolism (such as transport of xenobiotic conjugates across membranes, mercapturic acid formation, and DNA nucleotide excision repair) fall outside the Phase 1/Phase 2 system altogether. Our approach is to treat each enzymatic biotransformation much as one treats the reactions of intermediary metabolism, in terms of their stoichiometry, enzyme structure and mechanism, substrate specificity, and so on, drawing parallels and grouping enzymes as indicated by their biochemical characteristics.

In the third part, Molecular Principles Applied to Specific Toxicants, we apply the molecular logic of the first two parts to some chemicals of special significance as toxic agents, including the analgesic drug acetaminophen, the nitrogen and sulfur mustards, antimalaria drugs, and two families of chemical carcinogens, polycyclic aromatic hydrocarbons and aromatic amines.

The emphasis of this book is on the molecular and cellular levels, rather than the tissue, organ, organismal, or medical aspects of toxicology. We have deliberately avoided organizing our discussion of toxic agents around such headings as "hepatotoxicants," "neurotoxicants," etc. The organ system-oriented approach to toxicology is adopted by several other textbooks. Our roadmap is scaled to the molecular level; off-ramps leading to higher levels of organization are signposted, but not necessarily followed very far. As we progress along this route, we allow several excursions and detours. Most of these are marked as sidebars. The sidebars (many of which were written by specialists) usually deal with specific toxic agents, techniques, or applications of the central ideas. We also include a few historical "roadside plaques" which commemorate some of the individuals who have greatly influenced the development of the science of molecular toxicology.

Part One

▷

Toxicity

at

the

Cellular

Level

Toxicology

of

Oxygen

MOLECULAR OXYGEN AND OXIDATION— REDUCTION BIOCHEMISTRY

Molecular oxygen is required for aerobic life but it is also a toxicant (*1*). Obligate anaerobes, found among many phyla of the bacterial kingdom, are killed by exposure to oxygen and thrive only in anoxic ecological niches (*2*). Even organisms that depend on oxygen for survival cannot tolerate excessive exposure to the gas. Mice maintained in a pure oxygen atmosphere die within one week, due to massive lung damage (*3*). Premature infants treated with supplementary oxygen can develop pathologies including chronic lung disease and retinopathy (*4*). Beyond such acute toxic effects, *molecular oxygen imposes a chronic toxic stress on all aerobic cells.* Oxidative stress contributes to many physiological mechanisms, including immune defense and cell signaling (*5*), and pathological processes, such as neurodegeneration (*6*), diabetes (*7*), cardiovascular disease (*8*), and aging (*9, 10*). Our focus is on the toxicological aspects of oxidative stress.

Life Before Oxygen

About 50 years ago, Stanley Miller showed that the discharge of electrical energy into an atmosphere of reduced gases, such as ammonia, methane, hydrogen, and water, yields complex mixtures of organic compounds, including amino acids and sugars (*11*). The prebiotic chemical synthesis that made possible the origin of life probably took place under conditions dominated by such reduced gases (possibly with the involvement of partially oxidized compounds such as carbon monoxide (*12*)) and driven by sunlight, lightning, or other geological sources of energy. Molecular oxygen did not appear until a much later epoch, following the evolution of photosynthetic cells. The atmosphere of the earth today is (as far as we know) unique in containing molecular oxygen (O_2) as one of its chief components. This store of molecular oxygen is a reservoir of free energy that is continuously consumed by the oxidation of organic molecules and replenished from solar energy and water via photosynthesis.

The transformation of the atmosphere from reductive to oxidative conditions presented a new opportunity for—but also a great threat to—all forms of life. Oxidation of organic compounds could be exploited for the release of free energy far in excess of that yielded by anaerobic (fermentative) processes, but only if this energy could be harnessed and stored in a biologically useable form. Uncontrolled oxidation threatened the integrity of biomolecules. The peculiar chemical properties of the oxygen molecule permitted the evolution of biochemical processes that could realize the thermodynamic opportunity, without succumbing to the thermodynamic threat: playing with fire without getting burned. Aerobic organisms became dominant while anaerobic organisms retreated to a few anoxic sanctuaries, such as the mammalian intestinal tract or deep within the soil.

Redox Potentials

As discussed in any introductory chemistry course, the relative strengths of oxidants and reductants are described by *redox potentials*, which correspond (according to the Nernst equation) to the Gibbs free energy changes of redox reactions. Redox potentials for some biochemical redox couples can be measured by electrochemistry; that is, we construct an appropriate half-cell, with the redox-active species in solution, and measure its electrical potential relative to a standard electrode. However, electron transfer between a protein and, say, a platinum wire electrode may be very sluggish. Electrochemical measurements may be made possible by addition of redox-active small molecules, such as methylene blue or methyl viologen, which can catalyze electron transfer between the electrode and the protein redox couple (e.g., (13)). Alternatively, we can avoid electrochemical methods altogether, by measuring the equilibrium constant for a redox reaction with a known couple (e.g., by spectrophotometric analysis of the concentrations of the redox-active species; (14)); $\Delta E_0'$ can then be calculated from $\Delta G^{\circ\prime}$, via the Nernst equation (15, p. 495).

Reduction of Molecular Oxygen

The complete reduction of molecular oxygen to water requires four electrons $(O_2 + 4H^+ + 4e^- \rightarrow 2H_2O)$ and has a very large positive redox potential. Consequently, the reduction of oxygen to water by almost any biochemical reductant is thermodynamically favorable. Molecular oxygen is one of very few homonuclear diatomic species that exist as *ground-state triplet* molecules: the two highest-energy electrons occupy degenerate molecular orbitals (antibonding π^* orbitals) and have parallel spins.[1] Therefore, the ground-state O_2 molecule has net electron spin $= 1$: oxygen is paramagnetic. (An excited singlet state of molecular oxygen lies 94 kJ/mol above the triplet ground state (16).) The reaction of paramagnetic O_2 with diamagnetic organic molecules is hindered by the difference in spin states. *Molecular oxygen combines two characteristics that are often incompatible: thermodynamic potency and kinetic stability.* The free energy available from the reduction of O_2 can be released if this spin restriction is overcome. This can occur at high temperatures (combustion); by interaction with enzymes, especially those bearing transition metal ions; or by the *univalent* reduction of oxygen (17), which proceeds via partially reduced intermediates:

$$O_2 + e^- \rightarrow O_2^{\bullet-} \quad \text{(superoxide anion)}$$

$$O_2^{\bullet-} + e^- + 2H^+ \rightarrow H_2O_2 \quad \text{(hydrogen peroxide)}$$

$$H_2O_2 + e^- \rightarrow {}^\bullet OH + OH^- \quad \text{(hydroxyl radical)}$$

$${}^\bullet OH + e^- + H^+ \rightarrow H_2O \quad \text{(water)}$$

The values of these one-electron redox potentials are shown in figure 1-1 (18). This diagram shows that the thermodynamic potential inherent in the reduction of molecular oxygen is released mainly in the final step: reduction of the hydroxyl radical. The hydroxyl radical is an extremely potent oxidant and a highly reactive species. By comparison, with respect to

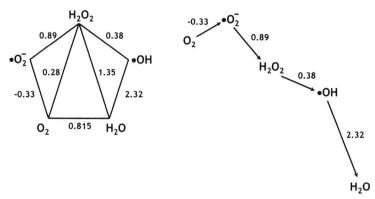

FIGURE 1-1.

Redox potentials (volts versus standard hydrogen electrode, pH 7) for the reduction of oxygen. (*Adapted from Hamilton, G. A. Mechanisms of biological oxidation reactions involving oxygen and reduced oxygen derivatives. In* Biological Oxidation Systems; *Reddy, C. C., Hamilton, G. A., Madyastha, K. M., Eds.; Academic Press: San Diego, 1990; Vol. I, pp. 3–15.*)

the reduction of oxygen to superoxide anion, oxygen is a rather poor oxidant; in fact, superoxide anion can reduce many biochemical couples, such as cytochrome c (*19*).

How are the redox potentials of reduced oxygen species measured experimentally? Hydrogen peroxide is a stable molecular species, so the redox potential for its reduction to water can be measured by electrochemistry. But superoxide anion and hydroxyl radical are unstable free radicals with very short lifetimes in aqueous solution. Special procedures are required to generate and study these species. The redox potential of superoxide can be measured by the use of *pulse radiolysis*. This technique (*20*) uses a brief (pico- to microsecond) burst of ionizing radiation from a linear accelerator to bombard a sample cell and generate radicals; the ensuing chemical reactions are monitored, usually by absorption spectrophotometry. A less reliable approach for evaluating redox potentials is to use data for gas-phase species, which are more stable and easier to study. However, it is then necessary to estimate hydration energies, to obtain values for the same species in solution.

The Roles of Pyridine and Flavin Coenzymes in Biochemistry

Pyridine and flavin cofactors (coenzymes) mediate most biochemical redox processes. The reduced forms of the pyridine cofactors NADH and NADPH are among the strongest reducing agents in the cell. The NADH/NAD$^+$ and NADPH/NADP$^+$ couples have almost identical redox potentials (-0.32 V) but play distinct roles in metabolism (very few enzymes can use them interchangeably). In most cases, NAD$^+$ is used in reactions that conserve respiratory energy for ATP generation via the electron transport chain, for example, glyceraldehyde-3-phosphate dehydrogenase (glycolysis) or β-hydroxyacyl-CoA dehydrogenase (β-oxidation of fatty acids). In contrast, NADPH provides reducing power for anabolic processes, for example, biosynthesis of fatty acids and steroids (*15*, p. 846).

Under typical cellular conditions, [NAD$^+$/NADH] is more abundant (about 1 mM) and mainly oxidized; [NADP$^+$/NADPH] is less abundant (about 0.1 mM) and mainly reduced. The maintenance of these two similar redox couples at very different redox poises—one mainly oxidized and the other mainly reduced—implies that the two couples are largely uncoupled from each other: exchange of reducing equivalents between the two systems is slow. This specialization of roles is essential, because cells must perform both oxidative (catabolic) and reductive (biosynthetic) tasks, simultaneously.

Pyridine cofactors are *freely diffusible substrates*, which can associate with/dissociate from the enzymes (e.g., dehydrogenases) that require them. In contrast, the flavin cofactors, $FAD/FADH_2$ and $FMN/FMNH_2$, are usually *prosthetic groups*, tightly bound to proteins to form *flavoenzymes*. The functional difference is that a coenzyme ($NAD^+/NADH$) is shuttled between different enzymes to complete a catalytic cycle, whereas a prosthetic group remains bound to the same protein during turnover. Since reduced nicotinamides are stronger reducing agents than reduced flavins, the path of electron flow in biological electron-transfer chains often goes from a nicotinamide-linked dehydrogenase to a flavoenzyme.

Flavoenzymes are versatile redox catalysts (*21*). If the apoprotein moiety of a flavoenzyme binds the reduced form of the flavin more tightly than the oxidized form, the protein stabilizes the *reduced* (bound) form, and the flavoenzyme will have a higher redox potential than the free flavin (the bound reduced form is a *weaker* reducing agent than the free reduced flavin). Conversely, if the protein stabilizes the *oxidized* (bound) form of the flavin more tightly, the flavoenzyme will have a lower redox potential than the free flavin (the bound reduced form is a *stronger* reducing agent than the free reduced flavin). Nature exploits the strong chemical interactions between protein and cofactor to "tune" the chemical behavior of the small molecule. Flavin coenzymes, unlike pyridine nucleotides, have relatively stable half-reduced (free radical) intermediates (figure 1-2); therefore, flavoenzymes are characteristically involved in one-electron transfer processes, such as the reduction of heme ferric iron in cytochromes.

Although the *direct* transfer of reducing equivalents from strong reductants (such as NADH) to strong oxidants (such as oxygen) is thermodynamically highly favorable, *nature always chooses a stepwise path*, via intermediate electron carriers: an *electron-transfer chain*. Why is this so? First, the direct route would release more free energy than can be stored in a chemical or chemiosmotic form. A heavy weight, lowered gradually, can be harnessed to do useful work (as in an old-fashioned clockworks); the same weight, allowed to drop freely, merely makes a crater when it hits the ground. Just as in this mechanical analogy, only the stepwise redox process can be controlled to meet changing metabolic requirements.

In the mitochondrial electron transport chain, NADH is produced by dehydrogenases in the mitochondrial matrix (e.g., the citric acid cycle enzymes isocitrate dehydrogenase and malate dehydrogenase). These reducing equivalents are passed on to the flavoenzyme *complex I*, then, via ubiquinone and cytochrome c, to oxygen. In the erythrocyte methemoglobin reductase system, reducing equivalents are passed from NADH to a flavoenzyme, cytochrome b_5 reductase, then to cytochrome b_5, and finally to (ferric) methemoglobin (*22*). A membrane-bound form of this chain drives the unsaturation of fatty acids in the fatty acyl-CoA desaturase system of the hepatic endoplasmic reticulum (*23*). In the microsomal

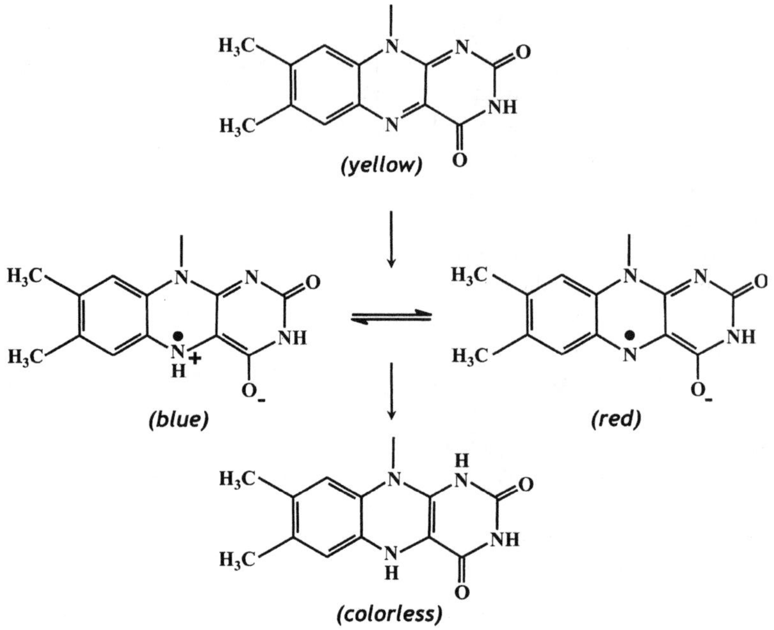

FIGURE 1-2.

Reduction of flavin nucleotides (FMN, FAD) via a radical intermediate. Two protonation states of the radical (neutral, anion) are shown; additional resonance structures can also be drawn. Only the dimethylisoalloxazine ring structure of the cofactor is shown.

cytochrome P450 system (chapter 7), electrons are passed from NADPH, via the flavoenzyme NADPH-cytochrome P450 reductase, to cytochrome P450.

Oxidation Mechanisms

From the time of Carl Wilhelm Scheele and Joseph Priestley, who discovered oxygen in the late 18th century, oxidation was understood to be a fundamental process for life: a mouse deprived of oxygen soon died. With the rise of quantitative experimental enzymology in the early 20th century, it became clear that biochemical oxidations could continue (albeit to a limited extent) even in anaerobic tissue extracts. Hence, the ultimate oxidant in such processes could not be oxygen itself. Heinrich Wieland (Nobel Prize in Chemistry, 1927) proposed, in the 1930s, that *enzymatic redox reactions involve transhydrogenations* (transfer of H^- equivalents) between organic donors (MH_2) and acceptors (*24*). The cofactors NAD^+, $NADP^+$, FMN, and FAD are the most important oxidizing agents in the reactions of intermediary metabolism. The Krebs (citric acid) cycle couples the complete oxidation of acetic acid (the product of carbohydrate and lipid catabolism) to carbon dioxide, with the stepwise generation of reduced cofactors, NADH and $FADH_2$. The β-oxidation of fatty acids proceeds by analogous biochemical steps. These oxidations are catalyzed by dehydrogenases:

$$MH_2 + Cofactor \rightarrow M + Cofactor \cdot H_2$$

The resulting reducing equivalents are subsequently reoxidized by the by respiratory electron-transport chains, using (in most cases) oxygen as the ultimate electron acceptor. This process provides the great majority of the energy yielded by aerobic catabolism. The direct involvement of oxygen in the catabolism of sugars and lipids is limited to a single important enzymatic reaction: the reduction of oxygen to water, at the final stage of the respiratory electron-transport chain. In the mitochondrion, this reaction is catalyzed by *cytochrome oxidase*. (We apply the term *oxidase* to any enzyme that catalyzes the reduction of molecular oxygen.)

The organization of the electron transport chain in the mitochondrial inner membrane allows the thermodynamically favorable flow of electrons (reducing equivalents) from reduced cofactors, through intermediary electron carriers, to oxygen, to be coupled to the vectorial transport of protons across the membrane. This transport establishes an electrochemical gradient and stores the free energy generated by the electron transport chain. Oxidative phosphorylation is driven by the return flow of protons across the membrane, down the electrochemical gradient (chemiosmotic energy transduction).

HYDROGEN PEROXIDE AND ITS DETOXICATION

Hydrogen peroxide was first prepared by the French chemist Louis-Jacques Thénard in 1818. Thénard soon noted the characteristic bubbling of hydrogen peroxide solutions in the presence of animal tissues, due to the evolution of oxygen gas. (His observation preceded, by many decades, the development of the enzyme concept.) The reaction that produces the oxygen is:

$$H_2O_2 + H_2O_2 \rightarrow 2H_2O + O_2$$

and the enzyme that catalyzes this reaction is called *catalase* (hydrogen peroxide: hydrogen peroxide oxidoreductase, EC 1.11.1.6; (*25*)). An early hypothesis held that hydrogen peroxide decomposition was a universal catalytic property of enzymes; this idea, while incorrect, accounts for the peculiar name of the enzyme. In nucleated eukaryotic cells, catalase is found in specialized organelles called *peroxisomes* (see sidebar).

Hydrogen peroxide can arise in the cell either directly (e.g., peroxisomal oxidase activities; see sidebar) or indirectly via the dismutation of superoxide (particularly as a byproduct of respiration), as discussed later in the chapter (*26, 27*). Hydrogen peroxide is a reactive oxidant that can pass through membranes readily, allowing it to diffuse between cellular compartments or between cells in a tissue. In addition to its toxic effects, hydrogen peroxide acts as a "second messenger" molecule that activates specific signal transduction pathways (*28*). Enzymes that catalyze hydrogen peroxide decomposition are ubiquitous in aerobic organisms.

Peroxidases (EC 1.11.1) are a second family of enzymes that catalyze hydrogen peroxide decomposition, according to the stoichiometry:

$$H_2O_2 + AH_2 \rightarrow 2H_2O + A$$

Hydrogen peroxide acts as both the oxidant and the reductant in the catalase-catalyzed reaction, whereas peroxidases use hydrogen peroxide

▶ **Peroxisomes**

Peroxisomes are organelles present in all nucleated eukaryotic cells (*29*). Like mitochondria, peroxisomes specialize in oxidative metabolic processes. Fatty acid β-oxidation occurs in both peroxisomes and mitochondria of mammalian cells. However, in contrast to mitochondria, peroxisomes are bounded by a single lipid bilayer membrane and do not produce ATP by chemiosmotic coupling. Peroxisomal oxidases (such as fatty acyl CoA oxidase, urate oxidase, and amino acid oxidase (*30*)) consume a substantial fraction of cellular oxygen (perhaps 20%), while reducing molecular oxygen to hydrogen peroxide. Peroxisomal catalase-catalyzed decomposition limits the release of this hydrogen peroxide into the cell (*31, 32*). (Chemical agents that induce the proliferation of hepatic peroxisomes, known as "peroxisome proliferators," are discussed in chapter 8.) ◀

to oxidize other organic or inorganic substrates. The term *hydroperoxidase* refers collectively to peroxidases and catalase.

Catalase

Mammalian catalase is a homotetrameric protein, with native molecular mass of 240 kDa. Each subunit has one heme group and one bound molecule of NADPH (*33, 34*). In fact, catalase is the major reservoir for erythrocyte NADPH. Catalase is found in erythrocyte cytosol; in liver and other tissues, the enzyme is localized in peroxisomes (*35*), reflecting the production of hydrogen peroxide by oxidases in these organelles. (In fact, catalase is typically used as a marker enzyme for detecting peroxisomes.)

Peroxidases

Mammals produce many peroxidase enzymes, each of which has unique characteristics, in terms of structure, expression patterns, substrate specificity, and biological role. Myeloperoxidase, lactoperoxidase, and eosinophil peroxidase comprise a family of human peroxidase enzymes, closely related in terms of DNA and amino acid sequence (*36*). Myeloperoxidase is discussed in detail later in the chapter, in connection with the respiratory burst.

Prostaglandin H synthase is the enzyme that catalyzes the first step in the biosynthesis of *prostaglandins* from polyunsaturated fatty acids. Prostaglandins are potent short-lived intercellular messengers that regulate vasoconstriction/vasodilatation, platelet aggregation, inflammation, and other physiological responses. This enzyme protein has two distinct activities: cyclooxygenase (conversion of arachidonic acid to PGG_2) and peroxidase (reduction of PGG_2 hydroperoxide to PGH_2 alcohol) (figure 1-3). Prostaglandin H synthase is an unusual peroxidase: the enzyme generates its own peroxide substrate, via the cyclooxygenase step, an enzyme-catalyzed lipid peroxidation reaction (see later discussion). Prostaglandin H synthase activity is found in many important target organs for chemical carcinogenesis, including the lung, kidney, skin, and bladder. The peroxidase activity of prostaglandin H synthase oxidizes many xenobiotic substrates, including aromatic amines and polycyclic aromatic hydrocarbons, to reactive intermediates (*37, 38*).

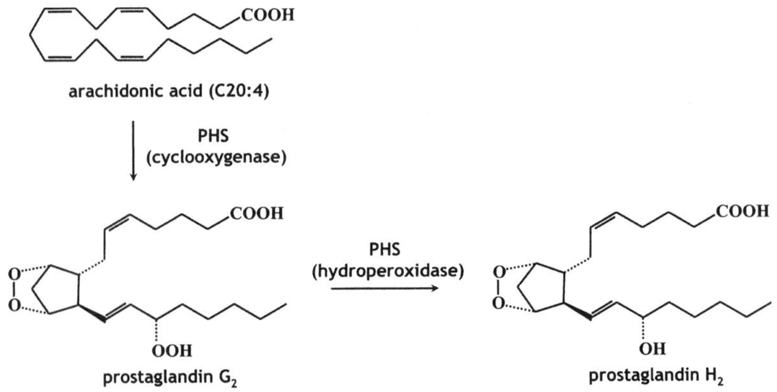

arachidonic acid (C20:4)

PHS
(cyclooxygenase)

prostaglandin G₂

PHS
(hydroperoxidase)

prostaglandin H₂

FIGURE 1-3.
Reactions catalyzed by prostaglandin H synthase.

Reaction Cycles of Catalase and Peroxidases

Beginning in the 1940s, Britton Chance (*39*) and his colleagues at the University of Pennsylvania applied the technique of fast-flow optical spectrophotometry to study the formation and decay of intermediates in the reaction cycles of catalase and peroxidases (*40, 41*). (These investigations were among the first studies to apply rapid-kinetics techniques to enzymes and characterize enzyme–substrate complexes.) The native state of catalase contains ferric (Fe^{3+}) heme. Chance identified a short-lived oxidized intermediate form of the enzyme, which he named "Compound I":

$$\text{Catalase} (Fe^{+3}) + H_2O_2 \rightarrow \text{Catalase Compound I} (Fe^{+5}O^{2-}) + H_2O$$
$$\text{Catalase Compound I} + H_2O_2 \rightarrow \text{Catalase} (Fe^{+3}) + O_2 + H_2O$$

The reaction cycle of peroxidases also begins with Compound I formation. However, with most organic reducing substrates, return to the resting (ferric) enzyme state occurs via one-electron steps; the half-oxidized enzyme state is known as Compound II, and has also been identified by optical spectroscopy:

$$\text{Peroxidase} (Fe^{+3}) + H_2O_2$$
$$\rightarrow \text{Peroxidase Compound I} (Fe^{+5}O^{2-}) + H_2O$$
$$\text{Peroxidase Compound I} (Fe^{+5}O^{2-}) + RH_2$$
$$\rightarrow \text{Peroxidase Compound II} (Fe^{+4}) + RH^{\bullet} + OH^{-}$$
$$\text{Peroxidase Compound II} (Fe^{+4}) + RH_2$$
$$\rightarrow \text{Peroxidase} (Fe^{+3}) + RH^{\bullet} + H^{+}$$
$$\text{Net: } H_2O_2 + 2RH_2 \rightarrow 2H_2O + 2RH^{\bullet}$$

The organic substrate is oxidized to a free radical. Substrate-derived radicals formed by peroxidases were first detected in 1960 by Isao Yamazaki and colleagues (*42*), using electron paramagnetic resonance (see below). Peroxidases can oxidize a wide variety of substrates, including ascorbate, hydroquinones, aminophenols, aromatic amines and diamines, and poly-cyclic aromatic hydrocarbons. These oxidations can generate toxic reactive intermediates (*43*), and human peroxidases, such as myeloperoxidase and prostaglandin H synthase, participate in metabolic activation of carcinogens (*44*).

Compound I, formed upon interaction of ferric catalase or peroxidase with hydrogen peroxide, represents a highly oxidized state of the protein active site. In the preceding equations, we have represented Compound I, for simplicity, by writing the nominal oxidation state Fe^{+5}. Spectroscopic and crystallographic studies (*45*) have shown that the heme iron in Compound I is oxy-ferryl (Fe^{+4}–O), with an additional oxidizing equivalent present as either a porphyrin π-cation radical (e.g., horseradish peroxidase) or a protein radical localized on an amino acid side chain near the heme (tryptophan, in the yeast mitochondrial enzyme cytochrome c peroxidase). The structure of Compound I also provides a model for the structure of the cytochrome P450 hydroxylating intermediate, which has a far shorter lifetime (see chapter 7).

Acatalasemia

The physiological importance of catalase is highlighted by an inborn error of metabolism: acatalasemia (46). This condition was discovered by an otolaryngologist at Okayama University Medical School, Shigeo Takahara, and is also known as Takahara's disease. Takahara routinely applied hydrogen peroxide solution as an antiseptic during oral surgery. One day in 1946, he undertook surgery on a girl suffering from oral gangrene. When he applied hydrogen peroxide to the wound, he was astonished to observe the patient's gums turning brown-black. Upon investigation, blood samples from four of the seven siblings in the family showed the same peculiar reaction to hydrogen peroxide and failed to "fizz" from the evolution of oxygen. Acatalasemia is an extremely rare condition. The oral gangrene that led to the discovery of acatalasemia is a common symptom. The lesions apparently result from the effects of hydrogen peroxide production by the metabolic action of bacteria, such as streptococcus, normally found on the gums. Aside from this, however, acatalasemic individuals get along normally and live full lifespans.

SUPEROXIDE AND SUPEROXIDE DISMUTASE

The scientific breakthrough that marks the beginning of the modern era of oxygen toxicology was the discovery of the enzyme superoxide dismutase in 1968. This discovery has had profound consequences for biochemistry and toxicology that could hardly have been envisaged at its beginnings, providing a fine illustration of the unexpected benefits of research driven purely by scientific curiosity (47–49).

Xanthine Oxidase

The purine nucleosides adenosine and guanosine are catabolized by convergent metabolic pathways. AMP is metabolized to hypoxanthine, GMP to xanthine (figure 1-4). Both of these purines are then converted into uric acid: hypoxanthine in two steps and xanthine in one. A single enzyme, xanthine oxidase, catalyzes the oxidation of hypoxanthine to xanthine, and of xanthine to uric acid, in the presence of oxygen.

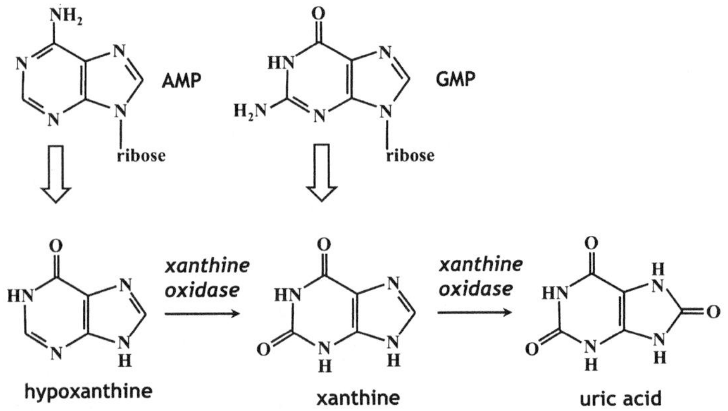

FIGURE 1-4.
The catabolism of purine nucleotides; oxidation of xanthine to uric acid catalyzed by xanthine oxidase.

▶ Uric Acid

Primates excrete uric acid (derived from nucleic acid turnover or dietary purines) in the urine. As suggested by Bruce Ames, the high levels of uric acid in human serum may serve an antioxidant role (50). For example, urate effectively inhibits protein tyrosine nitration by peroxynitrite, a reactive oxidant formed from the reaction of superoxide with nitric oxide (see later) (51). Uric acid is poorly soluble in water, and the deposition of uric acid crystals in the joints and kidney causes a painful condition called *gout*.

> A man can no more separate age and covetousness than he can part young limbs and lechery: but the gout galls the one and the pox pinches the other ...

> Falstaff, *King Henry IV, Part 2*; Act 1, Scene 2

Gout has been regarded as a "rich man's disease," associated with over-indulgence in fine food and wine. Today, followers of Falstaff have recourse to pharmacology: gout can be treated with *allopurinol*, a xanthine oxidase inhibitor (52). ◀

Xanthine oxidase (EC 1.2.3.2) is a flavoenzyme that contains molybdenum and four iron–sulfur centers (53). The enzyme can be isolated from milk (54), where it contributes to antibacterial activity (55). The transformation of hypoxanthine to xanthine is, stoichiometrically, a hydroxylation, followed by tautomerization from the enol to the keto form of the product. We can write a balanced equation:

$$\text{Hypoxanthine} + H_2O + O_2 \rightarrow \text{hypoxanthine} - OH + H_2O_2$$

and, indeed, hydrogen peroxide is produced by the xanthine/xanthine oxidase/O_2 or hypoxanthine/xanthine oxidase/O_2 systems. Oxidants other than oxygen, including $NADP^+$ (xanthine dehydrogenase activity) or organic nitro compounds, can drive the reaction. These alternative oxidants are, of course, reduced in the reaction. In 1949 Horecker and Heppel, investigating the ability of the xanthine/xanthine oxidase system to reduce such substrates, discovered that oxidized cytochrome c was reduced from the ferric to the ferrous form (56). But ferric cytochrome c could not replace oxygen in the reaction, so the reduction could not be a simple redox reaction between cytochrome c and xanthine. Apparently, the xanthine/xanthine oxidase/oxygen system was generating an unidentified reducing agent, which in turn could reduce cytochrome c. Irwin Fridovich (57) guessed that this reductant could be the superoxide radical, the one-electron reduction product of dioxygen. The concept of the superoxide radical as a chemical species had been developed by Linus Pauling (recipient of the 1954 Nobel Prize in Chemistry); see sidebar. But the possible involvement of superoxide in biological systems had been considered only in the context of ionizing radiation effects (see sidebar). The idea that an enzymatic reaction might produce superoxide, an unstable free radical, seemed extravagant, and Fridovich and Philip Handler speculated that an enzyme-bound form of superoxide might be formed.

Reports on the ability of cytochrome c to accept electrons from the xanthine/xanthine oxidase system were inconsistent, and Fridovich surmised that the irreproducibility of the results might be due to the varying purity of the cytochrome c preparations that had been used by different research groups. Perhaps an inhibitor of the reaction had been present in some of the preparations. Indeed, first myoglobin and then carbonic anhydrase, erythrocyte proteins that might well contaminate cytochrome c preparations, were found to be inhibitors of cytochrome c reduction (58).

▶ Potassium Superoxide

Since the 19th century, chemists were acquainted with a solid compound, formed by the high-temperature combustion of potassium, which was described by the formula K_2O_4 and called potassium tetroxide (59). When this substance is dissolved in water, it yields hydrogen peroxide and oxygen, following the stoichiometry:

$$K_2O_4 + 2H_2O \rightarrow O_2 + H_2O_2 + 2KOH$$

as determined by Harcourt in 1861 (60). Linus Pauling (61, 62) recognized that the textbook formula K_2O_4 might be an incorrect representation of the structure of this material:

> I knew that when potassium, rubidium and cesium burn in oxygen, higher oxides are formed which were called tetroxides ... in the reference books of inorganic chemistry. I also knew that the tetroxide ion, with the presumable structure of a chain containing three single oxygen–oxygen bonds, would be unstable ... It seemed likely, accordingly, that these substances ... in fact ... contain ... a unipositive alkali ion and the anion $O_2^{\bullet-}$. A test of this hypothesis could be made by measuring the magnetic susceptibility of the substances, because the tetroxides would be diamagnetic and the compounds MO_2, containing an anion with an odd number of electrons, would have the paramagnetism corresponding to one unpaired electron spin. I accordingly asked a postdoctoral fellow working with me, Edward W. Neuman, to prepare a sample of this oxide of potassium and to measure its magnetic susceptibility. He ... found the magnetic susceptibility to be that corresponding to an odd electron for every pair of oxygen atoms ... On 22 April 1933 in Berkeley ... I announced that Neuman had found the higher oxide of potassium to be paramagnetic ... I pointed out that KO_2 should not be called potassium dioxide, because the term dioxide is usually reserved for compounds of quadrivalent metals, as in PbO_2, lead dioxide ... Professor E.D. Eastman and Professor W.C. Bray ... suggested that the substance be called *potassium superoxide*, with the radical $O_2^{\bullet-}$ called the ... *superoxide radical*. I accepted this suggestion, and Dr. Neuman then published his paper ... with the title "Potassium Superoxide and the Three-Electron Bond." ◀

▶ Radiolysis of Water

The damaging effects of ionizing radiation on biological systems can be divided into two chemical mechanisms: *direct* damage results from the interaction of radiation with critical biological target molecules, such as DNA and protein; *indirect* damage is due to the effects of reactive species generated by radiolysis of water. Since water is by far the most common molecule in the cell, and since there are no radiation "chromophores," most of the absorbed radiation energy is absorbed by water, and indirect damage is probably a greater contributor to radiation effects than direct damage.

The interaction of ionizing radiation with water (63) generates energetic electrons and strips electrons from water molecules. The electrons rapidly become hydrated:

$$e^- + nH_2O \rightarrow e_{aq}^-$$

and then protonated:

$$e_{aq}^- + H_2O \rightarrow H^{\bullet} + OH^-$$

The water cation radicals yield hydroxyl radicals:

$$H_2O^{\bullet+} + H_2O \rightarrow {}^{\bullet}OH + H_3O^+$$

Thus, $H^{\bullet}$, ${}^{\bullet}OH$, and hydrated electrons, e_{aq}^-, are the major transient products of water, and comprise both oxidizing and reducing radicals. These radicals can recombine to give water, interact with one another to give H_2 and H_2O_2, or react with solutes.

In aerobic aqueous solutions, the reducing radicals (hydrated electron and hydrogen atom) can reduce molecular oxygen:

$$O_2 + e_{aq}^- \rightarrow O_2^{\bullet-} \; ; O_2 + H^{\bullet} \rightarrow HO_2^{\bullet}$$

yielding superoxide and *perhydroxyl radical*, respectively.

For experimental studies, it is often desirable to limit the radiation products to only one major product, so that its chemistry can be studied without interference by competing reactions. To produce a purely oxidizing system, nitrous oxide is useful:

$$e_{aq}^- + N_2O + H_2O \rightarrow N_2 + \, ^{\bullet}OH + OH^-$$

To generate superoxide alone, formate is added. Formate scavenges $^{\bullet}OH$, a potent oxidant, and the resulting anion radical, in turn, reduces oxygen:

$$^{\bullet}OH + HCO_2^- \rightarrow CO_2^{\bullet -} + H_2O; \; CO_2^{\bullet -} + O_2 \rightarrow CO_2 + O_2^{\bullet -}$$

In 1968 Joe McCord, a graduate student studying with Fridovich, set out to measure the binding of carbonic anhydrase to xanthine oxidase, reasoning that such binding must be the cause of the inhibitory effect. When these attempts came to nothing, he suddenly realized that the *real* inhibitor might not be carbonic anhydrase, myoglobin, or cytochrome c, but some other erythrocyte protein that had contaminated all of those preparations. An assay for this mysterious inhibitor was, of course, already at hand: inhibition of the xanthine/xanthine oxidase-catalyzed reduction of cytochrome c. So McCord went back to the original crude preparation (erythrocytes) and purified the inhibitory factor: indeed, it was different from any of the proteins that had been suspected. Precipitation with cold acetone, followed by ion-exchange chromatography, yielded a blue-green enzyme protein. Convinced that the mysterious reducing agent formed by the xanthine/xanthine oxidase/oxygen system was indeed superoxide anion, they named the enzyme *superoxide dismutase* (*64*). ("Dismutation" refers to the redox reaction of a compound with itself, such that one molecule is oxidized and one is reduced; the approved systematic name of the enzyme is superoxide: superoxide oxidoreductase, EC 1.15.1.1.) They recognized the enzyme to be identical to "hemocuprein," a copper-containing protein of unknown function that had been isolated from erythrocytes 30 years earlier.

Superoxide Dismutase: Assays

As with any enzyme, we can, in principle, assay superoxide dismutase by monitoring either disappearance of substrate or formation of product. Since the dismutation reaction can occur spontaneously, the formation of hydrogen peroxide does not afford a useful assay. Although superoxide absorbs ultraviolet light (below 300 nm), its concentration in enzymatic systems is usually far too small for direct detection. Consequently, any assay for superoxide dismutase is predicated on an assay for superoxide itself. The enzyme assays rely on the ability of superoxide dismutase to intercept $O_2^{\bullet -}$ and, hence, to inhibit alternative reactions of the form:

$$O_2^{\bullet -} + D \rightarrow O_2 + D^{\bullet -}$$

where D is a detector molecule and D^- is a readily detected product.

Many assays for superoxide dismutase activity have been devised (*65*). Superoxide dismutase-dependent inhibition of the reduction of cytochrome c was the basis for the discovery of the enzyme, and this assay is still widely used (*66*). The specificity of this assay relies on the inhibition by superoxide

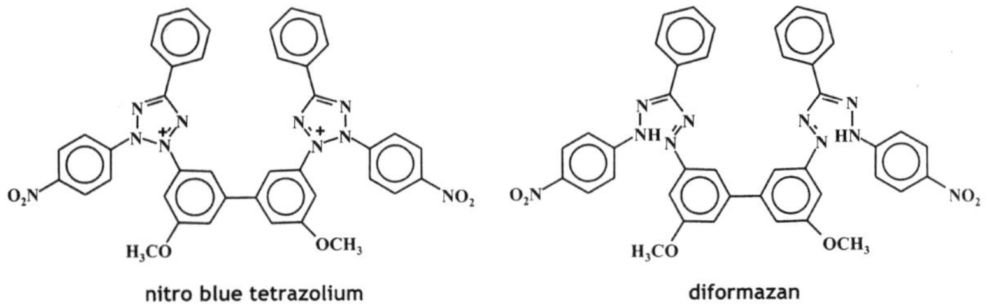

FIGURE 1-5.
Nitro blue tetrazolium and its formazan reduction product.

dismutase: superoxide-independent cytochrome c reduction is also possible, but is unaffected by superoxide dismutase.

Another widely used assay is based on the reduction of the chromogenic reagent nitro blue tetrazolium (NBT) (figure 1-5). Nitro blue tetrazolium is yellow, but, upon reduction, it yields a pigment called *formazan*, which is purple-blue colored (*67*). The pigment is insoluble; it precipitates and forms a stable colored band in a polyacrylamide gel. For detection of superoxide dismutase, the chromogen is incubated with a superoxide-generating system and enzyme activity is measured by the inhibition of color formation. Superoxide dismutase bands are visualized on gels as colorless bands visible against a blue background (*68*).

Superoxide dismutase can be assayed on the basis of inhibition of tetranitromethane reduction. Tetranitromethane is reduced by superoxide to the nitroform anion radical

$$O_2^{\bullet-} + C(NO_2)_4 \rightarrow O_2 + C(NO_2)_3^- + {}^{\bullet}NO_2$$

with a rate constant near the diffusion-controlled limit (*69*). The nitroform anion radical can be detected spectroscopically ($\lambda_{max} = 350$ nm).

EPR Spin Trapping

Electron paramagnetic resonance (EPR) spin trapping is a unique tool for the analysis of free radical processes in biochemical systems (*70–73*). Spin trapping provides qualitative and semiquantitative information about the kinds of reactive radicals formed in chemical systems. Free radicals are paramagnetic; that is, they align in a magnetic field. Just as in NMR, the different spin states of a paramagnetic molecule in a magnetic field are of different energies, and these energy differences can be measured by the resonant absorption of electromagnetic energy. This is the basis of EPR spectroscopy. In contrast to NMR, the energy differences involved in EPR are much larger, so EPR is inherently a very sensitive technique. Radical concentrations as low as 10^{-9} M may be detectable. Furthermore, diamagnetic molecules (i.e., those with no net spin) are EPR-silent. Minuscule populations of free radicals can be studied by EPR even in the presence of much greater numbers of nonradical molecules; this is invariably the situation in a biochemical system.

As with an NMR spectrum, the EPR spectrum provides detailed information about the structure of the molecules responsible for the signal. In the case of NMR, information is provided by the chemical shift values and spin–spin splitting (nucleus–nucleus magnetic interactions). In the case of EPR, information is provided by the *g*-value of the radical and by hyperfine splitting constants (electron–nucleus magnetic interactions). (The analysis of EPR spectra is discussed elsewhere (*74, 75*).)

For spectroscopic reasons that will not be discussed here, the superoxide radical cannot be detected directly in solution by the EPR technique. In any event, its steady-state concentration is usually below that required for detection of radicals by EPR. In the EPR spin-trapping technique, the primary radical is captured by a diamagnetic molecule, the spin trap, to yield a relatively stable free radical (a nitroxide), which can be detected by EPR:

Primary radical + spin trap → spin adduct

In favorable cases, the spectrum of the spin adduct (a nitroxide radical) will be characteristic of the primary radical, and thereby allow its identification. Increasingly, chromatographic separation and mass spectrometric analysis is being used in combination with EPR for the characterization of spin adducts (*76–78*).

Various classes of spin trap have been developed, including alkyl and aryl nitroso compounds and nitrones. A useful spin trap must meet many criteria, including rapid reaction with the primary radical; stability of the spin adduct; absence of unproductive side reactions; distinctive spectroscopic signature of the spin adducts; and good solubility.

The most useful spin traps for detection of reactive oxygen species such as superoxide and hydroxyl radical are *dimethylpyrroline-N-oxide* (DMPO) (*79*) and *phenyl-tert-butyl nitrone* (PBN) (*80*). DMPO reacts with superoxide to give a nitroxide spin adduct characterized by a six-line EPR spectrum (figure 1-6). The presence of this signal, and its sensitivity to

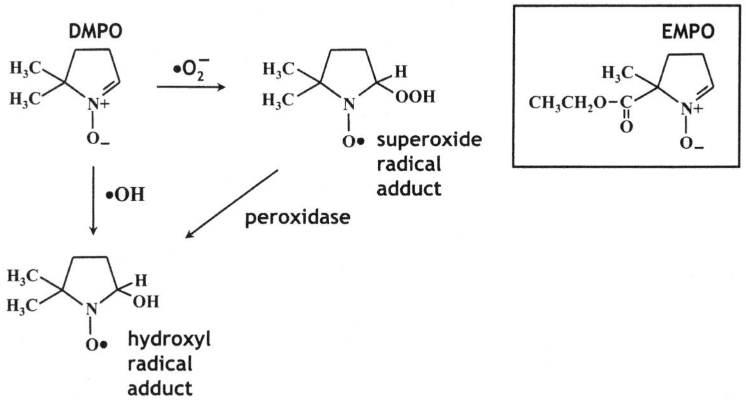

FIGURE 1-6.
Spin trapping of the hydroxyl radical and superoxide radical by DMPO. Peroxidase enzymes or other reductants may reduce the DMPO superoxide adduct to the hydroxyl radical adduct, possibly leading to the artifactual conclusion that hydroxyl radical has been formed in a reaction. This problem may be avoided by the use of the recently introduced congener EMPO (inset), which gives more stable superoxide spin adducts. (*Olive, G.; Mercier, A.; Le Moigne, F.; Rockenbauer, A.; Tordo, P. 2-Ethoxycarbonyl-2-methyl-3,4-dihydro-2H-pyrrole-1-oxide: evaluation of the spin trapping properties.* Free Radic. Biol. Med. **2000**, *28, 403–408.*)

inhibition by superoxide dismutase, is excellent evidence for the formation of superoxide, and the technique has been applied in many studies of biochemical and cellular systems suspected of generating oxygen radicals. Hydroxyl radical is also trapped by DMPO and yields an adduct with a distinctive four-line EPR spectrum (81). Scavengers such as dimethyl sulfoxide or ethanol react with the hydroxyl radical to produce methyl or hydroxyethyl radicals, respectively, and these secondary radicals can also be spin-trapped (71).

Superoxide Dismutase: Forms and Distribution

All superoxide dismutases (SODs) are metalloenzymes and share the same fundamental mechanism (82). A metal ion in the active site is first reduced by superoxide, releasing oxygen, and then oxidized by a second molecule of superoxide, releasing (upon protonation) hydrogen peroxide:

$$O_2^{\bullet-} + SOD\ Me^{n+} \rightarrow O_2 + SOD\ Me^{(n-1)+}$$
$$O_2^{\bullet-} + SOD\ Me^{(n-1)+} + 2H^+ \rightarrow H_2O_2 + SOD\ Me^{n+}$$

Three metalloprotein classes of SOD are widely distributed: Cu, Zn SOD (the enzyme first isolated by McCord and Fridovich), Mn SOD, and Fe SOD (83). (An unusual Ni SOD is found in certain Gram-positive bacteria (84, 85).) The Mn and Fe enzymes are homologous in both sequence and structure and presumably evolved from a common progenitor. Cu, Zn SOD must have arisen independently from the Mn SOD/Fe SOD family (83). The Mn enzyme occurs in many species of bacteria and in the mitochondria of eukaryotic cells, a distribution pattern that testifies to the endosymbiotic evolution of the mitochondrion (86). Fe SOD is the only form of the enzyme found in obligate-anaerobe bacteria. In most green plants, the chloroplasts contain Cu, Zn SOD and the mitochondria contain Mn SOD.

The E. coli chromosome (87) encodes three forms of the enzyme: Mn SOD (sodA, at 88.34 min. on the circular genetic map of E. coli), Fe SOD (sodB, 37.36 min.), and Cu, Zn SOD (sodC, 37.12 min.). The E. coli Cu, Zn SOD, which is localized to the periplasm and expressed only in the stationary phase of culture growth, was not discovered until the mid-1990s (88), long after the Fe and Mn enzymes had been characterized. Humans have three forms of superoxide dismutases: cytosolic Cu, Zn SOD (encoded by the gene SOD1 on chromosome 21), mitochondrial Mn SOD (SOD2, chromosome 6), and extracellular EC SOD (SOD3, chromosome 4).

Cu, Zn Superoxide Dismutase

The eukaryotic Cu, Zn SOD (89) can be purified from mammalian sources by treatment of erythrocytes with ethanol/chloroform, which denatures and precipitates hemoglobin and other unwanted proteins. Cu, Zn SOD is soluble in the organic phase; addition of acetone causes the enzyme to precipitate. Few other enzymes can survive such a protocol.

The protein has been studied as a holoenzyme and in metal-free form (e.g., (90)). The copper ion undergoes the catalytic redox state change and is essential for activity. (Small-molecule complexes of Cu(II), and even the free copper ion, are effective catalysts of superoxide dismutation (91).)

Human Cu, Zn SOD is a homodimer of 153 residue subunits. Each subunit contains one Cu and one Zn ion. The active site is located in a region of high electrostatic potential, due to the presence of lysine and arginine residues (and the metal ions themselves), and is located at the bottom of a channel, which is constructed as a sort of "molecular funnel" leading to the catalytic copper. Electrostatic facilitation of superoxide binding is an important contributor to the extraordinarily high catalytic efficiency of the Cu, Zn enzyme. The second-order rate constant for reaction of superoxide with the enzyme is near the diffusion-controlled limit. This means that most of the collisions with the substrate are productive, even though the active site occupies only a fraction of the volume of the protein. Negative surface charges prevent unproductive collisions and the positive potential in the channel pulls the substrate into the active site (92).

The copper ion is coordinated in a distorted square-planar geometry to the imidazole side-chain N atoms of four different histidine residues. The Zn^{2+} ion is buried within the protein, inaccessible to solvent, and is approximately tetrahedral in coordination, with three histidine imidazole N ligands and one aspartate oxygen. One histidine residue (his63 in the human enzyme) bridges the copper and zinc ions, with one N atom liganded to each (figure 1-7). Aside from Cu, Zn SOD, no other protein is known to have such a "histidine bridge."

Extracellular Superoxide Dismutase

The second mammalian Cu, Zn SOD was discovered in 1982. *Extracellular superoxide dismutase* (EC SOD) is secreted into blood plasma (93). The enzyme's polypeptide chain (94) is substantially longer (222 amino acid residues) than that of the cytosolic enzyme. The central section of the sequence of the EC SOD, encompassing the active site, is homologous to that of the cytosolic form, but there are extensions at both the amino

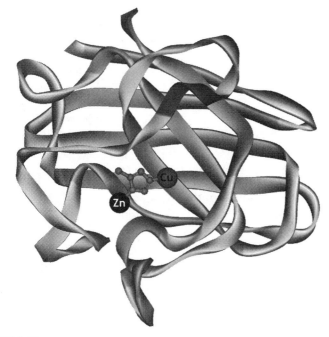

FIGURE 1-7.

Cu, Zn superoxide dismutase; 2sod.pdb. *Note*: A full-color version of this figure appears on the website.

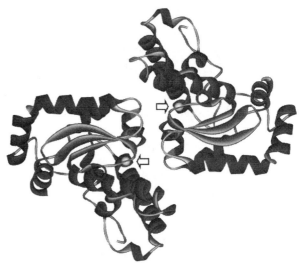

FIGURE 1-8.

Mn superoxide dismutase; 3mds.pdb. Arrows indicate positions of Mn(III) ions. *Note*: A full-color version of this figure appears on the website.

and carboxy termini. The N-terminal sequence mediates assembly of EC SOD tetramers, rather than the dimers formed by Cu, Zn SOD. The C-terminal region includes a domain that confers high-affinity binding to serum polysaccharides such as heparin and heparan sulfate (*95*), presumably keeping the enzyme sequestered in the serum and other extracellular compartments.

Mn and Fe Superoxide Dismutases

These enzymes occur as dimers or, in some cases, tetramers composed of subunits with about 190 amino acids; each subunit contains one metal ion. The Mn (*96, 97*) and Fe (*98*) SODs evolved from a common precursor and have very similar structures. The Mn(III) ion in the oxidized enzyme (*T. thermophilus*) (figure 1-8) is in a roughly trigonal bipyramidal coordination to three histidines, one aspartate, and a solvent water molecule. Despite the very different tertiary structure of these enzymes compared to the Cu, Zn SOD, some features are similar: the metal ion is located at the end of a funnel-like channel and positive charges (lysine and arginine residues) appear to attract anions into the funnel.

Spontaneous Superoxide Dismutation

Perhydroxyl radical, $pK_a = 4.8$, is an acid with strength comparable to that of acetic acid:

$$HO_2^\bullet \rightleftharpoons O_2^{\bullet-} + H^+$$

The dismutation of one superoxide anion with another is slow, due to electrostatic repulsion. The reaction goes fastest at the pK_a.

$$2HO_2^\bullet \rightarrow O_2 + H_2O_2 \qquad k_2 \approx 8 \times 10^5\ \mathrm{M^{-1}s^{-1}}$$
$$HO_2^\bullet + O_2^{\bullet-} + H^+ \rightarrow O_2 + H_2O_2 \quad k_2 \approx 8 \times 10^7\ \mathrm{M^{-1}s^{-1}}$$
$$2O_2^{\bullet-} + 2H^+ \rightarrow O_2 + H_2O_2 \qquad k_2 < 0.3\ \mathrm{M^{-1}s^{-1}}$$

▶ Kinetics of the Superoxide Dismutase-Catalyzed Reaction

The superoxide dismutase-catalyzed reaction follows "ping-pong" kinetics (65). Assuming that the reaction proceeds *via* two irreversible steps:

$$SOD^0 + O_2^{\bullet -} \xrightarrow{k_1} SOD^- + O_2$$

$$SOD^- + O_2^{\bullet -} + H^+ \xrightarrow{k_2} SOD^0 + H_2O_2$$

We make the steady-state approximation for the reduced-enzyme intermediate, SOD^-:

$$\frac{d}{dt}[SOD^-] = 0 = k_1[SOD^0][O_2^{\bullet -}] - k_2[SOD^-][O_2^{\bullet -}]$$

$$\therefore [SOD^-] = \frac{k_1[SOD^0]}{k_2}$$

$$\text{But} \quad [SOD]_{total} = [SOD^-] + [SOD^0] = [SOD^-] \times \frac{(k_1 + k_2)}{k_1}$$

The fraction of the enzyme found in the reduced form, at steady state, is given by this equation, and can be measured experimentally by observing the spectral bleaching of the cupric enzyme (99).

The overall reaction rate is equal to the rate of disappearance of superoxide:

$$\frac{d}{dt}[O_2^{\bullet -}] = k_1[SOD^0][O_2^{\bullet -}] + k_2[SOD^-][O_2^{\bullet -}]$$

$$= [SOD]_{total}[O_2^{\bullet -}] \times \frac{2(k_1 k_2)}{k_1 + k_2}$$

Thus, we can express the turnover number for the enzyme, k_{cat}, in terms of the rate constants for the two steps of the reaction:

$$k_{cat} = \frac{2(k_1 k_2)}{k_1 + k_2}$$

◀

Why is superoxide dismutase enzyme necessary, since the uncatalyzed dismutation of superoxide at physiological pH is already fast? As Fridovich has pointed out, the spontaneous dismutation is *second order* in the concentration of superoxide, whereas the enzymatic dismutation is *first order* (with respect to superoxide). Thus, at low prevailing concentrations of superoxide, the enzyme-catalyzed reaction dominates. Putting it another way, a superoxide radical is much more likely to encounter a molecule of superoxide dismutase than a second molecule of superoxide: the enzyme acts as the carrier of electrons from one superoxide radical to another. Calculations based on known rate constants and superoxide dismutase concentrations show that the enzyme maintains intracellular superoxide concentrations below 10^{-10} M.

Biological Sources of Superoxide

All aerobic organisms are exposed to superoxide and other reactive oxygen species. The most important source of superoxide in animal cells is usually the respiratory electron transport chain (*15*, p. 506). Although respiration is optimized for the complete four-electron reduction of oxygen to water, some reducing equivalents inevitably "leak" from the chain at intermediate stages, reducing molecular oxygen to superoxide or hydrogen peroxide (*100*). In the mammalian mitochondrion, complex III appears to be the most important site of reactive oxygen species generation, as determined by experiments using respiratory inhibitors such as antimycin and rotenone (*101*). The "respiratory burst" of phagocytic cells (neutrophils and macrophages), discussed in a later section of this chapter, is a unique biochemical system that consumes oxygen and generates reactive oxygen species for the purpose of destroying foreign cells, such as invading bacteria.

Green plant cells produce superoxide as a side-product of photosynthesis. Chloroplasts harvest solar light energy for the generation of NADPH reducing equivalents, which are then used for the reductive synthesis of carbohydrates from carbon dioxide. Upon exposure to light, chloroplasts generate superoxide, apparently from the autoxidation (i.e., oxidation by molecular oxygen) of components of photosystem I (*102*); chloroplast superoxide dismutase defends against this oxidative stress (*103*). (The genome of the flowering plant model organism *Arabidopsis thaliana* (*104*) encodes seven superoxide dismutases: three Cu, Zn, three Fe, and one Mn forms.)

Redox cycling agents are chemicals that undergo enzymatic one-electron reduction (usually catalyzed by a flavoenzyme), generating a transient radical; the radical is reoxidized by molecular oxygen, reducing it to superoxide (*105*) (figure 1-9). Redox cycling agents act as catalysts of superoxide formation, channeling reducing equivalents from NADH or NADPH to the univalent reduction of oxygen. Many compounds cause human toxicity by this oxidative stress mechanism. Paraquat (1,1'-dimethyl-4,4'-dipyridilium dichloride), a common herbicide used to control broadleaf weeds, is a pulmonary toxicant in humans (*106*). Fatal paraquat poisonings due to accidental, suicidal, or even homicidal exposures are often reported (*107, 108*). Paraquat redox cycling generates reactive oxygen species and depletes cellular NADPH (*109*); the particular sensitivity of the lung may result from its exposure to the highest levels of oxygen. Other agents that cause toxicity by redox cycling mechanisms include quinones (*110*); the cardiotoxic anticancer agent adriamycin (doxorubicin) (*111*); and nitroaromatic drugs such as nitrofurantoin (*112, 113*), which causes rare pulmonary and hepatic toxicity (*114*).

Ionizing radiation generates oxidizing radicals, as discussed earlier. The pathological effects of exposure to ionizing radiation (e.g., injury to neighboring normal tissues, following radiotherapy of solid tumors) are believed to result, in large measure, from oxidative damage (*115*).

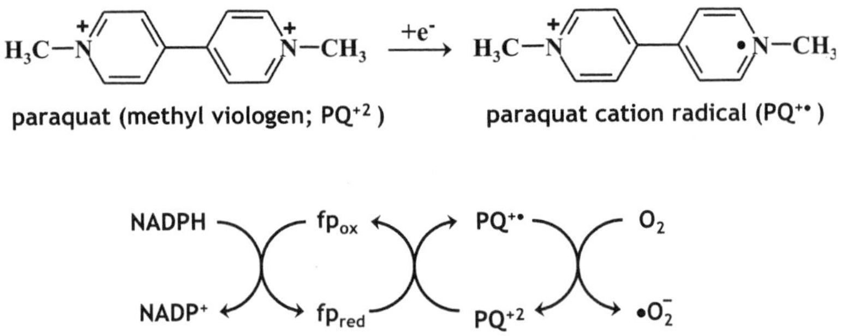

paraquat (methyl viologen; PQ^{+2})   paraquat cation radical ($PQ^{+\bullet}$)

FIGURE 1-9.

Upper: Reduction of paraquat to a cation free radical. Lower: Redox cycling action of paraquat; fp represents a flavoprotein.

Superoxide Dismutase Null Mutants

The physiological roles of superoxide dismutase enzymes have been examined by construction of organisms bearing null mutations in genes encoding the proteins. Such studies have been carried out in *E. coli* (*116, 117*), *Drosophila* (*118*), and other model organisms.

The role of superoxide in the toxicity of redox cycling agents is demonstrated by the results of a study of an engineered yeast (*Saccharomyces cerevisiae*) strain bearing a null mutation of the gene for Cu, Zn SOD. The SOD-minus mutant strain was killed by paraquat concentrations 100-fold lower than the levels required to have any toxic effect on the wild-type strain, *when the cells were challenged under aerobic conditions*. Under anaerobic conditions, in contrast, paraquat toxicity was very slight, and was similar in the two strains (*119*).

The technology for construction of "knockout mice" by insertional inactivation of genes in embryonic stem cells is described in chapter 8. This method has been used to generate homozygous-null mouse strains lacking each of the three mammalian superoxide dismutases. Either of the Cu, Zn superoxide dismutases (cytosolic *SOD1*, extracellular *SOD3*) could be inactivated without dramatic effects on viability; perhaps there is some complementation of function between the two enzymes, despite being localized in distinct compartments. *SOD1*-null mice, while viable, developed neurological deficiencies after the age of about six months (*120*). *SOD3*-null mice were found to be healthy and normal to at least one year of age (*121*). Only when the animals were challenged by exposure to a pure oxygen atmosphere did a difference between the wild-type and *SOD3*-null mice become apparent, with the latter group suffering greater lung damage and dying sooner than did the wild-type controls. The most drastic phenotype was seen in homozygous *SOD2*-null mice, deficient in Mn SOD (*122*). At birth, these animals appeared healthy but they failed to thrive, exhibited motor and behavioral defects, and died between one and three weeks of age. Ultrastructural examination showed damage or disintegration of mitochondria in the heart, neurons, bone marrow, and other tissues. These findings indicate that mitochondrial superoxide dismutases are not critical to the developing embryo, presumably due to lower ambient oxygen tension or reduced oxidative metabolism *in utero*. Postnatally, superoxide-mediated damage destroys mitochondria, especially in sensitive organs such as the heart.

Superoxide Dismutase and Familial Amyotrophic Lateral Sclerosis

Amyotrophic lateral sclerosis (ALS, also known as motor neuron disease and Lou Gehrig's disease) is a fatal and incurable degenerative condition marked by the progressive loss of control over the muscles (*123*). ALS is a consequence of the selective death of the motor neurons, probably by apoptosis (see the sidebar on apoptosis in chapter 5) (*124*). The effect is specific to motor neurons and does not affect cognition; the celebrated physicist Stephen Hawking continues his academic work despite his severe ALS disability. Most cases of ALS are sporadic, that is, they arise in individuals with no family history of the disease. About 10% of the cases of ALS are inherited (*familial amyotrophic lateral sclerosis*, FALS), almost

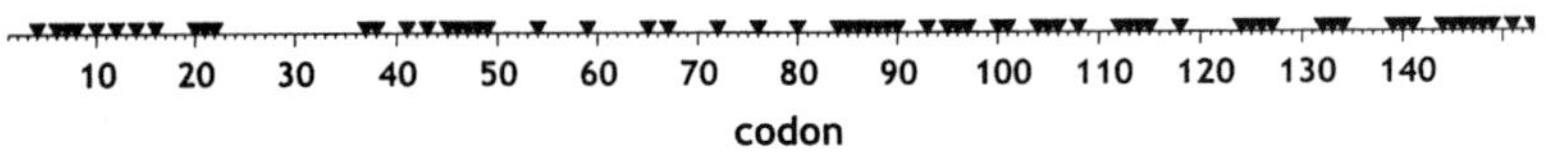

FIGURE 1-10.

Positions of amino acid substitutions associated with familial amyotrophic lateral sclerosis, in the sequence (153 amino acids) of human Cu, Zn superoxide dismutase.

always following an autosomal dominant Mendelian pattern (*125*). Several FALS genes have now been identified. One of these genes was determined, in 1993, to be *SOD1* (*126*), encoding Cu, Zn SOD. This landmark discovery has brought new impetus to research on oxidative stress. *SOD1* mutations account for about one-fifth of FALS cases, and therefore about one-fiftieth of all ALS cases.

At of the time of writing, 108 different mutations in *SOD1* associated with FALS have been identified (see the on-line database at: http://alsod1.iop.kcl.ac.uk/reports/mutations/ and (*127*)). These mutations encode amino acid substitutions at sites distributed almost uniformly along the whole primary structure (figure 1-10). The FALS-associated *SOD1* alleles are *not* inactivating missense mutations: the proteins encoded by FALS alleles have superoxide dismutase activities similar to that of the wild-type enzyme. Rather, the FALS alleles must confer a positive gain-of-function on the protein, resulting in the dominant pattern of Mendelian inheritance. The quest to discover the nature of this function, and thereby the mechanism by which the variant enzymes cause ALS, is being pursued assiduously by many research groups, but no definitive answer has been found (*128, 129*). One of the favored hypotheses is that the FALS-mutant forms of Cu, Zn SOD are structurally altered in a manner that predisposes the proteins to form insoluble fibrous aggregates; such aggregates are a common ultrastructural feature of ALS and several other neurodegenerative diseases.

Mechanisms of Superoxide Toxicity

The oxygen sensitivity of superoxide dismutase null mutants, discussed above, is strong evidence for the role of superoxide in oxidative stress and oxygen toxicity. But the difficult question remains: what is the chemical basis of superoxide toxicity? Superoxide anion is disconcertingly unreactive, although it can act as a reducing agent (as discussed earlier) or an oxidizing agent (oxidation of epinephrine, ascorbate, catecholamines, and other compounds).

Sources of superoxide are also sources of hydrogen peroxide, via dismutation. The so-called Haber–Weiss reaction

$$O_2^{\bullet-} + H^+ + H_2O_2 \rightarrow O_2 + {}^{\bullet}OH + H_2O$$

was proposed by Fritz Haber and others in the 1930s. Haber was investigating the earlier discovery that ferrous iron caused the decomposition of hydrogen peroxide and evolution of oxygen gas (*130*). This stoichiometry, the one-electron reduction of hydrogen peroxide by superoxide, represents a possible source of the reactive hydroxyl radical, and has occasionally been invoked to account for superoxide toxicity. However, subsequent

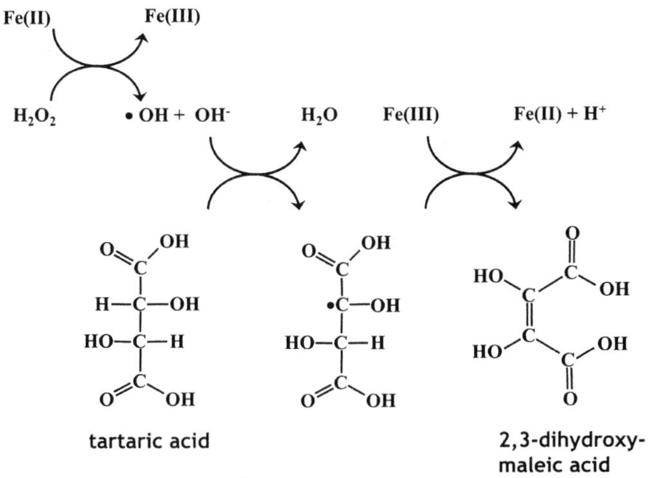

Fe(II)   Fe(III)

H$_2$O$_2$ • OH + OH$^-$ H$_2$O   Fe(III)   Fe(II) + H$^+$

tartaric acid

2,3-dihydroxy-maleic acid

FIGURE 1-11.

The Fenton reaction.

studies, including definitive measurements of rate constants by pulse radiolysis studies, showed that this proposed reaction does not occur at any appreciable rate. (Willem Koppenol (*130*) refers to the Haber–Weiss "non-reaction"!)

An alternative possibility, already recognized by Haber, is that metal ions catalyze the generation of hydroxyl radicals. As long ago as 1893, the English chemist Henry J.H. Fenton (*131*) showed that ferrous iron plus hydrogen peroxide oxidized tartaric acid to dihydroxymaleic acid (figure 1-11). Fenton developed several useful syntheses of carbohydrates by this route. The reduction of hydrogen peroxide by ferrous iron (the Fenton reaction) yields (at least on paper) the hydroxyl radical:

$$Fe^{2+} + H_2O_2 \rightarrow Fe^{3+} + OH^- + {}^{\bullet}OH$$

As predicted by this equation, the hydroxyl radical spin adduct is detected when ferrous sulfate is added to hydrogen peroxide in the presence of the spin trap DMPO (*132a*) and the oxygen atom of the trapped hydroxyl radical is derived from the peroxide, not from water (*81*). (The ferryl-oxo species $[Fe^{4+}=O]^{2+}$ has been suggested as an alternative to the hydroxyl radical, as the hydroxylating species in the Fenton reaction, but recent chemical studies have been interpreted as ruling out this possibility (*132b*).)

Ferrous iron is a stoichiometric reagent in Fenton chemistry. However, in the presence of superoxide, iron can act as a catalyst:

$$Fe^{3+} + O_2^{\bullet-} \rightarrow Fe^{2+} + O_2$$

$$Fe^{2+} + H_2O_2 \rightarrow Fe^{3+} + OH^- + {}^{\bullet}OH$$

$$Sum: O_2^{\bullet-} + H_2O_2 \rightarrow O_2 + {}^{\bullet}OH + OH^-$$

The net stoichiometry is equivalent to that of the Haber–Weiss "non-reaction." This so-called iron-catalyzed Haber–Weiss reaction (*133*) has been invoked to account for the synergistic toxicity of hydrogen peroxide plus superoxide (*134–136*). The hydroxyl radicals formed by this process can generate additional superoxide radicals by oxidizing hydrogen peroxide, setting up a chain reaction of hydrogen peroxide decomposition:

$$\cdot OH + H_2O_2 \rightarrow H_2O + O_2^{\bullet-} + H^+$$

$$O_2^{\bullet-} + H_2O_2 \rightarrow O_2 + \cdot OH + OH^-$$

$$Sum: 2H_2O_2 \rightarrow O_2 + 2H_2O$$

The chain reaction is terminated by reactions such as:

$$\cdot OH + Fe^{2+} \rightarrow Fe^{3+} + OH^-$$

Alternatively, the hydroxyl radicals can attack biomolecules such as protein, DNA, and lipid.

The mechanism proposed above requires the presence of free iron ions. How would these arise within the cell? A plausible answer was provided by the discovery that superoxide itself inactivates enzymes containing iron–sulfur clusters, such as aconitase (*137, 138*). This reaction releases free iron ions that can catalyze the Haber–Weiss reaction (*139*).

The biological significance of hydroxyl radical generation by the metal-catalyzed Haber–Weiss reaction is still controversial (*130, 135, 140*). However, the ability of metal ions such as chromium, nickel, and cadmium to catalyze the generation of reactive oxygen species, and thereby to damage macromolecules (*141, 142*), provides a plausible unifying explanation for their carcinogenicity (*143*).

Reactive Nitrogen Intermediates; Peroxynitrite

The study of free radicals in biology was transformed by the astonishing discovery, in 1987 (*144*), that nitric oxide is an important biological signaling molecule (*15*, pp. 686–687). The Nobel Prize in Physiology or Medicine, 1998, was awarded to Robert Furchgott, Louis Ignarro, and Ferid Murad in honor of this discovery (see also chapter 11). Nitric oxide ($NO^\bullet$), a diatomic free radical, is generated by the action of the enzyme *nitric oxide synthase* on arginine and molecular oxygen. Three forms of nitric oxide synthase are expressed in humans.

The recognition of the biochemical roles of nitric oxide has had a "radical" effect on the study of reactive oxygen species (*145*). Superoxide radical reacts rather sluggishly with most biomolecules, as noted earlier, but it reacts extremely rapidly (*146*) with nitric oxide (a radical–radical reaction (*147*)), forming the *peroxynitrite* anion:

$$NO^\bullet + O_2^{\bullet-} \rightarrow ONOO^-(O = N - O - O^-)$$

This reaction proceeds even more rapidly than that of superoxide with superoxide dismutase, which means that (depending on steady-state concentrations) nitric oxide may compete effectively with the enzyme as a trap for intracellular superoxide.

Peroxynitrite is not a radical; rather, it is a *reactive oxidizing agent* that can oxidize thiols, halide ions, phenols, and other functional groups (*148*). Nitric oxide and derived products such as peroxynitrite and nitrous acid are collectively labeled *reactive nitrogen intermediates* (*149*). The existence of peroxynitrite was inferred by Baeyer and Villiger in 1901, and it was synthesized from hydrogen peroxide and nitrous acid in 1935, but its chemistry was little studied until recently (*150–152*). Peroxynitrite anion is the conjugate base of peroxynitrous acid, $O=NOOH$, which dissociates with a pK slightly below neutrality. The acid slowly isomerizes to nitric acid (HNO_3). In 1990 Joseph Beckman and colleagues (*153*) suggested that superoxide toxicity could arise from its reaction with nitric oxide to form peroxynitrite, followed by homolysis of the N–O single bond of peroxynitrite to yield hydroxyl radical:

$$O = N - O - OH \rightarrow \,^{\bullet}NO_2 + \,^{\bullet}OH$$

This idea has major implications, because hydroxyl radical itself is so reactive that, if formed in a cell, it cannot travel beyond a few intermolecular distances before reacting. In contrast, peroxynitrite is relatively long-lived. Therefore, peroxynitrite can act as a semistable "carrier" of a hydroxyl radical equivalent.

Additional studies support a model (*154*) whereby homolytic decomposition of peroxynitrite yields a transient radical pair [$^{\bullet}OH-^{\bullet}NO_2$], which can either isomerize to nitric acid (HNO_3) or produce independent $^{\bullet}OH$ and $^{\bullet}NO_2$ radicals, which can react with other species in solution.

Peroxynitrite reacts rapidly with carbon dioxide to form nitrosoperoxocarboxylate, $O = NOOCO_2^-$, and this species can decompose (*155, 156*) to yield carbonate radical:

$$O = NOOCO_2^- \rightarrow \,^{\bullet}NO_2 + \,^{\bullet}CO_2^- \text{ (or } NO_3^- + CO_2)$$

In addition to the oxidations mentioned above, the many identified reactions of peroxynitrite with biomolecules include the initiation of lipid peroxidation (see below), oxidation and nitration of tyrosine residues in proteins, oxidation of guanine residues in DNA to yield 8-hydroxyguanine, 8-nitroguanine, and other products (*157, 158*), and nitration of glutathione (*159*). In summary, nitric oxide is expected to be a major intracellular target of the superoxide radical, and peroxynitrite may be a very important mediator of oxidative stress biochemistry.

THE PHAGOCYTE RESPIRATORY BURST

Phagocytosis

The toxicity of reactive oxygen intermediates is exploited as a defensive component of the immune system. Phagocytic white blood cells (including neutrophils, monocytes, and macrophages) kill microorganisms by generating large amounts of superoxide and oxidants derived from it.

The idea that white blood cells engulf and digest invading microorganisms was propounded by the Russian zoologist Ilya Ilyich Mechnikov (1845–1916; Nobel Prize in Medicine, 1908). When phagocytic cells encounter foreign antigens (such as surface antigens of microorganisms) that have been "tagged" by circulating antibodies (opsonization), they engulf the invader and wrap it in the phagocyte's plasma membrane. The membrane closes around the engulfed particle, forming a phagocytic *vacuole*. When a suspension of white blood cells is challenged by exposure to antigenic materials such as opsonized zymosan (yeast), a swift and massive increase in oxygen consumption ensues. This *respiratory burst* response, discovered in 1933, can be measured by manometric or electrochemical analysis of oxygen consumption. In 1959 Sbarra and Karnovsky (*160*) discovered that the usual inhibitors of respiration, such as cyanide and azide, had no effect on the respiratory burst. This result indicated that the respiratory burst is not simply an increase in the rate of normal cellular respiration. Bernard Babior and colleagues discovered that activated neutrophils produce large amounts of superoxide (*161*). The reduction of oxygen to superoxide is catalyzed by a multi-protein complex called the NADPH oxidase (*162*).

The NADPH Oxidase

The oxidase is assembled at the plasma membrane of the phagocytic cell, once it is activated by a signal transduction pathway triggered by exposure to opsonized antigen. At least five separate protein components comprise the oxidase. The reduction of oxygen is catalyzed by an unusual membrane-bound cytochrome called cytochrome b_{558} (the optical absorption spectrum of the protein shows an α-band peak at 558 nm). Cytochrome b_{558} is composed of two subunits, the smaller $p22^{PHOX}$ and the larger $gp91^{PHOX}$. (The superscript PHOX stands for "phagocyte oxidase"). Cytochrome b_{558} binds two heme groups and a flavin cofactor (*163*). The oxidase complex also contains the soluble proteins $p47^{PHOX}$ and $p67^{PHOX}$ and a cytosolic G protein (guanine nucleotide-binding protein; see chapter 5) called Rac (*164*). The $p47^{PHOX}$ and $p67^{PHOX}$ proteins interact via SH3 (src homology) domains, structural "modules" which are found in many signal-transduction proteins (*165*). Phosphorylation of $p47^{PHOX}$, causing a conformational change that exposes its SH3 domain, is an essential step in oxidase activation (*166*). The cytosolic components assemble with cytochrome b_{558} at the membrane, only upon activation of the phagocytic cell. As Babior has pointed out, this is a "fail-safe" system, is analogous to storing the individual components of a nuclear weapon in separate places: the respiratory burst "explosion" kills both the phagocytosed microorganism and the phagocyte itself.

Chronic granulomatous disease (CGD) is a rare, severe, inherited immunodeficiency (*167*). The diagnostic feature of this disease is the inability of neutrophils to generate the respiratory burst. (This can be tested by using a histochemical stain based on the superoxide-dependent reduction of nitro blue tetrazolium to formazan.) CGD patients suffer recurrent, chronic infections, beginning in infancy, and many patients die from untreatable bouts of bacterial or fungal infections. Many different microorganisms cause disease in CGD patients, including *S. aureus*, pseudomonas, fungi such as aspergillus and candida, and *M. tuberculosis*. Infections occur in the lungs, lymph nodes, liver, and other organs.

Myeloperoxidase

The production of superoxide by the NADPH oxidase is the first step in a series of reactions that generate bacteriocidal oxidants. The neutrophil contains several types of *granules*. Upon stimulation of the phagocyte, the primary (or azurophilic) granules migrate to, and fuse with, the phagosome, and release their contents into the vacuole. The granules deliver the enzyme *myeloperoxidase* (MPO; EC 1.11.1.7) (*168*). The name of the enzyme derives from the Greek *myelo* (bone marrow). Myeloperoxidase uses H_2O_2

produced from the respiratory burst (via superoxide dismutation) to oxidize halide ions (chloride and bromide):

$$H_2O_2 + X^- \rightarrow HOX + OH^-$$

The products are hypohalous acids (HOCl $\rightleftarrows$ OCl$^-$ and HOBr $\rightleftarrows$ OBr$^-$), very potent oxidants that kill bacterial cells (169). (Household bleach is sodium hypochlorite, NaOCl.) Myeloperoxidase also oxidizes thiocyanate (SCN$^-$) to hypothiocyanite (OSCN$^-$), another bacteriocidal oxidant (170).

Neutrophils are the major blood cell type expressing myeloperoxidase, and myeloperoxidase is the major protein expressed by these cells (171). The green color of myeloperoxidase is responsible for the typical color of pus secretions (172), which contain large numbers of leukocytes, primarily neutrophils. Myeloperoxidase is also expressed in blood monocytes (173) and liver Kupffer cells (174).

The human genes for myeloperoxidase, lactoperoxidase, and eosinophil peroxidase are closely linked, at chromosomal position 17q23.1 (175). The lactoperoxidase and myeloperoxidase genes are oriented tail-to-tail, separated by only 2.5 kb. Inherited myeloperoxidase deficiency is known (176), but the clinical features are not severe, presumably because myeloperoxidase-independent mechanisms for killing infectious agents are also effective.

Myeloperoxidase is a heme-containing peroxidase (177–179). The distinctive green color of myeloperoxidase is a consequence of the unusual covalent linkages between the heme group and the polypeptide, consisting of two ester bonds from the (modified) heme methyl groups to acidic residues on the protein, and a unique sulfonium ion linkage between a methionine residue and one of the heme vinyl groups (180). Myeloperoxidase is translated as a single 745 amino acid residue polypeptide that undergoes extensive posttranslational processing (181, 182). An amino-terminal signal peptide and a 125 amino acid propeptide are removed; another proteolytic step cleaves the remaining polypeptide into heavy and light chain fragments; the heavy and light chains become linked by a disulfide bridge; and two of these heavy + light units associate to form the dimeric mature enzyme.

LIPID PEROXIDATION

Lipid peroxidation[2] is a complex chemical process by which oxygen reacts with lipids, especially polyunsaturated fatty acids (PUFA). The earliest investigations of this process were carried out mainly by food scientists, since the peroxidation of lipids is responsible for the familiar deterioration (rancidity) of lipid-rich foodstuffs (such as butter, egg yolk, or vegetable oil) upon storage (183). More recently, researchers have recognized the wide importance of lipid peroxidation in toxicology and pathology.

Lipid peroxidation involves spontaneous free radical chain reactions and occurs in any membrane exposed to oxygen. However, peroxidation is accelerated by exposure to free radicals, including reactive oxygen species and some drug metabolites. The polyunsaturated fatty acyl (PUFA) chains of phospholipids in biological membranes are particularly susceptible to oxidative damage by free radicals. Uncontrolled lipid peroxidation is a toxic process resulting in the deterioration of biological membranes. The same chemical processes are harnessed, under enzymatic control, for the biosynthesis of eicosanoids (prostaglandins, leukotrienes, and related compounds). The biochemistry of PUFA peroxidation is the focus of the present discussion.

Reactive oxygen species can initiate peroxidation processes. As we have discussed, phagocytic cells, in response to infection, generate large fluxes of oxidants. Such phagocytic cells can also attack lipid-rich atherosclerotic plaques. The generation of reactive oxygen species plays a major role in the pathology of ischemia/reperfusion events, in which the supply of blood and oxygen to an organ is temporarily cut off, as can occur during a stroke, heart attack, or organ transplantation surgery. When the blood supply is restored, oxidative species are generated as a result of the activation of oxidase activities, and this *reperfusion injury* can damage the affected organ or tissue (*184*). Lipid peroxidation is also implicated in the pathology of neurodegenerative processes (*185, 186*) and may contribute to the development of diseases such as Alzheimer's disease (*187*), Parkinson's disease (*188*), and multiple sclerosis. Nerves and brain tissue are presumed to be especially sensitive to peroxidative damage because of the essential functional role of lipid membranes in nerve impulse conduction. Myelin, the lipid-rich "insulation" surrounding nerve fibers, is particularly vulnerable to oxidative damage (*189*).

In addition to redox cycling agents, mentioned earlier, many other exogenous agents can cause the generation of $O_2^{\bullet-}$ and $^\bullet OH$, such as CCl_4 (*190*), ethanol (*191*), and drugs such as acetaminophen (*192*), primaquine (*193*), cyclosporin A (*194*), and halothane. Lipid peroxidation is one of the toxic consequences of exposure to these compounds (*195*).

Products and Mechanisms of Lipid Peroxidation

Peroxidation produces a complex array of degradation products, even if we oxidize a single fatty acid (e.g., linolenic acid) in a test tube. Biological fats or membrane lipids contain many different unsaturated fatty acids and give even more complex product mixtures. The mechanisms of lipid peroxidation are still not completely characterized, but the process begins with a *free radical chain reaction*. Therefore, a single initiating event can trigger the peroxidation of a large number of lipid molecules.

Initiation of PUFA peroxidation occurs when an oxidizing free radical abstracts a hydrogen atom ($H^\bullet$) from a fatty acid (figure 1-12) (*196*). The ease of formation of the initial lipid radical product is determined by the bond dissociation energy of the C–H bond that is attacked. Since bis-allylic C–H bonds are weaker ($\sim$314 kJ/mol) than mono-allylic C–H bonds ($\sim$368 kJ/mol), *the methylene-bridged double bonds of common PUFA molecules (such as linoleic, linolenic, and arachidonic acids) are much more easily oxidized than are monounsaturated fatty acids* (*197*). The resulting resonance-stabilized pentadienyl radical can be viewed as a resonance hybrid of structures with the unpaired electron centered on one of three carbon atoms; the forms in which the two double bonds are conjugated (see figure) are the more important contributors. The pentadienyl radical intermediate, long assumed to be the initial product of PUFA peroxidation, has recently been detected by EPR, using the spin trap POBN (α-[4-pyridyl-1-oxide]-*N-tert*-butyl nitrone), in a linoleic acid peroxidation reaction (*198*).

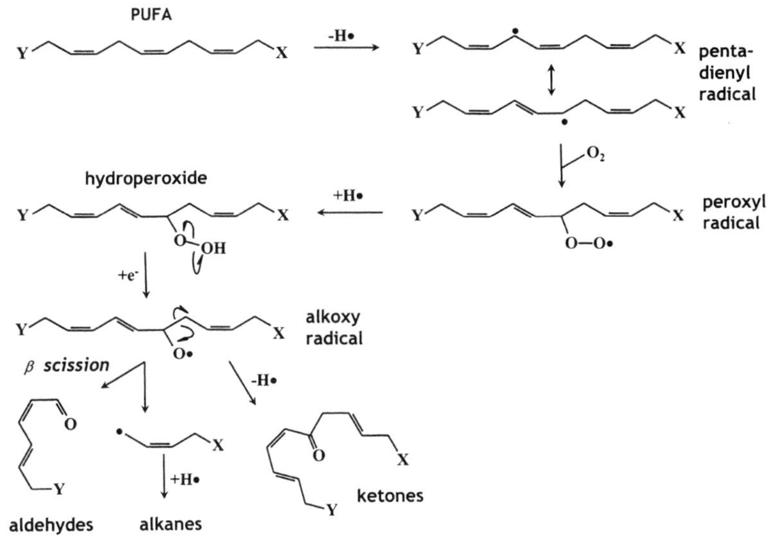

FIGURE 1-12.
Formation of the primary conjugated hydroperoxides and major secondary products from the peroxidation of a polyunsaturated fatty acid.

The multiple spin adduct products formed in the reaction were separated by on-line high-performance liquid chromatography (HPLC), and tandem mass spectrometry was used to confirm the identification of the products.

The peroxidation chain reaction is *propagated* by the extremely rapid reaction of the resulting *pentadienyl radical* with molecular oxygen, yielding a peroxyl radical: $R^{\bullet} + O_2 \rightarrow ROO^{\bullet}$. The peroxyl radical can then abstract $H^{\bullet}$ from another PUFA: $ROO^{\bullet} + RH \rightarrow ROOH + R^{\bullet}$. (By comparison, $H^{\bullet}$ abstraction from the O–H bond of a preformed hydroperoxide is relatively difficult and of minor importance.) The lipid peroxyl radical can then abstract a hydrogen atom from another PUFA, to form a metastable, conjugated lipid hydroperoxide and another fatty acyl free radical. The chain reaction *terminates* by the combination of any two free radicals to form non-radical products, especially by the process $ROO^{\bullet} + ROO^{\bullet} \rightarrow$ nonradical products.

The chain reaction can also be broken by the action of *antioxidants*, such as the lipid-soluble phenolic compounds vitamin E (tocopherol) and the synthetic preservatives BHA (*tert*-butyl hydroxyanisole) and BHT (di-*tert*-butyl hydroxytoluene) (figure 1-13). An antioxidant repairs the free radical by reduction: $ROO^{\bullet} + ArOH \rightarrow ROOH + ArO^{\bullet}$. The resulting phenolic radical is resonance-stabilized and insufficiently reactive to participate in further hydrogen atom abstraction reactions.

The second phase of the lipid peroxidation process converts the primary hydroperoxides into more stable end products. Reductive homolytic splitting of lipid hydroperoxide forms a lipid alkoxy radical ($RO^{\bullet}$). Alkoxy radicals are highly reactive alkyl analogues of the hydroxyl radical. Alkoxy radicals can undergo β-scission to form a shortened fatty acyl aldehyde and an alkyl radical; the alkyl radical may abstract another hydrogen atom to form an alkane. (Pentane and ethane are common products of lipid peroxidation of ω-6 and ω-3 fatty acids, respectively (*199*).) Acyl ketones are formed if an alkoxy radical loses a methinyl hydrogen atom.

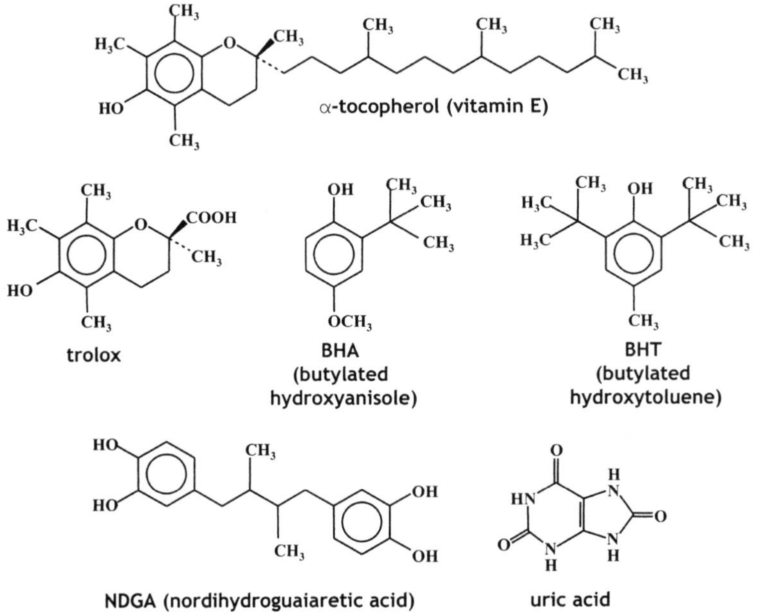

FIGURE 1-13.

Structures of some natural and synthetic antioxidants.

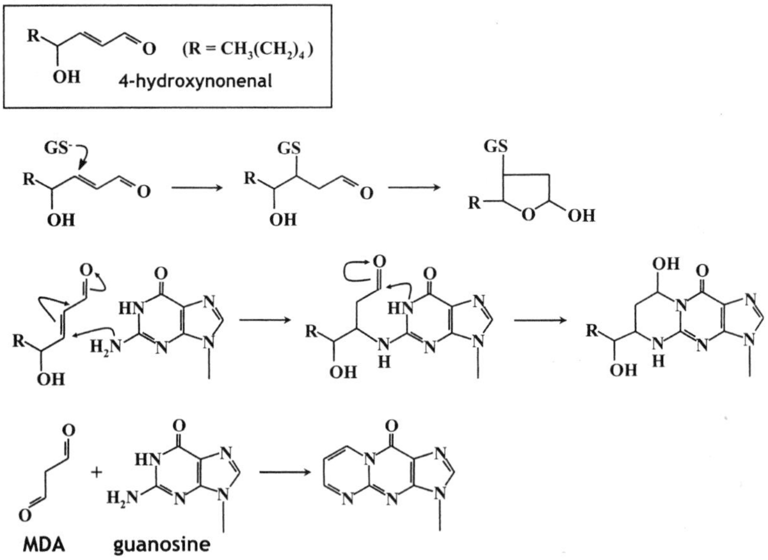

FIGURE 1-14.

From top: 4-Hydroxy-2-nonenal; reaction of 4-hydroxy-2-nonenal with glutathione (GSH); reaction of 4-hydroxy-2-nonenal with deoxyguanosine; reaction of malondialdehyde (MDA) with deoxyguanosine.

4-Hydroxynonenal, Malondialdehyde, and Other Biologically Active Lipid Peroxidation Products

In 1980 Hermann Esterbauer and colleagues identified *4-hydroxy-2-nonenal (200–202)* as a lipid peroxidation product (figure 1-14). This reactive unsaturated aldehyde may be one of the most important contributors to the toxic effects of lipid peroxidation products on cells (*203*). 4-Hydroxy-2-nonenal reacts with protein nucleophiles (such as cysteine, histidine, lysine) and with the tripeptide glutathione (chapter 9). It also binds to DNA, forming exocyclic adducts with deoxyguanosine residues. Exocyclic DNA adducts are discussed further in chapter 2. An even more reactive product of lipid peroxidation is the corresponding aldehyde-ketone, 4-oxo-2-nonenal (*204*). Additional secondary products are formed from the peroxidation of PUFA with more than two double bonds. Malonaldehyde (also known as malondialdehyde (MDA) or propanedial; figure 1-15), an end product of the peroxidation of arachidonic acid ($20:4\Omega6$), is often used as a chemical marker of lipid peroxidation. A possible mechanism of MDA formation has been suggested by William Pryor and colleagues. The key idea is that MDA is derived from a cyclic peroxide (endoperoxide) precursor, as illustrated in figure 1-16. This mechanism is similar to that of prostaglandin formation, catalyzed by the enzyme prostaglandin H synthase. The enzymatic process gives rise to a single product, with regio- and stereospecificity. In contrast, the nonenzymatic process gives rise to a wide range of isomers.

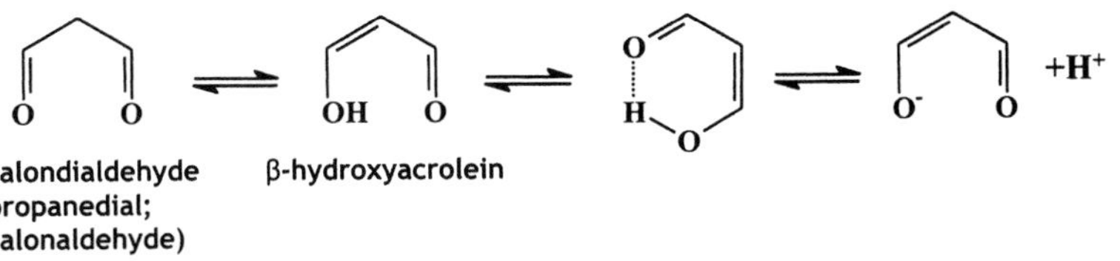

FIGURE 1-15.

Structure of malondialdehyde; tautomeric and acid–base equilibria.

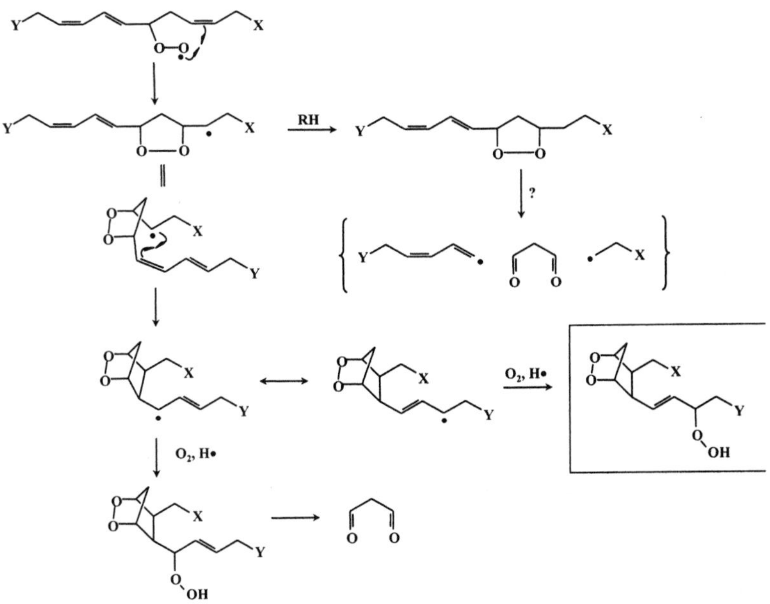

FIGURE 1-16.

Pathways for formation of malondialdehyde during lipid peroxidation. $X = (CH_2)_3CO_2^-$ and $Y = C_4H_9$. The PHS-catalyzed formation of a prostaglandin (boxed) is also shown for comparison.

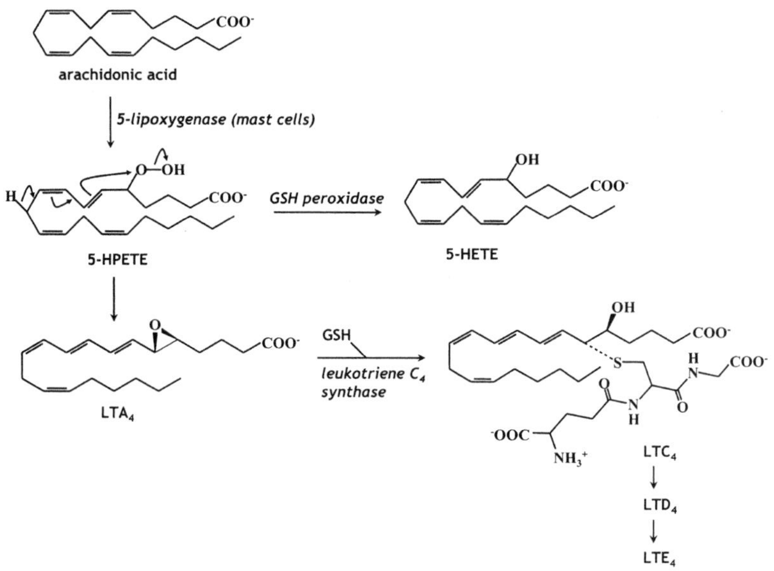

FIGURE 1-17.

Lipoxygenase-catalyzed oxidation of arachidonic acid generates HPETEs (hydroperoxyeicosatetraenoic acids), HETES (hydroxyeicosatetraenoic acids), and leukotrienes.

The action of *lipoxygenase* enzymes (EC 1.13.11.31) (*205*) on PUFA generates another series of biologically active peroxidized fatty acid derivatives, hydroperoxides and alcohols known as HPETEs (hydroperoxy-eicosatetraenoic acids) and HETEs (hydroxyeicosatetraenoic acids) (figure 1-17). Again, the enzymatic process is under regio- and stereo-specific control. 5-HPETE reacts with glutathione and is the precursor of the *leukotrienes* (*206*) (see chapter 9).

Assessment of Lipid Peroxidation

Many methods have been developed for the evaluation of lipid peroxidation (*207*). Oxygen uptake can be used to measure peroxidation kinetics in vitro, but is not applicable to the assessment of the extent of existing peroxida-tion in a biological sample. Even in cases of extensive lipid peroxidation, primary products may be hard to detect, due to their rapid conversion to secondary metabolites. Thus, the assessment of lipid peroxidation usually relies on the detection of secondary products. Monitoring of the loss of unsaturated lipids, or the formation of conjugated dienes (ultraviolet absorption at 232 nm), lipid hydroperoxides (detected by chemilumines-cence high-pressure liquid chromatography), fatty acyl alcohols, or alkanes (ethane, pentane; detected by gas chromatography/mass spectrometry) are all useful (*208*). By far the most popular of these methods, in both chemical and biological systems, remains the thiobarbituric acid (TBA) reactivity test. This test is based on the condensation of the lipid peroxidation product MDA (one molecule) with the analytical reagent TBA (two molecules), under acidic conditions (figure 1-18). The product of this reaction is a red pigment that can be quantitated by its light absorption at 532 nm. The validity of the TBA method rests on the assumptions that MDA formed during the TBA assay is diagnostic of

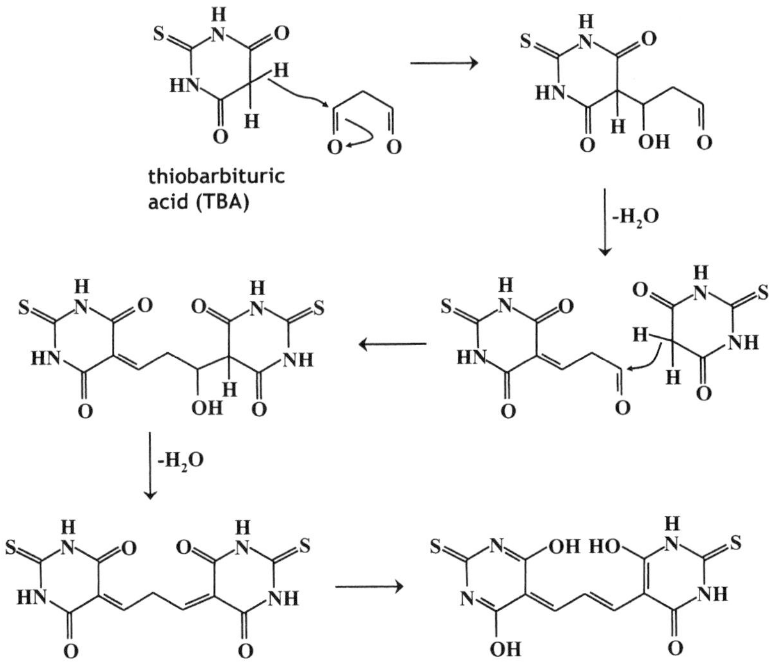

FIGURE 1-18.
The condensation of malondialdehyde with 2-thiobarbituric acid (TBA) yields the red pigment detectable at 532 nm.

the presence and amount of peroxides, and that a quantitative relationship exists between the extent of lipid peroxidation and the MDA detected. The MDA adduct is usually the main contributor to this absorption; TBA adducts formed by carbonyl compounds other than MDA have low absorption coefficients at 532 nm. However, since the assay is routinely used without definitive identification of the colored products, we often refer to the material detected by the test simply as "TBARS" ("thiobarbituric acid-reactive substances"). More recently, analytical techniques such as LC/MS have been applied to the chemical characterization of TBARS (209).

Cytotoxic Effects of Lipid Peroxidation

Lipid peroxidation degrades membrane lipids, shortening fatty acyl chains and leading to the formation of polar or charged acyl aldehydes, alcohols, ketones, carboxylic acids, and branched fatty acyl ethers. Both the degradation of the normal membrane components and the release of toxic reactive products, such as unsaturated aldehydes, can contribute to the toxic effects of lipid peroxidation.

Lipid peroxidation distorts the structure of the lipid bilayer and compromises its integrity and impermeability. All living cells maintain large transmembrane electrolyte concentration gradients. These gradients provide a source of free energy for transport processes that control cell turgor and mediate the import and export of metabolites. One of the primary biological effects of lipid peroxidation is membrane leakage: efflux of K^+, influx of Na^+, and concomitant influx of water into the cell. These functional impairments are probably caused by damages both to the membrane lipids themselves and to the transport activities of integral membrane proteins (*210*).

Apoptosis is a form of eukaryotic cell death characterized by the active degradation of the chromosomal DNA (see chapter 5). The release of the electron-transport chain hemeprotein cytochrome c from its normal mitochondrial compartment into the cytosol is a signal that the cell has undergone irreparable damage, and triggers apoptosis. Reactive products of lipid peroxidation, such as 4-hydroxynonenal, induce apoptosis by causing damage to the mitochondrial membrane (*211*). Thus, apoptosis may be, at least in part, a biological response that eliminates cells that have suffered excessive membrane damage due to the effects of oxidative stress (*212*).

Notes

1. Note that the commonly used "Lewis formula" representation of molecular oxygen :Ö=Ö: is inappropriate since it implies that all the electrons are paired.

2. The term *peroxidation* is most commonly applied to the incorporation of molecular oxygen into the polyunsaturated fatty acids (PUFA) of biological membranes. In studies of chemical model systems, the term *autoxidation* is preferred.

References

1. Carraway, M. S.; Piantadosi, C. A. Oxygen toxicity. *Respir. Care Clin. N. Am.* **1999,** *5*, 265–295.

2. Imlay, J. A. How oxygen damages microbes: oxygen tolerance and obligate anaerobiosis. *Adv. Microb. Physiol.* **2002,** *46*, 111–153.

3. Barazzone, C.; Horowitz, S.; Donati, Y. R.; Rodriguez, I.; Piguet, P. F. Oxygen toxicity in mouse lung: pathways to cell death. *Am. J. Respir. Cell Mol. Biol.* **1998,** *19*, 573–581.

4. Weinberger, B.; Laskin, D. L.; Heck, D. E.; Laskin, J. D. Oxygen toxicity in premature infants. *Toxicol. Appl. Pharmacol.* **2002,** *181*, 60–67.

5. Martindale, J. L.; Holbrook, N. J. Cellular response to oxidative stress: signaling for suicide and survival. *J. Cell Physiol.* **2002,** *192*, 1–15.

6. Contestabile, A. Oxidative stress in neurodegeneration: mechanisms and therapeutic perspectives. *Curr. Top. Med. Chem.* **2001,** *1*, 553–568.

7. Maritim, A. C.; Sanders, R. A.; Watkins, J. B., III. Diabetes, oxidative stress, and antioxidants: a review. *J. Biochem. Mol. Toxicol.* **2003,** *17*, 24–38.

8. Ceconi, C.; Boraso, A.; Cargnoni, A.; Ferrari, R. Oxidative stress in cardiovascular disease: myth or fact? *Arch. Biochem. Biophys.* **2003,** *420*, 217–221.

9. Finkel, T.; Holbrook, N. J. Oxidants, oxidative stress and the biology of ageing. *Nature* **2000,** *408*, 239–247.

10. Melov, S.; Ravenscroft, J.; Malik, S.; Gill, M. S.; Walker, D. W.; Clayton, P. E.; Wallace, D. C.; Malfroy, B.; Doctrow, S. R.; Lithgow, G. J. Extension of life-span with superoxide dismutase/catalase mimetics. *Science* **2000,** *289*, 1567–1569.

11. Bada, J. L.; Lazcano, A. Prebiotic soup: revisiting the Miller experiment. *Science* **2003,** *300*, 745–746.

12. Miyakawa, S.; Yamanashi, H.; Kobayashi, K.; Cleaves, H. J.; Miller, S. L. Prebiotic synthesis from CO atmospheres: implications for the origins of life. *Proc. Natl. Acad. Sci. USA* **2002,** *99*, 14628–14631.

13. Tatsumi, H.; Takagi, K.; Fujita, M.; Kano, K.; Ikeda, T. Electro-chemical study of reversible hydrogenase reaction of *Desulfovibrio vulgaris* cells with methyl viologen as an electron carrier. *Anal. Chem.* **1999,** *71*, 1753–1759.

14. Harris, D. C.; Rinehart, A. L.; Hereld, D.; Schwartz, R. W.; Burke, F. P.; Salvador, A. P. Reduction potential of iron in transferrin. *Biochim. Biophys. Acta* **1985,** *838*, 295–301.

15. Berg, J. M.; Tymoczko, J. L.; Stryer, L. *Biochemistry;* WH Freeman: New York, 2001.

16. Redmond, R. W.; Gamlin, J. N. A compilation of singlet oxygen yields from biologically relevant molecules. *Photochem. Photobiol.* **1999,** *70*, 391–475.

17. Malmström, B. G. Enzymology of oxygen. *Annu. Rev. Biochem.* **1982,** *51*, 21–59.

18. Wood, P. M. The potential diagram for oxygen at pH 7. *Biochem. J.* **1988,** *253*, 287–289.

19. Butler, J.; Jayson, G. G.; Swallow, A. J. The reaction between the superoxide anion radical and cytochrome c. *Biochim. Biophys. Acta* **1975,** *408*, 215–222.

20. Simic, M. G. Pulse radiolysis in study of oxygen radicals. *Methods Enzymol.* **1990,** *186*, 89–100.

21. Fraaije, M. W.; Mattevi, A. Flavoenzymes: diverse catalysts with recurrent features. *Trends Biochem. Sci.* **2000,** *25*, 126–132.

22. Percy, M. J.; Gillespie, M. J.; Savage, G.; Hughes, A. E.; McMullin, M. F.; Lappin, T. R. Familial idiopathic methemoglobinemia revisited: original cases reveal 2 novel mutations in NADH-cytochrome b$_5$ reductase. *Blood* **2002,** *100*, 3447–3449.

23. Tocher, D. R.; Leaver, M. J.; Hodgson, P. A. Recent advances in the biochemistry and molecular biology of fatty acyl desaturases. *Prog. Lipid Res.* **1998,** *37*, 73–117.

24. Witkop, B. Remembering Heinrich Wieland (1877–1957). Portrait of an organic chemist and founder of modern biochemistry. *Med. Res. Rev.* **1992,** *12*, 195–274.

25. Chelikani, P.; Fita, I.; Loewen, P. C. Diversity of structures and properties among catalases. *Cell Mol. Life Sci.* **2004,** *61*, 192–208.

26. Gonzalez-Flecha, B.; Boveris, A. Mitochondrial sites of hydrogen peroxide production in reperfused rat kidney cortex. *Biochim. Biophys. Acta* **1995,** *1243*, 361–366.

27. Gonzalez-Flecha, B.; Demple, B. Metabolic sources of hydrogen per-oxide in aerobically growing *Escherichia coli. J. Biol. Chem.* **1995,** *270*, 13681–13687.

28. Wood, Z. A.; Poole, L. B.; Karplus, P. A. Peroxiredoxin evolution and the regulation of hydrogen peroxide signaling. *Science* **2003,** *300*, 650–653.

29. Eckert, J. H.; Erdmann, R. Peroxisome biogenesis. *Rev. Physiol Biochem. Pharmacol.* **2003,** *147*, 75–121.

30. Yeldandi, A. V.; Rao, M. S.; Reddy, J. K. Hydrogen peroxide generation in peroxisome proliferator-induced oncogenesis. *Mutat. Res.* **2000,** *448*, 159–177.

31. Angermuller, S. Peroxisomal oxidases: cytochemical localization and biological relevance. *Prog. Histochem. Cytochem.* **1989,** *20*, 1–65.

32. Mueller, S.; Weber, A.; Fritz, R.; Mutze, S.; Rost, D.; Walczak, H.; Volkl, A.; Stremmel, W. Sensitive and realtime determination of H_2O_2 release from intact peroxisomes. *Biochem. J.* **2002,** *363*, 483–491.

33. Kirkman, H. N.; Gaetani, G. F. Catalase: a tetrameric enzyme with four tightly bound molecules of NADPH. *Proc. Natl. Acad. Sci. USA* **1984,** *81*, 4343–4347.

34. Kirkman, H. N.; Galiano, S.; Gaetani, G. F. The function of catalase-bound NADPH. *J. Biol. Chem.* **1987,** *262*, 660–666.

35. Purdue, P. E.; Castro, S. M.; Protopopov, V.; Lazarow, P. B. Targeting of human catalase to peroxisomes is dependent upon a novel C-terminal peroxisomal targeting sequence. *Ann. N.Y. Acad. Sci.* **1996,** *804*, 775–776.

36. Sakamaki, K.; Ueda, T.; Nagata, S. The evolutionary conservation of the mammalian peroxidase genes. *Cytogenet. Genome Res.* **2002,** *98*, 93–95.

37. O'Brien, P. J. Radical formation during the peroxidase catalyzed metabolism of carcinogens and xenobiotics: the reactivity of these radicals with GSH, DNA, and unsaturated lipid. *Free Radic. Biol. Med.* **1988,** *4*, 169–183.

38. Eling, T. E.; Thompson, D. C.; Foureman, G. L.; Curtis, J. F.; Hughes, M. F. Prostaglandin H synthase and xenobiotic oxidation. *Annu. Rev. Pharmacol. Toxicol.* **1990,** *30*, 1–45.

39. Yodh, A. G.; Tromberg, B. J. Celebrating Britton Chance. *J. Biomed. Opt.* **2000,** *5*, 114–118.

40. Chance, B. The kinetics of the enzyme–substrate compound of peroxidase. 1943. *Adv. Enzymol. Relat. Areas Mol. Biol.* **1999,** *73*, 3–23.

41. Chance, B. Kinetics of the enzyme–substrate compound of peroxidase. *J. Biol. Chem.* **1943,** *151*, 553–577.

42. Yamazaki, I.; Mason, H. S.; Piette, L. Identification, by electron paramagnetic resonance spectroscopy, of free radicals generated from substrates by peroxidase. *J. Biol. Chem.* **1960,** *235*, 2444–2449.

43. Aust, S. D.; Chignell, C. F.; Bray, T. M.; Kalyanaraman, B.; Mason, R. P. Free radicals in toxicology. *Toxicol. Appl. Pharmacol.* **1993,** *120*, 168–178.

44. Tafazoli, S.; O'Brien, P. J. Peroxidases: a role in the metabolism and side effects of drugs. *Drug Discov. Today* **2005,** *10*, 617–625.

45. Hiner, A. N.; Raven, E. L.; Thorneley, R. N.; Garcia-Canovas, F.; Rodriguez-Lopez, J. N. Mechanisms of compound I formation in heme peroxidases. *J. Inorg. Biochem.* **2002,** *91*, 27–34.

46. Ogata, M. Acatalasemia. *Hum. Genet.* **1991,** *86*, 331–340.

47. McCord, J. M.; Fridovich, I. Superoxide dismutase: the first twenty years (1968–1988). *Free Radic. Biol. Med.* **1988,** *5*, 363–369.

48. Bannister, W. H.; Bannister, J. V. Isolation and characterization of superoxide dismutase: a personal history and tribute to Joe McCord and Irwin Fridovich. *Free Radic. Biol. Med.* **1988,** *5*, 371–376.

49. Fridovich, I. Reflections of a fortunate biochemist. *J. Biol. Chem.* **2001,** *276*, 28629–28636.

50. Benzie, I. F. Evolution of antioxidant defence mechanisms. *Eur. J. Nutr.* **2000,** *39*, 53–61.

51. Robinson, K. M.; Morre, J. T.; Beckman, J. S. Triuret: a novel product of peroxynitrite-mediated oxidation of urate. *Arch. Biochem. Biophys.* **2004,** *423*, 213–217.

52. Bartels, E. C. Allopurinol (xanthine oxidase inhibitor) in the treatment of resistant gout. *JAMA* **1966,** *198*, 708–712.

53. Enroth, C.; Eger, B. T.; Okamoto, K.; Nishino, T.; Nishino, T.; Pai, E. F. Crystal structures of bovine milk xanthine dehydrogenase and xanthine oxidase: structure-based mechanism of conversion. *Proc. Natl. Acad. Sci. USA* **2000,** *97*, 10723–10728.

54. Massey, V.; Harris, C. M. Milk xanthine oxidoreductase: the first one hundred years. *Biochem. Soc. Trans.* **1997**, *25*, 750–755.

55. Stevens, C. R.; Millar, T. M.; Clinch, J. G.; Kanczler, J. M.; Bodamyali, T.; Blake, D. R. Antibacterial properties of xanthine oxidase in human milk. *Lancet* **2000**, *356*, 829–830.

56. Horecker, B. L.; Heppel, L. A. The reduction of cytochrome c by xanthine oxidase. *J. Biol. Chem.* **1949**, *178*, 683–690.

57. Fridovich, I. With the help of giants. *Annu. Rev. Biochem.* **2003**, *72*, 1–18.

58. Fridovich, I.; Handler, P. Xanthine oxidase: V. Differential inhibition of the reduction of various electron acceptors. *J. Biol. Chem.* **1962**, *237*, 916–921.

59. Pauling, L. *The Nature of the Chemical Bond;* Cornell University Press: Ithaca, NY, 1960.

60. Harcourt, A. V. On the peroxides of potassium and sodium. *J. Chem. Soc.* **1861**, *14*, 267.

61. Pauling, L. The discovery of the superoxide radical. *Trends Biochem. Sci.* **1979**, *4*, N270–N271.

62. Neuman, E. W. Potassium superoxide and the three-electron bond. *J. Chem. Phys.* **1934**, *2*, 31–33.

63. Schwarz, H. A. Free radicals generated by radiolysis of aqueous solutions. *J. Chem. Educ.* **1981**, *58*, 101–105.

64. McCord, J. M.; Fridovich, I. Superoxide dismutase. An enzymic function for erythrocuprein (hemocuprein). *J. Biol. Chem.* **1969**, *244*, 6049–6055.

65. Goldstein, S.; Michel, C.; Bors, W.; Saran, M.; Czapski, G. A critical reevaluation of some assay methods for superoxide dismutase activity. *Free Radic. Biol. Med.* **1988**, *4*, 295–303.

66. Kirby, T. W.; Fridovich, I. A picomolar spectrophotometric assay for superoxide dismutase. *Anal. Biochem.* **1982**, *127*, 435–440.

67. Picker, S. D.; Fridovich, I. On the mechanism of production of superoxide radical by reaction mixtures containing NADH, phenazine methosulfate, and nitroblue tetrazolium. *Arch. Biochem. Biophys.* **1984**, *228*, 155–158.

68. Beauchamp, C.; Fridovich, I. Superoxide dismutase: improved assays and an assay applicable to acrylamide gels. *Anal. Biochem.* **1971**, *44*, 276–287.

69. Hodgson, E. K.; Fridovich, I. Reversal of the superoxide dismutase reaction. *Biochem. Biophys. Res. Commun.* **1973**, *54*, 270–274.

70. Brackett, D. J.; Wallis, G.; Wilson, M. F.; McCay, P. B. Spin trapping and electron paramagnetic resonance spectroscopy. *Methods Mol. Biol.* **1998**, *108*, 15–25.

71. Mason, R. P.; Hanna, P. M.; Burkitt, M. J.; Kadiiska, M. B. Detection of oxygen-derived radicals in biological systems using electron spin resonance. *Environ. Health Perspect.* **1994**, *102* (Suppl. 10), 33–36.

72. Mason, R. P.; Knecht, K. T. In vivo detection of radical adducts by electron spin resonance. *Methods Enzymol.* **1994**, *233*, 112–117.

73. Knecht, K. T.; Mason, R. P. In vivo spin trapping of xenobiotic free radical metabolites. *Arch. Biochem. Biophys.* **1993**, *303*, 185–194.

74. Bunce, N. J. Introduction to the interpretation of electron spin resonance spectra of organic radicals. *J. Chem. Educ.* **1987**, *64*, 907–914.

75. Weil, J. A.; Bolton, J. R.; Wertz, J. E. *Electron Paramagnetic Resonance: Elementary Theory and Practical Applications;* Wiley-Interscience: New York, 2004.

76. Qian, S. Y.; Chen, Y. R.; Deterding, L. J.; Fann, Y. C.; Chignell, C. F.; Tomer, K. B.; Mason, R. P. Identification of protein-derived tyrosyl radical in the reaction of cytochrome c and hydrogen peroxide: characterization by ESR spin-trapping, HPLC and MS. *Biochem. J.* **2002**, *363*, 281–288.

77. Iwahashi, H.; Parker, C. E.; Mason, R. P.; Tomer, K. B. Radical identification by liquid chromatography/thermospray mass spectrometry. *Rapid Commun. Mass Spectrom.* **1990,** *4*, 352–354.

78. Deterding, L. J.; Ramirez, D. C.; Dubin, J. R.; Mason, R. P.; Tomer, K. B. Identification of free radicals on hemoglobin from its self-peroxidation using mass spectrometry and immuno-spin trapping: Observation of a histidinyl radical. *J. Biol. Chem.* **2004,** *279*, 11600–11607.

79. Janzen, E. G.; Jandrisits, L. T.; Shetty, R. V.; Haire, D. L.; Hilborn, J. W. Synthesis and purification of 5,5-dimethyl-1-pyrroline-N-oxide for biological applications. *Chem. Biol. Interact.* **1989,** *70*, 167–172.

80. Lown, J. W.; Sim, S. K.; Chen, H. H. Hydroxyl radical production by free and DNA-bound aminoquinone antibiotics and its role in DNA degradation. Electron spin resonance detection of hydroxyl radicals by spin trapping. *Can. J. Biochem.* **1978,** *56*, 1042–1047.

81. Lloyd, R. V.; Hanna, P. M.; Mason, R. P. The origin of the hydroxyl radical oxygen in the Fenton reaction. *Free Radic. Biol. Med.* **1997,** *22*, 885–888.

82. Hart, P. J.; Balbirnie, M. M.; Ogihara, N. L.; Nersissian, A. M.; Weiss, M. S.; Valentine, J. S.; Eisenberg, D. A structure-based mechanism for copper–zinc superoxide dismutase. *Biochemistry* **1999,** *38*, 2167–2178.

83. Zelko, I. N.; Mariani, T. J.; Folz, R. J. Superoxide dismutase multigene family: a comparison of the CuZn-SOD (SOD1), Mn-SOD (SOD2), and EC-SOD (SOD3) gene structures, evolution, and expression. *Free Radic. Biol. Med.* **2002,** *33*, 337–349.

84. Choudhury, S. B.; Lee, J. W.; Davidson, G.; Yim, Y. I.; Bose, K.; Sharma, M. L.; Kang, S. O.; Cabelli, D. E.; Maroney, M. J. Examination of the nickel site structure and reaction mechanism in *Streptomyces seoulensis* superoxide dismutase. *Biochemistry* **1999,** *38*, 3744–3752.

85. Barondeau, D. P.; Kassmann, C. J.; Bruns, C. K.; Tainer, J. A.; Getzoff, E. D. Nickel superoxide dismutase structure and mechanism. *Biochemistry* **2004,** *43*, 8038–8047.

86. Grace, S. C. Phylogenetic distribution of superoxide dismutase supports an endosymbiotic origin for chloroplasts and mitochondria. *Life Sci.* **1990,** *47*, 1875–1886.

87. Berlyn, M. K. Linkage map of *Escherichia coli* K-12, edition 10: the traditional map. *Microbiol. Mol. Biol. Rev.* **1998,** *62*, 814–984.

88. Imlay, K. R.; Imlay, J. A. Cloning and analysis of *sodC*, encoding the copper–zinc superoxide dismutase of *Escherichia coli*. *J. Bacteriol.* **1996,** *178*, 2564–2571.

89. Tainer, J. A.; Getzoff, E. D.; Richardson, J. S.; Richardson, D. C. Structure and mechanism of copper, zinc superoxide dismutase. *Nature* **1983,** *306*, 284–287.

90. Banci, L.; Bertini, I.; Cantini, F.; D'Onofrio, M.; Viezzoli, M. S. Structure and dynamics of copper-free SOD: the protein before binding copper. *Protein Sci.* **2002,** *11*, 2479–2492.

91. Kubota, S.; Yang, J. T. Bis[cyclo(histidylhistidine)]copper(II) complex that mimics the active center of superoxide dismutase has its catalytic activity. *Proc. Natl. Acad. Sci. USA* **1984,** *81*, 3283–3286.

92. Zhou, H. X.; Wong, K. Y.; Vijayakumar, M. Design of fast enzymes by optimizing interaction potential in active site. *Proc. Natl. Acad. Sci. USA* **1997,** *94*, 12372–12377.

93. Fattman, C. L.; Schaefer, L. M.; Oury, T. D. Extracellular superoxide dismutase in biology and medicine. *Free Radic. Biol. Med.* **2003,** *35,* 236–256.

94. Petersen, S. V.; Oury, T. D.; Valnickova, Z.; Thogersen, I. B.; Hojrup, P.; Crapo, J. D.; Enghild, J. J. The dual nature of human extracellular superoxide dismutase: one sequence and two structures. *Proc. Natl. Acad. Sci. USA* **2003,** *100,* 13875–13880.

95. Lookene, A.; Stenlund, P.; Tibell, L. A. Characterization of heparin binding of human extracellular superoxide dismutase. *Biochemistry* **2000,** *39,* 230–236.

96. Whittaker, J. W. Manganese superoxide dismutase. *Met. Ions Biol. Syst.* **2000,** *37,* 587–611.

97. Whittaker, J. W. Prokaryotic manganese superoxide dismutases. *Methods Enzymol.* **2002,** *349,* 80–90.

98. Lah, M. S.; Dixon, M. M.; Pattridge, K. A.; Stallings, W. C.; Fee, J. A.; Ludwig, M. L. Structure–function in *Escherichia coli* iron superoxide dismutase: comparisons with the manganese enzyme from *Thermus thermophilus. Biochemistry* **1995,** *34,* 1646–1660.

99. Klug, D.; Fridovich, I.; Rabani, J. Pulse radiolysis investigation of superoxide disproportionation: mechanism for bovine superoxide dismutase. *J. Am. Chem. Soc.* **1973,** *95,* 2786–2791.

100. Messner, K. R.; Imlay, J. A. The identification of primary sites of superoxide and hydrogen peroxide formation in the aerobic respiratory chain and sulfite reductase complex of *Escherichia coli. J. Biol. Chem.* **1999,** *274,* 10119–10128.

101. Chen, Q.; Vazquez, E. J.; Moghaddas, S.; Hoppel, C. L.; Lesnefsky, E. J. Production of reactive oxygen species by mitochondria: central role of complex III. *J. Biol. Chem.* **2003,** *278,* 36027–36031.

102. Tjus, S. E.; Scheller, H. V.; Andersson, B.; Møller, B. L. Active oxygen produced during selective excitation of photosystem I is damaging not only to photosystem I, but also to photosystem II. *Plant Physiol.* **2001,** *125,* 2007–2015.

103. Gupta, A. S.; Heinen, J. L.; Holaday, A. S.; Burke, J. J.; Allen, R. D. Increased resistance to oxidative stress in transgenic plants that overexpress chloroplastic Cu/Zn superoxide dismutase. *Proc. Natl. Acad. Sci. USA* **1993,** *90,* 1629–1633.

104. Kliebenstein, D. J.; Monde, R. A.; Last, R. L. Superoxide dismutase in *Arabidopsis*: an eclectic enzyme family with disparate regulation and protein localization. *Plant Physiol.* **1998,** *118,* 637–650.

105. Hassan, H. M.; Fridovich, I. Paraquat and *Escherichia coli.* Mechanism of production of extracellular superoxide radical. *J. Biol. Chem.* **1979,** *254,* 10846–10852.

106. Bus, J. S.; Gibson, J. E. Paraquat: model for oxidant-initiated toxicity. *Environ. Health Perspect.* **1984,** *55,* 37–46.

107. Daisley, H.; Simmons, V. Homicide by paraquat poisoning. *Med. Sci. Law* **1999,** *39,* 266–269.

108. Wesseling, C.; Hogstedt, C.; Picado, A.; Johansson, L. Unintentional fatal paraquat poisonings among agricultural workers in Costa Rica: report of 15 cases. *Am. J. Ind. Med.* **1997,** *32,* 433–441.

109. Suntres, Z. E. Role of antioxidants in paraquat toxicity. *Toxicology* **2002,** *180,* 65–77.

110. O'Brien, P. J. Molecular mechanisms of quinone cytotoxicity. *Chem. Biol. Interact.* **1991,** *80,* 1–41.

111. Wallace, K. B. Doxorubicin-induced cardiac mitochondrionopathy. *Pharmacol. Toxicol.* **2003,** *93,* 105–115.

112. Mason, R. P.; Holtzman, J. L. The role of catalytic superoxide formation in the O_2 inhibition of nitroreductase. *Biochem. Biophys. Res. Commun.* **1975,** *67,* 1267–1274.

113. Silva, J. M.; Khan, S.; O'Brien, P. J. Molecular mechanisms of nitrofurantoin-induced hepatocyte toxicity in aerobic versus hypoxic conditions. *Arch. Biochem. Biophys.* **1993,** *305,* 362–369.

114. Reinhart, H. H.; Reinhart, E.; Korlipara, P.; Peleman, R. Combined nitrofurantoin toxicity to liver and lung. *Gastroenterology* **1992,** *102,* 1396–1399.

115. Robbins, M. E. C.; Zhao, W. Chronic oxidative stress and radiation-induced late normal tissue injury: a review. *Int. J. Radiat. Biol.* **2004,** *80,* 251–259.

116. Touati, D. The molecular genetics of superoxide dismutase in *E. coli. Free Radic. Res. Commun.* **1991,** *12–13* (Pt. 1), 379–382.

117. Touati, D. Investigating phenotypes resulting from a lack of superoxide dismutase in bacterial null mutants. *Methods Enzymol.* **2002,** *349,* 145–154.

118. Parkes, T. L.; Kirby, K.; Phillips, J. P.; Hilliker, A. J. Transgenic analysis of the cSOD-null phenotypic syndrome in *Drosophila. Genome* **1998,** *41,* 642–651.

119. Gralla, E. B.; Valentine, J. S. Null mutants of *Saccharomyces cerevisiae* Cu, Zn superoxide dismutase: characterization and spontaneous mutation rates. *J. Bacteriol.* **1991,** *173,* 5918–5920.

120. Shefner, J. M.; Reaume, A. G.; Flood, D. G.; Scott, R. W.; Kowall, N. W.; Ferrante, R. J.; Siwek, D. F.; Upton-Rice, M.; Brown, R. H., Jr. Mice lacking cytosolic copper/zinc superoxide dismutase display a distinctive motor axonopathy. *Neurology* **1999,** *53,* 1239–1246.

121. Carlsson, L. M.; Jonsson, J.; Edlund, T.; Marklund, S. L. Mice lacking extracellular superoxide dismutase are more sensitive to hyperoxia. *Proc. Natl. Acad. Sci. USA* **1995,** *92,* 6264–6268.

122. Lebovitz, R. M.; Zhang, H.; Vogel, H.; Cartwright, J., Jr.; Dionne, L.; Lu, N.; Huang, S.; Matzuk, M. M. Neurodegeneration, myocardial injury, and perinatal death in mitochondrial superoxide dismutase-deficient mice. *Proc. Natl. Acad. Sci. USA* **1996,** *93,* 9782–9787.

123. Cleveland, D. W.; Rothstein, J. D. From Charcot to Lou Gehrig: deciphering selective motor neuron death in ALS. *Nat. Rev. Neurosci.* **2001,** *2,* 806–819.

124. Sathasivam, S.; Ince, P. G.; Shaw, P. J. Apoptosis in amyotrophic lateral sclerosis: a review of the evidence. *Neuropathol. Appl. Neurobiol.* **2001,** *27,* 257–274.

125. Siddique, T.; Nijhawan, D.; Hentati, A. Molecular genetic basis of familial ALS. *Neurology* **1996,** *47,* S27–S34.

126. Rosen, D. R.; Siddique, T.; Patterson, D.; Figlewicz, D. A.; Sapp, P.; Hentati, A.; Donaldson, D.; Goto, J.; O'Regan, J. P.; Deng, H. X. Mutations in Cu/Zn superoxide dismutase gene are associated with familial amyotrophic lateral sclerosis. *Nature* **1993,** *362,* 59–62.

127. Andersen, P. M.; Sims, K. B.; Xin, W. W.; Kiely, R.; O'Neill, G.; Ravits, J.; Pioro, E.; Harati, Y.; Brower, R. D.; Levine, J. S.; Heinicke, H. U.; Seltzer, W.; Boss, M.; Brown, R. H., Jr. Sixteen novel mutations in

the Cu/Zn superoxide dismutase gene in amyotrophic lateral sclerosis: a decade of discoveries, defects and disputes. *Amyotroph. Lateral. Scler. Other Motor Neuron Disord.* **2003,** *4,* 62–73.

128. Beckman, J. S.; Estevez, A. G.; Crow, J. P.; Barbeito, L. Superoxide dismutase and the death of motoneurons in ALS. *Trends Neurosci.* **2001,** *24,* S15–S20.

129. Cardoso, R. M.; Thayer, M. M.; DiDonato, M.; Lo, T. P.; Bruns, C. K.; Getzoff, E. D.; Tainer, J. A. Insights into Lou Gehrig's disease from the structure and instability of the A4V mutant of human Cu, Zn superoxide dismutase. *J. Mol. Biol.* **2002,** *324,* 247–256.

130. Koppenol, W. H. The Haber–Weiss cycle: 70 years later. *Redox. Rep.* **2001,** *6,* 229–234.

131. Koppenol, W. H. The centennial of the Fenton reaction. *Free Radic. Biol. Med.* **1993,** *15,* 645–651.

132. (a) Yamazaki, I.; Piette, L. H. ESR spin-trapping studies on the reaction of Fe^{2+} ions with H_2O_2-reactive species in oxygen toxicity in biology. *J. Biol. Chem.* **1990,** *265,* 13589–13594. (b) Pestovsky, O.; Stoian, S.; Bominaar, E. L.; Shan, X.-P.; Münck, E.; Que, Jr., L.; Bakac, A. Aqueous $Fe^{IV}=O$: spectroscopic identification and oxo-group exchange. *Angew. Chem.* **2005,** *44,* 6871–6874.

133. McCord, J. M.; Day, E. D., Jr. Superoxide-dependent production of hydroxyl radical catalyzed by iron-EDTA complex. *FEBS Lett.* **1978,** *86,* 139–142.

134. Liochev, S. I.; Fridovich, I. Superoxide and iron: partners in crime. *IUBMB Life* **1999,** *48,* 157–161.

135. Liochev, S. I.; Fridovich, I. The Haber–Weiss cycle: 70 years later: an alternative view. *Redox. Rep.* **2002,** *7,* 55–57.

136. Winterbourn, C. C. Toxicity of iron and hydrogen peroxide: the Fenton reaction. *Toxicol. Lett.* **1995,** *82–83,* 969–974.

137. Gardner, P. R.; Fridovich, I. Superoxide sensitivity of the *Escherichia coli* 6-phosphogluconate dehydratase. *J. Biol. Chem.* **1991,** *266,* 1478–1483.

138. Gardner, P. R.; Fridovich, I. Superoxide sensitivity of the *Escherichia coli* aconitase. *J. Biol. Chem.* **1991,** *266,* 19328–19333.

139. Keyer, K.; Imlay, J. A. Superoxide accelerates DNA damage by elevating free-iron levels. *Proc. Natl. Acad. Sci. USA* **1996,** *93,* 13635–13640.

140. Koppenol, W. H. The Haber–Weiss cycle: 71 years later. *Redox. Rep.* **2002,** *7,* 59–60.

141. Kasprzak, K. S. Oxidative DNA and protein damage in metal-induced toxicity and carcinogenesis. *Free Radic. Biol. Med.* **2002,** *32,* 958–967.

142. Bal, W.; Kasprzak, K. S. Induction of oxidative DNA damage by carcinogenic metals. *Toxicol. Lett.* **2002,** *127,* 55–62.

143. Galaris, D.; Evangelou, A. The role of oxidative stress in mechanisms of metal-induced carcinogenesis. *Crit. Rev. Oncol. Hematol.* **2002,** *42,* 93–103.

144. Ignarro, L. J.; Buga, G. M.; Wood, K. S.; Byrns, R. E.; Chaudhuri, G. Endothelium-derived relaxing factor produced and released from artery and vein is nitric oxide. *Proc. Natl. Acad. Sci. USA* **1987,** *84,* 9265–9269.

145. Hussain, S. P.; Hofseth, L. J.; Harris, C. C. Radical causes of cancer. *Nat. Rev. Cancer* **2003,** *3,* 276–285.

146. Kissner, R.; Nauser, T.; Bugnon, P.; Lye, P. G.; Koppenol, W. H. Formation and properties of peroxynitrite as studied by laser flash

photolysis, high-pressure stopped-flow technique, and pulse radiolysis. *Chem. Res. Toxicol.* **1997**, *10*, 1285–1292.

147. Winterbourn, C. C.; Kettle, A. J. Radical-radical reactions of superoxide: a potential route to toxicity. *Biochem. Biophys. Res. Commun.* **2003**, *305*, 729–736.

148. Szabo, C. Multiple pathways of peroxynitrite cytotoxicity. *Toxicol. Lett.* **2003**, *140–141*, 105–112.

149. Klebanoff, S. J. Reactive nitrogen intermediates and antimicrobial activity: role of nitrite. *Free Radic. Biol. Med.* **1993**, *14*, 351–360.

150. Pryor, W. A.; Squadrito, G. L. The chemistry of peroxynitrite: a product from the reaction of nitric oxide with superoxide. *Am. J. Physiol.* **1995**, *268*, L699–L722.

151. Squadrito, G. L.; Pryor, W. A. Oxidative chemistry of nitric oxide: the roles of superoxide, peroxynitrite, and carbon dioxide. *Free Radic. Biol. Med.* **1998**, *25*, 392–403.

152. Koppenol, W. H. 100 years of peroxynitrite chemistry and 11 years of peroxynitrite biochemistry. *Redox. Rep.* **2001**, *6*, 339–341.

153. Beckman, J. S.; Beckman, T. W.; Chen, J.; Marshall, P. A.; Freeman, B. A. Apparent hydroxyl radical production by peroxynitrite: implications for endothelial injury from nitric oxide and superoxide. *Proc. Natl. Acad. Sci. USA* **1990**, *87*, 1620–1624.

154. Lymar, S. V.; Khairutdinov, R. F.; Hurst, J. K. Hydroxyl radical formation by O–O bond homolysis in peroxynitrous acid. *Inorg. Chem.* **2003**, *42*, 5259–5266.

155. Bonini, M. G.; Radi, R.; Ferrer-Sueta, G.; Ferreira, A. M.; Augusto, O. Direct EPR detection of the carbonate radical anion produced from peroxynitrite and carbon dioxide. *J. Biol. Chem.* **1999**, *274*, 10802–10806.

156. Augusto, O.; Bonini, M. G.; Amanso, A. M.; Linares, E.; Santos, C. C.; De Menezes, S. L. Nitrogen dioxide and carbonate radical anion: two emerging radicals in biology. *Free Radic. Biol. Med.* **2002**, *32*, 841–859.

157. Burney, S.; Niles, J. C.; Dedon, P. C.; Tannenbaum, S. R. DNA damage in deoxynucleosides and oligonucleotides treated with peroxynitrite. *Chem. Res. Toxicol.* **1999**, *12*, 513–520.

158. Dedon, P. C.; Tannenbaum, S. R. Reactive nitrogen species in the chemical biology of inflammation. *Arch. Biochem. Biophys.* **2004**, *423*, 12–22.

159. Balazy, M.; Kaminski, P. M.; Mao, K.; Tan, J.; Wolin, M. S. S-Nitroglutathione, a product of the reaction between peroxynitrite and glutathione that generates nitric oxide. *J. Biol. Chem.* **1998**, *273*, 32009–32015.

160. Sbarra, A. J.; Karnovsky, M. L. The biochemical basis of phagocytosis: I. Metabolic changes during the ingestion of particles by polymorphonuclear leukocytes. *J. Biol. Chem.* **1959**, *234*, 1355–1362.

161. Curnutte, J. T.; Kuver, R.; Babior, B. M. Activation of the respiratory burst oxidase in a fully soluble system from human neutrophils. *J. Biol. Chem.* **1987**, *262*, 6450–6452.

162. Babior, B. M.; Lambeth, J. D.; Nauseef, W. The neutrophil NADPH oxidase. *Arch. Biochem. Biophys.* **2002**, *397*, 342–344.

163. Nisimoto, Y.; Otsuka-Murakami, H.; Lambeth, D. J. Reconstitution of flavin-depleted neutrophil flavocytochrome b_{558} with 8-mercapto-FAD and characterization of the flavin-reconstituted enzyme. *J. Biol. Chem.* **1995**, *270*, 16428–16434.

164. Dinauer, M. C. Regulation of neutrophil function by Rac GTPases. *Curr. Opin. Hematol.* **2003,** *10,* 8–15.

165. Mayer, B. J. SH3 domains: complexity in moderation. *J. Cell Sci.* **2001,** *114,* 1253–1263.

166. Ago, T.; Kuribayashi, F.; Hiroaki, H.; Takeya, R.; Ito, T.; Kohda, D.; Sumimoto, H. Phosphorylation of p47phox directs phox homology domain from SH3 domain toward phosphoinositides, leading to phagocyte NADPH oxidase activation. *Proc. Natl. Acad. Sci. USA* **2003,** *100,* 4474–4479.

167. Heyworth, P. G.; Cross, A. R.; Curnutte, J. T. Chronic granulomatous disease. *Curr. Opin. Immunol.* **2003,** *15,* 578–584.

168. Winterbourn, C. C.; Vissers, M. C.; Kettle, A. J. Myeloperoxidase. *Curr. Opin. Hematol.* **2000,** *7,* 53–58.

169. Winterbourn, C. C. Biological reactivity and biomarkers of the neutrophil oxidant, hypochlorous acid. *Toxicology* **2002,** *181–182,* 223–227.

170. van Dalen, C. J.; Whitehouse, M. W.; Winterbourn, C. C.; Kettle, A. J. Thiocyanate and chloride as competing substrates for myeloperoxidase. *Biochem. J.* **1997,** *327,* 487–492.

171. Weil, S. C.; Rosner, G. L.; Reid, M. S.; Chisholm, R. L.; Farber, N. M.; Spitznagel, J. K.; Swanson, M. S. cDNA cloning of human myeloperoxidase: decrease in myeloperoxidase mRNA upon induction of HL-60 cells. *Proc. Natl. Acad. Sci. USA* **1987,** *84,* 2057–2061.

172. Naskalski, J. W. Simple procedure of isolation of myeloperoxidase from leukocytes, pus and bone marrow cells. *Acta Med. Pol.* **1980,** *21,* 129–137.

173. Arkema, J. M.; Schadee-Eestermans, I. L.; Beelen, R. H.; Hoefsmit, E. C. A combined method for both endogenous myeloperoxidase and acid phosphatase cytochemistry as well as immunoperoxidase surface labelling discriminating human peripheral blood-derived dendritic cells and monocytes. *Histochemistry* **1991,** *95,* 573–578.

174. Brown, K. E.; Brunt, E. M.; Heinecke, J. W. Immunohistochemical detection of myeloperoxidase and its oxidation products in Kupffer cells of human liver. *Am. J. Pathol.* **2001,** *159,* 2081–2088.

175. Sakamaki, K.; Kanda, N.; Ueda, T.; Aikawa, E.; Nagata, S. The eosinophil peroxidase gene forms a cluster with the genes for myeloperoxidase and lactoperoxidase on human chromosome 17. *Cytogenet. Cell Genet.* **2000,** *88,* 246–248.

176. Kutter, D.; Devaquet, P.; Vanderstocken, G.; Paulus, J. M.; Marchal, V.; Gothot, A. Consequences of total and subtotal myeloperoxidase deficiency: risk or benefit? *Acta Haematol.* **2000,** *104,* 10–15.

177. Hope, H. R.; Remsen, E. E.; Lewis, C., Jr.; Heuvelman, D. M.; Walker, M. C.; Jennings, M.; Connolly, D. T. Large-scale purification of myeloperoxidase from HL60 promyelocytic cells: characterization and comparison to human neutrophil myeloperoxidase. *Protein Expr. Purif.* **2000,** *18,* 269–276.

178. Blair-Johnson, M.; Fiedler, T.; Fenna, R. Human myeloperoxidase: structure of a cyanide complex and its interaction with bromide and thiocyanate substrates at 1.9 A resolution. *Biochemistry* **2001,** *40,* 13990–13997.

179. Davey, C. A.; Fenna, R. E. 2.3 Å resolution X-ray crystal structure of the bisubstrate analogue inhibitor salicylhydroxamic acid bound to human

myeloperoxidase: a model for a prereaction complex with hydrogen peroxide. *Biochemistry* **1996,** *35,* 10967–10973.

180. Andersson, E.; Hellman, L.; Gullberg, U.; Olsson, I. The role of the propeptide for processing and sorting of human myeloperoxidase. *J. Biol. Chem.* **1998,** *273,* 4747–4753.

181. Hansson, M.; Olsson, I.; Nauseef, W. M. Biosynthesis, processing, and sorting of human myeloperoxidase. *Arch. Biochem. Biophys.* **2005,** in press.

182. Nauseef, W. M. Insights into myeloperoxidase biosynthesis from its inherited deficiency. *J. Mol. Med.* **1998,** *76,* 661–668.

183. German, J. B. Food processing and lipid oxidation. *Adv. Exp. Med. Biol.* **1999,** *459,* 23–50.

184. Black, S. C. In vivo models of myocardial ischemia and reperfusion injury: application to drug discovery and evaluation. *J. Pharmacol. Toxicol. Methods* **2000,** *43,* 153–167.

185. Keller, J. N.; Mattson, M. P. Roles of lipid peroxidation in modulation of cellular signaling pathways, cell dysfunction, and death in the nervous system. *Rev. Neurosci.* **1998,** *9,* 105–116.

186. Sayre, L. M.; Smith, M. A.; Perry, G. Chemistry and biochemistry of oxidative stress in neurodegenerative disease. *Curr. Med. Chem.* **2001,** *8,* 721–738.

187. Markesbery, W. R.; Carney, J. M. Oxidative alterations in Alzheimer's disease. *Brain Pathol.* **1999,** *9,* 133–146.

188. Jenner, P. Oxidative stress in Parkinson's disease. *Ann. Neurol.* **2003,** *53* (Suppl. 3), S26–S36.

189. Smith, K. J.; Kapoor, R.; Felts, P. A. Demyelination: the role of reactive oxygen and nitrogen species. *Brain Pathol.* **1999,** *9,* 69–92.

190. Weber, L. W.; Boll, M.; Stampfl, A. Hepatotoxicity and mechanism of action of haloalkanes: carbon tetrachloride as a toxicological model. *Crit. Rev. Toxicol.* **2003,** *33,* 105–136.

191. Reinke, L. A. Spin trapping evidence for alcohol-associated oxidative stress. *Free Radic. Biol. Med.* **2002,** *32,* 953–957.

192. Jaeschke, H.; Knight, T. R.; Bajt, M. L. The role of oxidant stress and reactive nitrogen species in acetaminophen hepatotoxicity. *Toxicol. Lett.* **2003,** *144,* 279–288.

193. Bolchoz, L. J.; Morrow, J. D.; Jollow, D. J.; McMillan, D. C. Primaquine-induced hemolytic anemia: effect of 6-methoxy-8-hydroxylaminoquinoline on rat erythrocyte sulfhydryl status, membrane lipids, cytoskeletal proteins, and morphology. *J. Pharmacol. Exp. Ther.* **2002,** *303,* 141–148.

194. Baliga, R.; Ueda, N.; Walker, P. D.; Shah, S. V. Oxidant mechanisms in toxic acute renal failure. *Drug Metab. Rev.* **1999,** *31,* 971–997.

195. Kappus, H. Oxidative stress in chemical toxicity. *Arch. Toxicol.* **1987,** *60,* 144–149.

196. Porter, N. A.; Caldwell, S. E.; Mills, K. A. Mechanisms of free radical oxidation of unsaturated lipids. *Lipids* **1995,** *30,* 277–290.

197. Gardner, H. W. Oxygen radical chemistry of polyunsaturated fatty acids. *Free Radic. Biol. Med.* **1989,** *7,* 65–86.

198. Yue, Q. S.; Tomer, K. B.; Yue, G. H.; Guo, Q.; Kadiiska, M. B.; Mason, R. P. Characterization of the initial carbon-centered pentadienyl radical and subsequent radicals in lipid peroxidation: identification via on-line high performance liquid chromatography/electron spin resonance and mass spectrometry. *Free Radic. Biol. Med.* **2002,** *33,* 998–1009.

199. Wade, C. R.; van Rij, A. M. In vivo lipid peroxidation in man as measured by the respiratory excretion of ethane, pentane, and other low-molecular-weight hydrocarbons. *Anal. Biochem.* **1985**, *150*, 1–7.

200. Benedetti, A.; Comporti, M.; Esterbauer, H. Identification of 4-hydroxynonenal as a cytotoxic product originating from the peroxidation of liver microsomal lipids. *Biochim. Biophys. Acta* **1980**, *620*, 281–296.

201. Schneider, C.; Tallman, K. A.; Porter, N. A.; Brash, A. R. Two distinct pathways of formation of 4-hydroxynonenal. Mechanisms of non-enzymatic transformation of the 9- and 13-hydroperoxides of linoleic acid to 4-hydroxyalkenals. *J. Biol. Chem.* **2001**, *276*, 20831–20838.

202. Schaur, R. J. Basic aspects of the biochemical reactivity of 4-hydroxynonenal. *Mol. Aspects Med.* **2003**, *24*, 149–159.

203. Uchida, K. 4-Hydroxy-2-nonenal: a product and mediator of oxidative stress. *Prog. Lipid Res.* **2003**, *42*, 318–343.

204. Lin, D.; Lee, H. G.; Liu, Q.; Perry, G.; Smith, M. A.; Sayre, L. M. 4-Oxo-2-nonenal is both more neurotoxic and more protein reactive than 4-hydroxy-2-nonenal. *Chem. Res. Toxicol.* **2005**, *18*, 1219–1231.

205. Brash, A. R. Lipoxygenases: occurrence, functions, catalysis, and acquisition of substrate. *J. Biol. Chem.* **1999**, *274*, 23679–23682.

206. Funk, C. D. Prostaglandins and leukotrienes: advances in eicosanoid biology. *Science* **2001**, *294*, 1871–1875.

207. Abuja, P. M.; Albertini, R. Methods for monitoring oxidative stress, lipid peroxidation and oxidation resistance of lipoproteins. *Clin. Chim. Acta* **2001**, *306*, 1–17.

208. Slater, T. F. Overview of methods used for detecting lipid peroxidation. *Methods Enzymol.* **1984**, *105*, 283–293.

209. Jardine, D.; Antolovich, M.; Prenzler, P. D.; Robards, K. Liquid chromatography-mass spectrometry (LC-MS) investigation of the thiobarbituric acid reactive substances (TBARS) reaction. *J. Agric. Food Chem.* **2002**, *50*, 1720–1724.

210. McConnell, E. J.; Bittelmeyer, A. M.; Raess, B. U. Irreversible inhibition of plasma membrane (Ca^{2+}/Mg^{2+})-ATPase and Ca^{2+} transport by 4-OH-2,3-trans-nonenal. *Arch. Biochem. Biophys.* **1999**, *361*, 252–256.

211. Ji, C.; Amarnath, V.; Pietenpol, J. A.; Marnett, L. J. 4-Hydroxynonenal induces apoptosis via caspase-3 activation and cytochrome c release. *Chem. Res. Toxicol.* **2001**, *14*, 1090–1096.

212. Higuchi, Y. Chromosomal DNA fragmentation in apoptosis and necrosis induced by oxidative stress. *Biochem. Pharmacol.* **2003**, *66*, 1527–1535.

2

Covalent Binding of Xenobiotics to DNA and Protein

COVALENT ADDUCTS TO MACROMOLECULES

Covalent adducts to DNA and protein mediate the toxic effects of many carcinogens and cytotoxic agents. Protein modification by xenobiotics can lead to cytotoxicity (1, 2), toxic immune-mediated reactions (3), and idiosyncratic reactions to drugs (4). DNA modifications (e.g., covalent adducts, strand breaks, loss of bases) may constitute *premutagenic lesions*, alterations that can result in mutations. Unrepaired DNA damage may kill the cell.

The earliest evidence for covalent modification of macromolecules by carcinogens[1] was obtained in the early 1950s. Researchers discovered that when animals or cells were exposed to radiolabeled carcinogens, radioactivity became bound to macromolecules. Even rigorous washing with solvents and buffers did not remove the bound radioactivity, indicating that covalent adduct formation had taken place. In subsequent decades of research, chemical mechanisms for the reaction of electrophiles with specific sites in DNA and protein have been deduced; the detailed structures of hundreds of macromolecular adducts have been elucidated; the effects of adduction on DNA conformation have been studied by high-resolution techniques; and highly sensitive techniques for the detection of DNA adducts have been developed and applied to human molecular epidemiology (5). We discuss the experimental approaches to detection (6) and identification of the chemical structures of DNA and protein adducts, and briefly consider some of the chemical mechanisms of their formation (7, 8). This chapter initiates a sequence of three chapters, exploring three closely related subjects: DNA damage, DNA repair, and chemical mutagenesis.

(Our discussion of the chemistry and biochemistry of macromolecular adduct formation will begin with the assumption that the reader is familiar with the covalent structures of DNA, RNA, and protein, including their monomer building blocks and the chemical linkages by which they form polymers. These topics are addressed in introductory biochemistry textbooks and are not reviewed here.)

In addition to the actions of xenobiotic chemicals, ultraviolet (UV) light and high-energy (ionizing) radiation also cause characteristic modifications to the DNA structure. Ionizing radiation damage may be *direct*, that is, due to the deposition of radiation energy in the DNA molecule itself, or *indirect*, due to the reactions of the free radicals formed by the radiolysis of water (9, 10). Free radical radiolysis products of water include reducing radicals, such as the solvated electron (e_{aq}^-) and the H$^•$ atom, and oxidizing radicals, especially the hydroxyl radical, $^•$OH. In the presence of molecular oxygen, solvated electrons react rapidly to form superoxide anion: $O_2 + e_{aq}^- \rightarrow O_2^{\bullet-}$ (see chapter 1; radiolysis sidebar). Thus, ionizing radiation damage and oxidative stress have much in common (11). The formation/repair of radiation-induced DNA damage is considered in chapter 3. Radiation can also, by similar mechanisms, damage RNA, protein, and other molecules in the cell.

A single toxic agent can induce many types of DNA damage. These various damages can induce a spectrum of mutational consequences. For example, alkylating agents react with all four DNA bases, especially guanine, and at multiple sites, including ring N and exocyclic O atoms (12). Patterns of DNA damages induced by an agent can serve as a distinctive "fingerprint" of exposure. We may be able to work backwards from an observed spectrum of DNA adducts to deduce the nature of the chemical agent responsible for them. Such analysis contributes to the science of molecular epidemiology (see sidebar, chapter 13). These themes are elaborated in subsequent chapters.

DNA ADDUCT IDENTIFICATION SCENARIOS

We may wish to detect and identify DNA adducts in a variety of chemical/biological contexts, and the nature of the context will affect our choice of experimental methods:

1. In vitro mechanistic studies. Here, we examine the reactions of purified DNA (or DNA constituents) with a carcinogen[2] in defined chemical systems. DNA modification levels are likely to be high and chemical interferences low. Direct chemical analysis (e.g., HPLC-MS) of the DNA hydrolysate may be possible.
2. Cellular or in vivo toxicology. A given agent (often radiolabeled) is applied to a cell or animal, and, after a time period, DNA is isolated and analyzed. Yield of adducts may be low; DNA purity and DNA yield may be limiting factors.
3. Molecular epidemiology. Prevalent DNA adducts are measured in DNA isolated from human donors. Here, the nature of the carcinogen may be poorly defined; adduct levels may be very low; complex mixtures of adducts may be anticipated.

NUCLEIC ACID TARGETS FOR ADDUCT FORMATION STUDIES

For in vitro mechanistic studies, several kinds of nucleic acids (or nucleic acid constituents) can be used for preparation of adducts (e.g., by in vitro reactions with activated metabolites of carcinogens). High-molecular-weight chromosomal DNA (isolated from sources such as calf thymus or salmon sperm, and commercially available) may seem the most obvious choice, and is indeed often used. Chromosomal DNA provides a great variety of local sequence contexts for adduct formation and may give very complex adduct profiles.

The monomer building blocks of nucleic acids (bases, ribonucleosides, ribonucleotides, deoxyribonucleosides, and deoxyribonucleotides) are chemically tractable targets, and are readily available, but, because of both electronic and steric factors, they may be poor models for the behavior of

DNA. Molecular-biological DNA constructs, such as plasmid or bacterio-phage DNA, are easily prepared and have well-defined sequence properties. These targets can also provide convenient bioassays. For example, we can assay the plaque-forming capacity of bacteriophage genomes (following in vitro packaging and infection of a bacterial host) or the yield of transformants (following transformation of suitable host cells by a plasmid) as a measure of DNA damage. Homopolymers offer the chemical simplicity of a single target base (13). Homopolyribonucleotides can be prepared by the action of the template-independent RNA polymerase, polynucleotide phosphorylase (14). Homopolydeoxyribonucleotides are prepared chemi-cally and can be annealed to produce synthetic double-stranded DNA molecules (poly [dT·dA] and poly [dG·dC]). One approach to analyzing the base specificity of a reactive species is to compare its binding among a series of RNA homopolyribonucleotides (15) or DNA homopolyde-oxyribonucleotides (16). For example, when synthetic ^{3}H-labeled 7-8-benzo[a]-pyrene dihydrodiol 9-10-epoxide (BPDE; see chapter 18) was incubated overnight with homopolyribonucleotides, the percentage of the BPDE bound covalently to the homopolymers was poly(G), 18%; poly(A), 2%; poly(C), 0.5% (17). This result shows that although purine bases are the major targets of BPDE binding, detectable binding to cytosine also occurs.

SYNTHETIC REACTIVE INTERMEDIATES

Some chemicals can form covalent adducts directly, whereas others require metabolic activation (18). Structural characterization of covalent adducts clarifies the nature of the activated intermediates that have reacted with DNA, and this information helps us to elucidate mechanisms of metabolic activation (a topic to which we will return in several later chapters). For in vitro studies, we can use metabolic activation systems (enzyme preparations; see chapter 4) to convert xenobiotics into reactive species. However, mechanistic and structural studies are easiest to perform if we can prepare the reactive intermediate chemically. DNA-reactive species include radicals, oxidants, and electrophiles. By definition, reactive intermediates are unstable species and they usually present challenging synthetic targets. In many cases, reactive intermediates were first postu-lated based on "paper chemistry" (intuition and speculation) and later prepared by synthetic organic chemistry. The adducts formed by reaction of DNA with a synthetic reactive intermediate, in vitro, can be compared with adducts formed from the corresponding enzymatically activated carcinogen, or with adducts formed in cells (figure 2-1), to test whether the synthetic molecule is identical to the product of metabolic activation. This approach was used to determine the metabolic activation pathway of benzo[a]pyrene, first ruling out the involvement of K-region epoxides and then verifying the important role of dihydrodiol epoxides (see chapter 18).

Among the classes of reactive intermediates/metabolically activated carcinogens that have been synthesized are the following. (i) The bay-region dihydrodiol epoxide derivatives of benzo[a]pyrene and other poly-cyclic aromatic hydrocarbons (PAHs) (see chapter 18); these are stable in dry organic solvents, but hydrolyze rapidly in water (19). (ii) N-Acetoxy esters of aromatic amines (see chapter 17) are isolable at low temperature, but

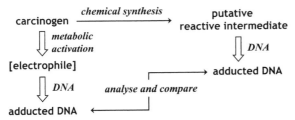

FIGURE 2-1.

Comparative analysis of patterns of DNA adduct formation by metabolically activated carcinogens (left) and synthetic reactive intermediates (right) can be used to test the involvement of specific electrophilic metabolites in DNA damage and toxicity.

decompose when warmed (20). In one case, N-acetoxysulfamethoxazole, an N-acetoxy ester proved to be stable even at room temperature (21). (iii) The α-hydroxy metabolites of dialkylnitrosamines are reactive species formed by P450-catalyzed oxidation (see chapter 7). Despite their instability (22), chemical synthesis was achieved in the early 1980s (23). Each of these classes of metabolites reacts spontaneously with DNA to give a spectrum of adducts similar to those observed following exposure of cells or animals to the parent carcinogen.

ISOLATION AND CHARACTERIZATION OF DNA ADDUCTS

The concentration of DNA in cells is low, relative to the abundance of protein and RNA. The level of cellular DNA adducts is correspondingly also low, even following exposure to large doses of a chemical mutagen or carcinogen. For molecular epidemiological studies, we may wish to measure specific adducts in humans who have not been exposed to specific occupational or therapeutic agents, and the background levels of such adducts may be extremely low. The detection of DNA adducts and their chemical characterization present major challenges (24). We consider several of the techniques that have been applied (see table 2-1 for an overview).

If a monomer target, such as a DNA base, is reacted with a synthetic electrophile, yielding few adducts in reasonable yields, adduct purification can be carried out by reversed-phase HPLC (e.g., (25)), capillary electrophoresis (26), or other methods. UV absorbance can be used to detect the products and structure determination can be achieved by standard organic methods, such as NMR spectroscopy (see later) and mass spectrometry.

The characterization of adducts formed with polydeoxyribonucleotide (DNA) targets, in vitro or in vivo, requires isolation of the DNA, followed by hydrolysis into its nucleotide, nucleoside, or base constituents. With in vitro systems, where the incubation mix is prepared with a large excess of DNA and little or no protein, DNA isolation is usually straightforward, but cellular systems offer a greater challenge. The chromosomal DNA is only a small fraction of the macromolecule mass of the cell, most of which is protein and RNA, and some of the protein is tightly complexed with the DNA.

TABLE 2-1.
Some Methods for Detection of Adducts in Cellular DNA

METHOD	ADVANTAGES	SENSITIVITY	DISADVANTAGES/REQUIREMENTS
Radiolabeled carcinogen/DNA isolation/ scintillation counting	Accurate quantitation	6	Radiolabeled carcinogen; does not provide chemical information; not applicable to endogenous adducts
Radiolabeled carcinogen/DNA isolation/ accelerator mass spectrometry	Ultrahigh sensitivity	11	Radiolabeled carcinogen; highly specialized instrumentation and relatively large DNA sample size
DNA isolation/hydrolysis/adduct separation/ specific detection (e.g., fluorescence, electrochemical)	Radiolabeled carcinogen not required; chemical identity verified by chromatography and chemical properties (e.g., fluorescence spectrum)	6	Limited application, depending on properties of carcinogen; sensitive to interferences
DNA isolation/hydrolysis/adduct separation/ chemical identification (e.g., mass spectrometry)	Radiolabeled carcinogen not required; universal applicability	7	Sophisticated instrumentation; sensitive to interferences
^{32}P postlabeling	Radiolabeled carcinogen not required; high sensitivity	9	Limited chemical information; some adducts may be difficult to label
Immunoassay	Radiolabeled carcinogen not required; high sensitivity	8	Limited chemical information; potential for interferences ("cross-reactivity"); semiquantitative only

Note: "carcinogen" refers to any DNA adduct-forming chemical. Sensitivity: typical method sensitivity, 1 adduct in 10^n nucleotides; e.g., "6" indicates a detection limit of approximately 1 adduct in 10^6 DNA nucleotides. Actual sensitivities may differ greatly, depending on the nature of the adduct and the experimental system.

A typical protocol for isolation of hepatic DNA is as follows (27). Tissue is homogenized in buffer, pH 8, containing EDTA (which chelates metal ions and inhibits DNAses) and SDS (sodium dodecyl sulfate); these conditions denature proteins, inhibit enzyme activity, and reduce the positive charge on histone proteins, decreasing their affinity for DNA. Incubation with *proteinase K* is performed, to degrade proteins. (Proteinase K (endopeptidase K, EC 3.4.21.64), a commercially available non-specific proteinase from the fungus *Tritirachium album*, is an unusually SDS-resistant enzyme (28).) Repeated two-phase extractions with buffer-saturated chloroform/isoamyl alcohol/phenol are performed. Chloroform and phenol are protein denaturants, and isoamyl alcohol reduces foaming at the aqueous–organic interface. These extractions cause much of the protein to denature, precipitate, and collect at the interface. The aqueous layer is retained and the DNA is precipitated by the addition of two volumes of ethanol, and cooling; the DNA is spooled out on a glass rod. To remove residual RNA, the crude DNA is redissolved in buffer and treated with RNAse at 37°C, followed by a repeat of the extraction and ethanol precipitation steps. Finally, the DNA is washed with alcohol and acetone and dried. Pure DNA is characterized by a ratio of $A_{260}/A_{280} = 1.8$; lower values indicate residual protein contamination, since protein absorbs more strongly at 280 than at 260 nm.

HYDROLYSIS OF DNA

As noted above, complete chemical characterization of DNA adducts is only possible once the adducted bases, deoxynucleosides, or deoxynucleotides have been released from the polymer. Hydrolysis in concentrated acid can cause extensive degradation of the adducted bases and sugars. The three common approaches to adduct release are (i) spontaneous release; (ii) mild acid hydrolysis; and (iii) enzymatic hydrolysis. Enzymatic hydrolysis is usually preferred (29). However, one must be cognizant of the possibility that the presence of covalently bound adducts will hinder enzymatic hydrolysis, leading to underestimation of the level of adducts (30).

Recovery of Adducted Bases

Since the bases are less polar than their sugar- or sugar–phosphate-bearing derivatives, they are likely to be more easily separated by reversed-phase HPLC methods and more suitable for analysis by mass spectrometry, although modern mass spectrometry techniques, such as electrospray ionization, are now making analysis of deoxynucleotides rather routine. Some DNA adducts "release themselves"; for example, N7-guanine adducts usually undergo spontaneous hydrolysis of the *N*-glycosylic bond, releasing the adduct as a modified base. Mild acid treatment (0.1 M HCl, 70°C) causes hydrolysis of the glycosylic bonds of purine bases, releasing (in addition to guanine and adenine) some purine adducts. Also, glycosylase enzymes (see chapter 3) that effect DNA base-excision repair release particular classes of adducted bases, which can be separated and quantitated (31). The *E. coli* repair enzyme formamidopyrimidine (Fapy) glycosylase (EC 3.2.2.23; see chapter 3) releases 8-oxoguanine from DNA. Formation of this oxidized base is as an indicator of oxidative stress (32).

Recovery of Adducted Deoxynucleosides and Deoxynucleotides

Complete hydrolysis of DNA requires the action of both an *endonuclease*, which cuts the polymer into oligonucleotide fragments, and an *exonuclease*, which completes the degradation to deoxynucleotides. Two distinct modes of nucleic acid hydrolysis are possible, since phosphodiester bonds can be hydrolyzed on either the 5′ or 3′ side. The most common approach is treatment with pancreatic deoxyribonuclease I (DNAse I; EC 3.1.21.1) and snake venom phosphodiesterase (exonuclease; EC 3.1.15.1) to yield deoxynucleoside 5′-monophosphates. These can then be converted to nucleosides, by the action of the nonspecific phosphatase, alkaline phosphatase (EC 3.1.3.1).

Alternatively, DNA degradation can be carried out with endonucleases such as micrococcal nuclease or spleen phosphodiesterase (EC 3.1.31.1), which yield deoxynucleoside 3′-monophosphates. This approach is used in the ^{32}P postlabeling method (discussed later in this chapter) that requires the presence of the 5′-OH group.

SEPARATION OF ADDUCTED DEOXYNUCLEOSIDES

Even after relatively extensive nucleic acid modification, nonadducted normal deoxynucleosides will outnumber adducts by orders of magnitude. The adducted deoxynucleosides must be purified from the DNA hydrolyzate, guided by an understanding of their expected chemical characteristics. Often, the analysis is done in two stages. First, adducts are separated, as a group, from normal deoxynucleosides. Second, the different adducts are separated from one another. Adducts of PAHs or aromatic amines, for example, are much more hydrophobic than normal deoxynucleosides. Preliminary purification on a hydrophobic matrix, such as Sephadex LH-20 (*33*) or short C-18 reversed-phase columns (*34*) is often very effective: the normal deoxynucleosides are eluted with water, and the adducts are eluted with methanol. Even adducted deoxynucleo*tides* can be separated this way (*35*). Another useful technique for separation of hydrophobic adducts is extraction into 1-butanol solvent (*36*). Separation of adducted deoxynucleosides usually relies on reversed-phase HPLC separation (e.g., (*37*)).

If the xenobiotic is radioactively labeled, the purification of the adducts can be monitored by scintillation counting. If labeled material is not available, spectroscopic detection methods such as UV absorption or fluorescence (e.g., (*38*)) may be applicable. For example, PAHs such as benzo[*a*]pyrene are strongly fluorescent. Benzo[*a*]pyrene is metabolically activated to the dihydrodiol epoxide metabolite (7*R*,8*S*)-dihydroxy-(9*S*,10*R*)-epoxy-7,8,9,10-tetrahydrobenzo[*a*]pyrene (BPDE), which forms covalent adducts to guanine and adenine bases in DNA (see chapter 18). Acid treatment of adducted DNA releases BP "tetrol," 7,8,9,10-tetrahydroxy-7,8,9,10-tetrahydrobenzo[*a*]pyrene, which is strongly fluorescent. HPLC with fluorescence detection can be used for analysis of BP tetrol as a marker of benzo[*a*]pyrene exposure (figure 2-2) (*39*).

In the absence of "tags" such as radioactivity or fluorescence, adduct detection may be difficult. Electrochemical detection (*40*) is applicable to

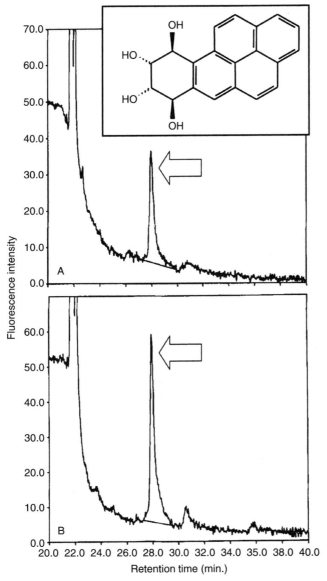

FIGURE 2-2.

BP "tetrol" is 7,8,9,10-tetrahydrobenzo[*a*]pyrene-7,8,9,10-tetrol (7*R*,8*S*,9*R*, 10*S*). The carcinogen benzo[*a*]pyrene (see chapter 18) is metabolically activated to (7*R*,8*S*)-dihydroxy-(9*S*,10*R*)-epoxy-7,8,9,10-tetrahydrobenzo[*a*]pyrene (BPDE), which reacts with DNA to form (among other adducts) an adduct at guanine N2. Mild acid hydrolysis of adducted DNA releases the bound BP from this site, in the form of BP tetrol. Adducted DNA was hydrolyzed (HCl) and then neutralized with NaOH. HPLC analysis was performed on a C18 analytical column eluted with 55% MeOH in H_2O at a flow rate of 1 ml/min. BP tetrol was quantified by fluorescence, $\lambda_{exc} = 344$ nm, $\lambda_{em} = 398$ nm. (A) Calf thymus DNA (100 µg) spiked with tetrol; (B) DNA (50 µg) isolated from HeLa cells after incubation (2 h) with BPDE, 50 nM. (*Source: Schwerdtle, T.; Seidel, A.; Hartwig, A. Effect of soluble and particulate nickel compounds on the formation and repair of stable benzo[*a*]pyrene DNA adducts in human lung cells.* Carcinogenesis **2002**, 23, 47–53. *Copyright Oxford University Press.*)

certain adducts. HPLC coupled to tandem mass spectrometry is now being applied successfully to the detection of DNA adducts (e.g., (*41*)) and this technology offers outstanding ability to overcome analytical interferences.

RADIOACTIVE LABELING AND ACCELERATOR MASS SPECTROMETRY

The biggest challenge in studies of DNA adduct formation is usually analytical sensitivity. In vitro reaction of synthetic reactive intermediates with purified DNA may give covalent binding as high as 1 adduct per 10^2 nucleotides. But in cellular studies, DNA is protected by multiple levels of defenses, and most of the dose of an applied reactive species will react with water, glutathione, protein, etc., so DNA binding will be much lower. In whole-animal studies or human monitoring, binding levels may be as low as "adducts per genome," that is, adducts per 10^9 nucleotides, and yet still have toxicological significance.

Many techniques have been applied to the problem of DNA adduct detection, as discussed above (*42*). With some carcinogens, we can take advantage of specific chemical properties such as fluorescence or electrochemical activity. However, these methods are limited in range of applicability and in sensitivity. The most universal detection methods use radioactive labeling. Three isotopes are of greatest importance: ^3H and ^{14}C are used to label organic carcinogens and ^{32}P is used to label nucleotides (in the postlabeling technique discussed in this chapter). These isotopes are produced artificially by bombardment of elemental targets with neutrons in a nuclear reactor. The desired labeled compounds are then synthesized from a radiolabeled elemental precursor.

The great advantages of radioactive labeling are specificity and sensitivity. Specificity derives from the fact that natural background levels of radioisotopes are very low, so any detected radioactivity probably derives from the administered labeled compound. In the case of ^{14}C, natural background is caused by cosmic ray bombardment of atmospheric nitrogen, which converts ^{14}N into ^{14}C. Ultimately, this atmospheric radiocarbon is incorporated into organic materials, giving a steady-state natural background level of about one part ^{14}C in 10^{12} parts ^{12}C. (After an organism dies, the assimilation of carbon ceases, and this radiocarbon decays with a half-life of 5760 years: this is the basis of the well-known radiocarbon dating method.)

Each decay of a radioactive nucleus releases a large amount of energy, that is, energy sufficient to cause multiple chemical bond cleavages or excitations. In the liquid scintillation counting technique, the radiolabeled sample is dissolved in a "cocktail" containing a fluorescent organic scintillant, and the energy released by each decay is converted into fluorescence energy. The bursts of fluorescence are detected by a photomultiplier and counted.

Ultimately, the sensitivity of detection of a radioactive compound by this approach is limited by two factors: the extent of incorporation of radiolabel into the compound and the rate of radioactive decay. In principle, every carbon atom of a compound could be replaced by ^{14}C but, in practice, the extent of incorporation is usually lower, and labeled compounds are usually diluted greatly with unlabeled "cold carrier."

TABLE 2-2.

Radioactive Decay Kinetics

	^{14}C	^3H	^{32}P
Half-life (y)	5760	12.3	—
Half-life (d)	$2.10 \times 10^{+6}$	$4.49 \times 10^{+3}$	14.3
Half-life (min)	$3.03 \times 10^{+9}$	$6.47 \times 10^{+6}$	$2.06 \times 10^{+4}$
λ (per min)	2.29×10^{-10}	1.07×10^{-7}	3.37×10^{-5}
Atoms (1 dpm)	$4.37 \times 10^{+9}$	$9.33 \times 10^{+6}$	$2.97 \times 10^{+4}$
Moles (1 dpm)	7.29×10^{-16}	1.56×10^{-18}	4.95×10^{-21}

The second and third rows give the half-life in years/days. This is converted to a half-life in minutes (fourth row). The decay rate λ is calculated from the relationship $\lambda \times t_{1/2} = \ln 2$. The sixth row shows the number of radiolabeled nuclei/atoms, N, required to yield one decay per minute (dpm), which is the reciprocal of λ (the probability of decay per minute per nucleus). 1 dpm is roughly the limit of detection by scintillation counting. Note that this quantity is several billion atoms of ^{14}C but only a few thousand atoms of ^{32}P. In the last row, N is expressed as a number of moles.

The kinetics of radioactive decay impose an unalterable constraint. The shorter the half-life of an isotope, then the more rapidly it decays, so a given number of radioactive nuclei will yield a higher count rate (counts per minute). However, experiments need to be done quickly if the half-life is only a few weeks, as with ^{32}P. Table 2-2 illustrates the relationship between half-life and decay rate for commonly used radioactive nuclei.

As an alternative to scintillation counting (or other methods that detect decay events, such as autoradiography), we can try to detect the radioisotope directly, by mass spectrometry, relying on the increased m/z value of the heavier nucleus. This idea carries the promise of greater sensitivity, especially for slow-decay isotopes such as ^{14}C. Since mass spectrometry weighs individual atoms (ions), and is extremely sensitive, we should be able to detect much less than the billion-atom-scale quantity of material needed for scintillation counting of ^{14}C. However, this approach means throwing away the greatest advantage of radiolabeling techniques, namely that nuclear decay events are so much more energetic than ordinary chemical reactions. Consequently, chemical interferences must be eliminated, or at least reduced, and sensitivity of detection of the isotopes must be maximized. Conventional mass spectrometry is inadequate, because its sensitivity is too low, and interferences from nonlabeled ions (e.g., ^{13}CH and $^{12}CH_2$, which have the same nominal mass as ^{14}C) are overwhelming. The specialized technique of *accelerator mass spectrometry* (AMS) was developed in the 1970s, initially driven by the demand for improved radiocarbon dating methods. Since about 1990, AMS has been applied in toxicology. Improvements in ^{14}C detection sensitivity amounting to many orders of magnitude have been achieved, making possible the detection of one DNA adduct per genome, or less. The carbon AMS technique is outlined here; for more details, see (43–45).

Carbon AMS is performed by analyzing *elemental* carbon. The carbon-containing sample[3] to be analyzed is converted to the elemental form by high-temperature combustion to CO_2, which is trapped and then reduced to graphite. The graphite sample is analyzed to determine the ^{14}C to ^{12}C ratio, using a dedicated AMS instrument. As in conventional mass spectrometry, the sample is first ionized in a vacuum, generating negative ions, which are accelerated and separated according to m/z in a magnetic field. This step generates a packet of ions of $m/z = -14$, but the packet contains interfering ions such as $^{13}CH^-$ in addition to the target analyte, $^{14}C^-$. In the next stage, the ions are accelerated to about 1 million volts in a van de Graaf generator. The resulting highly energetic ions collide with an extremely thin graphite foil target. The collision strips the electrons from the ions and fragments interfering molecular species such as $^{13}CH^-$. The resulting positive ions are then separated by a quadrupole analyzer and detected.

In a typical application of AMS to DNA adduct detection, Frantz et al. (46) administered ^{14}C-labeled 2-amino-3,8-dimethylimidazo[4,5-f]-quinoxaline (MeIQx), a heterocyclic amine food pyrolysis product (see chapter 17), to male Sprague-Dawley rats. Binding of MeIQx to hepatic DNA measured by AMS was found to be linear in applied dose over a range of about five orders of magnitude.

DNA ADDUCT STRUCTURE DETERMINATION

Determination of the structure of a purified deoxyribonucleoside or base adduct can be approached by the usual techniques of organic analysis. However, the amount of adduct that can be obtained from cells or tissues is often very limited. Most chemical characterization studies have been performed on adducts that were synthesized chemically or prepared in vitro by reaction of chemically activated xenobiotics with DNA, deoxyribonucleosides, etc. NMR is probably the most valuable tool for structure determination (47). High-field-strength NMR measurements can resolve every proton resonance on a nucleoside adduct. The resonances corresponding to protons on the adduct moiety can often be assigned by comparison of chemical shifts to those of the parent carcinogen, and the deoxyguanosine moiety resonances compared to those of the normal nucleoside. Table 2-3 lists chemical shift values for the guanine and deoxyribose protons in deoxyguanosine and some typical adducts (figure 2-3). Assignments can be confirmed by the use of decoupling or two-dimensional NMR techniques (48). ^{13}C-NMR has also been used. Mass spectrometry has also become increasingly useful for structure determination of nucleoside adducts, with the development of soft ionization modes, such as MALDI (matrix-assisted laser desorption ionization) and electrospray ionization, and tandem MS techniques (e.g., (49)).

Once a covalent adduct has been isolated and identified, the adduct can then be used as a standard for the identification, by co-chromatography, of adducts formed in vivo or in cells in vitro. The target of interest (such as hepatic DNA in vivo, or the chromosomal DNA of cultured hepatocytes) is exposed to the radiolabeled xenobiotic and DNA is isolated and hydrolyzed. The hydrolyzate is "spiked" by the addition of large amounts of *unlabeled* adduct standards. The spiked hydrolyzate is separated by HPLC, and the eluent is monitored for both UV absorbance (to detect

TABLE 2-3.
^{1}H-NMR Chemical Shifts of Deoxyribose and Guanine Protons in Deoxyguanosine and Some Representative Covalent Adducts

PROTON	A	B	C	D	E	F
	dG	dG-2AF	dG-6-AC	dG-6-BP	dG-AcAl	G-N7-GA
1'	6.1	6.36	6.33	5.42	6.08	—
2', 2''	2.46, 2.18	2.57, 2.05	2.24	2.87, 1.69	2.16	—
3'	4.31	4.45	4.39	3.98	4.31	—
4'	3.79	3.95	3.87	3.10–3.45	3.78	—
5', 5''	3.52, 3.49	3.80, 3.80	3.60, 3.50	3.49, 3.53	—	—
3'-OH	5.24	5.37	n.r.	4.74	5.2	—
5'-OH	4.92	6.02	n.r.	5.58–5.85	4.87	—
8	7.9	—	7.77	—	6.17	7.8
N1-H	10.58	10.59	10.81	10.95	—	10.84
2-NH$_2$	6.42	6.47	8.29	6.69	7.86	6.13

Sources: 2'-deoxyguanosine (A): (25); N-(deoxyguanosin-8-yl)-2-aminofluorene (B): (33, 107, 108); 5-(deoxyguanosin-N^2-yl)-6-aminochrysene (C): (109); 8-(benzo[a]-pyren-6-yl)-deoxyguanosine (D): (110); N7-(2-carbamoyl-2-hydroxyethyl)guanine (E): (111); 3-(2-deoxyribos-1-yl)-5,6,7,8-tetrahydro-8-hydroxy-6-methylpyrimido[1,2-a]purine-10(3H)one (F): (112). n.r. = not reported.

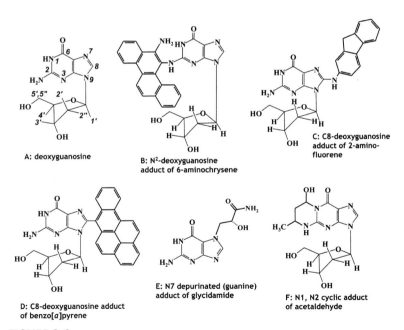

A: deoxyguanosine

B: N²-deoxyguanosine adduct of 6-aminochrysene

C: C8-deoxyguanosine adduct of 2-amino-fluorene

D: C8-deoxyguanosine adduct of benzo[a]pyrene

E: N7 depurinated (guanine) adduct of glycidamide

F: N1, N2 cyclic adduct of acetaldehyde

FIGURE 2-3.
Chemical structures of some deoxyguanosine and guanine adducts. NMR chemical shift data for these adducts are given in table 2-3. *Note*: A full-color version of this figure appears on the website.

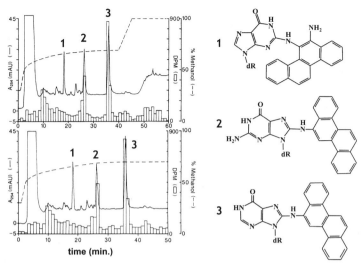

FIGURE 2-4.

Identification of DNA adducts by co-chromatography. Left panel: Reversed-phase HPLC analysis of DNA adducts. Rat hepatocytes were incubated with either ^{3}H-labeled 6-nitrochrysene (top) or 6-aminochrysene (bottom). DNA was isolated from the cells and hydrolyzed to nucleosides. Nonlabeled standards of adducts 1, 2, and 3 were added to the hydrolyzate, which was then separated by HPLC on a C-18 reversed-phase column using a methanol–water gradient (as indicated by the dashed line). The elution of the standards was monitored by absorbance at 254 nm (solid line), and the elution of the labeled DNA adducts was monitored by radioactivity (open bars). Co-elution with the unlabeled standards provides evidence for the identities of the adducts. Right panel: Structures of three major DNA adducts identified from the reaction of *N*-hydroxy-6-aminochrysene with calf thymus DNA in vitro. (Adduct 3, a deoxy*inosine* adduct, presumably arises from the deamination of a deoxyadenosine adduct precursor.) *Note*: A full-color version of this figure appears on the website. (*Source: Delclos, K. B.; Miller, D. W.; Lay, J. O., Jr.; Casciano, D. A.; Walker, R. P.; Fu, P. P.; Kadlubar, F. F. Identification of C8-modified deoxyinosine and N2- and C8-modified deoxyguanosine as major products of the in vitro reaction of N-hydroxy-6-aminochrysene with DNA and the formation of these adducts in isolated rat hepatocytes treated with 6-nitrochrysene and 6-aminochrysene. Carcinogenesis 1987, 8, 1703–1709. Copyright Oxford University Press.*)

the unlabeled standards) and radioactivity (to detect the radiolabeled adducts) (figure 2-4).

EXOCYCLIC DNA ADDUCTS

Exocyclic DNA adducts are adducts in which an additional ring has been incorporated into a base (dG, dA, or dC), by the reaction of a bifunctional electrophile with the base at two different sites. They form a structurally diverse class of DNA adducts. Important exocyclic adducts include ethenodeoxyadenosine (εdA) N^2,3-ethenodeoxyguanosine (εdG), ethenodeoxycytidine (εdC), pyrimidopurinone (M$_1$dG), and a series of hydroxypropanodeoxyguanosines (HO-PdG) (figure 2-5). Exocyclic adducts result from DNA modification by either exogenous or endogenous (50)

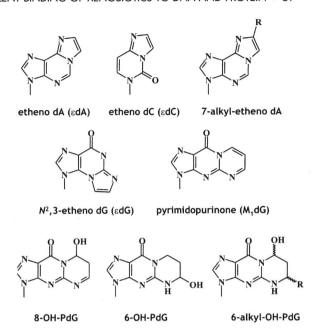

FIGURE 2-5.
Various exocyclic DNA adducts.

etheno dA (εdA)   etheno dC (εdC)   7-alkyl-etheno dA

N^2,3-etheno dG (εdG)   pyrimidopurinone (M$_1$dG)

8-OH-PdG   6-OH-PdG   6-alkyl-OH-PdG

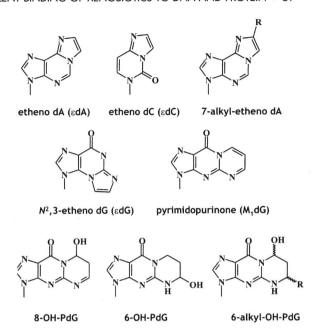

dA   malondi-aldehyde   − 2 H$_2$O   εdA

FIGURE 2-6.
Reaction of malondialdehyde with deoxyadenosine. *Note*: A full-color version of this figure appears on the website.

bifunctional electrophiles (figure 2-6). Bifunctional electrophiles can be generated by the cytochrome P450-catalyzed oxidation of xenobiotics (e.g., vinyl chloride → chloroethylene oxide) or by the oxidative degradation of cellular constituents, such as lipid peroxidation (threonine → acrolein; polyunsaturated fatty acids → malondialdehyde and 4-hydroxynonenal; deoxynucleotides → base propenals; see chapter 1) (*51*). εdA and εdG are produced via the reductive decomposition of hydroperoxy fatty acids (e.g., by ascorbic acid) or metabolism of the xenobiotic vinyl chloride. Levels of εdG in control hepatocytes and nonparenchymal liver tissue are in the range of 1 adduct in 10^7 to 10^8 nucleotides. Following exposure of rats to vinyl chloride, the levels increase approximately linearly with dose and time, to a limit of 10- to 15-fold above basal levels (*52*).

Exocyclic adducts block Watson-Crick base pairing and are therefore anticipated to be highly miscoding and mutagenic lesions. This has been verified by experiments such as in vitro replication of adduct-containing template-primers and in vivo replication of singly adducted viral genomes and shuttle vectors. However, mutagenic potency varies with adduct structure, sequence context, and the nature of the vector (e.g., single- vs. double-stranded) and the replication host (*53*). For example, M$_1$dG induces

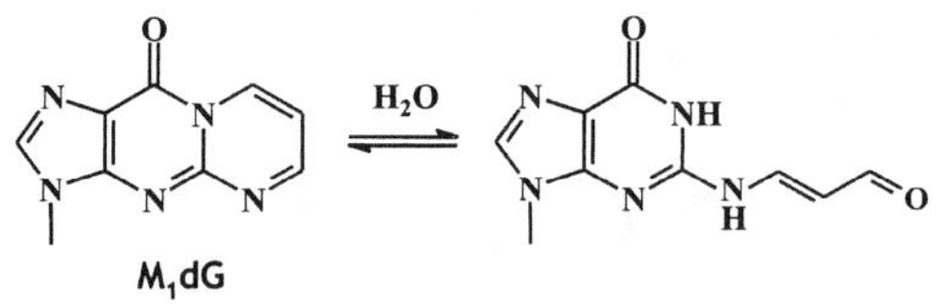

FIGURE 2-7.

Hydrolytic ring opening. *Note*: A full-color version of this figure appears on the website.

base pair substitution mutations in several sequence contexts in bacteria and mammalian cells but frameshift mutations only in reiterated $(CpG)_n$ sequences in either cell type. εdA is relatively weakly mutagenic in *E. coli* but strongly mutagenic when introduced in the same shuttle vector in COS-7 cells. These differences probably reflect processing by different DNA polymerases in different organisms (see chapter 4).

Exocyclic adducts may be repaired by base excision repair or nucleotide excision repair processes (see chapter 3) (*54*). εdA is an excellent alternative substrate for the base excision repair enzyme 3-methyladenine glycosylase whereas M_1dG and HO-PdG are removed by nucleotide excision repair. Consequently, M_1dG and HO-PdG lesions are more mutagenic when replicated in cells that are deficient in nucleotide excision repair. M_1dG and HO-PdG bind the mismatch repair protein MutS (*55*), which can lead to repair of the adducts but can also prevent nucleotide excision repair. The importance of this competition in mammalian cells has not yet been determined.

Some exocyclic adducts are chemically dynamic lesions. M_1dG undergoes hydrolytic ring opening to N^2-oxopropenyldeoxyguanosine (OPdG) in duplex DNA, but not in single-stranded DNA or in the nucleoside (figure 2-7) (*56*). Ring opening appears to be catalyzed during annealing of the duplex strands and requires a dC residue opposite the adduct. No ring opening is observed when duplexes containing M_1dG opposite T residues are annealed. Thermal denaturation of duplexes containing OPdG leads to rapid ring closure to give M_1dG. M_1dG is also directly reactive with nucleophiles and, in addition to water, will add certain amines, hydroxylamines, and hydrazines. The adduct is also rapidly reduced to a 5,6-dihydro derivative by sodium borohydride. Thus, M_1dG displays the hallmark features of a reactive electrophile in single- or double-stranded DNA. Note that the electrophilic carbon of M_1dG (carbon 8) is located in the major groove prior to reaction, whereas the electrophilic carbon of OPdG (the aldehyde) is present in the minor groove.

Similar interconversions and nucleophilic additions are observed with HO-PdG adducts in duplex DNA. However, these adducts exhibit the additional ability to cross-link with nucleophilic sites in DNA, producing interstrand DNA cross-links, and to react with proteins, forming DNA–protein cross-links. The formation of DNA–DNA cross-links is relatively slow and occurs from the ring-closed HO-PdG adducts, whereas DNA–protein cross-linking is rapid and results from reaction of the aliphatic aldehyde that lies in the minor groove. The latter reaction may account for the previously unexplained detection of DNA-protein cross-links in vivo. HO-PdG-mediated cross-links are acted upon by the nucleotide excision repair system.[4]

POSTLABELING ANALYSIS OF DNA ADDUCTS

The ^{32}P *postlabeling* technique for carcinogen–DNA adduct detection was introduced by Kurt Randerath and colleagues (*57, 58*). With this method, radiolabeled carcinogens are not required: instead, the label is introduced to the adduct *subsequent* to DNA hydrolysis. Since ^{32}P is used (half-life $= 14$ days), high specific activities, and, hence, high sensitivities, are achievable. The postlabeling technique is illustrated in figure 2-8. The DNA sample of interest (e.g., obtained from the tissue of a carcinogen-treated animal) is purified and hydrolyzed with micrococcal endonuclease plus spleen phosphodiesterase, yielding deoxyribonucleoside-3'-monophosphates (dNp). The hydrolyzate dNp mix will consist of a great excess of "normal" deoxynucleotides (dAp, dGp, dCp, Tp), a considerable amount of methylated normal deoxyribonucleotides (5-Me-dCp, 6-Me-dAp), plus a small amount of the adducted deoxyribonucleotides (dN*p) that we want to detect.

(It is often possible to enhance the sensitivity of the method by partially purifying the adducted deoxyribonucleotides at this stage, for example by solvent extraction of hydrophobic adducts into 1-butanol (*59*).)

The hydrolyzate (or 1-butanol extract) is treated with the enzyme polynucleotide kinase (polynucleotide 5'-hydroxy-kinase, EC 2.7.1.78) and [γ-^{32}P]-ATP. The kinase (encoded by bacteriophage T4) transfers the (labeled) γ-phosphate of ATP to the 5'-hydroxyl groups of the deoxyribonucleotides. The dNp are thus phosphorylated to give ^{32}P-labeled deoxyribonucleoside-3',5'-bisphosphates (^{32}pdNp). *As long as the adducted*

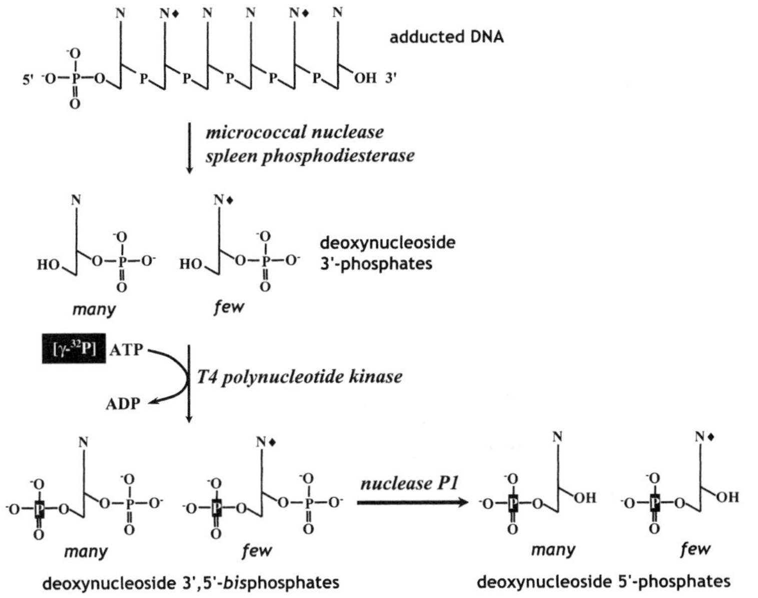

FIGURE 2-8.
The ^{32}P postlabeling method for detection of DNA adducts. Adducted DNA is hydrolyzed enzymatically to deoxyribonucleoside-3'-monophosphates. The hydrolyzate is labeled with [γ-^{32}P]-ATP and the resulting deoxyribonucleoside-3',5'-bisphosphates are separated by thin-layer chromatography or HPLC. Alternatively, they may be hydrolyzed to deoxyribonucleoside-5'-monophosphates prior to analysis. *Note*: A full-color version of this figure appears on the website.

deoxynucleosides have also been phosphorylated by the kinase enzyme, then the mixture will contain a small quantity of labeled adducts, ^{32}pdN*p.

A key step in the postlabeling method is *separation of the small quantity of radiolabeled adducted deoxynucleotides from the large excess of radiolabeled "normals."* If the chemical properties of the expected adducts are very different from the properties of the normal deoxyribonucleoside-3',5'-bisphosphates, this separation may be relatively straightforward. Just as in the case of direct analysis of adducts, discussed earlier, one may take advantage of the hydrophobicity of adducts bearing PAH moieties, for example, and effect a separation by reversed-phase adsorption chromatography. Even if the adducts are only slightly different from the normals, as in the case of alkylation damage, chromatographic separation may still be achievable. (Better separation can sometimes be achieved following hydrolysis of the deoxyribonucleoside-3',5'-bisphosphates to deoxyribonucleoside-5'-phosphates, using nuclease P1 (*60, 61*) (see figure 2-8). Nuclease P1 (EC 3.1.30.1), from *Penicillium citrinum*, is a phosphodiesterase that removes 3' phosphate groups from nucleotides (*62*).)

Chromatographic separation of the normal from the adducted deoxynucleotides is usually accomplished by multidimensional thin-layer chromatography (TLC) on polyethylene–imine–cellulose plates (*63*) or by HPLC. The pattern of adduct spots on the thin-layer plate is imaged by autoradiography. The result is a pattern of spots of varying intensities, representing the adducted bases, in the form of deoxyribonucleoside-3',5-bisphosphates (figure 2-9).

The sensitivity of the postlabeling technique relies on the high specific activity of [γ-^{32}P]-ATP. In favorable cases, as little as one adducted base per mammalian genome can be detected (*64*). However, the amount of material present is usually too small to permit direct chemical identification of the labeled species: unless authentic standards are available for comparison, the adducts can be identified only as numbered spots. (The TLC mobilities of the adducts may also provide some clues to their identities).

Another useful feature of the postlabeling technique is that it can be applied to analysis of DNA adduct formation by complex mixtures,

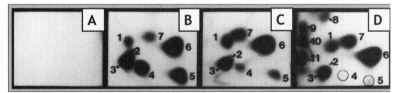

FIGURE 2-9.
^{32}P postlabeling detection of DNA adducts. The panels show maps of DNA adducts formed in mammary gland (B), lung (C), and liver (D) of rats treated with a single injection of the PAH carcinogen dibenzo[*a,l*]pyrene. Panel A shows vehicle (DMSO)-treated lung DNA. Adducts present in the ^{32}P-labeled digest (5 µg DNA) were resolved by multidirectional thin-layer chromatography on polyethylene–imine–cellulose sheets and visualized by autoradiography. *Note*: This figure also appears on the companion website. (*Source: Arif, J. M.; Smith, W. A.; Gupta, R. C. DNA adduct formation and persistence in rat tissues following exposure to the mammary carcinogen dibenzo*[a,l]*pyrene.* Carcinogenesis **1999**, 20, 1147–1150. Copyright Oxford University Press.*)

as well as pure compounds. Cigarette smoke (65) and coal tar (66) contain diverse PAHs. Postlabeling analysis of DNA adducts resulting from exposure to these mixtures shows a "diagonal zone" of radioactivity on polyethylene-imine-cellulose TLC plates, representing many partially resolved adduct spots.

IMMUNOASSAY OF DNA ADDUCTS

Carcinogen–nucleoside adducts and carcinogen-modified DNA can be antigenic, that is, eliciting an immune response in animals. (To raise antibodies, DNA adducts (haptens) are conjugated to protein carriers, such as albumin or keyhole limpet hemocyanin (67).) Both polyclonal and monoclonal antibodies to DNA adducts have been prepared successfully. Immunoassays exploit the tight and specific binding of antigen to antibody to permit the sensitive detection of adducts, even in complex mixtures. Miriam Poirier and colleagues have pioneered the application of immuno-assay techniques to the detection of DNA damage (68, 69).

The critical test of an immunoassay is specificity. For example, if the antibody to an adduct cross-reacts with normal deoxynucleosides, which are present in great excess over the adducts, reliable measurements will be impossible. An antiserum raised in rabbits to the aromatic amine RNA adduct guanosin-8-yl-acetylaminofluorene (see chapter 17) recognized the DNA adduct-derived deoxynucleosides deoxyguanosin-8-yl-acetyl-taminofluorene and deoxyguanosin-8-yl-aminofluorene (70), but did not cross-react with adduct-free DNA or with several other minor adducts. This antiserum was used for detection of these adducts by techniques including radioimmunoassay (RIA) and enzyme-linked immunosorbent assay (ELISA) (71). Immunoassays can be used to measure formation of carcinogen–DNA adducts in experimental animals or to detect adducts in human DNA samples. Antibodies against DNA adducts can also be applied to microscopic analysis of the distribution of a DNA adduct within a tissue (immunohistochemistry) (72) (figure 2-10).

Cigarette smokers are exposed to a complex mixture of PAHs, and an antiserum raised against BPDE-modified DNA will cross-react with adducts of some of these compounds. Nevertheless, relative exposure levels can be evaluated, even if the detailed chemical composition of the adduct mixture is unknown (73, 74).

Antibodies to DNA adducts can be used to prepare immunoaffinity columns for enrichment of the adducts from complex mixtures (75). Sub-sequently, the adducts can be separated and quantitated by chemical methods, such as ^{32}P postlabeling and chromatography.

POSITIONS OF ADDUCT FORMATION
ON DNA BASES

Reactive intermediates form characteristic patterns of DNA adducts. When double-stranded DNA is treated with alkylating agents in vitro, many sites on all four DNA bases are methylated (see chapter 15). In contrast, dihydrodiol epoxide metabolites of PAHs form adducts mainly at guanine N-2, a position that is spared by alkylating agents. Aromatic amines and nitro compounds, activated to nitrenium-ion reactive species, are highly selective for the guanine C-8 atom, as discussed in chapter 17.

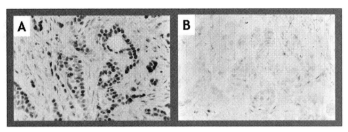

FIGURE 2-10.

Application of antibodies to DNA adducts in immunohistochemical analysis. Paraffin-embedded tissue blocks. Tissue slices (5 μm) were cut from human tumor tissue blocks and prepared on glass slides. Tissue slides were treated with RNase and proteinase K. To denature the DNA, slides were incubated with 4 N HCl for 7 min. Nonspecific antibody binding was blocked with 1.5% normal horse serum. Slides were incubated overnight at 4°C with anti-benzo[*a*]pyrene diol epoxide (BPDE)-DNA monoclonal antibody and then the antibody binding was visualized by standard protocols (see source reference for details). Methyl green was used as a counterstain. (A) Stage 1 breast cancer tissue showing intense nuclear staining. (B) Stage 2 breast cancer tissue showing low-level staining; ×400 magnification. *Note*: A full-color version of this figure appears on the website. (*Source: Rundle, A.; Tang, D.; Hibshoosh, H.; Estabrook, A.; Schnabel, F.; Cao, W.; Grumet, S.; Perera, F. P. The relationship between genetic damage from polycyclic aromatic hydrocarbons in breast tissue and breast cancer.* Carcinogenesis **2000**, 21, 1281–1289. Copyright Oxford University Press.)

Carcinogen-specific patterns of adduct formation have important biological consequences. Adducts at different positions are repaired differentially, have distinct effects on DNA conformation, and have differing propensities to lead to misincorporation/mutagenesis when the adducted DNA is replicated. All of these topics are dealt with at greater length in the following chapters.

What factors account for the patterns of adduct formation by various classes of reactive intermediates? The reactive intermediates are usually *electrophiles*: carbonium ion intermediates derived from the opening of the epoxide ring of a dihydrodiol epoxide (see chapter 18), arylnitrenium ions from the metabolism of aromatic amines (see chapter 17), alkyl cations from alkylating agents (see chapter 15), etc. The target sites on nucleic acids are nucleophilic atoms with lone pairs of electrons (exocyclic keto oxygen and amino nitrogens, and ring nitrogens of the bases) or negative charges (phosphate oxygens) (76). Some sites on the bases are particularly susceptible to electrophilic substitution, especially purine N-7.

"Hard" electrophiles (possessing highly localized positive charges), such as carbonium and nitrenium ions, react preferentially with "hard" nucleophilic centers, such as the lone pairs of amino nitrogen and keto oxygen atoms of the bases, rather than with "soft" (polarizable, delocalized negative charge) nucleophilic sites, such as thiol groups in protein and glutathione (77). These chemical considerations may contribute to determining the relative reactivities of, for example, the guanine O^6 and N^2 sites (78). However, the patterns of adduct formation in double-stranded DNA cannot be predicted from studies with monomers: the relative reactivities of sites in native DNA are often very different from those observed for the bases, deoxynucleosides, or deoxynucleotides. For example, the N-1 nitrogen atom is a major site (approximately 50% of total products) of alkylation of guanosine by methyl or ethyl iodide (79), but alkylation of this atom is usually undetectable in double-stranded DNA. There may be several reasons for such differences. The electrostatic potential developed by the high negative charge of the sugar–phosphate backbone of DNA (80) contributes to differences in reactivity when compared to bases of deoxynucleosides. Steric factors are probably the most important. In double-stranded DNA, only the "edges" of the bases are exposed to solvent, in the major and minor grooves of the double helix. Guanine N1, participating in Watson–Crick base pairing, is buried in the core of the double helix, whereas guanine N7 is exposed (figure 2-11). Since the major groove is wider and more accessible than the minor groove, one might expect sites exposed in the major groove to be particularly susceptible to adduction and, indeed, the guanine O^6, N7, and C8 positions are all prominent reaction positions (figure 2-12).

Both PAHs (81) and aromatic amines (82) have flat, hydrophobic structures that allow them to intercalate into DNA. (The familiar inter-calating fluorescent dye ethidium bromide is a substituted aromatic amine.) As discussed below, structural studies of DNA oligonucleotides adducted by these classes of carcinogens show that adducts derived from these carcinogens often adopt an intercalated conformation.

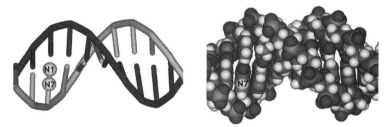

FIGURE 2-11.
Comparison of the N1 and N7 atoms of guanine in double-stranded DNA. Schematic view (left); space-filling model (right). The N1 atom cannot be seen in the view on the right. *Note*: A full-color version of this figure appears on the website.

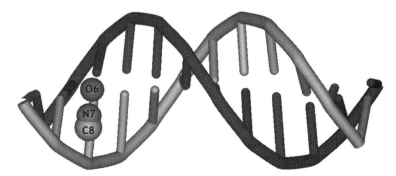

FIGURE 2-12.
Guanine atoms O6, N7, and C8 are relatively accessible to solvent in the major groove of double-stranded DNA. *Note*: A full-color version of this figure appears on the website.

Special Topic: **NMR METHODS FOR DNA STRUCTURE DETERMINATION**

Multidimensional NMR spectroscopy is a powerful method for determining the three-dimensional structures, dynamics, and interactions of biological macromolecules in the solution state. Following the discovery of the NMR phenomenon (Edwin Purcell, Nobel Prize in Physics, 1952), chemists quickly discovered the great value of NMR spectroscopy for characterization of the covalent structures of complex molecules (atom–atom connectivities and discrimination of stereoisomers). (We have already noted the importance of NMR for covalent structure elucidation of carcinogen–DNA adducts.)

A second NMR revolution followed the development of Fourier transform (Richard Ernst, Nobel Prize in Chemistry, 1991) and "multidimensional" spectroscopy techniques. One share of the Nobel Prize in Chemistry, 2002, was awarded to Kurt Wüthrich "for his development of NMR spectroscopy for determining the three-dimensional structure of biological macromolecules in solution." (Yet another Nobel prize-winning application of NMR has been the development of NMR imaging techniques, which are now among the most important methods for medical radiology.) These innovations have allowed NMR methods to be used to determine the three-dimensional structures (conformations) of many proteins and oligonucleotides and have provided insight into the effects of covalent adducts on DNA structure and dynamics.

In contrast to X-ray crystallography, NMR methods do not require crystallization of the macromolecule; the methods are applied to dissolved samples. This section provides a brief nonmathematical account of NMR principles and describes how NMR methods can provide structural information, specifically for DNA and DNA adducts. For the interested reader, comprehensive information about these methods can be obtained elsewhere (*83–85*).

Protons and neutrons have a magnetic moment (spin angular momentum) and can therefore interact with a magnetic field. Most elements have at least one isotope in which the magnetic moments of the neutrons and protons combine so as to give the nucleus a net magnetic moment (nonzero spin). In biological molecules, the most important nuclear spins are ^1H, ^2H, ^{13}C, ^{15}N, and ^{31}P. Interaction of the nuclear magnetic moment with a magnetic field produces different energy states, and transitions between these states occur at energies and frequencies determined by the equation $E = h\nu$, where h is Planck's constant and ν is the frequency. An NMR spectrum is a plot of energy absorbed versus frequency. Modern NMR spectrometers use large superconducting magnets to generate high magnetic field strengths, corresponding to ^1H spin transition frequencies of 400 MHz or higher.

Here, the application of NMR measurements to DNA structure determination is illustrated by following a specific example, the analysis of the structure of a DNA 11-mer duplex oligonucleotide. The sequence and numbering scheme of the DNA oligonucleotide duplex are shown in figure 2-13. The atom numbering schemes of Watson–Crick hydrogen bonded adenine–thymine and guanine–cytosine base pairs and a deoxyribose sugar are shown in figure 2-14. Each atom in a residue must be given a unique designation; hence the sugar atoms are labeled with a prime or

5′ C01–C02–A03–T04–A05–T06–G07–G08–C09–C10–C11 3′

3′ G22–G21–T20–A19–T18–A17–C16–C15–G14–G13–G12 5′

FIGURE 2-13.

DNA 11-mer duplex used as the example of NMR structure determination. See text for details.

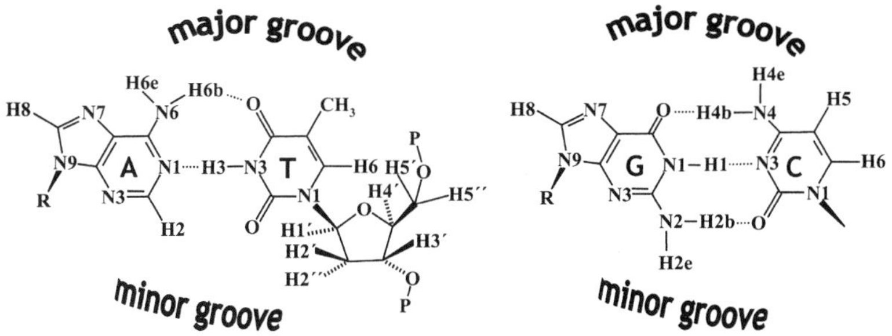

FIGURE 2-14.

Numbering schemes for Watson–Crick hydrogen bonded adenine–thymine and guanine–cytosine base pairs. The deoxyribose sugar ring is designated by R for all the bases except thymine, where the numbering scheme is provided.

asterisk to distinguish them from purine/pyrimidine ring atoms having the same number and type. In addition, the two amino protons of cytosine, adenine, and guanine are differentiated from one another either by using the letters "b" (hydrogen bonded) and "e" (exposed to solvent) or by the numbers 1 and 2.

Multidimensional NMR (figure 2-15) techniques make it possible to resolve spectral resonances very effectively, by spreading them out into a plane or a volume, and allow us to exploit spin properties in more subtle ways than can be done with the one-dimensional (1D) NMR experiment. 2D NMR is basically a series of 1D NMR experiments, each having a variable evolution period that creates different nonequilibrium spin states as a function of time. There are two main types of 2D NMR experiments, "through-bond" coupling and "through-space" dipolar coupling (figure 2-15). The through-bond experiments can be further subdivided into homonuclear (proton–proton) and heteronuclear (e.g., proton–carbon, proton–nitrogen, proton–phosphorus) classes. Heteronuclear experiments can even be expanded into 3D or 4D experiments, providing additional resolution of overlapped resonances. The diagonal in a proton–proton 2D experiment is equivalent to the 1D spectrum (figure 2-15). A "crosspeak" is an off-diagonal intersection of two (or more) resonances belonging to two (or more) interacting atoms in a multidimensional spectrum.

The concentration of protons in ordinary water (H_2O) is 110 M, whereas the concentration of the DNA sample is typically ∼0.5–1 mM. Therefore, the majority of the data collection is carried out for samples dissolved in D_2O buffer, in order to eliminate the overwhelming signal

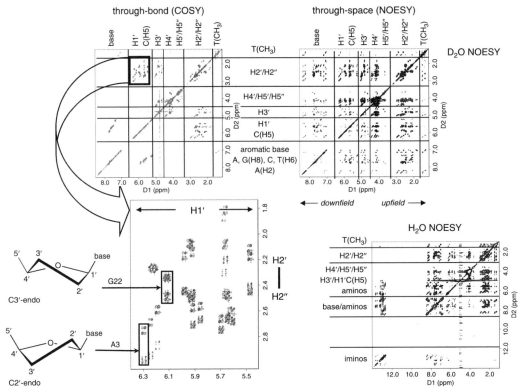

FIGURE 2-15.

Top: Side-by-side comparisons of the NMR correlation spectroscopy (COSY) data on the left (which provides through-bond connectivity information) with the nuclear Overhauser effect spectroscopy (NOESY) data on the right (which provides through-space connectivity information) of the DNA 11-mer duplex (D_2O buffer, pH 7.0, 25°C, 600 MHz). The chemical shift ranges found in typical B-DNA for different types of resonances are indicated above and to the side of the spectra. The diagonal in each spectrum is equivalent to a one-dimensional spectrum, while the off-diagonal crosspeaks correspond to two interacting protons. Bottom right: The chemical shift ranges for the amino and imino protons are designated in the NOESY spectrum of the DNA 11-mer duplex dissolved in H_2O buffer (pH 7.0, 1°C, 600 MHz). Bottom left: An expanded view of the sugar H1′ to H2′/H2″ region of the phase-sensitive COSY spectrum shows complicated patterns due to multiple splittings (e.g., H2′ is split by H2″, H1′, and H3′). The pattern for a C2′-endo sugar ring pucker conformation is demonstrated by the boxed region for the A3 residue. In this case, the downfield crosspeak corresponds to the H1′–H2″ coupling, while the upfield peak corresponds to the H1′–H2′ coupling. Often, the sugar ring of the 3′ residue (G22) exhibits a 3′-endo conformation (typically found in A-DNA and RNA), as evidenced by the inversion of the crosspeaks (H1′–H2″ is upfield of the H1′–H2′). Other sugar pucker conformations, such as O4′-endo and C1′-exo, are also found in B-DNA. *Note:* This figure also appears on the companion website.

from H_2O. However, G/T imino (NH) and A/C/G amino (NH_2) protons are exchangeable with H_2O; thus the sample has to be dissolved in H_2O buffer or else these protons would exchange with deuterium and not be observable. Several NMR experiments are available that have solvent-suppression routines built into them, to eliminate most of the water signal, either by saturation of the water signal or by selective excitation of only those signals of interest.

In an NMR spectrum, the position of a resonance depends on the NMR magnet's field strength (B_0) and the isotope's nuclear magnetic moment

(γ), parameters that are fixed for a given type of nucleus, as well as on the chemical environment of the specific nucleus. The position of the resonance in the spectrum is therefore referred to as the "chemical shift" (δ), and is measured in units of parts per million, ppm. When present in a strong magnetic field, the circulating electrons in an atom generate currents, which create an associated local magnetic field that opposes the applied field. Because the strength of this local field depends on local electron density (i.e., electronegativity of the bonded atoms), chemical shift data are used to assign functional groups in molecules for purposes of covalent structure determination (figure 2-15). For example, a proton bonded to an electronegative nitrogen atom has its electron density withdrawn (deshielding the nucleus), so that a smaller applied magnetic field is needed to achieve resonance; hence these protons exhibit a "downfield" chemical shift. This shift is illustrated by the hydrogen bonded imino protons of thymine (NH3) (T4, T6, T18, and T20) and guanine (NH1) (G7, G8, G12, G13, G14, G21, and G22), which resonate between 12 and 14 ppm. In contrast, the methyl protons of thymine experience a higher density of electrons that shield the nucleus and thus require a higher applied magnetic field for resonance; these protons exhibit an "upfield" chemical shift, typically 1–2 ppm. Ring current effects from aromatic rings also affect the chemical shift and provide information about base stacking in nucleic acids. Protons that stack over an aromatic ring experience upfield chemical shifts, while protons that are in the plane of an aromatic ring experience downfield chemical shifts. Typical chemical shift ranges for different types of protons in the DNA 11-mer duplex are shown in figure 2-15.

After acquisition of NMR data, the first step in analysis is assignment of the chemical shift of each resonance in the spectrum to a specific atom in the molecule. Once the proton chemical shifts are assigned, they are used to assign the ^{13}C and ^{31}P chemical shifts. (Due to its very low natural abundance (0.37%), ^{15}N is not readily observed, unless the DNA is specifically enriched with this isotope.) In the case of an oligonucleotide bearing a defined adduct, the proton and carbon chemical shifts for the resonances belonging to the adduct must also be assigned. In addition, the spectra of the adducted and adduct-free oligonucleotides are compared, noting the changes due to the presence of the adduct in the chemical shifts of the resonances belonging to the DNA. These types of studies are referred to as "chemical shift perturbation" experiments and they provide important information about the induced changes in DNA structure that occur upon covalent modification of the DNA.

Coupling constants (J) can be measured in proton NMR spectra by taking the difference (in Hz) between two peaks in a multiplet. The strength of the coupling is defined as J, which is dependent on the nuclear magnetic moments (H–C > H–N > C–C > N–C), hybridization (sp > sp^2 > sp^3), and torsion angle. The measurement of J provides information about dihedral angles, which can be derived using the Karplus equation: the three-bond proton-proton coupling constant and the torsion angle θ are related by $^3J = A\cos^2\theta - B\cos\theta + C$, where A, B, and C are empirical constants (86). Since J is based on an intrinsic property of the molecule, that is, chemical structure, it does not depend on B_0. In regards to DNA (and DNA adduct) structure, the COSY crosspeak patterns for deoxyribose proton-proton couplings enable the determination of the sugar ring conformation for each residue (e.g., C2′-*endo* or C3′-*endo*). Coupling constants, and thus dihedral angle information, about the adduct may also be measured if three-bond proton-proton coupling is present. Other types of NMR experiments, such as total correlation spectroscopy (TOCSY), are useful for providing long-range (>3 bonds) through-bond connectivity information.

The nuclear Overhauser effect (NOE) (*87*) monitors the transfer of magnetization through space as a result of cross-relaxation between adjacent pairs of spins located ~5 Å apart, and provides molecular structure information through the distance term ($1/r^6$). The NOE specifically measures the pairwise dipolar interactions between spins. In addition to the distance (r) between proton pairs, dipolar interactions depend on the magnetic moments of the nuclei, the angle between dipoles, and the correlation time, t_c.

In right-handed B-DNA helices, the base aromatic proton is stacked above the sugar of the preceding residue. Thus, interresidue NOEs between the aromatic base protons (A/G (H8) or C/T (H6)) and sugar protons (H1′, H2′, H2″, H3′, H4′, and H5′/H5″) can be observed. Since the intraresidue base-to-sugar proton NOE connectivities are also observed, it is possible to "step" from a base proton, to its own sugar proton, to the neighboring base proton, starting from one end of the DNA strand and proceeding in a "walk" to the opposite end of the strand. The assignment of the base to the H1′ region of a 2D NOESY spectrum for the DNA 11-mer duplex is described in figure 2-16.

NOESY and chemical shift information are used to determine whether the DNA base pairs are stacked over one another, as would be the case in duplex DNA, and if hydrogen bonding across a base pair is present. In a B-DNA duplex, crosspeaks from the G/T imino proton in each base pair to the G/T imino protons of the neighboring base pairs confirm the presence of base pair stacking (e.g., imino to imino proton "walk"). In some DNA adducts, this walk is disrupted if the covalently attached ligand intercalates between two adjacent DNA base pairs. For each Watson-Crick hydrogen bonded G:C base pair, NOE crosspeaks are observed between the G(NH1) imino proton and the cytosine hydrogen bonded (NH4b) and exposed (NH4e) protons (figure 2-15). For each A:T base pair, an NOE is observed between the thymine imino (NH3) and the adenine H2 proton. In cases where the hydrogen bonding of the base is disrupted by a covalent modification, or where the pairing is other than Watson-Crick (e.g., Hoogsteen hydrogen bonding), different NOE patterns will be observed.

Dynamics, in addition to the induced alterations in DNA structure resulting from the covalent modification, may play important roles in the biological activities of DNA adducts. The structures of several DNA adducts have been observed to interconvert between two distinct conformations (*88*, *89*), and this exchange process is influenced by DNA sequence. Conformational exchange can be evidenced by the presence of multiple sets of resonances belonging to the same atoms. The presence of two or more conformations of a DNA adduct may be important

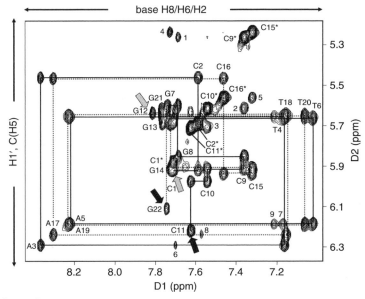

FIGURE 2-16.
We begin to assign specific crosspeaks to particular atoms in the molecule using information obtained from a through-space NOESY spectrum (300 ms mixing time, 600 MHz, 25°C). Starting at the 5′ residue, C1(H6) to its own C1(H1′) crosspeak, a horizontal line is drawn to the C1(H1″)–C2(H6) crosspeak. From this crosspeak, a vertical line is drawn to the C2(H6) to its own C2(H1′) crosspeak. The 5′ to 3′ walk continues moving from crosspeak to crosspeak until all the crosspeaks in the strand have been assigned. The 5′ and 3′ terminal base-H1′ crosspeaks are designated by gray and black arrows, respectively. Lines for the C1–C11 strand are solid, while the lines for the G12–G22 strand are dashed. Note that G12 has only one crosspeak in a vertical line while C1 has two crosspeaks. G12 begins at the 5′-end, so there is no 5′ residue from which to step. Cytosines have an additional C(H6) to C(H5) crosspeak, which is designated by *. There is a NOE present between the 5′-base proton and 3′-C(H5) proton (e.g., peak 1 is G8(H8)–C9(H5) connectivity, peak 2 is C9 (H6)–C10(H5), peak 3 is C10(H6)–C11(H5), peak 4 is G14(H6)–C15(H5), and peak 5 is C15(H6)–C16(H6)). There are four A(H2)s in the DNA sequence, and these are assigned by looking at the connectivities between the adenine H2 proton and nearby H1′ protons (e.g., peak 6, A3(H2)–A3(H1′); peak 7, A3(H2)–A3(H1′); peak 8, A17(H2)–A17(H1′); peak 9, A19(H2)– A19(H1′)). After all the crosspeaks in this region have been assigned, connectivities between base and base protons, base and other sugar protons (H3′, H4′, H2′, H2″), and sugar and sugar protons are assigned. *Note:* This figure also appears on the companion website.

for structure/function studies; different conformers may preferentially interact with different classes of proteins.

Once all the NMR data have been collected and analyzed, the next step is to use all this information to generate an ensemble of structures that satisfy all of the NMR-derived constraints and that have appropriate covalent geometries (bond lengths, angles, and van der Waals contacts). Unlike X-ray crystallography, where a single structure is determined, NMR data generate a family of structures, because the resolution only allows nuclear positions to be determined with respect to one another, and there is motion of the atoms when they are in solution. In addition, since DNA is proton-poor (when compared to proteins), regions of the DNA structure can be "under-determined" because of the limited number of NMR constraints available.

For structural calculations, the two basic sources of structural information are derived from the NOE intensities and the *J* coupling patterns. The NOEs provide proton–proton distance estimates, an assessment of whether a residue has *syn* or *anti* glycosidic torsion angles, and information on whether base pair hydrogen bonding and/or base pair stacking is intact or disrupted. *J* coupling patterns provide information about sugar ring pucker conformations. Additional structural information is derived from the linewidths of the resonances (providing information about dynamics), chemical shift data for ^{1}H, ^{31}P (providing information about the phosphodiester backbone), and ^{13}C (providing information about sugar ring pucker conformations), and chemical shift perturbation studies that compare differences in unmodified and modified DNA.

Computational methods are used to determine structures consistent with all of the NMR data. In general, a rough initial global model is generated from all the known distance and coupling information (*83–85, 90*). The initial models are then refined using a combination of iterative optimization of all the available input NMR data and energy minimization (typically by using a potential energy function, which includes electrostatics, hydrogen bonds, and van der Waals interactions).

The energy-minimized NMR structure of the DNA 11-mer duplex shown in figure 2-17 was calculated using the program DUPLEX, a molecular mechanics program that has been especially tailored for

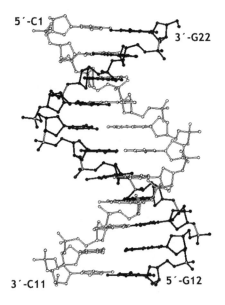

FIGURE 2-17.

The NMR structure of the example 11-mer duplex. The C1–C11 strand has outline bonds, while the G12–G22 strand is in black. *Note*: This figure also appears on the companion website.

investigating the conformations of modified nucleic acids (91). A key feature of DUPLEX is that it employs a consistent force field in the reduced variable domain of torsion angle space. A total of 298 NOE distant restraints, together with information from the NMR data on the hydrogen bonding pattern were used to calculate the structure. Full details of this approach, specifically as it applies to DNA adduct structure determination, can be found in earlier work (92).[5]

PROTEIN COVALENT ADDUCTS: TOXICITY MECHANISMS

Protein adducts have been less studied than DNA adducts, even though they are usually more abundant. There are both chemical and biological reasons for this bias. Unlike DNA, proteins are structurally highly diverse, making chemical analysis more difficult. DNA strands remain covalently intact from generation to generation, but proteins are degraded and resynthesized on a more or less rapid timescale, so one might expect that damage to proteins would not have lasting consequences. Arguing in the other direction, however, DNA is protected by an array of repair enzymes; proteins are not repaired (at least, not to any such extent).

Protein covalent adducts have attracted increasing attention in recent years. Protein damage has been implicated in cytotoxicity and immunotoxicity. The focus has been on protein-mediated toxicity induced by drugs, rather than by environmental pollutants or carcinogens, because drugs may be administered at levels high enough to cause substantial protein modification (93). Among the drugs for which covalent[6] protein binding has been demonstrated are acetaminophen; tamoxifen (antiestrogen (94)); halothane (anesthetic); tienilic acid (a diuretic agent withdrawn from sale due to hepatotoxic adverse reactions (95)); and cocaine, a drug of abuse. Covalent binding of acetaminophen (following P450-catalyzed oxidation to N-acetyl-p-benzoquinoneimine) to liver proteins, which has been studied intensively, is regarded as the major cause of liver necrosis following overdose exposure to this analgesic. Acetaminophen metabolism and toxicity are discussed further in chapter 19.

As mentioned earlier in this chapter, small molecules are usually poorly antigenic, so immune or allergic reactions to drugs are, thankfully, uncommon. Protein binding may lead to allergic responses, such as allergic contact dermatitis, following exposure to foreign chemicals (96). However, several drugs are associated with rare but potentially fatal adverse effects that appear to be *autoimmune* reactions. These clinical conditions include autoimmune hepatitis (97) and *systemic lupus erythematosus* (98). Regrettably, these reactions are both unpredictable and difficult to study experimentally, due to the lack of good animal or in vitro model systems. A widely accepted, although unproven, explanation (99) for these adverse reactions invokes protein binding, as follows. Recall that, to prepare antibodies to small molecules, immunologists usually couple the haptens to carrier proteins. Metabolic activation of a drug may generate reactive electrophilic intermediates that bind to proteins in an analogous manner. (Enzymes catalyzing the activation processes, such as cytochrome P450 enzymes, may be particularly susceptible to attack.) Covalent adduction by the drug metabolite modifies the structure of the protein, so that it is no longer recognized as "self" by the immune system. The patient then begins to produce antibodies against the protein.

PROTEIN COVALENT ADDUCTS: CHEMICAL MECHANISMS

Proteins have many nucleophilic sites that are potential targets for electrophiles. One target is the terminal amino group. Aside from the aliphatic side chains, most amino acid side chains have nucleophilic functional groups. Among the most important targets are: (i) cysteine thiol SH; (ii) histidine imidazole NH; (iii) lysine ε-NH$_2$; and (iv) tyrosine phenolic OH. As with DNA adduction, steric factors are important determinants of sites of damage. In a globular protein, only certain residues are exposed to solvent and likely to be adducted by a soluble electrophile. For example, in an in vitro study of hemoglobin modification by styrene oxide and ethylene oxide, the only amino acid residues found to be adducted were α-chain histidine 20 and β-chain histidines 77, 97, and 143 (*100*), although the hemoglobin α and β chains have 10 and 9 histidine residues, respectively.

Adducted proteins can be detected by gel electrophoretic separation of proteins, for example, following exposure of an animal to a radiolabeled drug. This analysis can reveal whether particular proteins are susceptible to modification. Adduction of highly abundant proteins, especially those that can be sampled in the blood, such as serum albumin and hemoglobin, have often been studied, with the hope that adduct analysis could be applied in biomonitoring of exposure, and this approach has been put into practice (*101*).

As with DNA binding, the chemical characterization of protein adducts usually requires degradation of the adducted macromolecule to monomers and this can be done chemically or enzymatically (*102*). Because of the diversity of protein structure, no single approach is sufficient. Specific chemical treatments can release certain classes of adducts (e.g., Raney nickel for release of cysteine sulfhydryl adducts (*103*)). Proteases can be used to hydrolyze polypeptides, followed by chromatographic isolation of nonstandard (adducted) amino acids from the hydrolyzate. As with the study of DNA adducts, HPLC/mass spectrometry methods are proving to be very powerful tools for detecting and analyzing drug-protein and carcinogen-protein adducts (*104*). For example, an HPLC/tandem mass spectrometric analysis method has been used to demonstrate the presence of serum albumin cysteine adducts derived from mustard gas (see chapter 15) in stored blood samples from individuals who suffered exposure to this alkylating agent during the Iran–Iraq War of the 1980s (*105*).

A recent study (*106*) has revealed that cocaine, a common drug of abuse, can bind to proteins (figure 2-18). In this case, the parent drug is active, and metabolism (hydrolysis of the methyl ester) prevents binding. In vitro experiments with amino acids suggested that the ε-amino group of lysine is the main target. Cocaine-adducted proteins were detected in blood plasma samples from cocaine users.

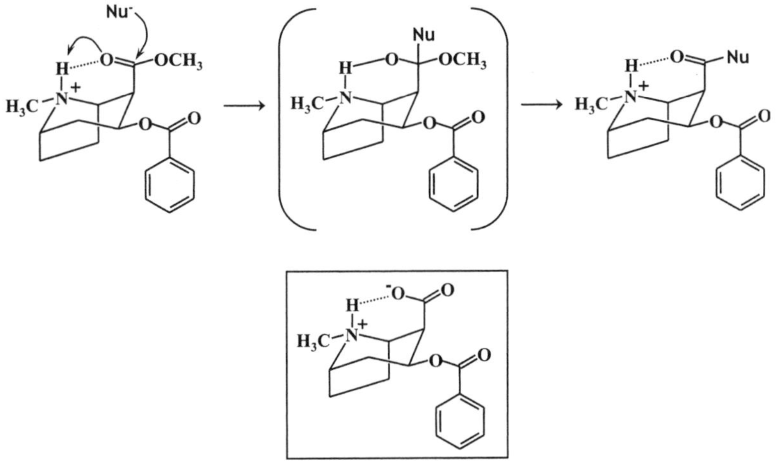

FIGURE 2-18.

Cocaine: protein binding mechanism. At top left, the attack of a nucleophile on cocaine hydrochloride is shown. The cocaine N atom hydrogen bonds to the methyl ester carbonyl, enhancing the electrophilicity of the ester carbon atom. At center is the tetrahedral intermediate. At right is the covalent adduct. Hydrolysis of the cocaine methyl ester yields a major cocaine metabolite; the acid metabolite is not reactive with protein, because the acid carboxylate replaces the methyl ester carbonyl as hydrogen bonding partner to the cocaine N atom (boxed structure at bottom). (*Adapted from Deng, S. X.; Bharat, N.; Fischman, M. C.; Landry, D. W. Covalent modification of proteins by cocaine.* Proc. Natl. Acad. Sci. USA **2002**, *99, 3412–3416*.)

Notes

1. In this chapter, we sometimes refer to compounds that form covalent DNA adducts as carcinogens, for simplicity, while recognizing that DNA binding activity is not truly synonymous with carcinogenicity.

2. For simplicity, in this discussion, we use the term "carcinogen" loosely, to refer to any chemical agent that may give rise to DNA adducts.

3. If the amount of material to be analyzed is $\ll 1$ mg, it is first mixed with "cold carrier" carbon.

4. Contributed by Lawrence J. Marnett, Vanderbilt University.

5. Contributed by Monique Cosman, Lawrence Livermore National Laboratory. This work was performed under the auspices of the U.S. Department of Energy by the University of California, Lawrence Livermore National Laboratory, W-7405-Eng-48.

6. Many xenobiotics bind reversibly (noncovalently) to proteins such as serum albumin and glutathione transferase.

References

1. Pumford, N. R.; Halmes, N. C. Protein targets of xenobiotic reactive intermediates. *Annu. Rev. Pharmacol. Toxicol.* **1997**, *37*, 91–117.
2. Pumford, N. R.; Halmes, N. C.; Hinson, J. A. Covalent binding of xenobiotics to specific proteins in the liver. *Drug Metab. Rev.* **1997**, *29*, 39–57.

3. Hess, D. A.; Rieder, M. J. The role of reactive drug metabolites in immune-mediated adverse drug reactions. *Ann. Pharmacother.* **1997,** *31,* 1378–1387.

4. Ju, C.; Uetrecht, J. P. Mechanism of idiosyncratic drug reactions: reactive metabolite formation, protein binding and the regulation of the immune system. *Curr. Drug Metab.* **2002,** *3,* 367–377.

5. Poirier, M. C.; Weston, A. DNA adduct determination in humans. *Prog. Clin. Biol. Res.* **1991,** *372,* 205–218.

6. Poirier, M. C.; Santella, R. M.; Weston, A. Carcinogen macromolecular adducts and their measurement. *Carcinogenesis* **2000,** *21,* 353–359.

7. Dipple, A. DNA adducts of chemical carcinogens. *Carcinogenesis* **1995,** *16,* 437–441.

8. Hemminki, K., Bartsch, H., Eds. *DNA Adducts of Carcinogenic and Mutagenic Agents: Chemistry, Identification, and Biological Significance;* International Agency for Research on Cancer: Lyons, 1993.

9. von Sonntag, C. *The Chemical Basis of Radiation Biology;* Taylor & Francis: London, 1987.

10. Dizdaroglu, M.; Jaruga, P.; Birincioglu, M.; Rodriguez, H. Free radical-induced damage to DNA: mechanisms and measurement. *Free Radic. Biol. Med.* **2002,** *32,* 1102–1115.

11. Riley, P. A. Free radicals in biology: oxidative stress and the effects of ionizing radiation. *Int. J. Radiat. Biol.* **1994,** *65,* 27–33.

12. Singer, B. Alkylation, mutagenesis and repair. *Mutat. Res.* **1990,** *233,* 289–290.

13. Chen, F. M. Covalent binding of benzo[*a*]pyrene diol epoxides to polynucleotides. *Biochemistry* **1985,** *24,* 5045–5052.

14. Marumo, G.; Noguchi, T.; Midorikawa, Y. Efficient method for the preparation of *Escherichia coli* polynucleotide phosphorylase suitable for the synthesis of polynucleotides. *Biosci. Biotechnol. Biochem.* **1993,** *57,* 513–514.

15. Subrahmanyam, V. V.; O'Brien, P. J. Peroxidase-catalysed binding of [U-^{14}C]phenol to DNA. *Xenobiotica* **1985,** *15,* 859–871.

16. Butler, J.; Hoey, B. M.; Ward, T. H. The alkylation of DNA *in vitro* by 2,5-*bis*(2-hydroxyethylamino)-3,6-diaziridinyl-1,4-benzoquinone. *Biochem. Pharmacol.* **1989,** *38,* 923–927.

17. Wolfe, A. R.; Smith, T. J.; Meehan, T. Benzo[*a*]pyrene diol epoxide forms covalent adducts with deoxycytidylic acid by alkylation at both exocyclic amino N(4) and ring imino N-3 positions. *Chem. Res. Toxicol.* **2004,** *17,* 476–491.

18. Lutz, W. K. Structural characteristics of compounds that can be activated to chemically reactive metabolites: use for a prediction of a carcinogenic potential. *Arch. Toxicol. Suppl.* **1984,** *7,* 194–207.

19. Keller, J. W.; Heidelberger, C.; Beland, F. A.; Harvey, R. G. Hydrolysis of *syn*- and *anti*-benzo[a]pyrene diol epoxides: stereochemistry, kinetics and the effect of an intramolecular hydrogen bond on the rate of *syn*-diol epoxide solvolysis. *J. Am. Chem. Soc.* **1976,** *98,* 8276–8277.

20. Bosold, F.; Boche, G. The ultimate carcinogen, O-acetyl-N-(2-fluorenyl)hydroxylamine ("N-acetoxy-2-aminofluorene"), and its reaction in vitro to form 2-N-(deoxyguanosin-8-yl)amino]fluorene. *Angew. Chem., Int. Ed. Engl.* **1990,** *29,* 63–64.

21. Nakamura, H.; Uetrecht, J.; Cribb, A. E.; Miller, M. A.; Zahid, N.; Hill, J.; Josephy, P. D.; Grant, D. M.; Spielberg, S. P. In vitro formation, disposition and toxicity of N-acetoxy-sulfamethoxazole, a potential mediator of sulfamethoxazole toxicity. *J. Pharmacol. Exp. Ther.* **1995,** *274,* 1099–1104.

22. Mesic, M.; Peuralahti, J.; Blans, P.; Fishbein, J. C. Mechanisms of decomposition of α-hydroxydialkylnitrosamines in aqueous solution. *Chem. Res. Toxicol.* **2000**, *13*, 983–992.

23. Mochizuki, M.; Anjo, T.; Takeda, K.; Suzuki, E.; Sekiguchi, N.; Huang, G. F.; Okada, M. Chemistry and mutagenicity of α-hydroxy nitrosamines. *IARC Sci. Publ.* **1982**, 553–559.

24. Phillips, D. H.; Farmer, P. B.; Beland, F. A.; Nath, R. G.; Poirier, M. C.; Reddy, M. V.; Turteltaub, K. W. Methods of DNA adduct determination and their application to testing compounds for genotoxicity. *Environ. Mol. Mutagen.* **2000**, *35*, 222–233.

25. Lakshmi, V. M.; Hsu, F. F.; McGarry, A. E.; Davis, B. B.; Zenser, T. V. Hypochlorous acid-mediated activation of N-acetylbenzidine to form N'-(3'-monophospho-deoxyguanosin-8-yl)-N-acetylbenzidine. *Toxicol. Sci.* **2000**, *53*, 202–212.

26. Esaka, Y.; Inagaki, S.; Goto, M. Separation procedures capable of revealing DNA adducts. *J. Chromatogr. B Analyt. Technol. Biomed. Life Sci.* **2003**, *797*, 321–329.

27. Snell, K.; Mullock, B. In *Biochemical Toxicology: A Practical Approach;* Snell, K., Mullock, B., Eds.; IRL Press: Oxford, 1987.

28. Goldenberger, D.; Perschil, I.; Ritzler, M.; Altwegg, M. A simple "universal" DNA extraction procedure using SDS and proteinase K is compatible with direct PCR amplification. *PCR Methods Appl.* **1995**, *4*, 368–370.

29. Martin, C. N.; Garner, R. C. The identification and assessment of covalent binding in vitro and in vivo. In *Biochemical Toxicology: A Practical Approach;* Snell, K., Mullock, B., Eds.; IRL Press: Oxford, 1987; pp. 109–128.

30. Dipple, A.; Pigott, M. A. Resistance of 7,12-dimethylbenz[a]anthracene-deoxyadenosine adducts in DNA to hydrolysis by snake venom phosphodiesterase. *Carcinogenesis* **1987**, *8*, 491–493.

31. Dong, Z. G.; Jeffrey, A. M. Hydrolysis of carcinogen–DNA adducts by three classes of deoxyribonucleosidase to their corresponding bases. *Carcinogenesis* **1991**, *12*, 1125–1128.

32. Beckman, K. B.; Saljoughi, S.; Mashiyama, S. T.; Ames, B. N. A simpler, more robust method for the analysis of 8-oxoguanine in DNA. *Free Radic. Biol. Med.* **2000**, *29*, 357–367.

33. Beland, F. A.; Allaben, W. T.; Evans, F. E. Acyltransferase-mediated binding of N-hydroxyarylamides to nucleic acids. *Cancer Res.* **1980**, *40*, 834–840.

34. Casale, G. P.; Singhal, M.; Bhattacharya, S.; RamaNathan, R.; Roberts, K. P.; Barbacci, D. C.; Zhao, J.; Jankowiak, R.; Gross, M. L.; Cavalieri, E. L.; Small, G. J.; Rennard, S. I.; Mumford, J. L.; Shen, M. Detection and quantification of depurinated benzo[a]pyrene-adducted DNA bases in the urine of cigarette smokers and women exposed to household coal smoke. *Chem. Res. Toxicol.* **2001**, *14*, 192–201.

35. Cheng, S. C.; Hilton, B. D.; Roman, J. M.; Dipple, A. DNA adducts from carcinogenic and noncarcinogenic enantiomers of benzo[a]pyrene dihydro-diol epoxide. *Chem. Res. Toxicol.* **1989**, *2*, 334–340.

36. Martin, C. N.; Beland, F. A.; Roth, R. W.; Kadlubar, F. F. Covalent binding of benzidine and N-acetylbenzidine to DNA at the C-8 atom of deoxyguanosine in vivo and in vitro. *Cancer Res.* **1982**, *42*, 2678–2686.

37. Upadhyaya, P.; Sturla, S. J.; Tretyakova, N.; Ziegel, R.; Villalta, P. W.; Wang, M.; Hecht, S. S. Identification of adducts produced by the reaction

of 4-(acetoxymethylnitrosamino)-1-(3-pyridyl)-1-butanol with deoxy-guanosine and DNA. *Chem. Res. Toxicol.* **2003,** *16,* 180–190.

38. Schwerdtle, T.; Seidel, A.; Hartwig, A. Effect of soluble and particulate nickel compounds on the formation and repair of stable benzo[*a*]pyrene DNA adducts in human lung cells. *Carcinogenesis* **2002,** *23,* 47–53.

39. Boysen, G.; Hecht, S. S. Analysis of DNA and protein adducts of benzo[a]pyrene in human tissues using structure-specific methods. *Mutat. Res.* **2003,** *543,* 17–30.

40. Bol, S. A.; de Groot, A. J.; Tijdens, R. B.; Meerman, J. H.; Mullenders, L. H.; van Zeeland, A. A. Electrochemical detection and quanti-fication of the acetylated and deacetylated C8-deoxyguanosine DNA adducts induced by 2-acetylaminofluorene. *Anal. Biochem.* **1997,** *251,* 24–31.

41. Paehler, A.; Richoz, J.; Soglia, J.; Vouros, P.; Turesky, R. J. Analysis and quantification of DNA adducts of 2-amino-3,8-dimethylimidazo[4,5-*f*] quinoxaline in liver of rats by liquid chromatography/electrospray tandem mass spectrometry. *Chem. Res. Toxicol.* **2002,** *15,* 551–561.

42. de Kok, T. M.; Moonen, H. J.; van Delft, J.; van Schooten, F. J. Methodologies for bulky DNA adduct analysis and biomonitoring of environmental and occupational exposures. *J. Chromatogr. B Analyt. Technol. Biomed. Life Sci.* **2002,** *778,* 345–355.

43. Vogel, J. S.; Turteltaub, K. W.; Finkel, R.; Nelson, D. E. Accelerator mass spectrometry. *Anal. Chem.* **1995,** *67,* 353A–359A.

44. Vogel, J. S.; Turteltaub, K. W. Accelerator mass spectrometry as a bioanalytical tool for nutritional research. *Adv. Exp. Med. Biol.* **1998,** *445,* 397–410.

45. Lappin, G.; Garner, R. C. Current perspectives of ^{14}C-isotope measure-ment in biomedical accelerator mass spectrometry. *Anal. Bioanal. Chem.* **2004,** *378,* 356–364.

46. Frantz, C. E.; Bangerter, C.; Fultz, E.; Mayer, K. M.; Vogel, J. S.; Turteltaub, K. W. Dose–response studies of MeIQx in rat liver and liver DNA at low doses. *Carcinogenesis* **1995,** *16,* 367–373.

47. Harris, T. M.; Stone, M. P.; Harris, C. M. Applications of NMR spectroscopy to studies of reactive intermediates and their interactions with nucleic acids. *Chem. Res. Toxicol.* **1988,** *1,* 79–96.

48. Koga, N.; Inskeep, P. B.; Harris, T. M.; Guengerich, F. P. S-[2-(N7-Guanyl)ethyl]glutathione, the major DNA adduct formed from 1,2-dibromoethane. *Biochemistry* **1986,** *25,* 2192–2198.

49. Van den Driessche, B.; Lemiere, F.; Van Dongen, W.; Esmans, E. L. Alkylation of DNA by melphalan: investigation of capillary liquid chromatography–electrospray ionization tandem mass spectrometry in the study of the adducts at the nucleoside level. *J. Chromatogr. B Analyt. Technol. Biomed. Life Sci.* **2003,** *785,* 21–37.

50. Nair, J.; Barbin, A.; Velic, I.; Bartsch, H. Etheno DNA-base adducts from endogenous reactive species. *Mutat. Res.* **1999,** *424,* 59–69.

51. el Ghissassi, F.; Barbin, A.; Nair, J.; Bartsch, H. Formation of 1,N6-ethenoadenine and 3,N4-ethenocytosine by lipid peroxidation products and nucleic acid bases. *Chem. Res. Toxicol.* **1995,** *8,* 278–283.

52. Morinello, E. J.; Ham, A. J.; Ranasinghe, A.; Nakamura, J.; Upton, P. B.; Swenberg, J. A. Molecular dosimetry and repair of N(2),3-ethenoguanine in rats exposed to vinyl chloride. *Cancer Res.* **2002,** *62,* 5189–5195.

53. Barbin, A. Etheno-adduct-forming chemicals: from mutagenicity testing to tumor mutation spectra. *Mutat. Res.* **2000,** *462,* 55–69.

54. Gros, L.; Ishchenko, A. A.; Saparbaev, M. Enzymology of repair of etheno-adducts. *Mutat. Res.* **2003,** *531,* 219–229.

55. Johnson, K. A.; Mierzwa, M. L.; Fink, S. P.; Marnett, L. J. MutS recognition of exocyclic DNA adducts that are endogenous products of lipid oxidation. *J. Biol. Chem.* **1999,** *274,* 27112–27118.

56. Mao, H.; Schnetz-Boutaud, N. C.; Weisenseel, J. P.; Marnett, L. J.; Stone, M. P. Duplex DNA catalyzes the chemical rearrangement of a malondialdehyde deoxyguanosine adduct. *Proc. Natl. Acad. Sci. USA* **1999,** *96,* 6615–6620.

57. Randerath, K.; Reddy, M. V.; Gupta, R. C. ^{32}P-labeling test for DNA damage. *Proc. Natl. Acad. Sci. USA* **1981,** *78,* 6126–6129.

58. Randerath, K.; Randerath, E.; Agrawal, H. P.; Gupta, R. C.; Schurdak, M. E.; Reddy, M. V. Postlabeling methods for carcinogen–DNA adduct analysis. *Environ. Health Perspect.* **1985,** *62,* 57–65.

59. Arlt, V. M.; Glatt, H.; Muckel, E.; Pabel, U.; Sorg, B. L.; Schmeiser, H. H.; Phillips, D. H. Metabolic activation of the environmental contaminant 3-nitrobenzanthrone by human acetyltransferases and sulfotransferase. *Carcinogenesis* **2002,** *23,* 1937–1945.

60. Reddy, M. V.; Randerath, K. Nuclease P1-mediated enhancement of sensitivity of ^{32}P-postlabeling test for structurally diverse DNA adducts. *Carcinogenesis* **1986,** *7,* 1543–1551.

61. Randerath, K.; Sriram, P.; Moorthy, B.; Aston, J. P.; Baan, R. A.; van den Berg, P. T.; Booth, E. D.; Watson, W. P. Comparison of immuno-affinity chromatography enrichment and nuclease P1 procedures for ^{32}P-postlabelling analysis of PAH–DNA adducts. *Chem. Biol. Interact.* **1998,** *110,* 85–102.

62. Romier, C.; Dominguez, R.; Lahm, A.; Dahl, O.; Suck, D. Recognition of single-stranded DNA by nuclease P1: high resolution crystal structures of complexes with substrate analogs. *Proteins* **1998,** *32,* 414–424.

63. Fullerton, P. D.; Finch, L. R. Use of polyethyleneimine–cellulose thin layers in assay of pyrophosphate–ATP exchange reactions. *Anal. Biochem.* **1969,** *29,* 544–547.

64. Keith, G.; Dirheimer, G. Postlabeling: a sensitive method for studying DNA adducts and their role in carcinogenesis. *Curr. Opin. Biotechnol.* **1995,** *6,* 3–11.

65. Randerath, E.; Avitts, T. A.; Reddy, M. V.; Miller, R. H.; Everson, R. B.; Randerath, K. Comparative ^{32}P-analysis of cigarette smoke-induced DNA damage in human tissues and mouse skin. *Cancer Res.* **1986,** *46,* 5869–5877.

66. Culp, S. J.; Warbritton, A. R.; Smith, B. A.; Li, E. E.; Beland, F. A. DNA adduct measurements, cell proliferation and tumor mutation induction in relation to tumor formation in B6C3F1 mice fed coal tar or benzo[a] pyrene. *Carcinogenesis* **2000,** *21,* 1433–1440.

67. Young, T. L.; Habraken, Y.; Ludlum, D. B.; Santella, R. M. Development of monoclonal antibodies recognizing 7-(2-hydroxyethyl)guanine and imidazole ring-opened 7-(2-hydroxyethyl)guanine. *Carcinogenesis* **1990,** *11,* 1685–1689.

68. Poirier, M. C.; Weston, A.; Gupta-Burt, S.; Reed, E. Measurement of DNA adducts by immunoassays. *Basic Life Sci.* **1990,** *53,* 1–11.

69. Poirier, M. C. Chemical-induced DNA damage and human cancer risk. *Nat. Rev. Cancer* **2004,** *4,* 630–637.

70. Poirier, M. C.; True, B. A.; Laishes, B. A. Determination of 2-acetyl-aminofluorene adducts by immunoassay. *Environ. Health Perspect.* **1982,** *49,* 93–99.

71. den Engelse, L.; Van Benthem, J.; Scherer, E. Immunocytochemical analysis of in vivo DNA modification. *Mutat. Res.* **1990**, *233*, 265–287.

72. Rundle, A.; Tang, D.; Hibshoosh, H.; Estabrook, A.; Schnabel, F.; Cao, W.; Grumet, S.; Perera, F. P. The relationship between genetic damage from polycyclic aromatic hydrocarbons in breast tissue and breast cancer. *Carcinogenesis* **2000**, *21*, 1281–1289.

73. Perera, F. P.; Hemminki, K.; Gryzbowska, E.; Motykiewicz, G.; Michalska, J.; Santella, R. M.; Young, T. L.; Dickey, C.; Brandt-Rauf, P.; De, V., I. Molecular and genetic damage in humans from environmental pollution in Poland. *Nature* **1992**, *360*, 256–258.

74. Kriek, E.; Rojas, M.; Alexandrov, K.; Bartsch, H. Polycyclic aromatic hydrocarbon–DNA adducts in humans: relevance as biomarkers for exposure and cancer risk. *Mutat. Res.* **1998**, *400*, 215–231.

75. Shuker, D. E.; Bartsch, H. Detection of human exposure to carcinogens by measurement of alkyl–DNA adducts using immunoaffinity clean-up in combination with gas chromatography–mass spectrometry and other methods of quantitation. *Mutat. Res.* **1994**, *313*, 263–268.

76. Coles, B. Effects of modifying structure on electrophilic reactions with biological nucleophiles. *Drug Metab. Rev.* **1984**, *15*, 1307–1334.

77. Carlson, R. M. Assessment of the propensity for covalent binding of electrophiles to biological substrates. *Environ. Health Perspect.* **1990**, *87*, 227–232.

78. Moschel, R. C.; Hudgins, W. R.; Dipple, A. Selectivity in nucleoside alkylation and arylation in relation to chemical carcinogenesis. *J. Org. Chem.* **1979**, *44*, 3324–3328.

79. Singer, B. Reaction of guanosine with ethylating agents. *Biochemistry* **1972**, *11*, 3939–3947.

80. Pullman, A.; Pullman, B. Electrostatic effect of the macromolecular structure on the biochemical reactivity of the nucleic acids. Significance for chemical carcinogenesis. *Int. J. Quantum Chem: Quantum Biol. Symp.* **1980**, *7*, 245–259.

81. Wolfe, A.; Shimer, G. H., Jr.; Meehan, T. Polycyclic aromatic hydrocarbons physically intercalate into duplex regions of denatured DNA. *Biochemistry* **1987**, *26*, 6392–6396.

82. Hong, S.; Piette, L. H. Electron spin resonance spin-label studies of intercalation of ethidium bromide and aromatic amine carcinogens in DNA. *Cancer Res.* **1976**, *36*, 1159–1171.

83. Wemmer, D. Structure and dynamics by NMR. In *Nucleic Acids: Structures, Properties, and Functions;* Bloomfield, V. A., Crothers, D. M., Tinoco, J. I., Eds.; University Science Books: Sausalito, CA, 2000; pp. 111–163.

84. Wüthrich, K. *NMR of Proteins and Nucleic Acids;* Wiley: New York, 1986.

85. Stassinopoulou, C. I. *NMR of Biological Macromolecules;* Springer: New York, 1994.

86. Karplus, M. Contact electron-spin coupling of nuclear magnetic moments. *J. Chem. Phys.* **1959**, *30*, 11–15.

87. Noggle, J. H.; Schirmer, R. G. *The Nuclear Overhauser Effect;* Academic Press: New York, 1983.

88. Geacintov, N. E.; Cosman, M.; Hingerty, B. E.; Amin, S.; Broyde, S.; Patel, D. J. NMR solution structures of stereoisometric covalent polycyclic aromatic carcinogen–DNA adducts: principles, patterns, and diversity. *Chem. Res. Toxicol.* **1997**, *10*, 111–146.

89. Brown, K.; Hingerty, B. E.; Guenther, E. A.; Krishnan, V. V.; Broyde, S.; Turteltaub, K. W.; Cosman, M. Solution structure of the

2-amino-1-methyl-6-phenylimidazo[4,5-*b*]pyridine C8-deoxyguanosine adduct in duplex DNA. *Proc. Natl. Acad. Sci. USA* **2001**, *98*, 8507–8512.

90. Clore, G. M.; Gronenborn, A. M. Determination of three-dimensional structures of proteins and nucleic acids in solution by nuclear magnetic resonance spectroscopy. *Crit. Rev. Biochem. Mol. Biol.* **1989**, *24*, 479–564.

91. Hingerty, B. E.; Figueroa, S.; Hayden, T. L.; Broyde, S. Prediction of DNA structure from sequence: a build-up technique. *Biopolymers* **1989**, *28*, 1195–1222.

92. Cosman, M.; Hingerty, B. E.; Geacintov, N. E.; Broyde, S.; Patel, D. J. Structural alignments of (+)- and (−)-*trans*-anti-benzo[*a*]pyrene-dG adducts positioned at a DNA template-primer junction. *Biochemistry* **1995**, *34*, 15334–15350.

93. Evans, D. C.; Watt, A. P.; Nicoll-Griffith, D. A.; Baillie, T. A. Drug–protein adducts: an industry perspective on minimizing the potential for drug bioactivation in drug discovery and development. *Chem. Res. Toxicol.* **2004**, *17*, 3–16.

94. Dehal, S. S.; Kupfer, D. Cytochrome P-450 3A and 2D6 catalyze ortho hydroxylation of 4-hydroxytamoxifen and 3-hydroxytamoxifen (droloxifene) yielding tamoxifen catechol: involvement of catechols in covalent binding to hepatic proteins. *Drug Metab. Dispos.* **1999**, *27*, 681–688.

95. Neuberger, J.; Williams, R. Immune mechanisms in tienilic acid associated hepatotoxicity. *Gut* **1989**, *30*, 515–519.

96. Ahlfors, S. R.; Sterner, O.; Hansson, C. Reactivity of contact allergenic haptens to amino acid residues in a model carrier peptide, and characterization of formed peptide–hapten adducts. *Skin Pharmacol. Appl. Skin Physiol.* **2003**, *16*, 59–68.

97. Obermayer-Straub, P.; Strassburg, C. P.; Manns, M. P. Autoimmune hepatitis. *J. Hepatol.* **2000**, *32*, 181–197.

98. Rubin, R. L. Etiology and mechanisms of drug-induced lupus. *Curr. Opin. Rheumatol.* **1999**, *11*, 357–363.

99. Rao, T.; Richardson, B. Environmentally induced autoimmune diseases: potential mechanisms. *Environ. Health Perspect.* **1999**, *107* (Suppl. 5), 737–742.

100. Badghisi, H.; Liebler, D. C. Sequence mapping of epoxide adducts in human hemoglobin with LC–tandem MS and the SALSA algorithm. *Chem. Res. Toxicol.* **2002**, *15*, 799–805.

101. Neumann, H. G.; van Dorp, C.; Zwirner-Baier, I. The implications for risk assessment of measuring the relative contribution to exposure from occupation, environment and lifestyle: hemoglobin adducts from amino- and nitro-arenes. *Toxicol. Lett.* **1995**, *82–83*, 771–778.

102. Törnqvist, M.; Fred, C.; Haglund, J.; Helleberg, H.; Paulsson, B.; Rydberg, P. Protein adducts: quantitative and qualitative aspects of their formation, analysis and applications. *J. Chromatogr. B Analyt. Technol. Biomed. Life Sci.* **2002**, *778*, 279–308.

103. Bechtold, W. E.; Strunk, M. R. S-Phenylcysteine in albumin as a benzene biomarker. *Environ. Health Perspect.* **1996**, *104* (Suppl. 6), 1147–1149.

104. Basile, A.; Ferranti, P.; Mamone, G.; Manco, I.; Pocsfalvi, G.; Malorni, A.; Acampora, A.; Sannolo, N. Structural analysis of styrene oxide/haemoglobin adducts by mass spectrometry: identification of suitable biomarkers for human exposure evaluation. *Rapid Commun. Mass Spectrom.* **2002**, *16*, 871–878.

105. Noort, D.; Hulst, A. G.; de Jong, L. P.; Benschop, H. P. Alkylation of human serum albumin by sulfur mustard in vitro and in vivo: mass spectrometric analysis of a cysteine adduct as a sensitive biomarker of exposure. *Chem. Res. Toxicol.* **1999,** *12,* 715–721.

106. Deng, S. X.; Bharat, N.; Fischman, M. C.; Landry, D. W. Covalent modification of proteins by cocaine. *Proc. Natl. Acad. Sci. USA* **2002,** *99,* 3412–3416.

107. Kriek, E.; Miller, J. A.; Juhl, U.; Miller, E. C. 8-(N-2-Fluorenyl-acetamido)guanosine, an arylamidation reaction product of guanosine and the carcinogen N-acetoxy-N-2-fluorenylacetamide in neutral solution. *Biochemistry* **1967,** *6,* 177–182.

108. Evans, F. E.; Miller, D. W.; Beland, F. A. Sensitivity of the conformation of deoxyguanosine to binding at the C-8 position by N-acetylated and unacetylated 2-aminofluorene. *Carcinogenesis* **1980,** *1,* 955–959.

109. Delclos, K. B.; Miller, D. W.; Lay, J. O., Jr.; Casciano, D. A.; Walker, R. P.; Fu, P. P.; Kadlubar, F. F. Identification of C8-modified deoxyinosine and N2- and C8-modified deoxyguanosine as major products of the in vitro reaction of N-hydroxy-6-aminochrysene with DNA and the formation of these adducts in isolated rat hepatocytes treated with 6-nitrochrysene and 6-aminochrysene. *Carcinogenesis* **1987,** *8,* 1703–1709.

110. Rogan, E. G.; Cavalieri, E. L.; Tibbels, S. R.; Cremonesi, P.; Warner, C. D.; Nagel, D. L.; Tomer, K. B.; Cerny, R. L.; Gross, M. L. Synthesis and identification of benzo[*a*]pyreneguanine nucleoside adducts formed by electrochemical oxidation and by horseradish peroxidase catalyzed reaction of benzo[*a*]pyrene with DNA. *J. Am. Chem. Soc.* **1988,** *110,* 4023–4029.

111. Gamboa da Costa, G.; Churchwell, M. I.; Hamilton, L. P.; Von Tungeln, L. S.; Beland, F. A.; Marques, M. M.; Doerge, D. R. DNA adduct formation from acrylamide via conversion to glycidamide in adult and neonatal mice. *Chem. Res. Toxicol.* **2003,** *16,* 1328–1337.

112. Wang, M.; McIntee, E. J.; Cheng, G.; Shi, Y.; Villalta, P. W.; Hecht, S. S. Identification of DNA adducts of acetaldehyde. *Chem. Res. Toxicol.* **2000,** *13,* 1149–1157.

INTRODUCTION: DNA DAMAGE AND REPAIR

All cellular macromolecules are vulnerable to chemical damage. The agents of such damage—oxidants, electrophiles, and even water itself—are ubiquitous. Protein, RNA, and structural components such as membrane lipids are turned over in the cell, so a biologically acceptable response to their damage is degradation and replacement (cellular "recycling"). But DNA is the irreplaceable genetic code. Not only its information content but also its physical structure is passed on from parent cell to daughter cell, since DNA replication is semiconservative. The chemical diversity of DNA damage is vast, including hydrolysis, alkylation, oxidation, and covalent adduction by xenobiotics, and these events can occur at many different sites on the bases, sugars, and phosphates. Views of the double helix secondary structure of DNA are shown in figures 3-1 and 3-2. The problem of recognizing and repairing an unlimited range of possible damages to DNA brings to mind the problem facing the enzymes of detoxication, which must recognize and metabolize an equally broad range of foreign compounds. We will later consider the ability of receptors (such as PXR, chapter 8) and enzymes (such as glutathione transferase, chapter 10) to recognize diverse xenobiotics by their hydrophobic binding to promiscuous active sites. Similarly, DNA repair proteins such as UvrB can recognize diverse DNA adducts, and, once again, hydrophobicity is probably the key structural recognition feature.

The stability of information transmission required for the evolution of complex genomes is only possible on the basis of the principle of

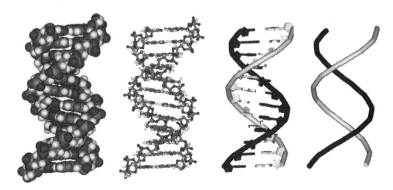

FIGURE 3-1.

The double helix structure of DNA, viewed at right angles to the helix axis. From left: space-filling representation; ball-and-stick representation; backbone strands with bases shown as plates; backbone strands only. *Note*: A full-color version of this figure appears on the website.

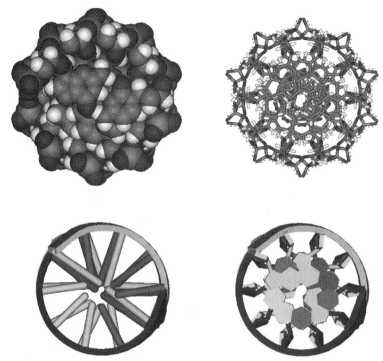

FIGURE 3-2.
The double helix structure of DNA, viewed along the helix axis. Top left: space-filling representation; top right: ball-and-stick representation; bottom left: backbone strands with bases shown as rods; bottom right: backbone strands with bases shown as plates. *Note*: A full-color version of this figure appears on the website.

self-complementarity: the redundant storage of genetic information. *DNA repair faithful to the information content of the gene is possible for the same reason.* The sequence of the damaged strand can be chemically deduced by enzymatic machinery that "reads" the complementary strand.[1]

A mutation is a heritable change in DNA sequence. Mutation is the raw material for natural selection, the driving force for the generation of biological diversity and evolutionary change. However, mutations are more likely to be deleterious than beneficial. Mutations arising in germ cells can lead to genetic diseases and mutations arising in somatic cells can lead to cancer. The relationship between DNA damage and mutation is subtle. A mutated DNA sequence is not "damaged" in a chemical sense; it simply carries genetic information that differs from that of the parental sequence to which we are comparing it. Mutation can occur in the absence of DNA damage, since the fidelity of DNA replication is not 100% (although it can be astoundingly close to that figure). All new DNA strands are synthesized from dNTP building blocks by the action of DNA polymerases, enzymes that "read" the sequence of the template strand and assemble the daughter strands following the Watson–Crick complementarity rules. Chemical damage to the template strand may interfere with this process, so DNA damages are often mutagenic, but not necessarily so. The levels of mutagenesis that would result from unrestrained chemical damage to DNA would be incompatible with the long-term stability of the genome. All organisms rely on DNA repair systems to maintain the integrity of their genetic information.

PROGRESS IN THE STUDY OF DNA REPAIR

All realms of biochemistry have been affected by the genomic and structural biology revolutions, but the study of DNA repair has been particularly transformed. DNA repair, DNA synthesis, and mutagenesis are complex biochemical/biological processes, often involving large numbers of interacting proteins. In some cases, we cannot assay the activity of a given protein until we have identified its partners, leaving us trapped in a vicious circle. Consequently, it has often been difficult to purify enzymes of DNA repair by standard assay-directed biochemical techniques. Cloning genes based on their ability to complement (correct) the DNA repair defects of mutation-prone cells provided one shortcut around this problem, and mapping the genes responsible for human inherited diseases of DNA repair provided another (1). With the availability of recombinant proteins of DNA repair, structural biology can provide insights into the molecular interactions that govern the recognition and repair of DNA damage. The biochemistry of DNA repair has grown into a very large subdiscipline, and we can only go into limited depth here. A textbook devoted exclusively to *DNA Repair and Mutagenesis* (2) and the review by Lindahl and Wood (3) are recommended for further reading.

DNA POLYMERASES

The *sine qua non* of faithful transmission of genetic information is the fidelity of DNA polymerase, the enzyme that assembles the daughter strands of DNA from dNTP precursors. DNA synthesis might appear to be a single operation, necessitating only a single piece of machinery. Actually, organisms express multiple DNA polymerases, with distinct biological roles and biochemical properties. Some of these enzymes are specialized for chromosome replication while others function primarily in DNA repair. The catalogue of DNA polymerases, both prokaryotic and eukaryotic, has expanded remarkably in recent years (4).

The action of a DNA polymerase enzyme synthesizing a new strand is an ordered, directional process, using dNTP building blocks as substrates, adding them as deoxyribonucleotides to the hydroxyl group at the 3' end, and extending the strand in the 5' to 3' direction. Since DNA duplexes are double stranded and antiparallel, one strand can be synthesized continuously, 5' to 3', at the replication fork. Synthesis of the complementary strand in the 3' to 5' direction, using 5'-dNTP substrates, is not possible. Instead, the complementary strand is synthesized in short stretches (Okazaki fragments), each assembled 5' to 3', that is, in the direction opposite to the progress of the replication fork. The Okazaki fragments are ligated into a continuous strand as the replication fork progresses.

In the simplest picture of DNA polymerase action, we can envisage a molecule of the enzyme attaching to the 3' end of a primer, remaining tightly bound to the growing strand, and extending it continuously until it reaches the end of the template strand. This mode of action is termed *processive* (5, p. 762). Alternatively, however, the polymerase might add only a few dNTPs to a given strand, and then dissociate from it. Further extension of the strand would not occur until the binding of another mole-cule of polymerase. This mode of action is termed *distributive*. We can rank DNA polymerases according to their degree of processivity, that is, the average number of dNTPs incorporated before enzyme dissociation.

E. coli

Five different DNA polymerases have been identified in *E. coli* to date (see table 3-1). The chief replicative enzyme is *DNA polymerase III* (Pol III) (*5, 6*, pp. 762–764). Pol III holoenzyme is a very large (nearly 1 MDa) molecular structure built from ten different types of polypeptide chains. The catalytic subunit is encoded by the *polC* gene. Additional subunits contribute proofreading (error-checking) activity and processivity func-tions. Pol III replicates both the leading and lagging strands of DNA at the replication fork. *E. coli* Pol I (*7*), the first DNA polymerase discovered, is a much smaller (103 kDa) single-polypeptide enzyme (*polA* gene). Pol I plays a secondary role in DNA replication, removing RNA primers via its 5′–3′ exonuclease activity; its DNA polymerase activity then replaces the RNA primer with DNA. Pol I's role in DNA repair is discussed later.

The function of Pol II remained obscure for many years following its discovery, but its induction as part of the SOS response (see below) indi-cated a role in DNA repair. (The gene designation *dinA* refers to d̲amage i̲nducible.) Ultraviolet (UV) irradiation causes a transient halt to DNA synthesis by *E. coli*, because Pol III "stalls" when it encounters UV-induced lesions (see below). Recent work has shown that Pol II is required for "replication restart" after such damage occurs (*8*). The "error-prone" poly-merases (Pol IV and Pol V), which are discussed further at the end of this chapter, allow replication to proceed through DNA lesions which would block the action of the replicative polymerase Pol III.

The most important determinant of replication fidelity in *E. coli* is that Pol III incorporates the correct (complementary) dNTP into the growing DNA chain. Formation of correct Watson–Crick hydrogen bonds between the base moiety of the incoming dNTP and the complementary base on the template strand was long believed to be required for polymerase fidel-ity. However, this assumption has been toppled by recent studies on the

TABLE 3-1.

E. coli DNA Polymerases

POLYMERASE	FUNCTION	GENE	MAP	ACCURACY	PROCESSIVITY
Housekeeping DNA polymerases					
Pol III	Replication	*dnaE* (*polC*)	4.42	Accurate	Processive
Pol I	DNA repair	*polA*	87.18	Accurate	Processive
DNA polymerases induced to higher levels by DNA damage					
Pol II	DNA repair	*polB* (*dinA*)	1.37	Accurate	Processive
Pol IV	Mutagenesis (?)	*dinB*	5.41	Error-prone	Distributive
Pol V	Lesion bypass	*umuDC*	26.51	Error-prone	Distributive

Map: position on the E. coli *genetic map, in minutes. Adapted from summaries provided by Patricia Foster and Takehiko Nohmi.*

incorporation into DNA of base analogues, notably the research of Eric Kool and collaborators (*9–12*). These experiments have shown that (at least in the case of certain DNA polymerases) the critical requirement is for a good steric fit, rather than for Watson–Crick hydrogen bonding interactions per se. In the absence of this fit, DNA polymerase is unable to undergo the conformational change required for catalysis of phosphodiester bond formation.

Occasional incorporation of an incorrect dNTP into the growing chain is inevitable, since the thermodynamic barrier to misincorporation is finite. However, in addition to its polymerization activity, Pol III also possesses a $3' \rightarrow 5'$ exonuclease activity, which can remove the last-inserted nucleotide, releasing it as a dNMP. This "proofreading" activity, associated with the epsilon subunit of the Pol III holoenzyme (*13*), double checks the action of the polymerase and removes most mismatched nucleotides immediately after they are inserted. The combination of faithful polymerization and proofreading reduces the in vitro error rate of Pol III to about one misincorporation event per million nucleotides. Note, however, that such a rate would still result in several mutations per *E. coli* cell division, in the absence of additional error-correcting processes (see below).

Eukaryotes

The major replicative DNA polymerase in eukaryotes is Pol δ (*14*), a complex of three polypeptide subunits (*15*) that replicates both the leading and lagging strands of the replication fork. At least two more polymerases, Pol α and Pol ε, are required for chromosome replication. Pol β participates in base excision repair (*16*); it is not essential for survival of mammalian cells in vitro (*16*) but knockout mice devoid of Pol β are nonviable (*17*). Additional error-prone eukaryotic DNA polymerases have been discovered recently, as discussed later in the chapter.

DEFECTIVE DNA REPAIR

Human Genetic Diseases

Defects in DNA repair are responsible for certain rare human genetic diseases, including xeroderma pigmentosum (XP) (*18*), ataxia telangiectasia (AT) (*19*), Fanconi's anemia (*20*), and Bloom's syndrome (*21*). Although these recessive diseases are very rare in the homozygous state, carriers (heterozygotes) are of course more common. For example, about one individual in 100 is an AT carrier. These carriers probably constitute a subpopulation at elevated risk of radiation-induced carcinogenesis (*22*).

XP patients suffer extreme sensitivity to UV radiation, resulting in severe sunburn and a very high incidence of skin cancer (*18*). This sensitivity is also observed in vitro: cultured cells from XP patients are sensitive to UV (and also to some chemical mutagens) relative to cells from control individuals. The XP defect can be demonstrated in individual cells by measuring clonogenic survival (colony-forming ability) or unscheduled DNA synthesis (UDS). In the UDS technique, cells are exposed to UV radiation and then incubated with the DNA precursor ^{3}H-thymidine. Normal cells will incorporate this labeled base into chromosomal DNA during repair, prior to mitosis, and the incorporation can be measured by scintillation counting or autoradiography. Such "unscheduled" repair synthesis can readily be distinguished from the much greater "scheduled" incorporation of thymidine during mitosis. (The discovery of UDS, in the 1960s, is recounted in a recent article by Cleaver (*23*).)

The sensitivity of XP cells in vitro provides a tool for molecular analysis of the disease. Cells from different individuals can be fused into hetero-karyon hybrids, by treatment with polyethylene glycol. When such heterokaryons are examined for UDS, it is observed that hybrids from certain pairs of individuals exhibit normal repair while other hybrids are defective. This method allows XP individuals to be classified into distinct *complementation groups*, representing lesions in different genes (encoding different proteins required for repair). Seven XP complementation groups are known (*24*).

Isolation of Repair-Defective Mammalian Cells In Vitro

Repair-defective mammalian cells can be generated in vitro. James Cleaver and colleagues isolated several UV-sensitive mutant derivatives of the CHO (Chinese hamster ovary) cell line. *Resistant* mutants can usually be isolated easily, by selecting for colonies that survive exposure to a toxic insult; but it is much more difficult to isolate *sensitive* mutants, since these are differentially *killed*. One must rely on the replica-plating technique and mass screening. Cleaver's group developed semiautomated methods for screening very large numbers of CHO colonies to identify UV-sensitive mutants (*25, 26*). Much effort has been directed to characterizing the complementation groups, enzymatic defects, and mutant genes in these clones. Transfection of repair-deficient cells with genomic DNA from a normal individual, followed by selection of UV-resistant transfectant clones, allows the cloning of normal genes that complement the cell line's repair defect (*27*). Extending this approach to human cells allowed the cloning of genes complementing the defects in several FA and XP cell lines (*28, 29*).

CLASSIFICATION OF DNA REPAIR PROCESSES

Cellular mechanisms for DNA repair can usefully be classified into five general categories (*30*) based on the type of biochemical processing that they effect. Each of these categories is briefly described in this preliminary section, and subsequently considered in greater detail.

Direct Reversal

Direct reversal mechanisms recognize altered DNA bases and chemically convert them back to the standard structures, without removing them from the double helix. Uniquely among DNA repair mechanisms, direct reversal does not depend on sequence information obtained from the complementary strand.

Base Excision Repair

The bases that encode the genetic information are attached to the sugar–phosphate backbone of DNA by *glycosylic* bonds from ring N atoms of the bases (pyrimidine N1, purine N9) to the anomeric C1′ hydroxyl groups of the deoxyribose sugar. Thus, in contrast to the role of amino acids in protein structure, *a base can be removed without breaking the covalent backbone of the nucleic acid*. Base excision repair mechanisms (*31, 32*) begin with the action of a glycosylase enzyme (*33*) that recognizes a damaged base and excises it from the strand, via hydrolysis of the glycosylic bond (*34*). Regardless of the nature of the damaged base, the immediate product of base removal is an abasic site (also called an AP = apurinic/apyrimidinic site) in DNA (*35*). Thus, *base excision repair is convergent*, with a family of repair enzymes converting several different forms of base damage into a single product, the abasic site. Abasic sites are then repaired by removal of a "patch" (a stretch of nucleotides from the damaged strand), repair synthesis by a polymerase, and resealing by DNA ligase.

Mismatch Repair

A *mismatch* is a site in a double-stranded DNA where an illegitimate (non-Watson–Crick) base pair is present. Perhaps we should not consider this to be a form of "DNA damage" per se, since both nucleotides are chemically normal. However, the presence of a mismatch may indicate that an error has been made by DNA polymerase. All organisms possess mismatch repair systems, which detect and correct such errors (*36–38*). A special case of base mismatching is the occurrence of G:U and G:T base pairs, which commonly arise by the deamination of cytosine or 5-methylcytosine bases, as discussed later. Mismatches are repaired by excision of a single-stranded oligonucleotide patch surrounding the mismatch, followed by resynthesis (*39*) of the strand.

The above classification system is (like most classifications) to some extent artificial. For example the categories of "mismatch repair" and "base excision repair" overlap, since some mismatch repair mechanisms rely on the action of glycosylase enzymes; and most types of DNA repair process require the action of DNA polymerase enzymes and ligases.

Nucleotide Excision Repair

As with base excision repair, nucleotide excision repair mechanisms recognize and remove the damaged portion of a DNA strand; DNA polymerase and DNA ligase fill and reseal the resulting gap. However, nucleotide excision repair mechanisms do not affect the glycosylic bond between the base and the backbone. Instead, an oligonucleotide segment including the damaged site is removed *in toto* by making cuts (i.e., hydrolyzing phosphodiester bonds) upstream (5′ direction) and downstream (3′ direction) of the damage site, releasing an oligonucleotide (between about 12 and 32 units long, depending on the system). Typically, *base excision repair mechanisms are relatively specific whereas nucleotide excision repair mechanisms are highly promiscuous*. Particular glycosylase enzymes recognize common damaged bases, such as 8-oxoguanine, which arise by oxidation or alkylation. In contrast, a single molecular machine, comprising multiple proteins, carries out nucleotide excision repair at a very wide range of damaged sites, including UV-induced thymine dimers and 6,4-photoproducts (discussed below) and bulky covalent adducts of aromatic amines, polycyclic aromatic hydrocarbons, psoralens, etc. (*40–42*).

As was first recognized by Phil Hanawalt and colleagues, there are two pathways of nucleotide excision repair. The first pathway, global genome repair, is the repair mechanism for dealing with stalled replication forks, which occur when DNA polymerase encounters a helix-distorting lesion. The second pathway, transcription-coupled repair (TCR), is the repair mechanism for dealing with stalled transcription complexes, which occur when RNA polymerase encounters DNA lesions. Global genome repair protects the genome against mutations and ensures that cell replication can be completed. TCR functions to protect actively transcribed genes. In the absence of such a repair process, lesions on the transcribed strands of highly expressed genes become cellular "traffic jams," blocking the production of critical proteins and leading to cell death (43a). Defects in TCR impair the viability of terminally differentiated cells and lead to the characteristic neurodegeneration seen in diseases such as Cockayne syndrome (43b).

Strand Break Repair

Damage to the deoxyribose sugars, for example by oxidation or radiation damage, often leads to breakage of the phosphodiester backbone of DNA; strand breakage by hydrolysis can occur even in the absence of chemical damage. Single-strand breaks are relatively easy to repair by ligation, since the complementary strand holds the double helix together.[2] But double-strand breaks, such as may be induced by ionizing radiation damage, are harder to repair, and likely to lead to clastogenic events (e.g., chromosome translocations or chromosome losses). The molecular mechanisms of double-strand break repair are only poorly understood.

DIRECT REVERSAL MECHANISMS

Certain DNA lesions are repaired in situ, that is, without removal of the damaged base/nucleotide. Bacteria, yeast, fish, and reptiles—but not mammals—possess light-dependent *photolyases* that repair UV-induced pyrimidine dimers. These remarkable enzymes harness light energy to effect the cleavage of the cyclobutane linkage joining adjacent pyrimidines in these lesions (44, 45). Alkylated bases are repaired by the action of DNA methyltransferase enzymes, which is discussed in chapter 15.

BASE EXCISION REPAIR MECHANISMS

As stated at the outset of this chapter, base excision repair systems (46–50) remove damaged bases by hydrolyzing the glycosylic bond between the damaged base and deoxyribose. Figure 3-3 illustrates some of the damaged bases that are known to be recognized and excised by base excision repair DNA glycosylase enzymes. Lindahl and Wood list eight human DNA repair glycosylases, four of which act on uracil residues in DNA. Krokan et al. have compiled a summary table of DNA repair glycosylases from all classes of organisms (32). Only a few examples will be presented here. The repair of DNA uracils, which is a special case of base excision repair (overlapping with mismatch repair), is discussed first. We then consider the repair of some oxidized bases. Finally, the repair of abasic sites, the common lesion generated by the action of all DNA glycosylases, is addressed.

Uracil DNA *N*-glycosylase

Uracil residues occur naturally in RNA but not in DNA, where thymine (5-methyluracil) replaces uracil as the partner for adenine. However, uracil bases in DNA continuously arise by the spontaneous (51) or chemically induced deamination of cytosine residues (figure 3-4) (or by the

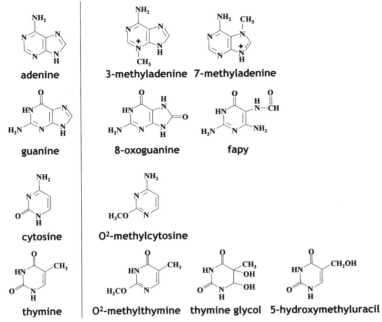

FIGURE 3-3.

The four normal DNA bases are shown on the left, and various damaged bases recognized by DNA base excision repair enzymes are shown to the right. (*Adapted from Krokan, H. E.; Standal, R.; Slupphaug, G. DNA glycosylases in the base excision repair of DNA. Biochem. J.* **1997**, *325, 1–16.*)

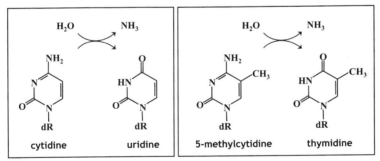

FIGURE 3-4.

Deamination of cytidine (left) and 5-methylcyidine (right).

misincorporation of dUTP into DNA (*52*)). The removal of uracil residues from DNA is an interesting case of base excision repair. DNA uracils are detected and excised by *uracil DNA N-glycosylase* (EC 3.2.2), an enzyme discovered by Tomas Lindahl in 1974. This discovery answers the riddle posed by the presence of thymine rather than uracil (the corresponding RNA base) in DNA. If DNA normally contained uracil, G–U base pairs resulting from cytosine deamination would give rise to A–U base pairs in one of the daughter strands at the time of replication. The spontaneous deamination of cytosine might lead to an unstoppable mutational drift from relatively chemically labile G–C base pairs toward A–U base pairs, and gradually erase the genetic code. Instead, because uracil is not normally present in DNA, uracil DNA *N*-glycosylase can safely remove any uracil residue that arises in DNA. The 5-methyl group of thymine provides a chemical "handle" that allows the enzyme to discriminate between uracil and thymine (53).

Nevertheless, thymine *can* arise directly in DNA, by the deamination of the modified pyrimidine base *5-methylcytosine*. 5-Methylcytosine base-pairs with guanine in exactly the same manner as does cytosine. *Deamination of 5-methylcytosine yields thymine, rather than uracil* (figure 3-4). 5-Methylcytosine is the most widely used epigenetic tag in biology. That is, organisms can modify the properties of DNA without changing its sequence, by methylation of cytosine residues, and the extent of such methylation can be used to distinguish the source of a DNA molecule. For example, methylation of cytosines in characteristic sequences is the mechanism that bacteria use to protect their own DNA against endogenous restriction enzymes, which degrade foreign (e.g., viral) DNA. In animals, methylation is the basis of "imprinting," the epigenetic mechanism that accounts for differential effects of maternal vs. paternal chromosomes (54).

In *E. coli*, the *dcm* (DNA cytosine methylation) gene product recognizes the sequences CCAGG and CCTGG and catalyzes the *S*-adenosylmethionine-dependent 5-methylation of the second cytosine. (This modification protects *E. coli* chromosomal DNA against digestion by the restriction endonuclease *Eco*RII, which recognizes the same DNA sequence (55); *dcm*-dependent cytosine methylation should not be confused with adenine methylation, discussed later in the chapter, which provides a signal for distinguishing parental and daughter DNA strands.) What are the consequences of deamination of such 5-methylcytosine residues? A thymine residue is formed, which, of course, is ignored by uracil DNA *N*-glycosylase, and the resulting G:T mismatch represents a possible premutagenic lesion. Upon replication, one daughter molecule would bear an A:T base pair in place of the original G:C base pair. Indeed, the second C residues in CCAGG sequences are major hotspots for spontaneous base-substitution mutations in the *lacI* gene of *E. coli*, and the mutations that occur are G:C → A:T transitions, as one would predict (56).

5-Methylcytosine-Dependent Mutagenesis in Mammalian Cells

As stated above, cytosine methylation is also an important epigenetic signal in eukaryotes (57, 58). A few percent of the C residues in human chromosomes are 5-methylated. The methylation is catalyzed by an enzyme that recognizes CpG sequences (59). *CpG sequences, which are potential sites for methylation, are highly underrepresented in the mammalian genome.* In a random DNA sequence, each dinucleotide XpY would occur at the same average frequency (6.25%). *In fact, the CpG sequence occurs in vertebrate genomes at a much lower frequency, as low as about 1% in the human genome (54, 60); this bias results from the highly non-random choice of codons for degenerately coded amino acid residues as well as from the characteristics of noncoding repetitive DNA sequences (61).* CpG sites may be relatively unstable due to their tendency to undergo 5-methylcytosine deamination-induced mutations to TpG.

The presence of 5-methylcytosines in specific genomic sequences cannot, of course, be measured by standard DNA sequencing, which does not distinguish between cytosine and 5-methylcytosine residues. However, some of the ^{me}CpG residues occur within the palindromic sequence

CCGG, and these residues can conveniently be detected by restriction analysis. The restriction enzymes *Msp*I and *Hpa*II are *isoschizomers*: that is, they both recognize the same sequence, CCGG. However, the former enzyme cuts at C-methylated sites, while the latter does not. Thus, comparisons of chromosomal DNA samples cut with these restriction enzymes, and then analyzed by Southern blotting or PCR amplification, can reveal sites of methylation in CCGG sequences (e.g., (*62*)).

Are 5-methylcytosine residues hotspots for mutagenesis in mammalian cells? Analysis of mutations occurring in the cII transgene of Big Blue mice (*63*) (see chapter 4 for a discussion of this experimental system) revealed that G:C to A:T transitions were the most common spontaneous base-substitution mutations, and more than three-quarters of these mutations occurred at CpG sites, consistent with a 5-methylcytosine deamination mechanism.

Josef Jiricny and colleagues discovered a *thymine DNA glycosylase* activity in human (HeLa) cell nuclei, which specifically recognizes G–T mispairs, the mismatch expected to result from deamination of 5-methylcytosine residues (*64, 65*). In fact, the enzyme is most effective on DNA substrates bearing a G–T mispair in a CpG:T sequence context, where they would be most likely to arise (*66*). (The enzyme also interacts with the nuclear receptors RAR, RXR and estrogen receptor alpha (see chapter 8), but the biological significance of this interaction is not yet known (*67*).)

Guanine Oxidation; 8-Oxoguanosine and Fapy

As the most easily oxidized group in DNA, guanine acts as a trap for oxidant radicals (*68*). In 1984 Hiroshi Kasai and Susumu Nishimura (*69*) reported the formation of 8-hydroxydeoxyguanosine (8-oxodeoxyguanosine) in DNA exposed to radiation or to chemical systems that generate hydroxyl radical (figure 3-5). Hydroxyl radical addition to the C8

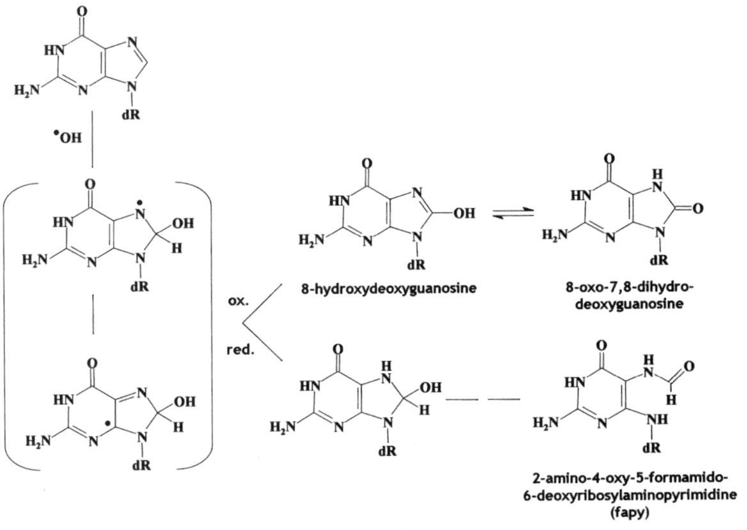

FIGURE 3-5.
Oxidative damage to deoxyguanosine and subsequent formation of 8-oxodeoxyguanosine and Fapy (2-amino-4-oxy-5-formamido-6-deoxyribosylaminopyrimidine).

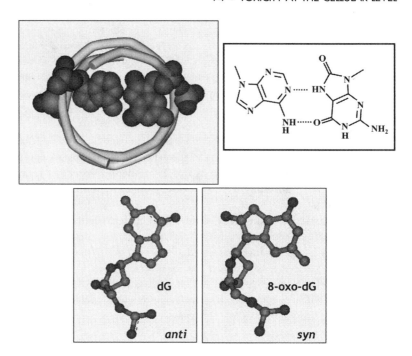

FIGURE 3-6.

Crystal structure of an oligonucleotide containing an 8-oxodeoxyguanosine mispair with adenine. Top left: view along the helix axis showing the 8-oxoG:A base pair. Top right: interpretive drawing of the base pair. Bottom left: normal *anti* conformation of the glycosylic bond of a guanine residue in DNA. Bottom right: *syn* conformation of the 8-oxoG base in the crystal structure. Structure file 178D.pbd. *Note*: A full-color version of this figure appears on the website.

position of deoxyguanosine gives a resonance-stabilized neutral radical. (The analogous reaction can also occur with adenosine, but this seems to be much less facile.) The guanine–OH adduct radical undergoes subsequent oxidation or reduction. Oxidation gives 8-hydroxydeoxyguanosine, which tautomerizes to the favored 6,8-diketo form (8-oxodeoxyguanosine). 8-Oxoguanine can be detected by HPLC-MS (*70*) in human urine as the base, ribonucleoside, and deoxyribonucleoside, and may represent a useful marker of oxidative stress. Reduction, followed by imidazole ring opening, gives the formamidopyrimidine product Fapy. Fapy has been observed as a product of radiation or oxidant damage to DNA (*71a*). 8-Oxoguanine readily undergoes further oxidation, yielding additional types of damaged bases with strongly mutagenic properties (*71b, 71c*). Structural analysis of an oligonucleotide containing an 8-oxodeoxyguanosine mispair with adenine (*72*) (figure 3-6) revealed that the glycosylic bond of the modified base flips from the normal *anti* conformation to the *syn* conformation, allowing the base to hydrogen bond to adenine by formation of so-called Hoogsteen (*73*, p. 340) base pairs (with purine N7 rather than N1 acting as the hydrogen bond acceptor). This mispairing propensity accounts for the fact that 8-oxodeoxyguanosine residues specifically and potently induce G:C → T:A transversion mutations (*74, 75*).

Base Excision Repair of 8-Oxoguanine

The multipronged defense against mutagenesis induced by guanine oxidation products, which includes several DNA repair enzymes, has been called the "GO" (guanine oxidation) system (74, 76, 77). In *E. coli*, the genes *mutM*, *mutT*, and *mutY* encode enzymes of the GO system (78). (The designation *mut* was chosen because strains bearing mutation in these genes have a *mutator* phenotype.) Jeffrey Miller and colleagues developed a set of *E. coli lacZ* strains that can be used to detect specific base-substitution mutations (see chapter 4). Using the strain from this set that detects G:C → T:A transversions, they screened pools of colonies for mutations that enhance the rate of this specific mutational event. This screen revealed the *mutY* and the *mutM* genes (79, 80).

Mapping of *mutM* revealed that it is the same gene, *fpg*, encoding a base excision repair enzyme that had already been characterized biochemically, formamidopyrimidine (Fapy)-DNA glycosylase (81). MutM (82) is a 30 kDa protein that acts as a glycosylase excising 8-oxoguanine, Fapy, and certain other modified bases from DNA. It also possesses β-lyase activity (see below). MutY (83) is an *adenine DNA glycosylase*, that is, it excises the *normal* adenine base from DNA, but only at sites where it is mispaired with 8-oxoguanine (or some other mispairs, such as adenine paired with undamaged guanine). MutY remains strongly bound to the abasic: 8-oxoguanine site that it creates (84), presumably to prevent removal of the 8-oxoguanine until the excised adenine has been replaced by cytosine.

The third member of the GO system family, MutT, is not a DNA repair enzyme per se. Rather, MutT (85) catalyzes hydrolysis of 8-oxoguanosine triphosphate (8-OH-dGTP) to 8-OH-dGMP + PP_i. This activity removes the oxidized base from the pool of dNTP precursors for DNA synthesis, preventing its incorporation into DNA.

The genome of the yeast *Saccharomyces cerevisiae* encodes two proteins with base excision repair activity for 8-oxoguanine residues, named Ogg1 and Ogg2 (86). Mammals also express an OGG1 enzyme. Knockout mice lacking OGG1 are viable (87) and apparently not cancer-prone, possibly because other repair systems back up OGG1. The X-ray crystal structure of the catalytic core of human OGG1, bound to a dsDNA oligonucleotide containing an 8-oxoG:C base pair, was published in 2000 (88). This structure provides a beautiful insight into the molecular recognition problem faced by a base excision repair enzyme. Truly, the enzyme searches for a needle in a haystack: it must detect a single oxygen atom altering the structure of one guanine base among thousands or millions of normal DNA guanines. The enzyme jams an aromatic residue (Tyr 203) into the double helix, adjacent to the "estranged" cytosine residue that would otherwise pair with the 8-oxoguanine, and this insertion drastically kinks the DNA backbone (figure 3-7). The 8-oxoguanine base is "flipped out" of the double helix altogether and grasped by the protein. The obvious way to discriminate between 8-oxoguanine and a normal guanine base would be by interactions with the extra O atom at C8—but the enzyme does not do the obvious! In fact, the C8 oxygen atom is a spectator, forming no strong interactions with the protein. Instead, the enzyme recognizes the N7 H atom present in 8-oxoguanine but absent in guanine. This NH forms a hydrogen bond with a main-chain C=O. This sole hydrogen bond is apparently the only "handle" by which the enzyme accepts 8-oxoguanine

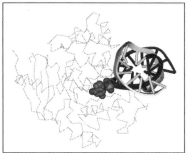
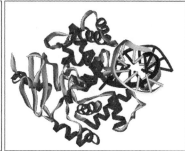
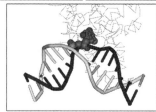

FIGURE 3-7.

Crystal structure of human OGG1 enzyme bound to a dsDNA oligonucleotide containing an 8-oxoG:C base pair. Top left: looking along the axis of the helix, with the protein shown as an alpha-carbon wire trace. The DNA bases are shown as rods, except for the space-filling view of the 8-oxoG base, which is flipped out of the helix and tightly bound to the protein. Top right: identical view to top left, but the protein is shown as a ribbon structure, with red representing alpha helices and cyan representing beta sheets. Bottom: as at top left, but showing a view perpendicular to the DNA helix axis. *Note*: A full-color version of this figure appears on the website.

and rejects guanines. A lysine residue at the active site attacks the C-1′ carbon atom of deoxyribose, forming a Schiff base linkage to the sugar and releasing the 8-oxoguanine base.

Generation of Abasic Sites

DNA bases are held to the phosphodiester backbone only by their glycosylic bonds; when this bond breaks, an abasic site (AP = apurinic/apyrimidinic site) is left behind. As we have just discussed, AP sites arise by the glycosylase-catalyzed removal of uracils or modified DNA bases (*89, 90*): the first step of base excision repair. But AP sites can arise in several other ways, too. The glycosylic bonds of pyrimidines and, especially, purines undergo spontaneous hydrolysis at a measurable rate, even in the absence of enzymatic catalysis. (Treatment of DNA with strong acid removes the purine bases quantitatively. In fact, Erwin Chargaff's pioneering studies of "apurinic acid" in the 1950s (*91*) led to the formulation of the base-pairing rules A = T and C = G.) Removal of the base leaves the deoxyribose sugar with a free 1′ hydroxyl group and allows the sugar to undergo mutarotation; the abasic site exists as a mixture of the anomeric hemiacetals, with trace amounts of the open chain aldehyde present (*92*). Spontaneous depurination may generate thousands of AP sites per human cell per day, but measurement of the steady-state level of abasic sites in DNA of mammalian cells is not easy, because of various analytical artifacts (see discussion in (*93*)).

Many forms of chemical adduction of DNA bases can labilize the glycosylic bond and induce apurinic sites. These reactions include guanine N7 adduction by alkylating agents (nitrosoureas (*94*), nitrogen and sulfur mustards (see chapter 15), activated metabolites of safrole, 1,3-butadiene, nitrosamines, etc.); polycyclic aromatic hydrocarbon metabolite binding to adenine N3 or N7 (*95*); and binding of catechol estrogen *ortho*-quinone metabolites to purines (*96*). In fact, for some of these agents, abasic (apurinic) sites may be more important lesions than are stable covalent adducts, although the relative significance of abasic sites and stable covalent adducts in carcinogenesis remains controversial (*97*).

Ionizing radiation and some xenobiotic chemicals can cause direct damage to the deoxyribose moeties of DNA. This can result not only in loss of the attached base but also in breakage of the phosphodiester linkage and degradation of the sugar, leaving a terminal structure such as a 3'-phosphoglycolate (figure 3-8). These oxidized abasic sites (*98*) represent even more serious lesions than the abasic site itself.

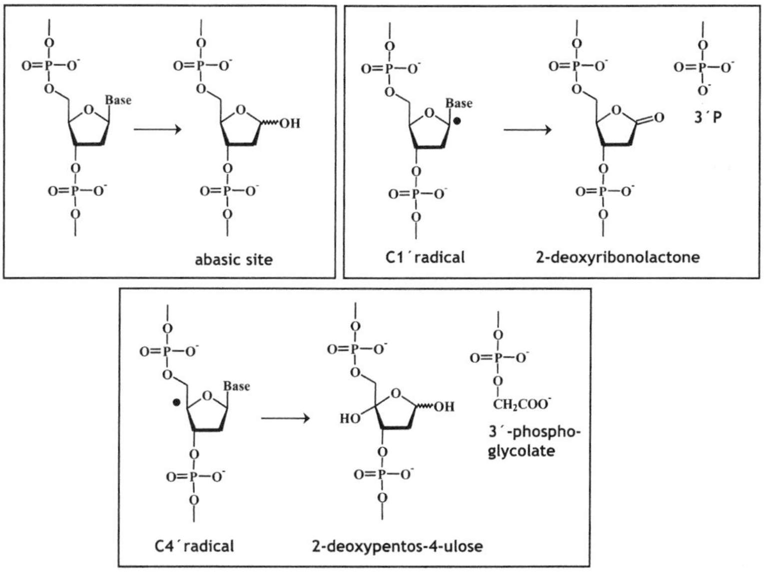

FIGURE 3-8.
Abasic sites (top left) arise from the removal of bases by hydrolysis of the *N*-glycosylic bond, catalyzed by base excision repair glycosylase enzymes, or by spontaneous depurination. Oxidative or radiolytic damage to DNA deoxyribose produces a host of products, some of which are shown here. Oxidation at C1' (top right) produces a carbon-centered radical that can give rise to a 2-deoxyribonolactone oxidized abasic site or a strand break terminating in a 3'-phosphate. Oxidation at C4' (bottom) produces a carbon-centered radical that can give rise to a 2-deoxypentose-4-ulose oxidized abasic site or a strand break terminating in a 3'-phosphoglycolate (a two-carbon remnant of the deoxyribose sugar). The detailed chemistry leading from the radicals to the oxidized abasic sites is not shown here. (*Adapted from Demple, B.; DeMott, M. S. Dynamics and diversions in base excision DNA repair of oxidized abasic lesions.* Oncogene **2002**, 21, 8926–8934.)

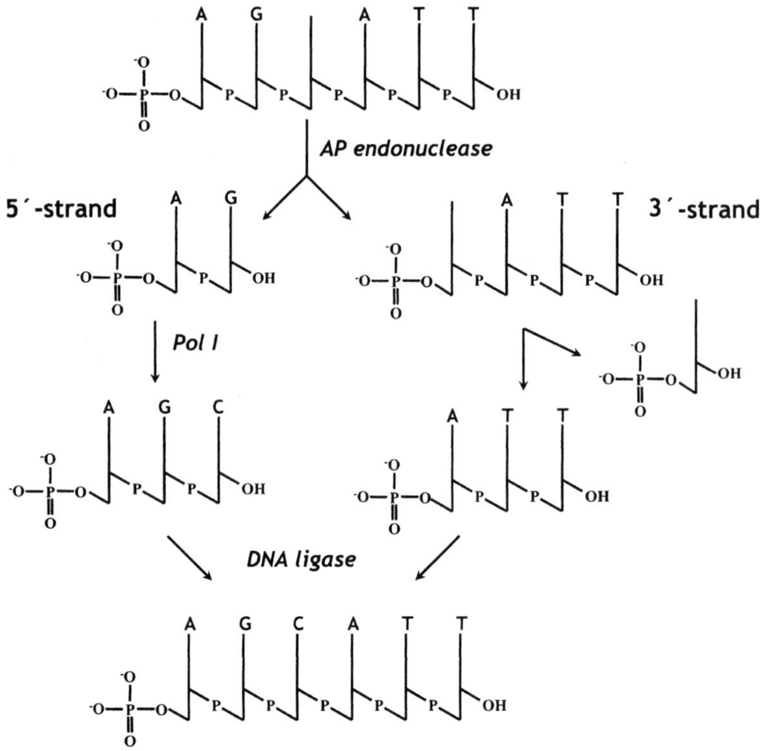

FIGURE 3-9.
Steps in the repair of an abasic site; see text for further discussion.

Repair of Abasic Sites

In the absence of repair mechanisms for AP sites, genetic information would quickly evaporate, by loss of the bases from DNA. AP sites are substrates for *AP endonucleases* (*99*), enzymes that hydrolyze an adjacent phosphodiester bond to create a single-strand break (figure 3-9). Most known AP endonucleases (e.g., *E. coli* endonuclease IV (*99*) and the major human AP endonuclease, APE1, also called Hap1 or Ref1 (*100, 101*)) are so-called "Type II" enzymes, which catalyze phosphodiester bond hydrolysis 5′ to the AP site. This cleavage leaves the 5′ strand bearing a normal 3′ hydroxyl group, and the 3′ strand bearing a 5′ phosphate plus abasic sugar (figure 3-10). The abasic site on the end of the 3′ strand is recognized and removed (*102*). The single nucleotide gap is filled by extension of the 5′ strand, catalyzed by Pol I (*E. coli*) or Pol β (eukaryotes (*16*)) and the 5′ strand is then rejoined to the 3′ strand by DNA ligase.

An alternative route for processing of AP sites is known. Some DNA glycosylases also possess a β-lyase (AP lyase) activity, which cleaves the phosphodiester bond to the 3′-hydroxyl of the abasic deoxyribose sugar by β-elimination from the open-chain aldehyde (figure 3-10). This leaves a normal 5′ phosphate on the 3′ strand and a damaged sugar (4-hydroxy-2-pentenal) residue blocking the 3′ terminus of the 5′ strand. The blocked 3′ terminus is processed by enzymatic 3′ "trimming" (an activity associated with many AP endonucleases) and ligase completes the repair by rejoining the two ends of the strand.

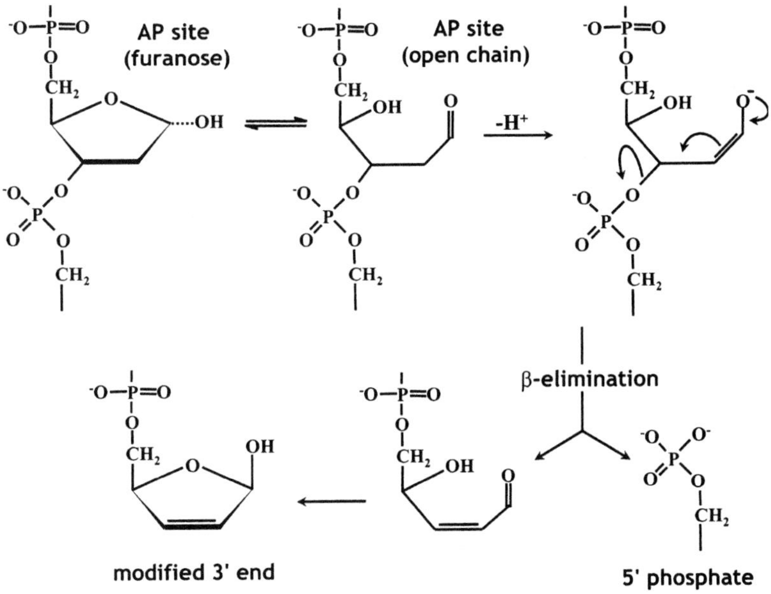

FIGURE 3-10.

Action of β-lyase at an abasic site; see text for further discussion.

MISMATCH REPAIR MECHANISMS

If DNA polymerase inserts an incorrect base during replication, then a mismatch arises: *normal DNA bases are present, but they are joined in a non-Watson–Crick pair.* As noted earlier, deamination of a 5-methylcytosine residue to form a thymine residue also induces a mismatch, and a second round of replication will fix this (i.e., make it permanent) as a G:C to A:T transition mutation. (Mismatches also arise as a consequence of recombination between nonidentical DNA sequences (*103*).) Mismatch repair systems detect and correct such base-pairing mismatches (*36–38*).

The existence of mismatch repair systems raises two profound questions. First, how can DNA mismatches be recognized? In contrast to the excision of chemically modified bases, all of the structural components of a mismatch are standard, unmodified components of DNA. Second, how does the repair machinery effect strand discrimination: deciding which of the two strands should be repaired and which should be used as template?

With respect to mismatch recognition, mismatches might induce a local distortion of the double helix; however, X-ray diffraction structural analysis of DNA oligonucleotides containing mismatches reveals little distortion of the helix backbone; instead, a "wobble" non-Watson–Crick hydrogen bonding of the mismatched bases occurs (*104, 105*). Rather, binding of the mismatch recognition protein (such as MutS; see below) to the mismatch site induces a large structural change (bending of the helix axis) by its interactions with the weakly bonded mismatched base. With respect to strand discrimination, if the goal of DNA repair is to restore the parental DNA sequence, then when a mismatch has arisen during replication, *the newly synthesized strand had best be repaired to complement the parental strand.*

E. coli

E. coli chromosomal DNA is modified by the Dam (DNA adenine methylase) enzyme that converts A residues in specific palindromic sequences (GATC) to N^6-methyladenines. Immediately following replication, *the newly synthesized daughter strand can be recognized by its low level of adenine methylation*, since insufficient time has elapsed for full *dam*-dependent modification to occur. Consequently, many GATC sites will be *hemimethylated*, that is, only the adenine on the parental strand will be N^6-methylated. The *E. coli* DNA repair system that reads this methylation signal is called *methyl-directed mismatch repair* (MMR). At least three proteins are involved: MutS, MutL, and MutH (*106, 107*). As with the base excision repair *mut* genes discussed earlier, strains bearing mutations in the genes encoding these proteins show a mutator phenotype (*108*). MutS protein binds to DNA mismatch sites, which it recognizes by inducing a sharp kink in the helix axis, widening the minor groove, reorienting the weakly bound mismatched base, and forming multiple contacts to it (*109*), notably a stacking hydrophobic interaction between the base and a phenylalanine residue. MutL binds to MutS at the site of the mismatch (*110*). MutH protein interacts with the MutLS complex, recognizes the hemimethylated GATC methylation site (*111*), and, acting as an endonuclease, specifically nicks the newly synthesized strand. A portion of the strand is then degraded and resynthesized by DNA polymerase III (figure 3-11).

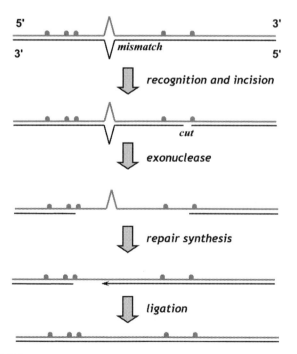

FIGURE 3-11.

Steps in methyl-directed mismatch repair in *E. coli*; see text for further discussion. *Note*: A full-color version of this figure appears on the website.

A second mismatch repair system, very-short-patch (VSP) repair (*112, 113*), specifically repairs G:T mismatches arising from deamination of 5-methylcytosine residues (see above). The Vsr endonuclease (*114*) coding sequence immediately follows the *dcm* gene on the *E. coli* chromosome; in fact, the genes actually overlap slightly (*115, 116*), presumably ensuring that the enzyme that creates the 5-methylcytosine residues is expressed in coordination with the enzyme that repairs the resulting mutagenic lesions.

Eukaryotes

Genes homologous to those encoding the *E. coli* mismatch repair proteins MutS and MutL—but not MutH—have been found in eukaryotes, including yeast and humans (*117, 118*). Apparently, the *recognition of mismatches in eukaryotes occurs by mechanisms homologous to those effective in prokaryotes, but the recognition of the newly synthesized strand occurs by different* (as yet unknown) *mechanisms*. As with nucleotide excision repair, the eukaryotic mismatch repair systems are more complicated than the corresponding prokaryotic ones (*119, 120*). There are five human MutS homologues (MSH2–MSH6); these proteins form heterodimers (e.g., MSH2–MSH6 and MSH2–MSH3) that recognize mispairs (*121*). Four human *mutL* gene homologues are known (MLH1, MLH3, PMS1, and PMS2);[3] these proteins also form active heterodimers.

Bert Vogelstein (Johns Hopkins University School of Medicine) and colleagues mapped and identified human genes responsible for *hereditary non-polyposis colorectal carcinoma* (HNPCC); they turned out to be genes for DNA mismatch repair proteins, principally MSH2 and MLH1 (*122–129*). Mouse knockouts of the corresponding murine genes are cancer-prone, developing lymphomas and other cancers. These discoveries further illustrate the relationship between mutagenesis and carcinogenesis, but the connection between the biochemical defect in a specific DNA repair pathway and the outcome in a specific tumor remains obscure. For example, the products of the murine genes *Mlh1* and *Pms2* form a heterodimer, but the spectra of tumors in *Mlh1* and *Pms2* knockout mice are different (*130*).

Mismatch repair defects are associated with *microsatellite instability*, a special class of mutations (see sidebar). Repeated sequences, such as those occurring in DNA microsatellites, are hot-spots for insertion or deletion mutations, which arise because of facile slippage (misregistration) between the parent and daughter DNA strands (the Streisinger slippage mechanism, as discussed again in chapter 4). HNPCC and some sporadic cancers display microsatellite instability resulting from defective mismatch repair ("microsatellite mutator phenotype") (*131*), and this instability accounts for oncogene-activating mutations observed in these tumors. For example, the third exon of the human *BAX* gene (which encodes a protein involved in the induction of apoptosis) contains the sequence . . . ATG GGG GGG GAG . . . and insertions or deletions of one base from the G_8 run are frequently present in mismatch repair-defective human cancer cell lines (*132*). Presumably the mismatch repair system is particularly effective in suppressing the occurrence of these insertion/deletion events.

▶ **Satellite DNA, Minisatellites, Microsatellites**

What are "microsatellites" (other than very small orbiting spacecraft!)? First, recall that nucleic acids can be highly purified by cesium chloride density-gradient centrifugation. In this technique (5, p. 123), the sample is dissolved in a high-density CsCl solution and spun in an ultracentrifuge. With time, a gradient of CsCl develops in the spinning tube, and this gradient eventually reaches a steady state, such that the rate of sedimentation of the salt toward the axis of rotation is exactly balanced by the rate of its diffusion in the opposite direction. Under these conditions, the nucleic acid will form a band at the position in the tube (i.e., in the density gradient) where the local density of the CsCl solution is the same as the density of the nucleic acid cesium salt. Even very slight differences in nucleic acid density can be detected by this technique. (Matthew Meselson and colleagues, in 1958, developed the technique to separate ^{15}N-labelled from natural (^{14}N) DNA, in the experiment that conclusively proved that DNA replication is semiconservative.)

The density of DNA varies slightly, depending on its G:C vs. A:T content. When bulk eukaryotic chromosomal DNA is prepared (undergoing random shearing and fragmentation in the process) and analyzed by the CsCl technique, it sediments as a single broad band, at a position corresponding to the average density/G:C content of chromosomal DNA. However, one or more minor bands are usually observed at slightly higher or lower densities (e.g., (133)). These small outlying bands are called "satellites"; satellites represent genomic regions of higher or lower than average G:C content, which arise due to *tandem-repeated sets of identical or nearly identical short* (approximately 10 bp) *DNA sequences*.

In 1985 Alec Jeffreys and colleagues (134) discovered the presence of large numbers of tandem-repeat short (typically 9–24 bp; as long as 70 bp) sequences in the human genome. These noncoding sequences are highly polymorphic: the number of tandem repeats at any particular locus varies among individuals. Consequently, when a Southern blot of human chromosomal DNA is analyzed with an oligonucleotide probe for these repeated sequences, one obtains a complex "fingerprint" pattern that varies from person to person. This approach is the basis for DNA fingerprinting to identify specific persons, as is now widely applied in forensic science. (The combination of such analysis with PCR amplification, in the 1990s, made it possible to identify an individual on the basis of microscopic amounts of blood, saliva, semen, etc.) Jeffreys called these short repetitive DNA sequences *minisatellites*, since they represented a shorter version of satellite DNA.

Michael Litt and Jeffrey A. Luty (135) extended this sequence analysis to *microsatellites*, that is, even shorter repeats, such as the dinucleotide repeat sequence $(TG)_n$, where n can be about 10–60 repeats. (For reasons discussed earlier in this chapter, $(CG)_n$ repeats are very rare.) Tens of thousands of such microsatellites occur, accounting for a fraction of 1% of the total genome; like minisatellites, they are highly polymorphic. Most microsatellites are located outside genes but some are found in protein coding sequences and have profound biological implications. Because of the propensity of DNA strands to slip (misregister) at repeated sequences, microsatellite sequences often show up as "stutters" on PCR or sequencing gels (136). Expansions of trinucleotide repeats in coding sequences are seen in several human genetic diseases (137), such as Huntington's disease and fragile X syndrome (138). ◀

NUCLEOTIDE EXCISION REPAIR MECHANISMS

E. coli

The origins of the science of DNA repair can be traced to the 1964 discovery by Carrier and Setlow (139) that thymine dimer photoproducts, formed during UV irradiation of *E. coli* cells (figures 3-12 and 3-13), are subsequently released in an acid-soluble (i.e., not macromolecular) form. Independently, Boyce and Howard-Flanders showed that such a process does not occur in a UV-sensitive (*uvrA*) strain (140). (These classic papers are reproduced, along with an historical account of the research, in a recent article by Cleaver (141).) These findings were the first evidence for the phenomenon of nucleotide excision repair. *E. coli* possesses only one excision repair system, effected by the UvrABC proteins in conjunction with DNA helicase II (encoded by *uvrD*), DNA polymerase I, and DNA ligase. Nevertheless, this single system has an extraordinary ability to recognize and excise a vast range of DNA damages, including UV irradiation products and most bulky covalent adducts (142–144). As we will see

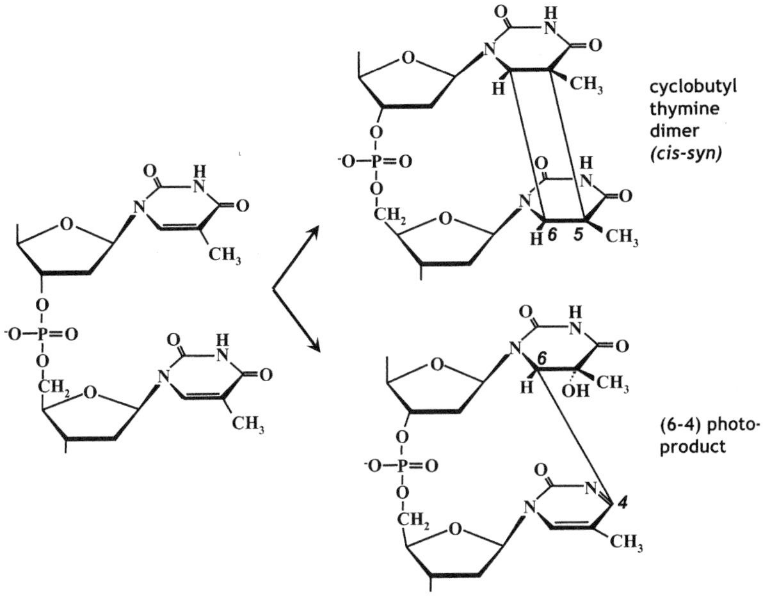

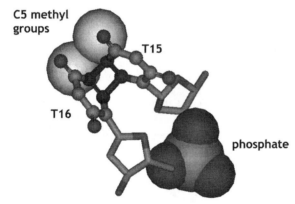

FIGURE 3-12.
Two thymine dimer products of UV irradiation of DNA at a TpT site. Top right: *cis-syn* cyclobutyl thymine dimer; bottom right: 6-4 photoproduct.

FIGURE 3-13.
Structure of the *cis-syn* cyclobutyl thymine dimer, extracted from crystal structure 1MV.pdb. The deoxyribose sugars are shown as sticks and the base atoms as balls. The four carbon atoms of the cyclobutane ring are darkened. The methyl groups of the thymines, to the left, are shown space filling, as is the bridging phosphate at the right. *Note*: A full-color version of this figure appears on the website.

in chapter 4, this repair system is so effective that its inactivation is essential for the construction of *E. coli* (or *S. typhimurium* Ames test) mutagenicity assay strains that can detect typical chemical carcinogens such as polycyclic aromatic hydrocarbons. In the presence of functional UvrABC, the resulting covalent adducts are repaired so completely that mutagenesis is almost undetectable.

Two of the most significant products of UV damage to DNA (*145*) are *thymine dimers*, in which two adjacent thymines dimerize to form a bridging cyclobutane ring (figure 3-12) (146), and thymine–cytosine "6-4" photo-products (147). The latter are believed to be the most important premuta-genic lesion induced by UV. UvrABC, which removes both of these lesions, is critical for bacterial resistance to UV radiation. The uvrA, uvrB, uvrC, and uvrD genes were first identified as genes mutated in UV-sensitive E. coli mutants.

The UvrA dimer binds to UvrB protein to form a complex, (UvrA)$_2$ UvrB, which scans along the double helix, recognizing and binding to damaged sites. How can this complex recognize a wide range of chemically different DNA lesions? As has been pointed out by Aziz Sancar, this bio-chemical problem is reminiscent of the need for detoxication enzymes to bind diverse xenobiotic substrates. The answer is probably that the enzyme halts at sites where the conformation of the double helix is distorted by the presence of an adduct, especially by the abnormal exposure to the outside of the helix of hydrophobic functionalities (the bases or the covalently adduc-ted xenobiotics) (148). Thus, the solution to the problem is comparable to that adopted by the enzymes of detoxication: a promiscuous binding site recognizes a variety of molecules based mainly on their hydrophobic character. At these sites, UvrB binds tightly, UvrA dissociates, UvrC binds to UvrB, and the DNA strand bearing the adduct is incised on either side of the damage site. The eighth phosphodiester bond 5′ to the DNA adduct and the fifth phosphodiester bond 3′ to the adduct[4] are hydrolyzed (149). DNA helicase II and DNA polymerase I displace the UvrABC complex, along with the excised damage-containing oligonucleotide (12 or 13 nucleotides long), and the polymerase fills in the gap. DNA ligase then seals the 3′ end of the newly synthesized oligonucleotide.

Eukaryotes

As noted earlier, UV- and radiation-sensitive yeast or mammalian cells can be isolated in vitro, and human diseases characterized by radiation sensitivity provide a source of human cells with presumptive DNA repair defects. Eukaryotic genes required for DNA excision repair have been identified by isolation of genes that complement such defects (i.e., restoring radiation resistance to sensitive cell lines) and also by positional cloning of genes responsible for inherited human diseases (151). These include the yeast RAD genes (more than 30 identified) (152), the ERCC (excision repair cross complementing) genes (which complement the defects of UV-sensitive rodent cell lines), and the human genes associated with radiation-sensitive diseases (153, 154). On this basis, at least 30 human gene products are known to play roles in nucleotide excision repair. We will not discuss the details of eukaryotic nucleotide excision repair (the inter-ested reader is referred to reviews by Sancar (40, 155) and by Lindahl and Wood (3)) but simply make some general observations. (i) The bacterial strategy of damage recognition, incisions at either side of a damage site, repair synthesis, and re-ligation, also applies in eukaryotes. (ii) The number of gene products involved is much greater in eukaryotes. (iii) The eukaryotic genes are unrelated, in terms of sequence, to the bacterial genes, suggesting independent evolution of the prokaryotic and eukaryotic systems. (iv) Each of the seven XP complementation groups (XP-A to XP-G) corresponds to a protein involved in nucleotide excision repair.

DNA STRAND BREAKS

DNA strand breaks can arise in various ways. The process of genetic recombination (which occurs, for example, during eukaryotic meiosis) depends on strand breakage as a mechanism for the interchange of genetic information between homologous chromosomes. Toxic agents that attack either the sugar or the phosphate of the DNA backbone can lead to strand breakage. Many classes of chemical carcinogens, including aromatic amines, polycyclic aromatic hydrocarbons, and alkylating agents, can cause strand breaks (e.g., in hepatocytes), and there is a correlation between carcinogenic potency and strand break induction. Some agents can cause strand breaks indirectly, via base damage followed by repair endonuclease action. Other agents (such as radiation, oxidants, and the chemotherapeutic drug bleomycin; see chapter 11) induce strand breaks directly, by attacking the DNA backbone itself. Strand breaks are also a characteristic consequence of the action of ionizing radiation on DNA.

Operationally, we can distinguish between single-strand breaks (SSB) and double-strand breaks (DSB): the former are measured in single-stranded (denatured) DNA and the latter are measured in native DNA. What this means in detail is less clear: how close must two breaks, on opposing strands, be, so that we have a DSB rather than two SSBs? This may depend on the way in which we measure the break.

> Clown: . . . I am resolv'd on two points.
> Maria: That if one break, the other will hold; or if both break, your gaskins fall.
>
> (*Twelfth Night*, Act 1, Scene V)

In the case of small "naked" DNA targets, such as defined oligonucleotides or restriction fragments in vitro, or plasmid DNA in bacterial cells, DSBs can be measured directly by electrophoresis. SSB can also be studied by electrophoresis of plasmid DNA, since the covalently closed circular (ccc) and open circular (nicked) molecules have different mobilities. The extremely long molecules of chromosomal DNA are so fragile that any standard protocol for DNA purification (as would be used to prepare genomic libraries, for example) will introduce large numbers of strand breaks. So, to examine strand breaks in chromosomal DNA, special techniques are needed. Analysis can be carried out under alkaline (pH > 12) or "neutral" conditions (pH < 10). Unlike protein or RNA, DNA resists hydrolysis by strong base, although the accumulation of negative charge on the DNA bases causes complete denaturation into single strands. Under alkaline conditions, then, one measures SSBs; more accurately, the sum of SSBs plus *alkali-labile sites*, that is, damages that are converted into SSBs by alkali treatment (abasic sites and some forms of base damage constitute alkali-labile sites). For the analysis of eukaryotic chromosomal DNA, the pulsed-field technique extends the applicability of gel electrophoresis methods into the megabase range, and can be used for the measurement of strand breaks induced by ionizing radiation (*156*).

Another method for electrophoretic analysis of DNA damage is the so-called "comet" assay (*157–159*). In this assay, individual cells are embedded in agarose and lyzed by immersion in detergent solution to release DNA. Electrophoresis is carried out, and the gel is then soaked

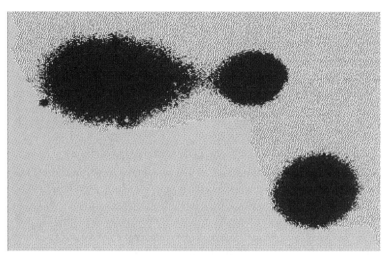

FIGURE 3-14.
The alkaline "comet" assay of DNA strand breakage. Two cells/comets from TK6 human lymphoblast cells are shown. The upper cell was exposed to 6 Gy and the lower cell is an unexposed control (6 Gy produces about 6000 DNA single strand breaks per cell). *Note*: A full-color version of this figure appears on the website. (*Courtesy of Dr. Peggy Olive, B.C. Cancer Research Centre, Vancouver, BC, Canada.*)

in a solution containing propidium iodide, a fluorescent stain for DNA (and RNA). The cells are then examined under a fluorescence microscope. The electrophoresed DNA gives the appearance of a "comet" streaming away from the cell (figure 3-14). Increasing DNA damage results in greater electrophoretic mobility and, hence, a longer comet "tail."

In the filter elution method (*160*), the DNA is deposited on a membrane filter with pore size of about 1 μm. The DNA is then slowly "squeezed" through the filter by pumping an eluting solution. The physical basis of the elution process is complicated and remains poorly understood. Intact cells can be applied to the gradients or filters. Lysis is accomplished by application of detergents (such as SDS) and treatment with nonspecific proteases (such as proteinase K). If an alkaline solution is used, noncovalent protein–DNA or DNA–RNA interactions, which might complicate the analysis, are broken. However, DNA-damaging treatments may induce forms of covalent damage, other than strand breaks, which could also greatly alter the molecular weight and conformation of the DNA molecules. These include covalent cross-links between separate DNA strands and protein–DNA cross-links, and might not be broken by detergent, enzyme, or alkali treatments.

Repair by Homologous Recombination

In contrast to a SSB, a DSB can fragment a DNA molecule into two separate pieces that lack complementary "sticky" ends. In the absence of mechanisms for repair of DSBs, chromosomes would gradually disintegrate into fragments, and complex genomes could not be maintained. If a homologous sister duplex DNA molecule is available to act as a template for repair synthesis (as will be the case, following the S phase of the cell cycle), *homologous recombination* (*161*) offers a potential mechanism for faithful

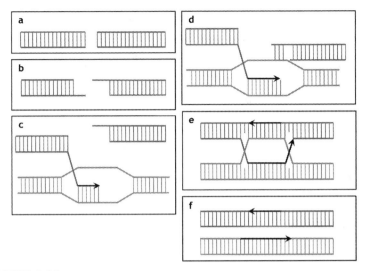

FIGURE 3-15.

Model for the repair of double-strand breaks (DSBs) by homologous recombination. (a) DSB in DNA. (b) Nucleases act at the DSB to expose single-stranded DNA. (c) One strand of the broken duplex invades an intact homologous duplex; repair synthesis begins. (d) The remaining strand of the broken duplex is captured into the repair complex. (e) Completion of repair synthesis leaves the restored duplexes involved in two "Holliday junction" (four-way DNA junction) intermediates. (f) Resolution of the two crossovers allows the repaired strands to separate. *Note*: A full-color version of this figure appears on the website. (*Adapted from West, S. C. Molecular views of recombination proteins and their control.* Nat. Rev. Mol. Cell Biol. **2003**, *4, 435–445.*)

repair of a DSB. As indicated in the model shown in figure 3-15, DSB repair by homologous recombination must involve the action of a nuclease that trims the broken end to expose a stretch of single-stranded DNA. This "tail" can then search for complementary sequences suitable for homologous recombination.

Elucidating the steps in enzymatic processing of DSBs has proved to be a very difficult challenge in molecular cell biology, but much progress has been made recently, using a combination of structural biology, genetics, and biochemical analysis (*162–165*). The MRN complex, formed from the proteins Mre11, Rad50, and Nbs1 (*166*), is the key player in DSB repair by homologous recombination (*167*). (The names of these proteins reflect the routes by which they were discovered. Mre11 was identified as a yeast gene resulting in defective meiotic recombination. Mutations in Rad genes confer radiation sensitivity, as noted earlier. Nbs refers to the human autosomal recessive disease "Nijmegen breakage syndrome," which results in extreme radiation sensitivity and elevated cancer incidence (*168*); Nijmegen is a city in Holland, where the condition was identified in 1981.) The Mre11 and Nbs1 (*169*) proteins contribute exonuclease activity and other functions required for recombination. Rad50 protein forms a very long alpha-helical coiled-coil fiber. Two of these fibers associate into a tightly bound dimer (figure 3-16), held together by a Zn^{2+} ion that is coordinated to the sulfur atoms of four conserved cysteine residues (two cysteines from each of the Rad50 monomers) (*170a*). The Rad50 dimer

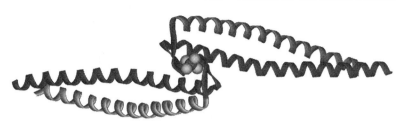

FIGURE 3-16.

The coiled coils of two Rad50 proteins are held together by coordination of four cysteines (two per Rad50 molecule) to a Zn^{2+} ion. Coordinates from structure file 1L8D.pdb. *Note*: A full-color version of this figure appears on the website.

probably plays the role of a molecular "bungee cord" or "fishing rod." Each monomer holds onto a DNA duplex, binding the two duplexes in proximity while recombination occurs (*170b*).

Nucleolytic resection at the site of a DSB exposes single-stranded DNA, which binds Rad51 protein, the human homologue of bacterial RecA. Rad51 recruits another important player in DSB repair, Rad52 (*171*). Other proteins involved in DSB repair by homologous recombination include the protein kinase ATM (*172–174*) (identified as the protein encoded by the human gene for ataxia telangiectasia, mentioned earlier in the chapter; ATM interacts with the MRN complex (*175*)) and the proteins encoded by the genes responsible for Fanconi's anemia (*176*) and breast cancer susceptibility (*BRCA1* and *BRCA2*).

Repair by Nonhomologous End Joining

Prior to the S phase, a homologous DNA template is unlikely to be available, excluding the option of DSB repair by homologous recombination. However, DSB repair can still be achieved under these conditions, by the *nonhomologous end-joining* (NHEJ) mechanism (*177, 178*). This process can reseal the frayed ends of the chromosome, but at the risk of creating deleterious gene fusions. NHEJ is also the route whereby breaks are repaired during the recombinational process that occurs in cells of the immune system, in the generation of antibody diversity (V(D)J recombination) (*179*). Early in the NHEJ process, the Ku70/Ku80[5] dimer (*181*) recognizes and binds to the broken DNA ends. DNA ligase IV and Xrcc4 proteins then act to reseal the breaks. (Recent work in the bacterium *M. tuberculosis* has shown that two mycobacterial proteins, a Ku protein and a DNA ligase, are sufficient to effect NHEJ repair (*182*). Although the eukaryotic NHEJ systems are more complex, this simpler bacterial system should provide mechanistic insight into the repair process.)

REPLICATION OF DAMAGED DNA

We have discussed some of the manifold pathways for the faithful repair of DNA damage. However, all defense systems can be overwhelmed. DNA damage that escapes repair, and persists until the next round of replication, presents a challenge to DNA polymerase. DNA lesions may also arise at the time of replication, giving the cell no opportunity for timely repair. What happens when DNA polymerase encounters a damage site? Some polymerases can replicate past some types of damage, although possibly with reduced fidelity; these are *error-promoting* lesions. Other damages strongly inhibit DNA replication; these are *replication-blocking* lesions. In vitro studies reveal that synthesis of the nascent strand by *E. coli* Pol III stops at (or near) template lesions such as abasic sites or pyrimidine dimers. *Such replication blocks are potentially catastrophic, since DNA replication is essential for cell division.*

How can cells resume DNA synthesis on templates with replication blocks? One way is to reinitiate DNA synthesis farther along the template. This leaves a gap in the daughter strand, which may be filled after replication (postreplication repair). Alternatively, *the cell may switch to the use of an alternative DNA polymerase that is more tolerant of DNA template damage, at the cost of an increased rate of replication errors.* Replication-blocking (lethal) lesions become, instead, error-promoting (mutagenic) lesions. Put simply, it is better to mutate than to die.

E. coli possesses a sophisticated defense mechanism that is invoked when the bacterium faces overwhelming DNA damage, such as results from intense UV exposure. This mechanism is known as the "SOS" (save our souls!) response, in which a large number of genes throughout the *E. coli* chromosome are simultaneously induced (i.e., a regulon) (*183–185*).

The RecA and LexA proteins are components of the switch that activates the SOS response (*73*, p. 1094). Single-stranded DNA regions are continuously exposed during replication; replication-blocking DNA lesions cause accumulation of such ssDNA regions. The RecA protein binds to these ssDNA regions, and the ssDNA-RecA complex initiates the SOS response. LexA is the repressor of the genes in the SOS regulon, which includes (among about 40 genes) *recA*, *lexA* itself, *uvrA* and *uvrB*, etc. LexA protein binds to a consensus sequence present in the operators of these genes. Interaction with the ssDNA-RecA complex converts LexA into a protease that degrades other LexA molecules (*186, 187*), triggering a catalytic cascade that inactivates the LexA repressor and thereby switches on the SOS response genes.

The chromosomal genes *umuD* and *umuC* (which are co-transcribed) are part of the SOS regulon. These genes (UV mutable) were identified as greatly enhancing *E. coli* mutability by UV radiation (*188*). This function was described as "error-prone repair" of DNA, although, as we will see, a more appropriate term is "error-prone replication." *umuD* and *umuC* are homologous to the *mucA* and *mucB* genes (mutagenesis, UV and chemical) identified on plasmid pKM101. (This plasmid, described in more detail in chapter 4, was found to increase greatly the yield of mutations in *E. coli* cells treated with UV or chemical mutagens and was subsequently used to enhance the sensitivity of the Ames mutation assay.) The biochemical function of the UmuDC and MucAB proteins remained mysterious; they were thought to interact with Pol III in some manner that enabled the polymerase to bypass replication-blocking lesions (*189*). However, in the late 1990s translesion replication activity was reconstituted in vitro, with the use of purified recombinant Umu proteins, and it became evident that the UmuDC protein complex is actually an alternative *E. coli* DNA polymerase, pol V, whose activity had previously been overlooked (*190–192*). UmuC is the catalytic component; UmuD undergoes proteolytic self-cleavage, removing an N-terminal peptide fragment, to produce UmuD', an activator of UmuC function (figure 3-17). UmuC is, in fact,

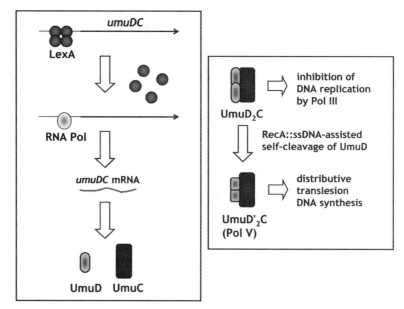

FIGURE 3-17.

The UmuDC operon; see text for details. *Note*: A full-color version of this figure appears on the website. (*Adapted from Ferentz, A. E.; Walker, G. C.; Wagner, G. Converting a DNA damage checkpoint effector (UmuD₂C) into a lesion bypass polymerase (UmuD′₂C). EMBO J. **2001**, 20, 4287–4298.*)

only one member of a large family of DNA polymerases, now called the "Y-family" (*193–196*). This family includes another newly defined *E. coli* polymerase, DinB or pol IV (*197*), and three new human DNA polymerases, Pol η (eta), Pol κ (kappa), and Pol ι (iota) (*198*). Mutations in the gene encoding Pol η are responsible for the so-called "variant" (XP-V) form of xeroderma pigmentosum (*199*). Y-family polymerases are not, strictly speaking, repair proteins; rather, they enable a cell to survive DNA damage, but at the cost of the induction of mutations.

The biology of these polymerases is still being explored, but they share the properties of surprisingly poor replication fidelity combined with the ability to replicate past template lesions. Y-family polymerases are *distributive* (*197*): that is, as discussed earlier in this chapter, the enzymes bind to a DNA template, catalyze incorporation of only a few dNTPs, and then dissociate. This is the appropriate catalytic strategy for enzymes that act at multiple sites of damage within the genome, rather than participating in the replication of the bulk of the chromosome.

Notes

1. This may not be possible in cases where both strands are damaged simultaneously, for example by ionizing radiation.

2. However, single-strand breaks formed by oxidants or radiation are often accompanied by damage to the terminal deoxyribose sugar/phosphate, and this must be repaired before ligation can take place.

3. *Pms* genes were first characterized as genes involved in postmeiotic segregation in the yeast *Saccharomyces cerevisiae*.

4. How were the positions of the cut sites determined? Sancar and Rupp (*149*) did not yet have access to technology for incorporating damaged bases at specific sites in oligonucleotides. Instead, they used ^{32}P-end-labeled, UV-irradiated, plasmid DNA restriction fragments as substrates. They then compared, on sequencing gels, the sizes of the fragments formed by incubation with purified UvrABC vs. T4 endonuclease V. The latter enzyme cuts right at the site of the UV damage (*150*).

5. Autoantibodies to Ku are produced in patients with scleroderma-polymyositis overlap syndrome (*180*). "Ku" is derived from the name of one of these patients.

References

1. Wood, R. W.; Mitchell, M.; Lindahl, T. Human DNA repair genes, 2005. *Mutat. Res.* **2005,** *577,* 275–283.

2. Friedberg, E. C.; Walker, G. C.; Siede, W.; Wood, R. D.; Schultz, R. A.; Ellenberger, T. *DNA Repair and Mutagenesis,* 2nd ed.; ASM Press: Washington, DC, 2005.

3. Lindahl, T.; Wood, R. D. Quality control by DNA repair. *Science* **1999,** *286,* 1897–1905.

4. Hubscher, U.; Maga, G.; Spadari, S. Eukaryotic DNA polymerases. *Annu. Rev. Biochem.* **2002,** *71,* 133–163.

5. Berg, J. M.; Tymoczko, J. L.; Stryer, L. *Biochemistry;* WH Freeman: New York, 2001.

6. Sutton, M. D.; Walker, G. C. Managing DNA polymerases: coordinating DNA replication, DNA repair, and DNA recombination. *Proc. Natl. Acad. Sci. USA* **2001,** *98,* 8342–8349.

7. Patel, P. H.; Suzuki, M.; Adman, E.; Shinkai, A.; Loeb, L. A. Prokaryotic DNA polymerase: I. Evolution, structure, and "base flipping" mechanism for nucleotide selection. *J. Mol. Biol.* **2001,** *308,* 823–837.

8. Rangarajan, S.; Woodgate, R.; Goodman, M. F. A phenotype for enigmatic DNA polymerase: II. A pivotal role for pol II in replication restart in UV-irradiated *Escherichia coli. Proc. Natl. Acad. Sci. USA* **1999,** *96,* 9224–9229.

9. Kool, E. T. Active site tightness and substrate fit in DNA replication. *Annu. Rev. Biochem.* **2002,** *71,* 191–219.

10. Kool, E. T. Hydrogen bonding, base stacking, and steric effects in DNA replication. *Annu. Rev. Biophys. Biomol. Struct.* **2001,** *30,* 1–22.

11. Kool, E. T. Synthetically modified DNAs as substrates for polymerases. *Curr. Opin. Chem. Biol.* **2000,** *4,* 602–608.

12. Delaney, J. C.; Henderson, P. T.; Helquist, S. A.; Morales, J. C.; Essigmann, J. M.; Kool, E. T. High-fidelity in vivo replication of DNA base shape mimics without Watson–Crick hydrogen bonds. *Proc. Natl. Acad. Sci. USA* **2003,** *100,* 4469–4473.

13. Hamdan, S.; Carr, P. D.; Brown, S. E.; Ollis, D. L.; Dixon, N. E. Structural basis for proofreading during replication of the *Escherichia coli* chromosome. *Structure (Camb.)* **2002,** *10,* 535–546.

14. Hindges, R.; Hubscher, U. DNA polymerase delta, an essential enzyme for DNA transactions. *Biol. Chem.* **1997,** *378,* 345–362.

15. Johansson, E.; Majka, J.; Burgers, P. M. Structure of DNA polymerase delta from *Saccharomyces cerevisiae. J. Biol. Chem.* **2001,** *276,* 43824–43828.

16. Sobol, R. W.; Horton, J. K.; Kuhn, R.; Gu, H.; Singhal, R. K.; Prasad, R.; Rajewsky, K.; Wilson, S. H. Requirement of mammalian DNA polymerase-beta in base-excision repair. *Nature* **1996,** *379,* 183–186.

17. Wilson, D. M., III; Thompson, L. H. Life without DNA repair. *Proc. Natl. Acad. Sci. USA* **1997**, *94*, 12754–12757.

18. Cleaver, J. E. Cancer in xeroderma pigmentosum and related disorders of DNA repair. *Nat. Rev. Cancer* **2005**, *5*, 564–573.

19. Spacey, S. D.; Gatti, R. A.; Bebb, G. The molecular basis and clinical management of ataxia telangiectasia. *Can. J. Neurol. Sci.* **2000**, *27*, 184–191.

20. Carreau, M.; Buchwald, M. Fanconi's anemia: what have we learned from the genes so far? *Mol. Med. Today* **1998**, *4*, 201–206.

21. German, J. Bloom's syndrome. *Dermatol. Clin.* **1995**, *13*, 7–18.

22. Smilenov, L. B.; Brenner, D. J.; Hall, E. J. Modest increased sensitivity to radiation oncogenesis in ATM heterozygous versus wild-type mammalian cells. *Cancer Res.* **2001**, *61*, 5710–5713.

23. Cleaver, J. E. Excision repair: the first steps into mammalian cells. 1968. *DNA Repair (Amst.)* **2004**, *3*, 91–99.

24. Francis, M. A.; Bagga, P.; Athwal, R.; Rainbow, A. J. Partial complementation of the DNA repair defects in cells from xeroderma pigmentosum groups A, C, D and F but not G by the denV gene from bacteriophage T4. *Photochem. Photobiol.* **2000**, *72*, 365–373.

25. Busch, D. B.; Cleaver, J. E.; Glaser, D. A. Large-scale isolation of UV-sensitive clones of CHO cells. *Somatic. Cell Genet.* **1980**, *6*, 407–418.

26. Busch, D.; Greiner, C.; Lewis, K.; Ford, R.; Adair, G.; Thompson, L. Summary of complementation groups of UV-sensitive CHO cell mutants isolated by large-scale screening. *Mutagenesis* **1989**, *4*, 349–354.

27. Tanaka, K.; Satokata, I.; Ogita, Z.; Uchida, T.; Okada, Y. Molecular cloning of a mouse DNA repair gene that complements the defect of group-A xeroderma pigmentosum. *Proc. Natl. Acad. Sci. USA* **1989**, *86*, 5512–5516.

28. Barnes, D. E. DNA repair. Damage-limitation exercises. *Nature* **1992**, *359*, 12–13.

29. Boulikas, T. Xeroderma pigmentosum and molecular cloning of DNA repair genes. *Anticancer Res.* **1996**, *16*, 693–708.

30. Pegg, A. E. DNA repair pathways and cancer prevention. *Adv. Exp. Med. Biol.* **1999**, *472*, 253–267.

31. Seeberg, E.; Eide, L.; Bjoras, M. The base excision repair pathway. *Trends Biochem. Sci.* **1995**, *20*, 391–397.

32. Krokan, H. E.; Standal, R.; Slupphaug, G. DNA glycosylases in the base excision repair of DNA. *Biochem. J.* **1997**, *325*, 1–16.

33. Hang, B.; Singer, B. Protein–protein interactions involving DNA glycosylases. *Chem. Res. Toxicol.* **2003**, *16*, 1181–1195.

34. McCullough, A. K.; Dodson, M. L.; Lloyd, R. S. Initiation of base excision repair: glycosylase mechanisms and structures. *Annu. Rev. Biochem.* **1999**, *68*, 255–285.

35. Wilson, D. M., III; Barsky, D. The major human abasic endonuclease: formation, consequences and repair of abasic lesions in DNA. *Mutat. Res.* **2001**, *485*, 283–307.

36. Schofield, M. J.; Hsieh, P. DNA mismatch repair: molecular mechanisms and biological function. *Annu. Rev. Microbiol.* **2003**, *57*, 579–608.

37. Hsieh, P. Molecular mechanisms of DNA mismatch repair. *Mutat. Res.* **2001**, *486*, 71–87.

38. Harfe, B. D.; Jinks-Robertson, S. DNA mismatch repair and genetic instability. *Annu. Rev. Genet.* **2000**, *34*, 359–399.

39. Modrich, P. Strand-specific mismatch repair in mammalian cells. *J. Biol. Chem.* **1997**, *272*, 24727–24730.

40. Petit, C.; Sancar, A. Nucleotide excision repair: from *E. coli* to man. *Biochimie* **1999**, *81*, 15–25.

41. de Laat, W. L.; Jaspers, N. G.; Hoeijmakers, J. H. Molecular mechanism of nucleotide excision repair. *Genes Dev.* **1999**, *13*, 768–785.

42. Jaspers, N. G.; Hoeijmakers, J. H. DNA repair. Nucleotide excision-repair in the test tube. *Curr. Biol.* **1995**, *5*, 700–702.

43. (a) Mellon, I. Transcription-coupled repair: a complex affair. *Mutat. Res.* **2005**, *577*, 155–161. (b) Spivak, G. The many faces of Cockayne syndrome. *Proc. Natl. Acad. Sci. USA* **2004**, *101*, 15273–15274.

44. Carell, T.; Burgdorf, L. T.; Kundu, L. M.; Cichon, M. The mechanism of action of DNA photolyases. *Curr. Opin. Chem. Biol.* **2001**, *5*, 491–498.

45. Mees, A.; Klar, T.; Gnau, P.; Hennecke, U.; Eker, A. P.; Carell, T.; Essen, L. O. Crystal structure of a photolyase bound to a CPD-like DNA lesion after in situ repair. *Science* **2004**, *306*, 1789–1793.

46. Scharer, O. D.; Jiricny, J. Recent progress in the biology, chemistry and structural biology of DNA glycosylases. *Bioessays* **2001**, *23*, 270–281.

47. Lindahl, T. Past, present, and future aspects of base excision repair. *Prog. Nucleic Acid Res. Mol. Biol.* **2001**, *68*, xvii–xxxx.

48. Huffman, J. L.; Sundheim, O.; Tainer, J. A. DNA base damage recognition and removal: new twists and grooves. *Mutat. Res.* **2005**, *577*, 55–76.

49. Fromme, J. C.; Verdine, G. L. Base excision repair. *Adv. Protein Chem.* **2004**, *69*, 1–41.

50. Zharkov, D. O.; Grollman, A. P. The DNA trackwalkers: principles of lesion search and recognition by DNA glycosylases. *Mutat. Res.* **2005**, *577*, 24–54.

51. Shapiro, R.; Klein, R. S. The deamination of cytidine and cytosine by acidic buffer solutions. Mutagenic implications. *Biochemistry* **1966**, *5*, 2358–2362.

52. Duthie, S. J.; McMillan, P. Uracil misincorporation in human DNA detected using single cell gel electrophoresis. *Carcinogenesis* **1997**, *18*, 1709–1714.

53. Savva, R.; McAuley-Hecht, K.; Brown, T.; Pearl, L. The structural basis of specific base-excision repair by uracil-DNA glycosylase. *Nature* **1995**, *373*, 487–493.

54. Jones, P. A.; Takai, D. The role of DNA methylation in mammalian epigenetics. *Science* **2001**, *293*, 1068–1070.

55. Takahashi, N.; Naito, Y.; Handa, N.; Kobayashi, I. A DNA methyltransferase can protect the genome from postdisturbance attack by a restriction-modification gene complex. *J. Bacteriol.* **2002**, *184*, 6100–6108.

56. Coulondre, C.; Miller, J. H.; Farabaugh, P. J.; Gilbert, W. Molecular basis of base substitution hotspots in *Escherichia coli*. *Nature* **1978**, *274*, 775–780.

57. El Osta, A.; Wolffe, A. P. DNA methylation and histone deacetylation in the control of gene expression: basic biochemistry to human development and disease. *Gene Expr.* **2000**, *9*, 63–75.

58. Robertson, K. D.; Wolffe, A. P. DNA methylation in health and disease. *Nat. Rev. Genet.* **2000**, *1*, 11–19.

59. Cedar, H. DNA methylation and gene activity. *Cell* **1988**, *53*, 3–4.

60. Takai, D.; Jones, P. A. Comprehensive analysis of CpG islands in human chromosomes 21 and 22. *Proc. Natl. Acad. Sci. USA* **2002**, *99*, 3740–3745.

61. Lathe, R. Synthetic oligonucleotide probes deduced from amino acid sequence data. Theoretical and practical considerations. *J. Mol. Biol.* **1985**, *183*, 1–12.

62. Kuismanen, S. A.; Holmberg, M. T.; Salovaara, R.; Schweizer, P.; Aaltonen, L. A.; de la, C. A.; Nyström-Lahti, M.; Peltomäki, P. Epigenetic phenotypes distinguish microsatellite-stable and -unstable colorectal cancers. *Proc. Natl. Acad. Sci. USA* **1999**, *96*, 12661–12666.

63. Harbach, P. R.; Zimmer, D. M.; Filipunas, A. L.; Mattes, W. B.; Aaron, C. S. Spontaneous mutation spectrum at the lambda *cII* locus in liver, lung, and spleen tissue of Big Blue transgenic mice. *Environ. Mol. Mutagen.* **1999**, *33*, 132–143.

64. Hardeland, U.; Bentele, M.; Jiricny, J.; Schar, P. The versatile thymine DNA-glycosylase: a comparative characterization of the human, Drosophila and fission yeast orthologs. *Nucleic Acids Res.* **2003**, *31*, 2261–2271.

65. Hardeland, U.; Bentele, M.; Lettieri, T.; Steinacher, R.; Jiricny, J.; Schar, P. Thymine DNA glycosylase. *Prog. Nucleic Acid Res. Mol. Biol.* **2001**, *68*, 235–253.

66. Sibghat, U.; Gallinari, P.; Xu, Y. Z.; Goodman, M. F.; Bloom, L. B.; Jiricny, J.; Day, R. S., III. Base analog and neighboring base effects on substrate specificity of recombinant human G:T mismatch-specific thymine DNA-glycosylase. *Biochemistry* **1996**, *35*, 12926–12932.

67. Chen, D.; Lucey, M. J.; Phoenix, F.; Lopez-Garcia, J.; Hart, S. M.; Losson, R.; Buluwela, L.; Coombes, R. C.; Chambon, P.; Schar, P.; Ali, S. T:G mismatch-specific thymine-DNA glycosylase potentiates transcription of estrogen-regulated genes through direct interaction with estrogen receptor alpha. *J. Biol. Chem.* **2003**, *278*, 38586–38592.

68. Steenken, S. Purine bases, nucleosides, and nucleotides: aqueous solution redox chemistry and transformation reactions of their radical cations and e$^-$ and OH adducts. *Chem. Rev.* **1989**, *89*, 503–520.

69. Kasai, H.; Tanooka, H.; Nishimura, S. Formation of 8-hydroxyguanine residues in DNA by X-irradiation. *Gann* **1984**, *75*, 1037–1039.

70. Weimann, A.; Belling, D.; Poulsen, H. E. Quantification of 8-oxo-guanine and guanine as the nucleobase, nucleoside and deoxynucleoside forms in human urine by high-performance liquid chromatography–electrospray tandem mass spectrometry. *Nucleic Acids Res.* **2002**, *30*, E7.

71. (a) Tudek, B. Imidazole ring-opened DNA purines and their biological significance. *J. Biochem. Mol. Biol.* **2003**, *36*, 12–19. (b) Henderson, P. T.; Delaney, J. C.; Muller, J. G.; Neeley, W. L.; Tannenbaum, S. R.; Burrows, C. J.; Essigmann, J. M. The hydantoin lesions formed from oxidation of 7,8-dihydro-8-oxoguanine are potent sources of replication errors in vivo. *Biochemistry* **2003**, *42*, 9257–9262. (c) Jia, L.; Shafirovich, V.; Shapiro, R.; Geacintov, N. E.; Broyde, S. Spiroiminodihydantoin lesions derived from guanine oxidation: structures, energetics, and functional implications. *Biochemistry* **2005**, *44*, 6043–6051.

72. McAuley-Hecht, K. E.; Leonard, G. A.; Gibson, N. J.; Thomson, J. B.; Watson, W. P.; Hunter, W. N.; Brown, T. Crystal structure of a DNA duplex containing 8-hydroxydeoxyguanine-adenine base pairs. *Biochemistry* **1994**, *33*, 10266–10270.

73. Nelson, D. L.; Cox, M. M. *Lehninger Principles of Biochemistry;* Worth Publishers: New York, 2004.

74. Grollman, A. P.; Moriya, M. Mutagenesis by 8-oxoguanine: an enemy within. *Trends Genet.* **1993**, *9*, 246–249.

75. Wallace, S. S. Biological consequences of free radical-damaged DNA bases. *Free Radic. Biol. Med.* **2002**, *33*, 1–14.

76. Michaels, M. L.; Miller, J. H. The GO system protects organisms from the mutagenic effect of the spontaneous lesion 8-hydroxyguanine (7,8-dihydro-8-oxoguanine). *J. Bacteriol.* **1992**, *174*, 6321–6325.

77. Slupphaug, G.; Kavli, B.; Krokan, H. E. The interacting pathways for prevention and repair of oxidative DNA damage. *Mutat. Res.* **2003**, *531*, 231–251.

78. Tajiri, T.; Maki, H.; Sekiguchi, M. Functional cooperation of MutT, MutM and MutY proteins in preventing mutations caused by spontaneous oxidation of guanine nucleotide in *Escherichia coli*. *Mutat. Res.* **1995**, *336*, 257–267.

79. Nghiem, Y.; Cabrera, M.; Cupples, C. G.; Miller, J. H. The *mutY* gene: a mutator locus in *Escherichia coli* that generates G.C-T.A transversions. *Proc. Natl. Acad. Sci. USA* **1988**, *85*, 2709–2713.

80. Cabrera, M.; Nghiem, Y.; Miller, J. H. *mutM*, a second mutator locus in *Escherichia coli* that generates G.C-T.A transversions. *J. Bacteriol.* **1988**, *170*, 5405–5407.

81. Boiteux, S.; O'Connor, T. R.; Laval, J. Formamidopyrimidine-DNA glycosylase of *Escherichia coli*: cloning and sequencing of the fpg structural gene and overproduction of the protein. *EMBO J.* **1987**, *6*, 3177–3183.

82. Fromme, J. C.; Verdine, G. L. DNA lesion recognition by the bacterial repair enzyme MutM. *J. Biol. Chem.* **2003**, *278*, 51543–51548.

83. Fromme, J. C.; Banerjee, A.; Huang, S. J.; Verdine, G. L. Structural basis for removal of adenine mispaired with 8-oxoguanine by MutY adenine DNA glycosylase. *Nature* **2004**, *427*, 652–656.

84. Li, X.; Wright, P. M.; Lu, A. L. The C-terminal domain of MutY glycosylase determines the 7,8-dihydro-8-oxo-guanine specificity and is crucial for mutation avoidance. *J. Biol. Chem.* **2000**, *275*, 8448–8455.

85. Tassotto, M. L.; Mathews, C. K. Assessing the metabolic function of the MutT 8-oxodeoxyguanosine triphosphatase in *Escherichia coli* by nucleotide pool analysis. *J. Biol. Chem.* **2002**, *277*, 15807–15812.

86. Nash, H. M.; Bruner, S. D.; Scharer, O. D.; Kawate, T.; Addona, T. A.; Spooner, E.; Lane, W. S.; Verdine, G. L. Cloning of a yeast 8-oxoguanine DNA glycosylase reveals the existence of a base-excision DNA-repair protein superfamily. *Curr. Biol.* **1996**, *6*, 968–980.

87. Klungland, A.; Rosewell, I.; Hollenbach, S.; Larsen, E.; Daly, G.; Epe, B.; Seeberg, E.; Lindahl, T.; Barnes, D. E. Accumulation of premutagenic DNA lesions in mice defective in removal of oxidative base damage. *Proc. Natl. Acad. Sci. USA* **1999**, *96*, 13300–13305.

88. Bruner, S. D.; Norman, D. P.; Verdine, G. L. Structural basis for recognition and repair of the endogenous mutagen 8-oxoguanine in DNA. *Nature* **2000**, *403*, 859–866.

89. Kasai, H. Chemistry-based studies on oxidative DNA damage: formation, repair, and mutagenesis. *Free Radic. Biol. Med.* **2002**, *33*, 450–456.

90. Lu, A. L.; Li, X.; Gu, Y.; Wright, P. M.; Chang, D. Y. Repair of oxidative DNA damage: mechanisms and functions. *Cell Biochem. Biophys.* **2001**, *35*, 141–170.

91. Tamm, C.; Chargaff, E. Physical and chemical properties of the apurinic acid of calf thymus. *J. Biol. Chem.* **1953**, *203*, 689–694.

92. Manoharan, M.; Ransom, S. C.; Mazumder, A.; Gerlt, J. A.; Wilde, J. A.; Withka, J. A.; Bolton, P. H. The characterization of abasic sites in DNA heteroduplexes by site specific labeling with carbon-13. *J. Am. Chem. Soc.* **1998**, *110*, 1620–1622.

93. Atamna, H.; Cheung, I.; Ames, B. N. A method for detecting abasic sites in living cells: age-dependent changes in base excision repair. *Proc. Natl. Acad. Sci. USA* **2000**, *97*, 686–691.

94. Prakash, A. S.; Gibson, N. W. Sequence-selective depurination, DNA interstrand cross-linking and DNA strand break formation associated with alkylated DNA. *Carcinogenesis* **1992**, *13*, 425–431.

95. Chakravarti, D.; Pelling, J. C.; Cavalieri, E. L.; Rogan, E. G. Relating aromatic hydrocarbon-induced DNA adducts and c-H-ras mutations in mouse skin papillomas: the role of apurinic sites. *Proc. Natl. Acad. Sci. USA* **1995**, *92*, 10422–10426.

96. Zhang, F.; Swanson, S. M.; van Breemen, R. B.; Liu, X.; Yang, Y.; Gu, C.; Bolton, J. L. Equine estrogen metabolite 4-hydroxyequilenin induces DNA damage in the rat mammary tissues: formation of single-strand breaks, apurinic sites, stable adducts, and oxidized bases. *Chem. Res. Toxicol.* **2001**, *14*, 1654–1659.

97. Melendez-Colon, V. J.; Luch, A.; Seidel, A.; Baird, W. M. Cancer initiation by polycyclic aromatic hydrocarbons results from formation of stable DNA adducts rather than apurinic sites. *Carcinogenesis* **1999**, *20*, 1885–1891.

98. Demple, B.; DeMott, M. S. Dynamics and diversions in base excision DNA repair of oxidized abasic lesions. *Oncogene* **2002**, *21*, 8926–8934.

99. Ramotar, D. The apurinic-apyrimidinic endonuclease IV family of DNA repair enzymes. *Biochem. Cell Biol.* **1997**, *75*, 327–336.

100. Evans, A. R.; Limp-Foster, M.; Kelley, M. R. Going APE over ref-1. *Mutat. Res.* **2000**, *461*, 83–108.

101. Wilson, D. M., III; Takeshita, M.; Demple, B. Abasic site binding by the human apurinic endonuclease, Ape, and determination of the DNA contact sites. *Nucleic Acids Res.* **1997**, *25*, 933–939.

102. Piersen, C. E.; McCullough, A. K.; Lloyd, R. S. AP lyases and dRPases: commonality of mechanism. *Mutat. Res.* **2000**, *459*, 43–53.

103. Evans, E.; Alani, E. Roles for mismatch repair factors in regulating genetic recombination. *Mol. Cell Biol.* **2000**, *20*, 7839–7844.

104. Brown, T.; Kennard, O.; Kneale, G.; Rabinovich, D. High-resolution structure of a DNA helix containing mismatched base pairs. *Nature* **1985**, *315*, 604–606.

105. Hunter, W. N.; Brown, T.; Kneale, G.; Anand, N. N.; Rabinovich, D.; Kennard, O. The structure of guanosine–thymidine mismatches in B-DNA at 2.5-Å resolution. *J. Biol. Chem.* **1987**, *262*, 9962–9970.

106. Smith, J.; Modrich, P. Mutation detection with MutH, MutL, and MutS mismatch repair proteins. *Proc. Natl. Acad. Sci. USA* **1996**, *93*, 4374–4379.

107. Yang, W. Structure and function of mismatch repair proteins. *Mutat. Res.* **2000**, *460*, 245–256.

108. Glickman, B. W.; Radman, M. *Escherichia coli* mutator mutants deficient in methylation-instructed DNA mismatch correction. *Proc. Natl. Acad. Sci. USA* **1980**, *77*, 1063–1067.

109. Natrajan, G.; Lamers, M. H.; Enzlin, J. H.; Winterwerp, H. H.; Perrakis, A.; Sixma, T. K. Structures of *Escherichia coli* DNA mismatch repair enzyme MutS in complex with different mismatches: a common recognition mode for diverse substrates. *Nucleic Acids Res.* **2003**, *31*, 4814–4821.

110. Schofield, M. J.; Nayak, S.; Scott, T. H.; Du, C.; Hsieh, P. Interaction of *Escherichia coli* MutS and MutL at a DNA mismatch. *J. Biol. Chem.* **2001**, *276*, 28291–28299.

111. Friedhoff, P.; Thomas, E.; Pingoud, A. Tyr212: a key residue involved in strand discrimination by the DNA mismatch repair endonuclease MutH. *J. Mol. Biol.* **2003**, *325*, 285–297.

112. Bhagwat, A. S.; Lieb, M. Cooperation and competition in mismatch repair: very short-patch repair and methyl-directed mismatch repair in Escherichia coli. *Mol. Microbiol.* **2002**, *44*, 1421–1428.

113. Lieb, M.; Bhagwat, A. S. Very short patch repair: reducing the cost of cytosine methylation. *Mol. Microbiol.* **1996**, *20*, 467–473.

114. Tsutakawa, S. E.; Morikawa, K. The structural basis of damaged DNA recognition and endonucleolytic cleavage for very short patch repair endonuclease. *Nucleic Acids Res.* **2001**, *29*, 3775–3783.

115. Sohail, A.; Lieb, M.; Dar, M.; Bhagwat, A. S. A gene required for very short patch repair in *Escherichia coli* is adjacent to the DNA cytosine methylase gene. *J. Bacteriol.* **1990**, *172*, 4214–4221.

116. Dar, M. E.; Bhagwat, A. S. Mechanism of expression of DNA repair gene *vsr*, an *Escherichia coli* gene that overlaps the DNA cytosine methylase gene, *dcm*. *Mol. Microbiol.* **1993**, *9*, 823–833.

117. Buermeyer, A. B.; Deschenes, S. M.; Baker, S. M.; Liskay, R. M. Mammalian DNA mismatch repair. *Annu. Rev. Genet.* **1999**, *33*, 533–564.

118. Jiricny, J. Mediating mismatch repair. *Nat. Genet.* **2000**, *24*, 6–8.

119. Marti, T. M.; Kunz, C.; Fleck, O. DNA mismatch repair and mutation avoidance pathways. *J. Cell Physiol.* **2002**, *191*, 28–41.

120. Kolodner, R. D.; Marsischky, G. T. Eukaryotic DNA mismatch repair. *Curr. Opin. Genet. Dev.* **1999**, *9*, 89–96.

121. Lau, P. J.; Kolodner, R. D. Transfer of the MSH2.MSH6 complex from proliferating cell nuclear antigen to mispaired bases in DNA. *J. Biol. Chem.* **2003**, *278*, 14–17.

122. Peltomäki, P.; Aaltonen, L. A.; Sistonen, P.; Pylkkanen, L.; Mecklin, J. P.; Järvinen, H.; Green, J. S.; Jass, J. R.; Weber, J. L.; Leach, F. S. Genetic mapping of a locus predisposing to human colorectal cancer. *Science* **1993**, *260*, 810–812.

123. Leach, F. S.; Nicolaides, N. C.; Papadopoulos, N.; Liu, B.; Jen, J.; Parsons, R.; Peltomäki, P.; Sistonen, P.; Aaltonen, L. A.; Nyström-Lahti, M. Mutations of a *mutS* homolog in hereditary nonpolyposis colorectal cancer. *Cell* **1993**, *75*, 1215–1225.

124. Papadopoulos, N.; Nicolaides, N. C.; Wei, Y. F.; Ruben, S. M.; Carter, K. C.; Rosen, C. A.; Haseltine, W. A.; Fleischmann, R. D.; Fraser, C. M.; Adams, M. D. Mutation of a *mutL* homolog in hereditary colon cancer. *Science* **1994**, *263*, 1625–1629.

125. Nicolaides, N. C.; Papadopoulos, N.; Liu, B.; Wei, Y. F.; Carter, K. C.; Ruben, S. M.; Rosen, C. A.; Haseltine, W. A.; Fleischmann, R. D.; Fraser, C. M. Mutations of two PMS homologues in hereditary non-polyposis colon cancer. *Nature* **1994**, *371*, 75–80.

126. Fishel, R.; Lescoe, M. K.; Rao, M. R.; Copeland, N. G.; Jenkins, N. A.; Garber, J.; Kane, M.; Kolodner, R. The human mutator gene homolog MSH2 and its association with hereditary nonpolyposis colon cancer. *Cell* **1993**, *75*, 1027–1038.

127. Fishel, R.; Wilson, T. MutS homologs in mammalian cells. *Curr. Opin. Genet. Dev.* **1997**, *7*, 105–113.

128. Muller, A.; Fishel, R. Mismatch repair and the hereditary non-polyposis colorectal cancer syndrome (HNPCC). *Cancer Invest.* **2002**, *20*, 102–109.

129. Jacob, S.; Praz, F. DNA mismatch repair defects: role in colorectal carcinogenesis. *Biochimie* **2002**, *84*, 27–47.

130. Yao, X.; Buermeyer, A. B.; Narayanan, L.; Tran, D.; Baker, S. M.; Prolla, T. A.; Glazer, P. M.; Liskay, R. M.; Arnheim, N. Different mutator phenotypes in Mlh1- versus Pms2-deficient mice. *Proc. Natl. Acad. Sci. USA* **1999**, *96*, 6850–6855.

131. Perucho, M. Cancer of the microsatellite mutator phenotype. *Biol. Chem.* **1996**, *377*, 675–684.

132. Rampino, N.; Yamamoto, H.; Ionov, Y.; Li, Y.; Sawai, H.; Reed, J. C.; Perucho, M. Somatic frameshift mutations in the BAX gene in colon cancers of the microsatellite mutator phenotype. *Science* **1997**, *275*, 967–969.

133. Lohe, A. R.; Brutlag, D. L. Multiplicity of satellite DNA sequences in *Drosophila melanogaster*. *Proc. Natl. Acad. Sci. USA* **1986**, *83*, 696–700.

134. Jeffreys, A. J.; Wilson, V.; Thein, S. L. Hypervariable "minisatellite" regions in human DNA. *Nature* **1985**, *314*, 67–73.

135. Litt, M.; Luty, J. A. A hypervariable microsatellite revealed by in vitro amplification of a dinucleotide repeat within the cardiac muscle actin gene. *Am. J. Hum. Genet.* **1989**, *44*, 397–401.

136. Miller, M. J.; Yuan, B. Z. Semiautomated resolution of overlapping stutter patterns in genomic microsatellite analysis. *Anal. Biochem.* **1997**, *251*, 50–56.

137. Ashley, C. T., Jr.; Warren, S. T. Trinucleotide repeat expansion and human disease. *Annu. Rev. Genet.* **1995**, *29*, 703–728.

138. Oostra, B. A.; Chiurazzi, P. The fragile X gene and its function. *Clin. Genet.* **2001**, *60*, 399–408.

139. Cleaver, J. E. Richard B. Setlow, a commentary on seminal contributions and scientific controversies. *Environ. Mol. Mutagen.* **2001**, *38*, 122–131.

140. Boyce, R. P.; Howard-Flanders, P. Release of ultraviolet light-induced thymine dimers from DNA in *E. coli* K-12. *Proc. Natl. Acad. Sci. USA* **1964**, *51*, 293–300.

141. Cleaver, J. E. Excision repair: its bacterial beginnings. 1963. 1964. *DNA Repair (Amst.)* **2003**, *2*, 1273–1287.

142. Lin, J. J.; Sancar, A. (A)BC excinuclease: the *Escherichia coli* nucleotide excision repair enzyme. *Mol. Microbiol.* **1992**, *6*, 2219–2224.

143. Van Houten, B.; Snowden, A. Mechanism of action of the *Escherichia coli* UvrABC nuclease: clues to the damage recognition problem. *Bioessays* **1993**, *15*, 51–59.

144. Van Houten, B.; Croteau, D. L.; DellaVecchia, M. J.; Wang, H.; Kisker, C. "Close-fitting sleeves": DNA damage recognition and repair by the UvrABC nuclease system. *Mutat. Res.* **2005**, *577*, 92–117.

145. Sinha, R. P.; Hader, D. P. UV-induced DNA damage and repair: a review. *Photochem. Photobiol. Sci.* **2002**, *1*, 225–236.

146. Park, H.; Zhang, K.; Ren, Y.; Nadji, S.; Sinha, N.; Taylor, J. S.; Kang, C. Crystal structure of a DNA decamer containing a cis–syn thymine dimer. *Proc. Natl. Acad. Sci. USA* **2002**, *99*, 15965–15970.

147. Franklin, W. A.; Doetsch, P. W.; Haseltine, W. A. Structural determination of the ultraviolet light-induced thymine–cytosine pyrimidine–pyrimidone 6-4) photoproduct. *Nucleic Acids Res.* **1985**, *13*, 5317–5325.

148. Orren, D. K.; Sancar, A. Formation and enzymatic properties of the UvrB.DNA complex. *J. Biol. Chem.* **1990**, *265*, 15796–15803.

149. Sancar, A.; Rupp, W. D. A novel repair enzyme: UVRABC excision nuclease of *Escherichia coli* cuts a DNA strand on both sides of the damaged region. *Cell* **1983**, *33*, 249–260.

150. Nakabeppu, Y.; Sekiguchi, M. Physical association of pyrimidine dimer DNA glycosylase and apurinic/apyrimidinic DNA endonuclease essential for repair of ultraviolet-damaged DNA. *Proc. Natl. Acad. Sci. USA* **1981,** *78,* 2742–2746.

151. Savitsky, K.; Bar-Shira, A.; Gilad, S.; Rotman, G.; Ziv, Y.; Vanagaite, L.; Tagle, D. A.; Smith, S.; Uziel, T.; Sfez, S. A single ataxia telangiectasia gene with a product similar to PI-3 kinase. *Science* **1995,** *268,* 1749–1753.

152. He, Z.; Wong, J. M.; Maniar, H. S.; Brill, S. J.; Ingles, C. J. Assessing the requirements for nucleotide excision repair proteins of *Saccharomyces cerevisiae* in an in vitro system. *J. Biol. Chem.* **1996,** *271,* 28243–28249.

153. Tanaka, K.; Wood, R. D. Xeroderma pigmentosum and nucleotide excision repair of DNA. *Trends Biochem. Sci.* **1994,** *19,* 83–86.

154. de Boer, J.; Hoeijmakers, J. H. Nucleotide excision repair and human syndromes. *Carcinogenesis* **2000,** *21,* 453–460.

155. Sancar, A.; Reardon, J. T. Nucleotide excision repair in *E. coli* and man. *Adv. Protein Chem.* **2004,** *69,* 43–71.

156. Ruiz de Almodovar, J. M.; Steel, G. G.; Whitaker, S. J.; McMillan, T. J. A comparison of methods for calculating DNA double-strand break induction frequency in mammalian cells by pulsed-field gel electrophoresis. *Int. J. Radiat. Biol.* **1994,** *65,* 641–649.

157. Fairbairn, D. W.; Olive, P. L.; O'Neill, K. L. The comet assay: a comprehensive review. *Mutat. Res.* **1995,** *339,* 37–59.

158. Olive, P. L. The comet assay. An overview of techniques. *Methods Mol. Biol.* **2002,** *203,* 179–194.

159. Olive, P. L. DNA damage and repair in individual cells: applications of the comet assay in radiobiology. *Int. J. Radiat. Biol.* **1999,** *75,* 395–405.

160. Hutchinson, F. On the measurement of DNA double-strand breaks by neutral elution. *Radiat. Res.* **1989,** *120,* 182–186.

161. West, S. C. Molecular views of recombination proteins and their control. *Nat. Rev. Mol. Cell Biol.* **2003,** *4,* 435–445.

162. Krejci, L.; Chen, L.; Van Komen, S.; Sung, P.; Tomkinson, A. Mending the break: two DNA double-strand break repair machines in eukaryotes. *Prog. Nucleic Acid Res. Mol. Biol.* **2003,** *74,* 159–201.

163. Valerie, K.; Povirk, L. F. Regulation and mechanisms of mammalian double-strand break repair. *Oncogene* **2003,** *22,* 5792–5812.

164. Hopfner, K. P.; Putnam, C. D.; Tainer, J. A. DNA double-strand break repair from head to tail. *Curr. Opin. Struct. Biol.* **2002,** *12,* 115–122.

165. Shin, D. S.; Chahwan, C.; Huffman, J. L.; Tainer, J. A. Structure and function of the double-strand break repair machinery. *DNA Repair (Amst.)* **2004,** *3,* 863–873.

166. Stracker, T. H.; Theunissen, J. W.; Morales, M.; Petrini, J. H. The Mre11 complex and the metabolism of chromosome breaks: the importance of communicating and holding things together. *DNA Repair (Amst.)* **2004,** *3,* 845–854.

167. Assenmacher, N.; Hopfner, K. P. MRE11/RAD50/NBS1: complex activities. *Chromosoma* **2004,** *113,* 157–166.

168. Digweed, M.; Reis, A.; Sperling, K. Nijmegen breakage syndrome: consequences of defective DNA double strand break repair. *Bioessays* **1999,** *21,* 649–656.

169. Tauchi, H.; Kobayashi, J.; Morishima, K.; Van, G.; Shiraishi, T.; Verkaik, N. S.; vanHeems, D.; Ito, E.; Nakamura, A.; Sonoda, E.; Takata, M.; Takeda, S.; Matsuura, S.; Komatsu, K. Nbs1 is essential for DNA repair

by homologous recombination in higher vertebrate cells. *Nature* **2002**, *420*, 93–98.

170. (a) Hopfner, K. P.; Craig, L.; Moncalian, G.; Zinkel, R. A.; Usui, T.; Owen, B. A.; Karcher, A.; Henderson, B.; Bodmer, J. L.; McMurray, C. T.; Carney, J. P.; Petrini, J. H.; Tainer, J. A. The Rad50 zinc-hook is a structure joining Mre11 complexes in DNA recombination and repair. *Nature* **2002**, *418*, 562–566. (b) Moreno-Herrero, F.; de Jager, M.; Dekker, N. H.; Kanaar, R.; Wyman, C.; Dekker, C. Mesoscale conformational changes in the DNA-repair complex Rad50/Mre11/Nbs1 upon binding DNA. *Nature* **2005**, *437*, 440–443.

171. Kumar, J. K.; Gupta, R. C. Strand exchange activity of human recombination protein Rad52. *Proc. Natl. Acad. Sci. USA* **2004**, *101*, 9562–9567.

172. Savitsky, K.; Sfez, S.; Tagle, D. A.; Ziv, Y.; Sartiel, A.; Collins, F. S.; Shiloh, Y.; Rotman, G. The complete sequence of the coding region of the ATM gene reveals similarity to cell cycle regulators in different species. *Hum. Mol. Genet.* **1995**, *4*, 2025–2032.

173. Rotman, G.; Shiloh, Y. ATM: a mediator of multiple responses to genotoxic stress. *Oncogene* **1999**, *18*, 6135–6144.

174. Shiloh, Y. ATM and related protein kinases: safeguarding genome integrity. *Nat. Rev. Cancer* **2003**, *3*, 155–168.

175. Lee, J. H.; Paull, T. T. Direct activation of the ATM protein kinase by the Mre11/Rad50/Nbs1 complex. *Science* **2004**, *304*, 93–96.

176. Donahue, S. L.; Lundberg, R.; Saplis, R.; Campbell, C. Deficient regulation of DNA double-strand break repair in Fanconi anemia fibroblasts. *J. Biol. Chem.* **2003**, *278*, 29487–29495.

177. Lees-Miller, S. P.; Meek, K. Repair of DNA double strand breaks by non-homologous end joining. *Biochimie* **2003**, *85*, 1161–1173.

178. Weterings, E.; Van, G. The mechanism of non-homologous end-joining: a synopsis of synapsis. *DNA Repair (Amst.)* **2004**, *3*, 1425–1435.

179. Lieber, M. R.; Ma, Y.; Pannicke, U.; Schwarz, K. The mechanism of vertebrate nonhomologous DNA end joining and its role in V(D)J recombination. *DNA Repair (Amst.)* **2004**, *3*, 817–826.

180. Takeda, Y.; Dynan, W. S. Autoantibodies against DNA double-strand break repair proteins. *Front Biosci.* **2001**, *6*, D1412–D1422.

181. Walker, J. R.; Corpina, R. A.; Goldberg, J. Structure of the Ku heterodimer bound to DNA and its implications for double-strand break repair. *Nature* **2001**, *412*, 607–614.

182. Della, M.; Palmbos, P. L.; Tseng, H. M.; Tonkin, L. M.; Daley, J. M.; Topper, L. M.; Pitcher, R. S.; Tomkinson, A. E.; Wilson, T. E.; Doherty, A. J. Mycobacterial Ku and ligase proteins constitute a two-component NHEJ repair machine. *Science* **2004**, *306*, 683–685.

183. Sutton, M. D.; Smith, B. T.; Godoy, V. G.; Walker, G. C. The SOS response: recent insights into *umuDC*-dependent mutagenesis and DNA damage tolerance. *Annu. Rev. Genet.* **2000**, *34*, 479–497.

184. Smith, B. T.; Walker, G. C. Mutagenesis and more: *umuDC* and the *Escherichia coli* SOS response. *Genetics* **1998**, *148*, 1599–1610.

185. Hannon, G. J. RNA interference. *Nature* **2002**, *418*, 244–251.

186. Devoret, R. At the birth of molecular radiation biology. *Environ. Mol. Mutagen.* **2001**, *38*, 135–143.

187. Walker, G. C. To cleave or not to cleave? Insights from the LexA crystal structure. *Mol. Cell* **2001**, *8*, 486–487.

188. Kato, T.; Shinoura, Y. Isolation and characterization of mutants of *Escherichia coli* deficient in induction of mutations by ultraviolet light. *Mol. Gen. Genet.* **1977,** *156,* 121–131.

189. Rajagopalan, M.; Lu, C.; Woodgate, R.; O'Donnell, M.; Goodman, M. F.; Echols, H. Activity of the purified mutagenesis proteins UmuC, UmuD', and RecA in replicative bypass of an abasic DNA lesion by DNA polymerase III. *Proc. Natl. Acad. Sci. USA* **1992,** *89,* 10777–10781.

190. Reuven, N. B.; Arad, G.; Maor-Shoshani, A.; Livneh, Z. The mutagenesis protein UmuC is a DNA polymerase activated by UmuD', RecA, and SSB and is specialized for translesion replication. *J. Biol. Chem.* **1999,** *274,* 31763–31766.

191. Tang, M.; Shen, X.; Frank, E. G.; O'Donnell, M.; Woodgate, R.; Goodman, M. F. UmuD'(2)C is an error-prone DNA polymerase, *Escherichia coli* pol V. *Proc. Natl. Acad. Sci. USA* **1999,** *96,* 8919–8924.

192. Ferentz, A. E.; Walker, G. C.; Wagner, G. Converting a DNA damage checkpoint effector (UmuD2C) into a lesion bypass polymerase (UmuD'2C). *EMBO J.* **2001,** *20,* 4287–4298.

193. Yang, W. Damage repair DNA polymerases Y. *Curr. Opin. Struct. Biol.* **2003,** *13,* 23–30.

194. Ohmori, H.; Friedberg, E. C.; Fuchs, R. P.; Goodman, M. F.; Hanaoka, F.; Hinkle, D.; Kunkel, T. A.; Lawrence, C. W.; Livneh, Z.; Nohmi, T.; Prakash, L.; Prakash, S.; Todo, T.; Walker, G. C.; Wang, Z.; Woodgate, R. The Y-family of DNA polymerases. *Mol. Cell* **2001,** *8,* 7–8.

195. Goodman, M. F. Error-prone repair DNA polymerases in prokaryotes and eukaryotes. *Annu. Rev. Biochem.* **2002,** *71,* 17–50.

196. Prakash, S.; Johnson, R.E.; Prakash, L. Eukaryotic translesion synthesis DNA polymerases: specificity of structure and function. *Annu. Rev. Biochem.* **2005,** *74,* 317–353.

197. Wagner, J.; Gruz, P.; Kim, S. R.; Yamada, M.; Matsui, K.; Fuchs, R. P.; Nohmi, T. The *dinB* gene encodes a novel E. coli DNA polymerase, DNA pol IV, involved in mutagenesis. *Mol. Cell* **1999,** *4,* 281–286.

198. Kunkel, T. A.; Pavlov, Y. I.; Bebenek, K. Functions of human DNA polymerases eta, kappa and iota suggested by their properties, including fidelity with undamaged DNA templates. *DNA Repair (Amst.)* **2003,** *2,* 135–149.

199. Broughton, B. C.; Cordonnier, A.; Kleijer, W. J.; Jaspers, N. G.; Fawcett, H.; Raams, A.; Garritsen, V. H.; Stary, A.; Avril, M. F.; Boudsocq, F.; Masutani, C.; Hanaoka, F.; Fuchs, R. P.; Sarasin, A.; Lehmann, A. R. Molecular analysis of mutations in DNA polymerase eta in xeroderma pigmentosum-variant patients. *Proc. Natl. Acad. Sci. USA* **2002,** *99,* 815–820.

4

Chemical

Mutagenesis

BASE SUBSTITUTIONS

Mutations are heritable changes in genetic sequences. There is a close analogy between mutations in the base sequence of DNA and typographical errors in a string of alphabetic text. The DNA alphabet has only four letters; all "words" (codons in coding sequences) have three letters; and there are no "punctuation marks," other than the start/stop/splicing signals encoded in the base sequence itself. But the biggest difference between DNA "text" and alphabetic text is that DNA is double-stranded, so the functional unit is the base pair, not the individual letter (base).

A *base-substitution* mutation is the replacement of one base pair by another. Twelve base-substitution mutations are possible on a single strand: each of the four bases can be replaced by any of the other three. The requirement of self-complementarity of double-stranded DNA reduces the number of possibilities by half, that is, six base substitutions are distinguishable.

(Some viruses, such as the filamentous bacteriophage M13, carry single-stranded DNA genomes ("viral strand"), which are converted into dsDNA ("replicative form") after infection of *E. coli*. (M13 was once widely used to prepare ssDNA for sequencing.) Mutation assays (*1*) based on M13 or other ssDNA constructs allow all 12 base substitutions to be enumerated.)

Base substitutions are classified as *transversions* (purine replaced by pyrimidine, or vice versa):

$$G{:}C \rightarrow T{:}A; \ G{:}C \rightarrow C{:}G; \ A{:}T \rightarrow T{:}A; \ A{:}T \rightarrow C{:}G$$

and *transitions* (purine replaced by purine, or pyrimidine replaced by pyrimidine):

$$G{:}C \rightarrow A{:}T; \ A{:}T \rightarrow G{:}C$$

An A:T → C:G transversion (for example) could arise by misinsertion of a G across from an A or, to the same effect, by the misinsertion of a C across from a T.

INSERTIONS AND DELETIONS

Beside base-substitution events, other types of mutations can occur. *Insertions* give rise to daughter DNA molecules with additional base pairs; *deletions*, fewer. If the change in the number of bases is not a multiple of three, then an insertion/deletion ("indel") event causes a *frameshift* of the triplet reading frame for the genetic code. Such mutations are very likely to result in truncation of a protein-coding sequence due to premature occurrence of a nonsense (stop) codon. For example, many instances of inherited breast cancer result from nonsense mutations in the *BRCA1* gene, which can be detected by a "protein truncation test" (*2*). Cystic fibrosis is caused by inherited defects in the cystic fibrosis transmembrane conductance regulator (CFTR) gene. In this well-characterized case, the most common mutation is an in-frame three-base-pair deletion, which eliminates residue Phe-508 without altering the remainder of the protein sequence. Hundreds of other sequence alterations are known, including nonsense and frameshift mutations (*3*).

Complex mutations combine more than one sequence change, for example an insertion accompanied by a base substitution.

IS MUTATION "RANDOM"?

We sometimes see the noun "mutation" prefaced by the adjective "random." The Russian-American population geneticist Theodosius Dobzhansky (1900–1975) explained how we should interpret "randomness" in this context (*4*, p. 92):

> Mutations are often described as accidental, random, undirected, chance events. Just what do these epithets mean?...Mutations are undirected with respect to the adaptive needs of the species. They arise regardless of their actual or potential usefulness. It may seem a deplorable imperfection of nature that mutability is not restricted to changes that enhance the adaptedness of their carriers. However, only a vitalist Pangloss[1] could imagine that the genes know how and when it is good for them to mutate.

Undirected with respect to the adaptive needs of the species: this is the correct Darwinian interpretation of the word "random" as applied to mutation. But we should not construe the word "random" to imply that there are no discernable patterns to the kinds of mutations that occur, or the positions where they are most likely to arise. As Lynn Ripley observed (*5*):

> All experimental measures of mutagenesis demonstrate that spontaneous mutagenesis is not random...Although a portion of observed nonrandomness in most measurements of mutation is due to the phenotypic properties of the mutants, mutant spectra still reveal that mutations are distributed in genes in highly biased patterns... Apparent differences in mutation rates per gene are far smaller than are the differences in mutation rates between sites within a gene. Indeed, one or a few hotspots often comprise as much as two-thirds of the total inactivating mutations in a spontaneous mutant spectrum.

The nonrandomness of mutations arises from many factors. For example, the four bases of DNA are differentially susceptible to attack by specific agents, as discussed many times in this book. Local (and even global) DNA sequence properties influence mutational mechanisms; an important example is the "Streisinger slippage" mechanism, discussed later in this chapter, which occurs far more readily at repeated sequences. Genes that are actively transcribed may be more exposed to damaging agents than silent genes, but they are also more readily repaired ("transcription-coupled repair") (*6*, *7*) as discussed in the previous chapter.

MUTATION AND SELECTION

When we survey the prevalent alleles of a particular gene in a given population, we are not examining the process of mutagenesis as such, although we garner evidence that mutations have occurred. The same is true when we perform a mutagenesis assay, such as the Ames test: we are examining a population of mutants that are *products* of the process of mutagenesis. But we observe such populations through the "filter" of natural (or artificial) selection: only those mutants that grow (and in the laboratory, growth is usually measured under specific selective conditions) are observed. If these selective conditions are very stringent (such as the requirement that a mutant allele revert to functionality), only a small fraction of the mutants will be observed.

Sequence analysis of the gene encoding the protein cytochrome c (8, p. 507) reveals that about one-quarter of its amino acid residues have remained invariant since the evolutionary divergence of yeast and animals. Surely the main factor dictating this sequence conservation is natural selection: mutations at highly conserved sites are probably incompatible with survival. But highly conserved (vs. highly variant) sites within a gene could also reflect intrinsically low (vs. intrinsically high) rates of mutagenesis at those positions, as we discuss later.

In 1998 the National Institute of Environmental Health Sciences, USA, began the Environmental Genome Project (EGP; http://www.niehs.nih.gov/envgenom/). The goal of this major initiative is to compile a database on human genetic polymorphisms occurring in genes that influence individual response to environmental exposures and thereby affect disease risk. A list of over 500 target genes was assembled, encompassing genes/proteins involved in carcinogen metabolism, DNA repair, cell cycle control, cell division, signaling, DNA repair, and other relevant cellular functions. To date, almost 10,000 single nucleotide polymorphisms (SNPs) have been catalogued by the EGP. As we learn more about the interindividual variability of gene sequences on a genome-wide scale, new insights into patterns of mutagenesis are sure to arise.

TRANSITION BIAS

There are twice as many possible transversions (four) as transitions (two). However, statistical comparative analysis of mammalian genome sequence data indicates that *transitions occur much more commonly* (several-fold) than do transversions during molecular evolution (*9, 10*). Why would this be so? G:C to A:T transitions at CpG sites occur readily, because of spontaneous deamination of 5-methylcytosine residues, a mutational mechanism that we discussed in chapter 3. However, CpG is the rarest dinucleotide combination in the human genome and the "transition bias" remains strong, even when these events are excluded from the analysis.

Mutations are fixed (i.e., made permanent) by mispairing events during DNA replication or repair. A transition would arise from mispairing of a purine with a pyrimidine, for example, G:C → G:T → A:T; a transversion would arise from mispairing of a purine with a purine, or a pyrimidine with a pyrimidine, for example, G:C → G:A → T:A. The major reason for the bias towards transitions is probably that a purine–purine or pyrimidine–pyrimidine mispairing causes greater structural distortion of the double helix, and, consequently, is more easily recognized and repaired. When a damaged base (e.g., O^6-methylguanine, as discussed later) is present in the template, DNA polymerase may still prefer to insert a pyrimidine opposite a purine, and a purine opposite a pyrimidine—although it may insert the incorrect base (e.g., T rather than C opposite O^6-methyl-G).

MUTATION ASSAYS

DNA replication is usually faithful, and spontaneous mutations are infrequent events. Even when a cell is treated with high doses of mutagens, selectable mutations in specific target genes are rare. E. coli (strain K-12) has a genome of 4.6 million base pairs, encoding genes for about 4300 proteins. If mutations are distributed randomly throughout the chromosome, then only 1 in about 4000 mutations will affect a particular gene of interest: and not all of these will confer a selectable mutant phenotype. The dose of mutagen that can be applied in a mutation assay is also limited: if the cell's burden of DNA damage is too high, it may be unable to replicate its DNA; and if too many mutations occur, its progeny may die from their functional consequences. Not surprisingly, then, any mutagen is toxic or growth inhibitory at high concentrations. (Solubility also limits doses.) The study of molecular mutagenesis requires the development of sensitive assays for mutations.

Usually, in genetic analysis of mutagenesis, we rely on phenotypic selection to detect the progeny of the mutant organism (e.g., a bacterial strain, yeast strain, or mammalian cell line). That is, we establish selective conditions in which the parent phenotype cannot grow, but the mutant can. With bacterial mutation assays, very large numbers of cells ($>10^8$) can be plated on a single Petri dish. If strong selection for mutant survival can be achieved, even rare events can be detected. With mammalian cells in vitro, the number of cells that can be plated per dish is perhaps 100-fold lower; the number of genes is at least 10-fold higher; and the total genomic DNA content is about 100-fold greater, compared to E. coli. Each of these factors tends to reduce the sensitivity of mutagenicity assays with mammalian cells, relative to bacteria.

FORWARD AND REVERSE MUTATIONS

Forward mutations convert a gene coding for a wild-type (functional) protein product into a mutant form that codes for an altered or nonfunctional product. Some forward mutations may confer resistance to a toxic agent, such as an antibiotic, or permit growth on a substrate that does not normally support the organism. For example, wild-type E. coli cells are sensitive to the antibiotic rifampicin, which inhibits RNA polymerase activity (11). Rifampicin-resistant mutants have an altered RNA polymerase, which is less susceptible to inhibition.

Mutation of a biosynthetic gene may give rise to an auxotrophic mutant, an organism dependent, for colony growth, upon supply of a particular nutrient (e.g., an amino acid or nucleic acid base). Wild-type E. coli grows on minimal medium (salts plus glucose), and so auxotrophic mutants can be detected by replica plating.[2]

In contrast to forward mutations, *reversion* mutations restore biological function to a nonfunctional gene. Revertants are usually selected by their (regained) ability to grow on minimal media (*prototrophy*). For example, the various strains of *Salmonella typhimurium* used in the *Ames assay* are auxotrophic for histidine, and revertants are selected by their ability to grow in the absence of this amino acid (see below). Ease of selection is often an advantage of reversion assays, but their sensitivity is inherently lower than for forward assays, since mutations are more likely to inactivate genes than to reactivate them.

Mechanisms of Reversion

Reversion of, say, a base-substitution mutation could occur by the precise reversal of the original (forward) mutation. However, a reversion mutation does not necessarily restore the original DNA sequence. Suppose the wild-type gene has a codon AAG, specifying lysine at, say, residue 142, and, in the mutant allele, this is replaced by UAG, a stop codon; the protein is truncated and nonfunctional. A second mutation from UAG to UAC, specifying tyrosine, might yield a phenotypic revertant, if the protein remains active with a tyrosine residue at position 142, in place of the wild-type lysine.

The reversion mutation might even occur in a different codon. This situation is illustrated by the *hisD3052* mutation (figure 4-1) found in *S. typhimurium* Ames test strains such as TA98 (described below). *hisD3052* carries a −1 frameshift mutation in the histidinol dehydrogenase gene.

```
wild-type hisD
LEU ALA GLU LEU PRO ARG ALA ASP THR ALA AR
CTG GCG GAA CTG CCG CGC GCG GAC ACC GCC CG
                                        ⇧

hisD3052
CTG GCG GAA CTG CCG CGC GCG GAC ACC GCC -G

LEU ALA GLU LEU PRO ARG ALA ASP THR ALA GLY ARG
CTG GCG GAA CTG CCG CGC GCG GAC ACC GCC GGC AGG CC

most common revertant
CTG GCG GAA CTG C-- CGC GCG GAC ACC GCC GG

LEU ALA GLU LEU PRO ARG GLY HIS ARG ARG GLN ALA
CTG GCG GAA CTG CCG CGC GGA CAC CGC CGG CA
```

FIGURE 4-1.
The target in Ames test strains TA1538 and TA98 is an allele of the histidinol dehydrogenase (*hisD*) gene. The target segment of the gene is shown here. Top: the wild-type DNA and protein sequence; the arrow indicates the site of the mutation in *hisD3052*, a deletion of a C base. Middle: the *hisD3052* mutant sequence is shown aligned with the wild-type sequence (upper) and frameshifted (lower); the mutant amino acid sequence is shown, with the first two altered residues shown in purple. A premature stop codon arises downstream (not shown). The hot-spot (CG)4 sequence is shown in red, underlined. Bottom: the most common reversion mutation is a deletion of CpG from the hotspot, as indicated. The revertant protein has three missense codons (amino acids indicated in purple). *Note*: A full-color version of this figure appears on the website.

The frameshift (loss of a C residue) creates a string of missense codons, closely followed by a stop codon, and therefore results in a truncated, nonfunctional protein product. Many *hisD3052* revertants have been characterized by DNA sequencing (*12*). Very few of these are original-site revertants (insertion of the missing C). The most common revertant results from loss of two more base pairs, GC, from a repeated sequence CGCGCGCG that lies just upstream from the site of the original mutation. For example, 99.9% of the mutations induced by 4-aminobiphenyl in strain TA1538 occur at this hot-spot (*13*). The revertant sequence is one codon shorter than the wild-type one. Between the site of the original mutation and the site of the reversion, codons for four residues of the wild-type protein (ala-asp-thr-ala) have been replaced by codons for three residues of the revertant protein (gly-his-arg); beyond the site of the original mutation, the reading frame is restored and the remaining amino acid sequence is identical to the wild-type one. The altered amino acids are not essential for enzyme activity and the revertants are phenotypically His$^+$.

Each mutation assay has advantages, disadvantages, and peculiarities. In the following sections, we will examine a forward mutation assay and a reversion mutation assay based on genes of the *E. coli lac* operon; the widely used Ames test, which is a reversion assay using *S. typhimurium*; some mammalian mutation assays with endogenous genes; and transgenic rodent mutation assays.

MUTATION ASSAY SYSTEMS BASED ON THE *E. coli lac* OPERON GENES

The *lac* Operon

The *lacI* and *lacZ* genes of *E. coli* are important targets used in mutation research. In this section, we briefly introduce the genetics and biochemistry of the *lac* operon system (*14, 15*). Benno Müller-Hill, one of the pioneers of *lac* biology, has written an entertaining historical account that is highly recommended (*16*).

Lactose (milk sugar) is a disaccharide composed of galactose and glucose linked by a β-glycosidic bond. Wild-type *E. coli* can grow on *lactose* as sole carbon source. The elements of the lactose utilization system consist of a regulatory gene (*lacI*), control sites (*lacP*, promoter; and *lacO*, operator), and structural genes (*lacZ, lacY*, and *lacA*). Together, these units comprise the *lac* operon. The operation of the *lac* operon as a negative-control mechanism was first explained in the early 1960s by Jacques Monod (1910–1976; Nobel prize, 1965) and co-workers.

The enzymes encoded by the structural genes of the *lac* operon make possible the cell's utilization of lactose. *lacZ* codes for β-galactosidase, the enzyme that catalyzes cleavage of the glycosidic bond in lactose, releasing galactose and glucose, which can be used for energy metabolism and biosynthesis. *lacY* codes for galactoside permease, which is required for lactose uptake (transport through the cell membrane). *lacA* encodes the enzyme galactoside acetyltransferase; this enzyme is not required for lactose metabolism and its biological role remains unclear (*17*). All three genes are coordinately expressed: they are transcribed as a single polycistronic mRNA.

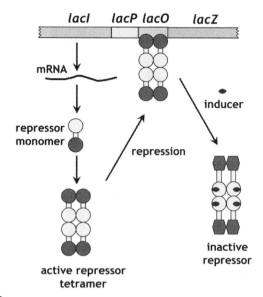

FIGURE 4-2.

The start of the *lac* operon of *E. coli*; see text for details. *lacI* encodes the lac repressor; *lacP* is the promoter of the *lac* operon; *lacO* is the operator (the sequence to which LacI protein binds); *lacZ* is the first structural gene of the operon, encoding β-galactosidase. *Note*: A full-color version of this figure appears on the website.

The *lac* Repressor

lacI encodes the *lac repressor* protein, which is a DNA-binding regulatory protein, not an enzyme. The *lac* repressor binds with high affinity to a specific region of DNA, near the beginning of the *lacZ* gene, which is termed the *operator* (figure 4-2). The presence of repressor protein bound to the operator blocks RNA polymerase from initiating transcription at the nearby *lac* promoter. This negative control prevents the cell from synthesizing the enzymes when they are not required, that is, in the absence of the substrate (lactose). The repressor, operator, and promoter are the control elements of a "genetic switch," which turns on the synthesis of the enzymes only in the presence of compounds called *inducers*. Lactose itself is an inducer, as are many lactose analogues (see sidebar). How does this "genetic switch" (*18*) work?

The *lac* repressor protein is composed of four identical subunits. The repressor is the "transducer" that senses the concentration of lactose in the cell, and acts, on the basis of this information, to regulate the transcription of the *lac* operon structural genes. Each repressor subunit consists of two functionally independent domains. The N-terminal DNA-binding domain (approximately the first 60 amino acids) mediates operator binding (*19*). The remaining "core" domain (amino acids 61–330) (*20*) contains sites for aggregation (formation of repressor tetramers), inducer binding, and transmission of the induction signal from the inducer-binding site to the DNA-binding domain. The binding of inducer to the repressor is highly cooperative (*21*), just as in the case of oxygen binding to hemoglobin: inducer binding to one monomer facilitates binding to the other monomers. Furthermore, *lac* repressor binding to the operator is also highly cooperative

▶ *lac* **Operon Substrates and Inducers**

Lactose, the (presumed) natural substrate of the *lac* operon, is both an inducer[3] of *lac* operon gene expression and a substrate for β-galactosidase, as already noted. Beginning in about 1950, Monod examined a large number of glycosides, testing them as possible substrates or inducers of the (yet-to-be-named) *lac* operon. These studies, which have had a lasting influence on molecular biology, were made possible by the development of the synthetic substrate o-nitrophenyl-β-D-galactoside (ONPG). ONPG is hydrolyzed by β-galactosidase, producing the yellow product o-nitrophenol. With this substrate, β-galactosidase activity could be measured sensitively and quantitatively. Monod's studies identified "gratuitous" inducers, compounds that induce β-galactosidase activity but are not substrates for metabolism by β-galactosidase. The best known of these is isopropyl-β-D-thiogalactopyranoside (IPTG; first synthesized at Monod's suggestion). IPTG is an even more potent inducer than natural lactose; the fact that it is not broken down by β-galactosidase makes it a stable and very useful reagent for *lac* induction, and it is still widely used for that purpose. In contrast, phenyl-β-D-galactoside (P-gal) is a substrate for β-galactosidase (yielding phenol and galactose) but is *not* an inducer. (It was Monod's discovery of compounds such as P-gal and IPTG that convinced him that inducers must interact with a receptor different from β-galactosidase, and started the search for the *lac* repressor.) 5-Bromo-4-chloro-3-indolyl-β-D-galactopyranoside (24) (X-gal) is a synthetic β-galactosidase substrate that, like ONPG, produces a colored product. However, the product of X-gal hydrolysis is an insoluble blue pigment, so X-gal is useful for staining colonies or tissues expressing β-galactosidase. ◀

(*22*): the operator site has two-fold sequence symmetry, and binds cooperatively to two subunits of the repressor. (In fact, all four subunits can bind simultaneously, since there is a second nearby operator site, which is located within the *lacZ* coding sequence (*23*).)

Inducers such as lactose bind to the C-terminal subunits of the repressor, causing a change in the conformation of the repressor, including changes to its DNA-binding region (*25*). This conformational change prevents repressor binding to the operator. Consequently, *over a narrow range of inducer concentration, the repressor switches from the operator-binding conformation to the nonbinding conformation.* The repressor protein falls off the operator; RNA polymerase can now bind to the promoter sequence and initiate the expression of the genes of the *lac* operon: the lactose utilization enzymes are produced.

The binding of *lac* repressor to the operator site on the chromosome is mediated by highly specific contacts between the protein's N-terminal domain and the DNA bases of the operator site. Even a single amino acid residue change in the repressor sequence can greatly weaken its binding to the operator. Such a mutation will lead to *constitutive* synthesis of the *lac* genes, that is, expression of the genes in the absence of inducer. We can establish conditions under which only constitutive mutants will form colonies (see below), so *most mutations occurring in the DNA-binding domain of lacI can be selected phenotypically.*

The *lacI* Forward Mutagenicity Assay

The *lacI* mutation assay (*14*) is performed by incubating a culture of a *lacI* wild-type strain with mutagen, and then plating the cultures onto agar plates containing P-gal (see sidebar). P-gal is a substrate for β-galactosidase, providing a carbon source for the bacteria, but it is *not* an inducer of the *lac* operon. Consequently, only constitutive mutants—those that express β-galactosidase even in the absence of inducer—will grow, and these are mainly *lacI* mutants, in which the repressor fails to bind to the *lac* operator. This *E. coli* mutation assay has been used in many studies of

```
              XXX HIS
          CYS XXX ARG SER GLY
      GLY PHE CYS PRO ILE ALA
  VAL ALA TYR SER LEU ASN ASP
  ASP ASP ALA PHE GLU ALA LEU
  ARG LEU PRO ASP XXX PRO PHE
  CYS ILE THR ILE LYS SER ILE

  GLY VAL SER TYR GLN THR VAL
  GGT GTC TCT TAT CAG ACC GTT

  A   AA  AA  A  A   A    A   AA
  TT      T   T  TTT TT   T
  C   CC  C      C   C    C   CC
      G   GG  GGG GG  GG       G
```

FIGURE 4-3.

A small section of the *lacI* gene is shown (as both a DNA sequence and an amino acid sequence) boxed at the center. The red letters in the lower box indicate base substitutions that have been observed in lacI⁻ mutants, aligned with the corresponding positions in the wild-type sequence. The upper box shows the corresponding altered amino acid residues. XXX represents a stop codon. Note that every codon and almost every base is a possible target site, although the third base in each codon is usually "cold," because the degeneracy of the genetic code is greatest at the third position in the codon. *Note*: A full-color version of this figure appears on the website. (*Data from de Boer, J. G.; Glickman, B. W. The* lacI *gene as a target for mutation in transgenic rodents and* Escherichia coli. Genetics *1998*, 148, *1441–1451.*)

chemical and spontaneous mutagenesis. De Boer and Glickman (*15*) have compiled the results of sequencing studies on thousands of *E. coli lacI* mutants, allowing a detailed examination of the nature and distribution of mutations that yield a constitutive (and hence selectable) phenotype. The distribution of mutations is particularly dense in the part of the gene encoding the N-terminal DNA-binding domain, because, as noted earlier, even a single amino acid change in this region can greatly reduce the affinity of repressor for operator. In fact, of the 177 base pairs from positions 29–205, 134 are mutated in a reported *lacI* mutant (*15*). Since many mutations at the third base of a codon are silent, this means that almost all amino acid changes in this region of the protein are selectable (figure 4-3). This very high density of selectable mutations gives the *lacI* assay great sensitivity and makes it highly informative with regard to mutational specificity.

The N-terminal 60 amino acids of Lac repressor define the protein's DNA-binding domain, as mentioned above. Mutations in this region of *lacI* (*lacI⁻ᵈ*) have a characteristic property: they are *dominant negatives*. A merodiploid (partial diploid) *E. coli* strain constructed by moving a *lacI⁻ᵈ* allele (carried on an episome) into a *lacI* wild-type host cell is phenotypically *constitutive*. That is, the nonfunctional Lac repressor appears to inactivate the functional one. This occurs because the *lacI⁻ᵈ* gene product aggregates with the wild-type repressor protein to form mixed tetramers, but these tetramers are missing one or more functional DNA-binding domains. Since repressor-DNA binding is highly cooperative, these mixed tetramers bind poorly to the operator, resulting in a constitutive phenotype. Such *lacI⁻ᵈ* mutants can be readily identified by a complementation test. Many studies of *lacI* mutational spectra have focused on the *lacI*$^{-d}$ subset, so this part of the *lacI* gene (approximately the first 200 base pairs) has been analyzed in particular detail (*15*).

The *lacI* target has also been incorporated into bacteriophage λ constructs used in transgenic rodent mutation assays, to be discussed later.

The *lacZ* Reversion Mutagenicity Assay

β-Galactosidase (*26, 27*) is the enzyme that catalyzes lactose hydrolysis. It is a large protein: a 1023 amino acid polypeptide chain that aggregates to form the active holoenzyme, a homotetramer. *lacZ* mutants, having no functional β-galactosidase, cannot grow on lactose medium.[4] Revertants to *lacZ*$^+$ can be selected by their ability to grow on lactose. This is the simple phenotypic basis of the *lacZ* reversion assay.

Jeffrey Miller and co-workers designed a set of *E. coli lacZ* tester strains that revert by specific DNA sequence changes. As we have already discussed, mutations (e.g., Ames test *hisD3052*) can, in general, revert at more than one site. In such cases, we can only determine the DNA sequence change that has taken place by molecular analysis (e.g., PCR amplification and sequencing). Miller recognized the value of having a mutant that could only revert by a precise reversal of the original mutation: the DNA sequence change could be inferred reliably from the observation of a phenotypic revertant, without need for DNA sequencing. The key to achieving this goal is to generate mutants at codons corresponding to amino acid residues at the active site of an enzyme, where any variation from the wild-type sequence is almost certain to destroy enzyme activity. The target he chose was the well-understood *lacZ* gene. The codon (GAA) for an essential catalytic-site residue in the enzyme, Glu461, was altered in various ways, by site-directed mutagenesis. The *lacZ* mutant strains are, of course, unable to grow on lactose and revertants are selected by growth on lactose plates. Six different strains were constructed; each strain can revert to a glutamate codon by one (and only one) of the six possible base substitution mutations. Thus, a chemical can be tested against this set of six strains to analyze the base substitution specificity of the mutations that it induces (*29, 30*). (However, the precaution to be borne in mind is that only a single local DNA sequence context is examined in this manner.) The sequence targets are shown in table 4-1.

A set of frameshift-detection strains was also assembled (*31*). Each frameshift is located in a run of repeated single bases or alternating bases, to

TABLE 4-1.

Base-Substitution Targets in the Miller *E. coli lacZ* Reversion Assay

F'	TARGET CODON	MUTATION DETECTED	AA CHANGE
CC101	TAG	A:T → C:G	amber → E
CC102	GGG	G:C → A:T	G → E
CC103	CAG	G:C → C:G	Q → E
CC104	GCG	G:C → T:A	A → E
CC105	GTG	A:T → T:A	V → E
CC106	AAG	A:T → G:C	K → E

The mutant alleles are carried on F' episomes, which can be moved between E. coli *strains by conjugation.*

maximize the likelihood of mutagenesis by the Streisinger slippage mechanism (*31*) (see below).

THE AMES MUTAGENICITY ASSAY

Strain Construction

The Ames assay, developed in the early 1970s by Bruce Ames and co-workers (University of California, Berkeley), encompasses a series of strains for the detection of mutagens, all of which are histidine-requiring strains of *Salmonella typhimurium* (*32–35*). Despite the subsequent development of many other systems, based on organisms ranging from *E. coli* to mice, the Ames assay remains the most widely used mutagenicity assay. Regulatory agencies continue to require Ames test data as part of the new chemical entity approval process. One reason for the continuing importance of the Ames test is simply the value of the knowledge base on chemical mutagenicity that has been accumulated through 30 years of experimentation. However, one should bear in mind that the Ames test was developed by a series of empirical steps and historical happenstances, in the era before DNA sequencing and modern molecular biology. This accounts for some peculiarities of the system, such as the choice of the murine pathogen *S. typhimurium* rather than the more familiar enteric Gram-negative bacterium *E. coli*.

The Ames assay is a reversion assay: the mutants are prototrophic colonies derived from histidine-auxotrophic mutants (tester strains); only the revertant colonies can grow on minimal agar plates. (A small amount of histidine is incorporated in these plates, to support a few rounds of division of the auxotrophic cells, sufficient to permit expression of the phenotype in the induced mutants.) After incubation for about two days, revertant colonies are counted.

The Ames assay strains are derived from several mutants of *S. typhimurium* strain LT-2, chosen from a large collection of histidine-requiring mutants accumulated by Philip Hartman (*36*), Bruce Ames, and their fellow "histidinologists" in the 1960s. Mutants were chosen for high frequencies of chemically induced reversion and low (or, at least, tolerable) rates of spontaneous reversion. The development of the two most widely used tester strains[5] is summarized in figure 4-4 (*38*). The objective of these additional steps in strain construction was increased sensitivity to induced mutations.

Δ*uvrB* strains lack functional nucleotide excision repair (see chapter 3) and are far more sensitive to mutagens that form bulky DNA adducts, such as aromatic amines and polycyclic aromatic hydrocarbons (PAHs). The lipopolysaccharide (LPS) coat of the Gram-negative bacterial cell serves as a protective barrier against the entry of foreign compounds. Strain LT-2 is phenotypically "smooth": it possesses a complete LPS coat. Ames and colleagues introduced either the *gal* (galactose synthesis) mutation, which prevents biosynthesis of the O-antigen component of LPS, or the *rfa* ("deep rough") phenotype (selected on the basis of bacteriophage C21 resistance). Deep rough strains retain little of the LPS coat beyond the lipid A core, and are more sensitive to some mutagens, presumably due to increased uptake of the compounds from the external medium.

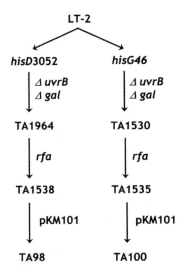

FIGURE 4-4.

The stepwise construction of the *S. typhimurium* Ames test strains TA98 and TA100; see text for details. *Note*: This figure also appears on the companion website.

Plasmid pKM101, a derivative of a naturally occurring R-factor (antibiotic resistance factor), was constructed by Kristien Mortelmans in the laboratory of Donald MacPhee (*39*). The presence of this plasmid was observed to enhance the mutagenic response to ultraviolet (UV) light and some chemical mutagens. Ames and colleagues introduced plasmid pKM101 into the salmonella tester strains, and found that it dramatically increased the mutagenicity of many compounds, such as aflatoxin B_1 and benzyl chloride (*34*). Graham Walker and colleagues, at the Massachusetts Institute of Technology (*40*), used molecular biological methods to map and dissect the genes encoded on this large plasmid. The critical genes for enhancement of chemical mutagenesis were named *mucAB* (mutagenesis; UV and chemical). Much later, these genes were shown to encode Y-class error-prone DNA polymerases (see chapter 3).

Metabolic Activation

The capacity of bacteria to bioactivate mutagenic chemicals is very restricted (although *S. typhimurium* bacteria do express NAT enzyme activity; see below), so most classes of chemical carcinogens do not mutagenize bacteria directly. One early solution to the challenge of combining mammalian metabolic activation with a bacterial mutagenicity was the "host-mediated" assay (*41, 42*). In this protocol, an aliquot of the test bacteria is injected into a rat (e.g., via the tail vein) and then the test chemical is administered (e.g., intraperitoneal injection). After a period of a few hours, the animal is sacrificed and bacteria are recovered from the liver (by homogenization, low-speed centrifugation to remove debris, and medium-speed centrifugation to recover the bacteria). The bacteria are then plated on nonselective media to enumerate survivors and selective media to determine mutants (*43*). Clearly, an in vitro alternative to such an invasive assay is preferable. Heinrich Malling discovered that rat hepatic microsomes can convert dialkylnitrosamines to bacterial mutagens in an in vitro incubation (*44, 45*). Ames asked Malling to send him some of the microsomal preparations, and Ames then combined this activation system with *S. typhimurium* strains sensitive to chemically induced reversion mutations (*46*), resulting in the short-term assay that became known as the Ames test (*47, 48*). In routine Ames tests, mammalian liver homogenate (or, occasionally, microsomal preparation) is prepared from rats pretreated with Aroclor 1254 (polychlorinated biphenyls) or other P450 inducers (*49*). The test chemical is usually preincubated with the tester strain bacteria and the S9,[6] before the entire mix is plated onto the selective (minimal) medium plates.

Some mutagens are positive in the Ames test even in the absence of S9; certainly, DNA-reactive alkylating agents such as *N*-ethyl-*N*-nitrosourea (ENU; see chapter 15) fall into this class. Such compounds are often called "direct-acting" mutagens. This terminology can be misleading, however, because some S9-independent mutagens undergo metabolic activation catalyzed by enzymes present in the *S. typhimurium* strain bacteria. *S. typhimurium* Ames test strains express substantial levels of NAT enzyme activity, contributing to the high sensitivity of the Ames test to mutagens such as aromatic amines and nitroaromatic compounds (see following section); in contrast, NAT activity in *E. coli* is much less (*50*).

The target sequences for reversion of the *his* mutations in the Ames test strains were determined (*51*) long after the test was established. The *hisD3052* mutation in strain TA98 is a −1 frameshift; the high sensitivity of this strain is primarily due to the presence of a hot-spot, as discussed earlier. When these hot-spot revertants are eliminated from consideration, by preliminary hybridization screening, the patterns of mutations among the remaining revertants induced by particular mutagens can be distinctive and mechanistically informative. An example is shown in figure 4-5. In this way, the Ames test with strain TA98, although a reversion assay, can be used to probe mutational specificity in a manner more commonly associated with forward mutation assays.

The *hisG46* target allele in strain TA100 is a missense codon base substitution (CTC (leu) → CCC (pro)) and can revert by base substitutions at either the first or second positions (note that all four CCX codons encode proline). Tandem double base substitutions and tRNA suppressor mutations are also observed (*52*).

DETECTION AND IDENTIFICATION OF ENVIRONMENTAL MUTAGENS

Bacterial mutation assays, especially the Ames test, proved to be valuable tools for detecting environmental mutagens. The sensitivity and flexibility of the Ames test allow it to be used to test not only pure chemicals, but environmental samples and complex mixtures of many kinds, including soil, foods, airborne particulates, substances leached from solids such as fabrics, volatile gases, and biofluids such as urine. When active test samples are discovered, bioassay-directed fractionation may be possible, using the mutagenicity assay to guide the purification of active compounds. A few examples of the application of the Ames test in this manner are given in the following.

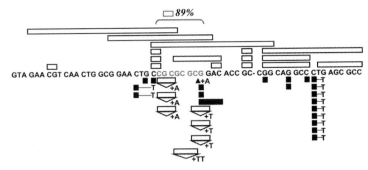

FIGURE 4-5.

Mutation spectrum of S9-activated cigarette smoke condensate in Ames test strain TA98. Each symbol represents the mutation present in a single revertant. Of 398 revertants examined, 356 (89%) carried the hotspot −GpC deletion; these clones were identified by colony hybridization and the remaining clones were then characterized by DNA sequencing. The one-nucleotide deletion in the *hisD3052* allele is represented by a dash. The reversion mutations are represented by the following symbols: open bars, deletions; solid bars, duplications; open bars plus triangles, complex mutations (deletion or addition combined with base substitution); solid bars connected to a letter by a line indicate duplications combined with a base substitution at the indicated site. Note that the net effect of each mutation is to restore the reading frame, for example insertion of 1 base, deletion of 2, 5, 8, etc., bases. *Note*: A full-color version of this figure appears on the website. (*Adapted from DeMarini, D. M.; Shelton, M. L.; Levine, J. G. Mutation spectrum of cigarette smoke condensate in* Salmonella: *comparison to mutations in smoking-associated tumors.* Carcinogenesis *1995, 16, 2535–2542.*)

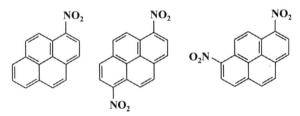

1-nitropyrene	1,6-dinitropyrene	1,8-dinitropyrene

FIGURE 4-6.

1-Nitropyrene and dinitropyrene mutagens.

Nitropyrenes

In 1980 two research groups independently discovered mutagenic activity in "toner" (the black powder used to form the image in photocopiers/laser printers) (*53, 54*). In one case, an air sampler was being used to collect particulate material, which was then extracted and tested for mutagenic activity. The target samples were collected from a sampler placed on top of a tall building in downtown Stockholm, Sweden; as a control, samples were collected inside one of the offices. The inside samples were the more mutagenic, and the source was traced to a nearby photocopier. Herbert Rosenkranz (*54a*) and colleagues purified the active constituents, which proved to be nitrated PAHs (*54b*), particularly 1,6- and 1,8-dinitropyrene (DNP; figure 4-6). Nitrated PAHs were formed during the treatment

▶ Bacterial Nitroreductase and NAT Enzymes

Research on the mutagenicity of dinitropyrene led to new insights concerning the metabolic capacity of *Salmonella* to activate mutagens. Nitropyrenes are activated by reduction to intermediates such as nitroso- and hydroxylamino-aromatics. The "classic" nitroreductase enzyme in *S. typhimurium* is encoded by the *cnr* gene (57). Disruption of *cnr* greatly reduces the mutagenicity of 1-nitropyrene in strain TA98, but has no effect on the mutagenicity of 1,8-dinitropyrene, which must be reduced by other enzymes. A second *Salmonella* nitroreductase, encoded by *snrA*, has been cloned (58); however, *snrA* is deleted in strain TA98, which carries a particularly large Δ*uvrB* deletion, so the mechanism of 1,8-dinitropyrene reduction remains to be determined.

Following growth of Ames tester strain TA98 on agar plates containing bacteriotoxic levels of 1,8-DNP, a derivative strain was isolated that proved to be highly resistant to 1,8-DNP mutagenicity (59). This strain (TA98/1,8-DNP$_6$) was initially thought to be nitroreductase-deficient. In fact, it lacks acetyl CoA:*N*-hydroxyarylamine *O*-acetyltransferase (OAT) activity (60). The OAT enzyme activates hydroxylamine metabolites of nitro compounds and arylamines, within the bacterial cell, to form reactive *N*-acetoxy esters (see chapters 13 and 17).

Takehiko Nohmi and colleagues, National Institute of Health Sciences, Tokyo, cloned the gene encoding *Salmonella* OAT (which also possesses acetyl CoA:aromatic amine *N*-acetyltransferase (NAT) activity) by screening on the basis of the gene's enhancement of 1,8-DNP toxicity. The gene was reintroduced into TA98/1,8-DNP$_6$ on a multicopy plasmid. The resulting strains are much more sensitive than TA98 to the mutagenicity of aromatic nitro and amino compounds (61). The genes encoding two forms of the human enzyme have also been introduced into Ames test strains (62). This innovation allows the consequences of biotransformation by mammalian hepatic enzymes to be studied in bacterial mutagenicity assay systems (63). ◀

of the carbon black powder with nitric acid during the toner production process. Manufacturers of toner responded quickly, finding alternative procedures that eliminated the formation of these mutagenic impurities. However, nitropyrenes and other nitrated PAHs are also formed in diesel engines and other combustion processes (*55*) and may be found at levels as high as parts per billion in soil from urban areas (*56*). The discovery of this previously unknown class of mutagens demonstrated the practical value of the Ames test in environmental toxicology.

Flame Retardants

A swatch from a pair of child's pyjamas proved to be mutagenic in the Ames test, and the cause was soon tracked down: the fabric had been treated with the flame-retardant chemical tris: tris(2,3-dibromopropyl) phosphate (TDBP; figure 4-7) (*64–67*). TDBP has also been used as a flame-retardant additive in polystyrene and polyurethane foams. Both TDBP and its metabolite 2-bromoacrolein are mutagens in Ames strain TA100. TDBP proved to be a carcinogen in rats and mice. Use of TDBP in children's sleepwear was banned (USA) in 1977.

Another important class of environmental mutagens that was first detected by application of the Ames test to complex mixtures, the protein pyrolysis product heterocyclic amines, is discussed in chapter 17.

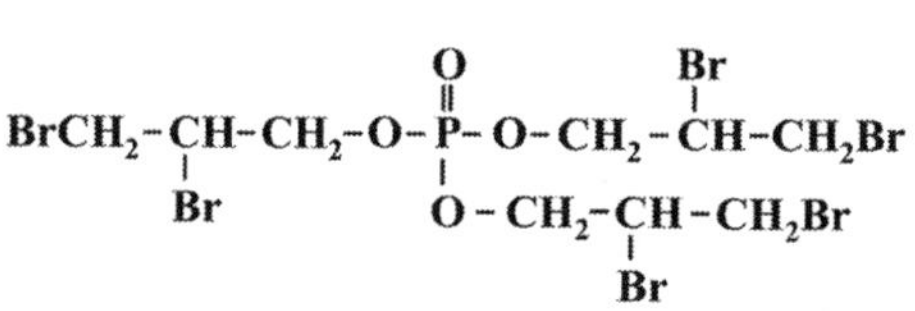

$$BrCH_2-\underset{\underset{Br}{|}}{CH}-CH_2-O-\underset{\underset{O-CH_2-\underset{\underset{Br}{|}}{CH}-CH_2Br}{|}}{\overset{\overset{O}{\|}}{P}}-O-CH_2-\underset{\underset{Br}{|}}{CH}-CH_2Br$$

FIGURE 4-7.

The mutagenic flame-retardant chemical tris: tris(2,3-dibromopropyl) phosphate.

MUTATION ASSAYS: DNA SEQUENCE
ANALYSIS OF MUTANTS

DNA sequencing is now so routine that it is hard to imagine how mutation research was conducted without access to it. But the Ames test, for example, was established by phenotypic screening of histidine-requiring bacterial mutants, without knowledge of the DNA sequences of the target genes. (In fact, the first evidence concerning the nature of the frameshift mutational target in *S. typhimurium hisD3052*, the allele present in TA98, was obtained by purifying histidinol dehydrogenase enzyme and sequencing the protein (*68*). This approach is now antiquated.) The discovery of the PCR, and the rapid decline in cost (and improvement in reliability) of DNA sequencing, driven by the requirements of the Human Genome Project during the 1990s, have opened up the study of mutagenesis at the molecular level.

MUTATIONAL FINGERPRINTS

As stated at the outset of this chapter, even spontaneous mutagenic events are not "random": their distribution is strongly influenced by the nature of the DNA sequence target. Such effects are even more strongly apparent when we examine mutations induced by specific chemical agents. We refer to a "spectrum" or "fingerprint" characterizing the mutagenic effects of a specific chemical. Many mutagens have been examined for their mutational specificity. Why has so much effort been put into these studies? Investigations of mutational specificity probe the molecular mechanisms of mutagenesis, examining the interactions between DNA polymerases and mutagen-derived DNA damages. Furthermore, as molecular detectives, we may be able to recognize the fingerprint of a mutagen that we have "on file." This is being tested by cataloguing the mutations seen in tumor suppressor genes and oncogenes in human tumors and comparing them to fingerprints of mutagens that might have induced the tumors, such as aflatoxin and liver cancer (*69*), or UV light and skin cancer (*70*). Similarity of a tumor spectrum and a known mutational fingerprint does not prove causation (eyewitnesses to crimes can also be confused by multiple suspects with similar appearances), but at least it is suggestive evidence.

A particularly clear mutational fingerprint is demonstrated by alkylating agents: induction of G:C → A:T transitions accounts for almost all of the base substitutions induced by these agents. This example is discussed in detail in chapter 15. Other mutagens can give rise to very different patterns of mutation. Ohta and colleagues used the *lacZ* assay system to study the mutational specificities of several DNA cross-linking agents. Like alkylating agents, *cis*-platinum mainly induced G:C → A:T transitions. Mitomycin C induced only G:C → T:A transversions; psoralen plus UV radiation induced A:T → G:C transitions (*71*). In chapter 3, we noted that 8-oxodeoxyguanosine damage induces G:C → T:A transversion mutations. These base-substitutions and G:C → C:G transversions dominate the mutational spectra of oxidants such as ozone (*72*) and other agents that induce oxidative stress (*73*).

SITE SPECIFICITY OF MUTAGENESIS

In addition to specificity in the induction of particular classes of mutational events, mutagens may also be *site specific*. That is, the positional distribution of mutations within a genetic target is nonuniform. Particularly mutable sites are known as hot-spots; we saw a striking example of a hot-spot in the *hisD3052* reversion spectrum presented earlier. Hot-spots were first observed in Seymour Benzer's early experiments on the fine-structure genetic mapping of *rII* mutants in bacteriophage T4 (*74*), which proved that the base pair is the smallest unit of mutation and recombination.

Many factors influence the distribution of hot-spots within a gene. First, phenotypic selection may induce a bias: certain codons within the gene correspond to critical amino acid residues, whose alteration causes profound changes in protein structure and function. Other codons correspond to residues that may be substituted without significant effects on the protein's function. Different mutagens can target different hot-spots. The local DNA sequence may influence the susceptibility of a particular base to chemical damage, via local secondary structure effects. For similar reasons, lesions in different sites may be repaired with different efficiencies. Local sequences, such as palindromes or runs of repeated bases, may also influence mutational mechanisms, as discussed below.

▶ The Streisinger Slippage Mechanism

A simple and yet deep insight into the process of mutagenesis was achieved by George Streisinger (75) in 1966 (76, 77). Streisinger realized that repeated sequences along a DNA molecule would be "slippery," especially at the time of replication, when the strands separate. When repeated sequences are present, one strand (template or daughter strand) can slip and reanneal to the complementary strand, offset by an integral number of repeats. Replication from such a slipped intermediate would result in gain or loss of an integral number of repeats, depending on which strand of the duplex slips (figure 4-8). Streisinger predicted—long before DNA sequencing or the PCR was invented—that *repeated sequences would be hot-spots for frameshift mutations* and that *the resulting frameshifts would represent gain or loss of an integral number of repeat units*. This prediction has been fully verified, as exemplified by the $(CpG)_4$ hot-spot in the Ames test strain TA98 (see above) and by the trinucleotide-repeat expansions observed in certain human genetic diseases (see chapter 3). ◀

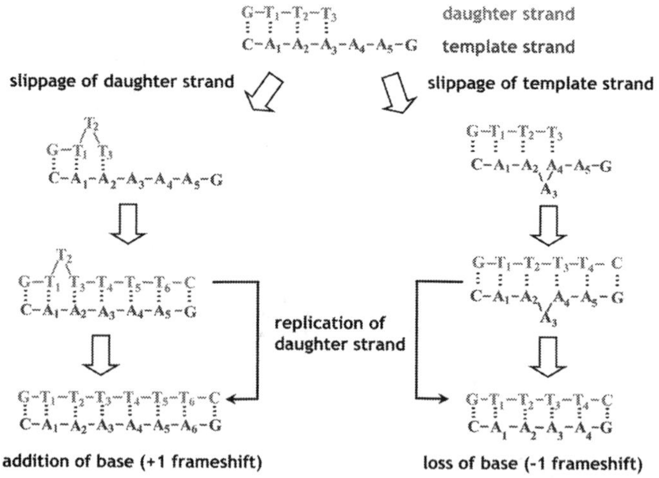

FIGURE 4-8.

The frameshift mutation mechanism proposed by Streisinger. Insertion of an additional A into a run of A residues is illustrated. *Note*: A full-color version of this figure appears on the website.

MAMMALIAN MUTAGENICITY ASSAY SYSTEMS

Since eukaryotic cells are diploid, many mutations arising in mammalian cells cannot be selected directly, since the second copy of the gene complements the first. To circumvent this problem, we can study hemizygous (or functionally hemizygous) genes, such as the X-linked *hprt* gene (*78*) or heterozygous cell lines, such as $tk^{+/-}$ (thymidine kinase) human lymphoblastoid cells (*79*). These assays are most often conducted with fibroblasts, which grow well in vitro but may be poor surrogates for the target cells for human cancer.

Indirect genotoxicity endpoints are also commonly used in mammalian cell studies, including unscheduled DNA synthesis (UDS), a measure of DNA repair (*80*); sister chromatid exchange, a measure of chromosome breakage (*81*); and the "comet" assay for DNA strand breakage, already discussed in chapter 3 (*82–84*).

TRANSGENIC RODENT MUTATION ASSAYS

In the 1990s a new type of mutation assay was developed, based on transgenic rodent technology (*85–88*). Bacterial "reporter" genes, which can serve as targets for detecting mutations, are incorporated into the chromosomes of transgenic mice or rats. The reporter genes are present in all cells of the animal, allowing mutagenesis to be measured even in tissues or cells in which no good endogenous endpoints are available (*89*). Although it may be argued that such transgenes (which are usually nontranscribed) are imperfect surrogates for the behavior of endogenous mammalian genes, the sensitivity and generality of the transgene mutation assays have made them important tools in mutation research.

Two obstacles had to be overcome to construct such assays: getting the transgenes into the animals, and getting them back out again. The first obstacle was removed when techniques for construction of transgenic rodents were invented, as discussed in chapter 8. To examine the transgene for mutations, the corresponding DNA must be recovered from the huge excess of endogenous rodent DNA in each cell. There are several ways to accomplish this, but the most common method is to exploit the bacteriophage λ cos site system, as explained below. An *E. coli* target gene is carried on a modified bacteriophage λ genome that, in turn, is introduced into one of the rodent chromosomes. In a mutagenesis assay, the transgenic rodent is treated with a suspected mutagen and the transgene is subsequently recovered from the rodent cells and tested for mutagenesis using an *E. coli* assay.

Let us recall some features of bacteriophage λ biology. The λ genome is "bracketed" by cohesive ends (*cos* sites). These are short DNA sequences recognized by the enzymatic machinery of bacteriophage λ. When the virus infects *E. coli*, it directs the cell to make λ-encoded proteins (which constitute, and assemble, bacteriophage "heads" and "tails") and, of course, to replicate λ chromosomes. The λ DNA is synthesized by "rolling circle" replication as a linear concatemer of many tandemly repeated λ genomes. Protein factors encoded by λ recognize and bind to the *cos* sites that bracket each copy of the λ genome, cut the DNA at these sites, and then stuff the λ DNA into the λ heads to form infective virus particles.

Bacteriophage λ-based vectors are widely used in molecular biology, and the mechanics of obtaining virus particles from λ DNA are well established. "Packaging extract," a protein preparation obtained from λ-infected *E. coli*, is mixed with λ DNA, and infectious virus particles self-assemble in vitro. The same strategy is used to rescue the transgene from the mammalian genome. Chromosomal DNA is purified and mixed with packaging extract, which recognizes the λ *cos* sites bracketing the transgene, excises the insert from the chromosome, and packages it into virus particles. Mutations in the transgene carried on the bacteriophage λ genome can be scored following infection of bacteria. An important feature of this system is that it allows one to separate the mutagenic event (which occurs in the mammalian cells) from mutation selection (which occurs in the bacteria). The absence of selection pressure in the rodent makes it possible to study mutagenesis in any rodent tissue using these systems.

Another strategy for recovery of a transgene insert from mammalian cells is plasmid rescue (*90, 91*). This is another technique based on *lac* operon biology: in this case, taking advantage of the very high binding affinity of Lac repressor protein for *lac* operator. The transgene construct is an *E. coli* plasmid that carries *lacZ* as a mutational target, along with *lac* operator sequences. The chromosomal DNA is digested with a restriction enzyme. LacI repressor protein (which binds the plasmid fragments via the *lac* operator sequence) is conjugated to magnetic beads and used for affinity purification of the transgene DNA. The plasmids are then introduced into *E. coli* (by electroporation) for mutation analysis.

Now let us examine some transgene mutation assay constructs in more detail. The two most widely used systems, the Big Blue™ mouse (and rat) and the Muta™ mouse, are based on *E. coli lacI* and *lacZ* transgenes, respectively.

Big Blue™ Mouse and Rat

In the Big Blue™ transgenic mouse system, the marker transgene is *lacI*, contained in a λ vector present in a concatemer (approximately 40 copies), in a C57Bl mouse genetic background. The Big Blue™ insert (figure 4-9) includes the *lacI* gene along with required λ genes. When the λ particles incorporating the transgene DNA are assembled and infected into *lacI*⁻ *E. coli* cells, bacteriophage carrying wild-type *lacI* repress the lac operon and bacteriophage carrying mutated *lacI* do not. In either case, the bacteriophage infection forms a plaque on the bacterial lawn (figure 4-10).

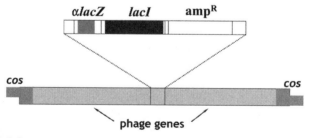

FIGURE 4-9.

The λ transgene construct in the Big Blue™ mouse and rat (schematic). The cos sites are separated by about 45 kb. See text for details. *Note*: A full-color version of this figure appears on the website.

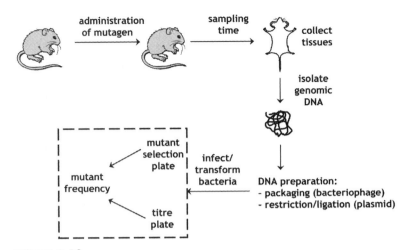

FIGURE 4-10.

Flow chart of experimental protocol for determining chemical mutagenesis in vivo with a transgenic assay.

The indicator substrate X-gal (see earlier discussion of the *lac* operon) is incorporated in the plates, so the wild-type plaques are clear and the rare mutant plaques are blue, and can be counted by eye.

That was the original plan for the Big Blue™ system. However, it was soon recognized that since induced mutant frequencies are typically on the order of 10^{-5}, experiments required the scanning of very large numbers of plaques, making the assay both tedious and expensive. John Jakubczak et al. (*92*) noted that the Big Blue™ λ construct also carries the λ *cII* transgene. *cII* protein is involved in the lytic vs. lysogenic decision process, that is, it is required for λ, a temperate bacteriophage, to escape from the lytic replication mode that kills the host cell (*18*). Of course, the *cII* transgene is susceptible to mutagenesis, just as is *lacI*. Under appropriate conditions and with appropriate *E. coli* host strains, only bacteriophage carrying mutant *cII* transgenes will form plaques. This permits a selective plaque-forming assay, in which mutants can be scored directly by enumerating plaques. This variation on the Big Blue™ assay has become preferred to the originally planned *lacI*-based analysis. (Another advantage of the *cII* assay is the small size of the gene, which can easily be sequenced in a single run.)

Muta Mouse

This transgenic mouse line is based on a recombinant λgt10 bacteriophage vector containing the entire *E. coli lacZ* gene. Mutations occurring in the *lacZ* gene are measured by positive selection of *lacZ⁻* mutants on P-gal-containing medium (*93*).

In the following is an illustration of the application of the Big Blue™ system to the study of chemically induced mutagenesis in the rat. Mugimane Manjanatha and colleagues (*94*) examined the effects of the PAH mammary carcinogen 7,12-dimethylbenz[*a*]anthracene (DMBA; see chapter 18) on the mammary glands of female Big Blue™ rats. The seven-week-old animals were treated (gavage) with 130 mg/kg DMBA in 2 mL sesame oil, or with vehicle alone. After a given number of weeks, rats were sacrificed, mammary gland tissues were removed, and chromosomal DNA

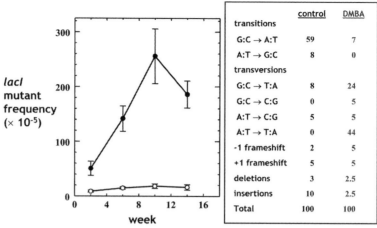

FIGURE 4-11.

7,12-Dimethylbenz[*a*]anthracene-induced mutagenesis in the *lacI* transgene, female Big Blue™ rat mammary gland. The graph shows mutant frequency as a function of time after administration of DMBA (solid circles) or vehicle alone (open circles). The table at right gives the % of each category of mutation observed in lacI mutations from control and treated animals. (*Data from Manjanatha, M. G.; Shelton, S. D.; Culp, S. J.; Blankenship, L. R.; Casciano, D. A. DNA adduct formation and molecular analysis of in vivo lacI mutations in the mammary tissue of Big Blue rats treated with 7,12-dimethylbenz[a]anthracene.* Carcinogenesis **2000**, *21, 265–273.*)

was purified and processed for determination of *lacI* mutant[7] frequency. The results are shown in figure 4-11. The mutagenic activity of DMBA in the rat mammary gland is clearly apparent, increasing with time over a period of many weeks after dosing. This increase may indicate both the continuing systemic mobilization and activation of the hydrophobic PAH, and the ongoing process of cell division and mutagenesis in the target tissue. *lacI* mutants were also sequenced, and data on mutational specificity are also shown in the figure. The difference between the spontaneous (no-DMBA animals) and induced mutational specificity is also striking (table is shown in figure 4-11). G:C → A:T transitions dominate the spontaneous spectrum and 70% of these occur at CpG hot-spot sites. Relatively few G:C → A:T transitions are observed among the mutations in the DMBA-treated animals. The DMBA-induced mutants are mainly G:C → T:A and A:T → T:A transversions.

CONSTRUCTION OF ADDUCTED OLIGONUCLEOTIDES

The processes leading from mutagen exposure to mutations are highly divergent. Even a single chemical agent may be metabolized to multiple reactive species; each such species may yield several different adducts;[8] and DNA adducts can be formed at an almost limitless number of positions within the genome (figure 4-12). Consequently, many different molecular mechanisms may contribute to mutagenesis by any given chemical. Rather than trying to disentangle these processes, we can use chemical and

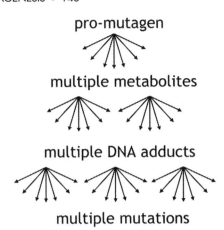

FIGURE 4-12.
Divergent pathways of mutagenesis by a single chemical; see text.

biochemical methods to place a *defined DNA alteration* (e.g., a specific modified base) at a *predetermined position* in a piece of DNA (e.g., a cloning vector), and then examine the mutations that result from its replication in a host cell. This approach, pioneered by John Essigman (*95*), has been applied to a wide variety of mutagens, including alkylating agents (*95*), thymine dimers, aminofluorene adducts, 8-hydroxyguanine, etc.

Even a cloning vector is too large to be modified directly in a site-specific manner, so the modification is performed on an oligonucleotide, which is subsequently ligated into the chosen vector. Once the site-specifically adducted oligonucleotide is in hand, it can be annealed with a complementary oligonucleotide (containing a mismatched base opposite the adducted base, if desired) and structural analysis (X-ray crystallography or NMR) can be performed to study the effect of the modified base on base pairing and DNA conformation.

How can we prepare an oligonucleotide containing a defined adduct, in a defined position? Two distinct strategies are as follows. (i) *Oligonucleotide first.* Many mutagens are selectively reactive with a single type of base, as we have already seen (e.g., aromatic amine C8 guanine adducts). A single-strand oligonucleotide is synthesized, containing only a single residue of that (target) base (*96, 97*), and is then treated with the reagent; adduct formation should occur exclusively (or predominantly) at that single site, although purification may be needed to obtain a homogeneous product. (ii) *Adduct first.* The modified base of interest is synthesized and converted to a phosphoramidite, suitable for use in solid-phase DNA synthesis; the oligonucleotide is then assembled, substituting the modified base at the desired site. Chemical protection/deprotection of the modified base may be necessary (*98, 99*). A variation on this strategy is incorporation of a modified base that can subsequently be converted into the adduct of interest (*100*).

MUTAGENICITY ASSAYS WITH SITE-SPECIFICALLY MODIFIED VECTORS

Adducted DNA prepared as described above can be used in mutagenesis assays. An in vitro approach is to prepare a labeled primer and allow DNA

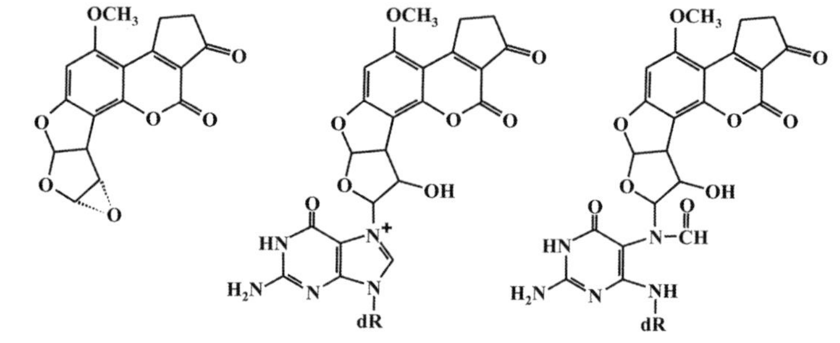

FIGURE 4-13.
Left: aflatoxin B_1 exo-8,9-epoxide; centre: AFB_1 N7–guanine adduct; right: AFB1–fapy adduct.

polymerase to extend it, using the adduct-containing single strand as template; frequencies of misincorporation opposite the adduct are measured by sequencing the extended primer strand. The adducted oligonucleotide can also be incorporated into a plasmid, viral genome, or shuttle vector, which can be propagated in cells; mutant progeny are selected phenotypically.

Let us illustrate the application of this technology by examining a recent study[9] of the mutagenicity of the carcinogenic fungal toxin aflatoxin B_1 (AFB_1; see also chapters 7 and 11). AFB_1 is implicated in human hepatocellular carcinoma, especially in tropical regions where *Aspergillus flavus* commonly contaminates stored grain. The tumor suppressor gene *p53* is often mutated in these cancers, and the mutational "signature" believed to be associated with AFB_1 is a G:C → T:A transversion at the third position of *p53* codon 249 (*101*). Indeed, this mutation is commonly induced by aflatoxin in short-term mutation assays. But what is the premutagenic lesion that induces this mutation? P450-catalyzed oxidation of AFB_1 produces the *exo*-8,9-epoxide derivative, which forms an adduct at the N7 nitrogen atom of guanine (figure 4-13). This primary N7 adduct can decompose to form a ring-opened adduct similar to fapy (see chapter 3). Also, as with other guanine N7 adducts, facile hydrolysis of the glycosylic bond generates apurinic sites. Which of these damages is the most biologically important? Smela et al. (*102*) compared the mutational consequences of site-specific AFB_1 fapy vs. AFB_1 N7 adducts. The M13 single-stranded bacteriophage vector was used as the carrier of the adduct. The oligonucleotide CCTCTTCGAACTC, containing a single guanine, was prepared and treated with AFB_1 epoxide, yielding AFB_1 guanine N7. Treatment with pH 10 buffer was used to convert the N7 adduct partially to the fapy adduct, and the two adducts were separated and purified by HPLC. The AFB_1 fapy or AFB_1 N7 adducts were ligated into M13 vectors; the oligonucleotide sequence is within the *lacI* gene, as discussed below.

The adduct-containing M13 ssDNA genome was introduced into *E. coli* strains (several strains were studied, with or without expression of the error-prone polymerases MucAB and UmuDC; see chapter 3). The yield of infective M13 particles following introduction (by electroporation) of the adducted bacteriophage genomes into *E. coli* is a measure of the ability of the bacterial DNA polymerases to replicate the adducted DNA, and provides information about the *replication-blocking* characteristics of the adducts. Indeed, adducted M13 DNA was replicated less efficiently (by as much as three orders of magnitude) than a nonadducted control, and the AFB_1 fapy adduct blocked replication much more severely than did the AFB_1 N7 adduct.

The M13-based mutation assay used in this study also exploits *lac* operon biology. The adducted oligonucleotide lies within the coding sequence of the *E. coli lacZ* gene carried on the recombinant M13 construct. Progeny phage carrying the wild-type *lacZ* sequence produce functional β-galactosidase and give dark-blue plaques on X-gal (see discussion of lac operon earlier in this chapter) plates. The guanine bearing the adduct is the first base of a *lacZ* codon specifying a glutamate residue (GAA). If the anticipated G:C → T:A transversion mutation occurs at this site, the codon is changed to TAA, which is an "ochre" stop codon. One would expect a truncated, nonfunctional β-galactosidase product and a colorless plaque— but this phenotype could not be distinguished from other classes of *lacZ⁻* mutants (base substitutions at other sites, deletions, etc.). To pick out the G:C → T:A transversion mutants, the assay was performed in an *E. coli* strain that partially suppresses (i.e., reads through) ochre codons. A small amount of active enzyme is produced, despite the ochre mutation, and light-blue plaques result. The key finding of the mutagenesis study was that the AFB_1 fapy adduct was approximately six times as effective as the AFB_1 N7 adduct at the induction of G:C → T:A transversions.

SPONTANEOUS MUTATIONS

As we have already noted, mutations arise even in the absence of treatment with chemical mutagens. What are the molecular origins of spontaneous mutations (*103*)? DNA polymerases misincorporate bases at a low but nonzero rate; proofreading activity and mismatch repair correct most, but not all of these errors. Natural background radiation and endogenous production of reactive oxygen species cause DNA damage, as discussed previously. One should bear in mind, too, that even the most carefully composed growth medium or animal feed will contain some traces of environmental mutagens, so "control" samples are not necessarily free of mutagen exposure.

DNA bases exist in equilibrium between the common keto/imino and rare enol/amino tautomers; the rare tautomers can form mismatched base pairs that may "fool" DNA polymerase into inserting the incorrect base in the daughter strand. The biological significance of this mechanism has been disputed, however, since there is very little direct evidence concerning the prevalence of rare tautomers in DNA (as opposed to monomeric bases or nucleosides) (*104*). Studies of mutational specificity can provide some insight into the factors contributing to spontaneous mutagenesis.

▶ Do Environmental Chemicals Cause Heritable Damage to the Genome?

Many examples of chemically induced cancers are described in this text; particularly prominent environmental carcinogens are tobacco-related toxicants, estimated to cause 30% of all human cancers. Experiments in mice, *Drosophila*, and other model organisms have demonstrated the ability of genotoxins to damage both males and female germ cells (*105*). Do environmental chemicals cause mutations in human germ cells, such that environmental exposures account for a measurable proportion of human genetic diseases? Definitive evidence for environmentally induced genetic disease in humans is still lacking, but advances in genomics and molecular

continues next page

continued from previous page

biology may soon provide answers to this important question (*106, 107*) and screening of the population for clinically significant mutations should be feasible in the near future.

By definition, a genetic disease results from one or more heritable mutations. However, variant alleles have been accumulating in the human population for as long as our species has existed, and it is far from easy to ascertain the mechanisms (spontaneous or environmentally induced) by which they originally arose. Most of the common human birth defects, such as spina bifida and cleft palate, are developmental rather than genetic in origin. Genetic defects may be inherited or they may arise as new ("de novo") mutations, either in the parents' gametes or during the development of the embryo. The molecular basis of such defects may be cytogenetic (chromosomal damage, particularly whole or partial chromosome aneuploidies) or small scale (e.g., point mutations). Animal experiments indicate that germ cells are less sensitive to the action of DNA damaging agents than are somatic cells. Whether this reflects more active/more faithful DNA repair in germ cells or pharmacological sequestering of such cells from chemical exposure is not clear.

We observe a wide spectrum of different genetic diseases in the population, and the incidence of each disease is small; most of them are not monogenic in origin, but depend on several genes. Because of this complexity, it is very difficult to correlate adverse outcomes with particular environmental exposures. (This situation can be contrasted with the relatively high incidence of, for example, smoking-induced lung cancer.) Nevertheless, it may be time to renew the search for chemical causes of human genetic disease, with the aid of improved human monitoring and genetic analysis.

The on-line human mutation database (*108*) gathers data on mutations causing inherited disease in humans. As of January 2005, the database contains more than 44,000 mutations in more than 1700 different human genes. However, each mutation identified is entered into the database only once. Therefore, this database does not provide information about mutation rates or potential mutation hot-spots.

Analyses of mutations in the hemophilia B gene factor IX, which is a potential sentinel gene for germline genetic damage, have been performed by Steve Sommer and colleagues (City of Hope Medical Center, Duarte, California) (*109*). Approximately 80% of the mutations causing this form of hemophilia were found to have been inherited; 20% were new mutations. Improvements in medical care have increased the reproductive (Darwinian) fitness of hemophiliacs, and most of the inherited mutations probably occurred in recent generations. Sommer's group observed that factor IX mutation patterns did not vary greatly among different ethnic groups or geographic regions, and they concluded that the mechanisms of germline mutation in the factor IX gene are primarily endogenous rather than environmental.

Can we identify specific "sentinel" genetic diseases appropriate for germ cell monitoring? Which genetic diseases would be the best such sentinels (*110*)? Since all genetic diseases are rare, we would be well advised to look at the most common, particularly those with a substantial proportion of de novo mutations; possible candidates include NF1 (neurofibromatosis), HemB (hemophilia), HFE (hereditary hemochromatosis), and PKU (phenylketonuria). In order to relate germ cell mutations to environmental exposures, it would be necessary to differentiate new from inherited mutations, a task that is now feasible. The effects of the sentinel genes should be highly penetrant (i.e., give rise to obvious phenotypes). Mutations in genes for dominant or X-linked diseases would provide a phenotype after one hit. Among the more common examples are the genetically dominant diseases Duchenne muscular dystrophy (DMD), NF1, ACH (achondroplasia), and recessive hemophilia. Common recessive diseases for which a second hit could be readily identified might also be informative. For example, cystic fibrosis (CF) is the most common inherited disease among populations of European background (*111*), and this disease is likely to be monitored routinely, by genotyping, in the near future. Standard genetic testing would reveal cases of de novo mutations.

The genes for DMD and NF1 are very large, making molecular analysis difficult. Some gene targets (e.g., ACH) are too small to provide an adequate target for analysis of diverse types of DNA–chemical interactions. Diverse spectra of mutations have been recovered from LDLR (low-density lipoprotein receptor gene, causing familial hypercholesterolemia), NF1, CF, and the hemophilia genes HemA and Hem B. Genes already monitored routinely at birth could provide important data on de novo mutations. PKU is in this category, although the current test for the condition is biochemical rather than genetic.

What are the likely sources of exposure to environmental mutagens, and what types of damage should we expect to see? Tobacco smoke probably represents one of the major sources of environmental genotoxins involved in the causation of human genetic disease. As discussed elsewhere (e.g., chapters 5 and 18), tobacco smoke contains hundreds of toxic and mutagenic compounds, such as polycyclic aromatic hydrocarbons and nitrosamines. Andrew Wyrobek and his colleagues (University of California, Berkeley) have obtained cytogenetic evidence of damage to human sperm induced by environmental agents, such as cancer chemotherapeutic drugs (*112*) and cigarette smoke. Perhaps surprisingly, however, the smoking status of the parents of children born with birth defects is not yet routinely recorded.[10] ◀

Notes

1. Pangloss, the fictional philosopher in Volatire's *Candide*, could convince you that even the worst tragedy was actually a blessing in disguise.

2. *Replica plating:* a sample of a bacterial or yeast culture is mutagenized, diluted, and plated on Petri dishes containing minimal (salts + glucose) agar medium supplemented with a nutrient, such as a particular amino acid. Once colonies have started to grow, a piece of sterile velvet stretched over a wooden block is pressed onto the Petri dish, and then pressed onto a second ("replica") dish. The replica dish contains minimal agar medium only. Auxotrophic mutants will grow on the first dish, but not on the replica.

3. To be precise, the inducer is *allolactose,* an isomer of lactose formed, in part, by the action of β-galactosidase.

4. An unusual feature of this enzyme is *alpha complementation.* This phenomenon, like so many aspects of *lac* biology, was discovered by Monod and co-workers. Mutants expressing a β-galactosidase protein that is missing a small section of peptide near the amino-terminus are inactive (e.g., *lacZΔM15*, which lacks the codons for residues 12–42). But when such a mutant protein is combined with a short (and, obviously, inactive) peptide fragment corresponding to only the first 60 residues of β-galactosidase, enzyme activity is restored! The short peptide binds noncovalently to the large one and re-forms an active tetrameric holoenzyme. This circumstance is exploited in many vectors used in molecular biology. The coding sequence for the short fragment (*lacZα* peptide) is carried on the vector. When such a vector is introduced into an *E. coli lacZΔM15* strain, the strain is converted to *lacZ*$^+$. But if the *lacZα* peptide sequence on the vector has been disrupted by insertion of a recombinant gene, alpha complementation no longer occurs and the resulting strain remains *lacZ*$^-$. The two types of strains can be distinguished by plating on X-gal medium, the well-known "blue/white" screening technique (*28*).

5. Note that the characteristics of the various strains subsequent to the histidine mutations were introduced independently; the Δ*uvrB* deletions in strains TA98 and TA100 removed 125 kb and 50 kb of neighboring chromosomal DNA, respectively (*37*).

6. An "S9 mix" is prepared, containing S9 (post-mitochondrial supernatant), NADP$^+$, and glucose-6-phosphate, which drives NADP$^+$ reduction via the activity of glucose-6-phosphate dehydrogenase.

7. We refer to mutant, rather than mutation, frequency, since the assay measures the proportion of mutations prevalent at a given time, not necessarily the frequency of induction of new mutations.

8. Alkylating agents, for example, probably react to some extent with every nucleophilic site in DNA: ring and exocyclic N atoms and exocyclic O atoms of all the bases, phosphodiester O atoms, etc.

9. Some details of the work have been simplified in this summary.

10. Rosalie Elespuru, Division of Biology, Office of Science & Engineering Laboratories, Center for Devices & Radiological Health, US Food and Drug Administration. (Disclaimer: The views expressed are those of the author and do not represent FDA policy.)

References

1. Brandenburger, A.; Godson, G. N.; Radman, M.; Glickman, B. W.; van Sluis, C. A.; Doubleday, O. P. Radiation-induced base substitution mutagenesis in single-stranded DNA phage M13. *Nature* **1981,** *294,* 180–182.

2. Hogervorst, F. B.; Cornelis, R. S.; Bout, M.; van Vliet, M.; Oosterwijk, J. C.; Olmer, R.; Bakker, B.; Klijn, J. G.; Vasen, H. F.; Meijers-Heijboer, H. Rapid detection of BRCA1 mutations by the protein truncation test. *Nat. Genet.* **1995,** *10,* 208–212.

3. Tsui, L. C. The cystic fibrosis transmembrane conductance regulator gene. *Am. J. Respir. Crit. Care Med.* **1995,** *151,* S47–S53.

4. Dobzhansky, T. *Genetics of the Evolutionary Process;* Columbia University Press: New York, 1970.

5. Ripley, L. S. Predictability of mutant sequences. Relationships between mutational mechanisms and mutant specificity. *Ann. N.Y. Acad. Sci.* **1999,** *870,* 159–172.

6. Surralles, J.; Ramirez, M. J.; Marcos, R.; Natarajan, A. T.; Mullenders, L. H. Clusters of transcription-coupled repair in the human genome. *Proc. Natl. Acad. Sci. USA* **2002,** *99,* 10571–10574.

7. Svejstrup, J. Q. Mechanisms of transcription-coupled DNA repair. *Nat. Rev. Mol. Cell Biol.* **2002,** *3,* 21–29.

8. Berg, J. M.; Tymoczko, J. L.; Stryer, L. *Biochemistry;* WH Freeman: New York, 2001.

9. Rosenberg, M. S.; Subramanian, S.; Kumar, S. Patterns of transitional mutation biases within and among mammalian genomes. *Mol. Biol. Evol.* **2003,** *20,* 988–993.

10. Zhang, Z.; Gerstein, M. Patterns of nucleotide substitution, insertion and deletion in the human genome inferred from pseudogenes. *Nucleic Acids Res.* **2003,** *31,* 5338–5348.

11. Campbell, E. A.; Korzheva, N.; Mustaev, A.; Murakami, K.; Nair, S.; Goldfarb, A.; Darst, S. A. Structural mechanism for rifampicin inhibition of bacterial RNA polymerase. *Cell* **2001,** *104,* 901–912.

12. DeMarini, D. M.; Shelton, M. L.; Abu-Shakra, A.; Szakmary, A.; Levine, J. G. Spectra of spontaneous frameshift mutations at the *hisD3052* allele of *Salmonella typhimurium* in four DNA repair backgrounds. *Genetics* **1998,** *149,* 17–36.

13. Levine, J. G.; Schaaper, R. M.; DeMarini, D. M. Complex frameshift mutations mediated by plasmid pKM101: mutational mechanisms deduced from 4-aminobiphenyl-induced mutation spectra in *Salmonella. Genetics* **1994,** *136,* 731–746.

14. Coulondre, C.; Miller, J. H. Genetic studies of the lac repressor. IV. Mutagenic specificity in the *lacI* gene of *Escherichia coli. J. Mol. Biol.* **1977,** *117,* 577–606.

15. de Boer, J. G.; Glickman, B. W. The lacI gene as a target for mutation in transgenic rodents and *Escherichia coli. Genetics* **1998,** *148,* 1441–1451.

16. Müller-Hill, B. *The lac Operon: A Short History of a Genetic Paradigm;* de Gruyter: Berlin, 1996.

17. Wang, X. G.; Olsen, L. R.; Roderick, S. L. Structure of the lac operon galactoside acetyltransferase. *Structure (Camb.)* **2002,** *10,* 581–588.

18. Ptashne, M. *A Genetic Switch: Gene Control and Phage λ;* Blackwell Scientific: Palo Alto, CA, 1987.

19. Bell, C. E.; Lewis, M. The Lac repressor: a second generation of structural and functional studies. *Curr. Opin. Struct. Biol.* **2001,** *11,* 19–25.

20. Markiewicz, P.; Kleina, L. G.; Cruz, C.; Ehret, S.; Miller, J. H. Genetic studies of the lac repressor: XIV. Analysis of 4000 altered *Escherichia coli lac* repressors reveals essential and non-essential residues, as well as "spacers" which do not require a specific sequence. *J. Mol. Biol.* **1994,** *240*, 421–433.

21. Barry, J. K.; Matthews, K. S. Ligand-induced conformational changes in lactose repressor: a fluorescence study of single tryptophan mutants. *Biochemistry* **1997,** *36*, 15632–15642.

22. Oehler, S.; Amouyal, M.; Kolkhof, P.; Wilcken-Bergmann, B.; Müller-Hill, B. Quality and position of the three *lac* operators of *E. coli* define efficiency of repression. *EMBO J.* **1994,** *13*, 3348–3355.

23. Reznikoff, W. S. The lactose operon-controlling elements: a complex paradigm. *Mol. Microbiol.* **1992,** 6, 2419–2422.

24. Horwitz, J. P.; Chua, J.; Curby, R. J.; Tomson, A. J.; Darooge, M. A.; Fisher, B. E.; Mauricio, J.; Klundt, I. Substrates for cytochemical demonstration of enzyme activity: i. Some substituted 3-indolyl-beta-D-glycopyranosides. *J. Med. Chem.* **1964,** *53*, 574–575.

25. Lewis, M.; Chang, G.; Horton, N. C.; Kercher, M. A.; Pace, H. C.; Schumacher, M. A.; Brennan, R. G.; Lu, P. Crystal structure of the lactose operon repressor and its complexes with DNA and inducer. *Science* **1996,** *271*, 1247–1254.

26. Jacobson, R. H.; Zhang, X. J.; DuBose, R. F.; Matthews, B. W. Three-dimensional structure of beta-galactosidase from *E. coli*. *Nature* **1994,** *369*, 761–766.

27. Juers, D. H.; Jacobson, R. H.; Wigley, D.; Zhang, X. J.; Huber, R. E.; Tronrud, D. E.; Matthews, B. W. High resolution refinement of beta-galactosidase in a new crystal form reveals multiple metal-binding sites and provides a structural basis for alpha-complementation. *Protein Sci.* **2000,** *9*, 1685–1699.

28. Slilaty, S. N.; Lebel, S. Accurate insertional inactivation of lacZα: construction of pTrueBlue and M13TrueBlue cloning vectors. *Gene* **1998,** *213*, 83–91.

29. Cupples, C. G.; Miller, J. H. A set of *lacZ* mutations in *Escherichia coli* that allow rapid detection of each of the six base substitutions. *Proc. Natl. Acad. Sci. USA* **1989,** *86*, 5345–5349.

30. Josephy, P. D. The *Escherichia coli lacZ* reversion mutagenicity assay. *Mutat. Res.* **2000,** *455*, 71–80.

31. Cupples, C. G.; Cabrera, M.; Cruz, C.; Miller, J. H. A set of *lacZ* mutations in *Escherichia coli* that allow rapid detection of specific frameshift mutations. *Genetics* **1990,** *125*, 275–280.

32. Ames, B. N. The detection of chemical mutagens with enteric bacteria. In *Chemical Mutagens: Principles and Methods for their Detection;* Hollaender, A., Ed.; Plenum: New York, 1971; pp. 267–282.

33. Ames, B. N.; Durston, W. E.; Yamasaki, E.; Lee, F. D. Carcinogens are mutagens: a simple test system combining liver homogenates for activation and bacteria for detection. *Proc. Natl. Acad. Sci. USA* **1973,** *70*, 2281–2285.

34. McCann, J.; Spingarn, N. E.; Kobori, J.; Ames, B. N. Detection of carcinogens as mutagens: bacterial tester strains with R factor plasmids. *Proc. Natl. Acad. Sci. USA* **1975,** *72*, 979–983.

35. Maron, D. M.; Ames, B. N. Revised methods for the *Salmonella* mutagenicity test. *Mutat. Res.* **1983,** *113*, 173–215.

36. Cebula, T. A. Remembering Philip E. Hartman. *Environ. Mol. Mutagen.* **2003,** *42*, 125–126.

37. Porwollik, S.; Wong, R. M.; Sims, S. H.; Schaaper, R. M.; DeMarini, D. M.; McClelland, M. The Δ*uvrB* mutations in the Ames strains of *Salmonella* span 15 to 119 genes. *Mutat. Res.* **2001**, *483*, 1–11.

38. Busch, D. B.; Archer, J.; Amos, E. A.; Hatcher, J. F.; Bryan, G. T. A protocol for the combined biochemical and serological identification of the Ames mutagen tester strains as *Salmonella typhimurium*. *Environ. Mutagen.* **1986**, *8*, 741–751.

39. MacPhee, D. G. Development of bacterial mutagenicity tests: a view from afar. *Environ. Mol. Mutagen.* **1989**, *14* (Suppl. 16), 35–38.

40. Perry, K. L.; Walker, G. C. Identification of plasmid (pKM101)-coded proteins involved in mutagenesis and UV resistance. *Nature* **1982**, *300*, 278–281.

41. Gabridge, M. G.; Denunzio, A.; Legator, M. S. Microbial mutagenicity of streptozotocin in animal-mediated assays. *Nature* **1969**, *221*, 68–70.

42. Gabridge, M. G.; Legator, M. S. A host-mediated microbial assay for the detection of mutagenic compounds. *Proc. Soc. Exp. Biol. Med.* **1969**, *130*, 831–834.

43. Prieto-Alamo, M. J.; Jurado, J.; Abril, N.; Diaz-Pohl, C.; Bolcsfoldi, G.; Pueyo, C. Mutational specificity of aflatoxin B1. Comparison of in vivo host-mediated assay with in vitro S9 metabolic activation. *Carcinogenesis* **1996**, *17*, 1997–2002.

44. Malling, H. V. Dimethylnitrosamine: formation of mutagenic compounds by interaction with mouse liver microsomes. *Mutat. Res.* **1971**, *13*, 425–429.

45. Malling, H. V. Incorporation of mammalian metabolism into mutagenicity testing. *Mutat. Res.* **2004**, *566*, 183–189.

46. Malling, H. V. History of the science of mutagenesis from a personal perspective. *Environ. Mol. Mutagen.* **2004**, *44*, 372–386.

47. Malling, H. V.; Frantz, C. N. In vitro versus in vivo metabolic activation of mutagens. *Environ. Health Perspect.* **1973**, *6*, 71–82.

48. Zeiger, E. History and rationale of genetic toxicity testing: an impersonal, and sometimes personal, view. Environ. *Mol. Mutagen.* **2004**, *44*, 363–371.

49. Elliott, B. M.; Combes, R. D.; Elcombe, C. R.; Gatehouse, D. G.; Gibson, G. G.; Mackay, J. M.; Wolf, R. C. Alternatives to Aroclor 1254-induced S9 in in vitro genotoxicity assays. *Mutagenesis* **1992**, *7*, 175–177.

50. Josephy, P. D.; Summerscales, J.; DeBruin, L. S.; Schlaeger, C.; Ho, J. *N*-hydroxyarylamine *O*-acetyltransferase-deficient *Escherichia coli* strains are resistant to the mutagenicity of nitro compounds. *Biol. Chem.* **2002**, *383*, 977–982.

51. Hartman, P. E.; Ames, B. N.; Roth, J. R.; Barnes, W. M.; Levin, D. E. Target sequences for mutagenesis in *Salmonella* histidine-requiring mutants. *Environ. Mutagen.* **1986**, *8*, 631–641.

52. Koch, W. H.; Henrikson, E. N.; Kupchella, E.; Cebula, T. A. *Salmonella typhimurium* strain TA100 differentiates several classes of carcinogens and mutagens by base substitution specificity. *Carcinogenesis* **1994**, *15*, 79–88.

53. Löfroth, G.; Hefner, E.; Alfheim, I.; Møller, M. Mutagenic activity in photocopies. *Science* **1980**, *209*, 1037–1039.

54. (a) Zeiger, E. Herbert, S. Rosenkranz, a fond remembrance. *Environ. Mol. Mutagen.* **2005**, *45*, 407–408. (b) Rosenkranz, H. S.; McCoy, E. C.; Sanders, D. R.; Butler, M.; Kiriazides, D. K.; Mermelstein, R. Nitropyrenes: isolation, identification, and reduction of mutagenic impurities in carbon black and toners. *Science* **1980**, *209*, 1039–1043.

55. Hayakawa, K.; Nakamura, A.; Terai, N.; Kizu, R.; Ando, K. Nitroarene concentrations and direct-acting mutagenicity of diesel exhaust particulates fractionated by silica-gel column chromatography. *Chem. Pharm. Bull. (Tokyo)* **1997**, *45*, 1820–1822.

56. Watanabe, T.; Hasei, T.; Takahashi, Y.; Otake, S.; Murahashi, T.; Takamura, T.; Hirayama, T.; Wakabayashi, K. Mutagenic activity and quantification of nitroarenes in surface soil in the Kinki region of Japan. *Mutat. Res.* **2003**, *538*, 121–131.

57. Yamada, M.; Espinosa-Aguirre, J. J.; Watanabe, M.; Matsui, K.; Sofuni, T.; Nohmi, T. Targeted disruption of the gene encoding the classical nitroreductase enzyme in *Salmonella typhimurium* Ames test strains TA1535 and TA1538. *Mutat. Res.* **1997**, *375*, 9–17.

58. Nokhbeh, M. R.; Boroumandi, S.; Pokorny, N.; Koziarz, P.; Paterson, E. S.; Lambert, I. B. Identification and characterization of SnrA, an inducible oxygen-insensitive nitroreductase in *Salmonella enterica* serovar Typhimurium TA1535. *Mutat. Res.* **2002**, *508*, 59–70.

59. McCoy, E. C.; Rosenkranz, H. S.; Mermelstein, R. Evidence for the existence of a family of bacterial nitroreductases capable of activating nitrated polycyclics to mutagens. *Environ. Mutagen.* **1981**, *3*, 421–427.

60. Josephy, P. D. New developments in the Ames assay: high-sensitivity detection of mutagenic arylamines. *Bioessays* **1989**, *11*, 108–112.

61. Einisto, P.; Watanabe, M.; Ishidate, M., Jr.; Nohmi, T. Mutagenicity of 30 chemicals in *Salmonella typhimurium* strains possessing different nitroreductase or O-acetyltransferase activities. *Mutat. Res.* **1991**, *259*, 95–102.

62. Grant, D. M.; Josephy, P. D.; Lord, H. L.; Morrison, L. D. *Salmonella typhimurium* strains expressing human arylamine N-acetyltransferases: metabolism and mutagenic activation of aromatic amines. *Cancer Res.* **1992**, *52*, 3961–3964.

63. Josephy, P. D. Genetically engineered bacteria expressing human enzymes and their use in the study of mutagens and mutagenesis. *Toxicology* **2002**, *181–182*, 255–260.

64. Prival, M. J.; McCoy, E. C.; Gutter, B.; Rosenkranz, H. S. Tris(2,3-dibromopropyl) phosphate: mutagenicity of a widely used flame retardant. *Science* **1977**, *195*, 76–78.

65. Gold, M. D.; Blum, A.; Ames, B. N. Another flame retardant, tris(1,3-dichloro-2-propyl)-phosphate, and its expected metabolites are mutagens. *Science* **1978**, *200*, 785–787.

66. Blum, A.; Gold, M. D.; Ames, B. N.; Jones, F. R.; Hett, E. A.; Dougherty, R. C.; Horning, E. C.; Dzidic, I.; Carroll, D. I.; Stillwell, R. N.; Thenot, J. P. Children absorb tris-BP flame retardant from sleepwear: urine contains the mutagenic metabolite, 2,3-dibromopropanol. *Science* **1978**, *201*, 1020–1023.

67. Van Beerendonk, G. J.; Nelson, S. D.; Meerman, J. H. Metabolism and genotoxicity of the halogenated alkyl compound tris(2,3-dibromopropyl)-phosphate. *Hum. Exp. Toxicol.* **1994**, *13*, 861–865.

68. Isono, K.; Yourno, J. Chemical carcinogens as frameshift mutagens: *Salmonella* DNA sequence sensitive to mutagenesis by polycyclic carcinogens. *Proc. Natl. Acad. Sci. USA* **1974**, *71*, 1612–1617.

69. Lunn, R. M.; Zhang, Y. J.; Wang, L. Y.; Chen, C. J.; Lee, P. H.; Lee, C. S.; Tsai, W. Y.; Santella, R. M. p53 mutations, chronic hepatitis B virus infection, and aflatoxin exposure in hepatocellular carcinoma in Taiwan. *Cancer Res.* **1997**, *57*, 3471–3477.

70. Brash, D. E.; Rudolph, J. A.; Simon, J. A.; Lin, A.; McKenna, G. J.; Baden, H. P.; Halperin, A. J.; Ponten, J. A role for sunlight in skin cancer: UV-induced p53 mutations in squamous cell carcinoma. *Proc. Natl. Acad. Sci. USA* **1991,** *88,* 10124–10128.

71. Ohta, T.; Ohmae, S.; Yamaya, K.; Kanemichi, Y.; Tokishita, S.; Yamagata, H. Characterization of the mutational specificity of DNA cross-linking mutagens by the Lac+ reversion assay with *Escherichia coli. Teratog. Carcinog. Mutagen.* **2001,** *21,* 275–282.

72. Jorge, S. A.; Menck, C. F.; Sies, H.; Osborne, M. R.; Phillips, D. H.; Sarasin, A.; Stary, A. Mutagenic fingerprint of ozone in human cells. *DNA Repair (Amst.)* **2002,** *1,* 369–378.

73. Schulz, I.; Mahler, H. C.; Boiteux, S.; Epe, B. Oxidative DNA base damage induced by singlet oxygen and photosensitization: recognition by repair endonucleases and mutagenicity. *Mutat. Res.* **2000,** *461,* 145–156.

74. Benzer, S. On the topography of the genetic fine structure. *Proc. Natl. Acad. Sci. USA* **1961,** *47,* 403–415.

75. Stahl, F. W. George Streisinger (December 27, 1927–August 11, 1984). *Genetics* **1985,** *109,* 1–2.

76. Streisinger, G.; Okada, Y.; Emrich, J.; Newton, J.; Tsugita, A.; Terzaghi, E.; Inouye, M. Frameshift mutations and the genetic code. *Cold Spring Harb. Symp. Quant. Biol.* **1966,** *31,* 77–84.

77. Drake, J. W.; Glickman, B. W.; Ripley, L. S. Updating the theory of mutation. *Am. Scient.* **1983,** *71,* 621–630.

78. Dobo, K. L.; Eastmond, D. A.; Grosovsky, A. J. Sequence specific mutations induced by N-nitrosodimethylamine at two marker loci in metabolically competent human lymphoblastoid cells. *Carcinogenesis* **1998,** *19,* 755–764.

79. Busby, W. F., Jr.; Penman, B. W.; Crespi, C. L. Human cell mutagenicity of mono- and dinitropyrenes in metabolically competent MCL-5 cells. *Mutat. Res.* **1994,** *322,* 233–242.

80. Furihata, C.; Matsushima, T. Use of in vivo/in vitro unscheduled DNA synthesis for identification of organ-specific carcinogens. *Crit. Rev. Toxicol.* **1987,** *17,* 245–277.

81. Tucker, J. D.; Auletta, A.; Cimino, M. C.; Dearfield, K. L.; Jacobson-Kram, D.; Tice, R. R.; Carrano, A. V. Sister-chromatid exchange: second report of the Gene-Tox Program. *Mutat. Res.* **1993,** *297,* 101–180.

82. Fairbairn, D. W.; Olive, P. L.; O'Neill, K. L. The comet assay: a comprehensive review. *Mutat. Res.* **1995,** *339,* 37–59.

83. Olive, P. L. The comet assay. An overview of techniques. *Methods Mol. Biol.* **2002,** *203,* 179–194.

84. Olive, P. L. DNA damage and repair in individual cells: applications of the comet assay in radiobiology. *Int. J. Radiat. Biol.* **1999,** *75,* 395–405.

85. Vijg, J.; van Steeg, H. Transgenic assays for mutations and cancer: current status and future perspectives. *Mutat. Res.* **1998,** *400,* 337–354.

86. Gossen, J. A.; de Leeuw, W. J.; Vijg, J. LacZ transgenic mouse models: their application in genetic toxicology. *Mutat. Res.* **1994,** *307,* 451–459.

87. Hoorn, A. J.; Custer, L. L.; Myhr, B. C.; Brusick, D.; Gossen, J.; Vijg, J. Detection of chemical mutagens using Muta Mouse: a transgenic mouse model. *Mutagenesis* **1993,** *8,* 7–10.

88. Gossen, J. A.; de Leeuw, W. J.; Verwest, M.; Vijg, J. Analysis of spontaneous and induced mutation frequencies in transgenic mice using a lambda shuttle vector system. *Prog. Clin. Biol. Res.* **1991,** *372,* 313–318.

89. Thybaud, V.; Dean, S.; Nohmi, T.; de Boer, J.; Douglas, G. R.; Glickman, B. W.; Gorelick, N. J.; Heddle, J. A.; Heflich, R. H.; Lambert, I.; Martus, H. J.; Mirsalis, J. C.; Suzuki, T.; Yajima, N. In vivo transgenic mutation assays. *Mutat. Res.* **2003,** *540,* 141–151. Lambert, I. B.; Singer, T. M.; Boucher, S. E.; Douglas, G. R. Detailed review of transgenic rodent mutation assays. *Mutat. Res.* **2005,** *590,* 1–280.

90. Gossen, J. A.; de Leeuw, W. J.; Molijn, A. C.; Vijg, J. Plasmid rescue from transgenic mouse DNA using LacI repressor protein conjugated to magnetic beads. *Biotechniques* **1993,** *14,* 624–629.

91. Dolle, M. E.; Martus, H. J.; Gossen, J. A.; Boerrigter, M. E.; Vijg, J. Evaluation of a plasmid-based transgenic mouse model for detecting in vivo mutations. *Mutagenesis* **1996,** *11,* 111–118.

92. Jakubczak, J. L.; Merlino, G.; French, J. E.; Muller, W. J.; Paul, B.; Adhya, S.; Garges, S. Analysis of genetic instability during mammary tumor progression using a novel selection-based assay for in vivo mutations in a bacteriophage lambda transgene target. *Proc. Natl. Acad. Sci. USA* **1996,** *93,* 9073–9078.

93. Gossen, J. A.; Molijn, A. C.; Douglas, G. R.; Vijg, J. Application of galactose-sensitive *E. coli* strains as selective hosts for LacZ⁻ plasmids. *Nucleic Acids Res.* **1992,** *20,* 3254.

94. Manjanatha, M. G.; Shelton, S. D.; Culp, S. J.; Blankenship, L. R.; Casciano, D. A. DNA adduct formation and molecular analysis of in vivo *lacI* mutations in the mammary tissue of Big Blue rats treated with 7,12-dimethylbenz[a]anthracene. *Carcinogenesis* **2000,** *21,* 265–273.

95. Loechler, E. L.; Green, C. L.; Essigmann, J. M. In vivo mutagenesis by O6-methylguanine built into a unique site in a viral genome. *Proc. Natl. Acad. Sci. USA* **1984,** *81,* 6271–6275.

96. Cosman, M.; Hingerty, B. E.; Luneva, N.; Amin, S.; Geacintov, N. E.; Broyde, S.; Patel, D. J. Solution conformation of the (−)-*cis*-anti-benzo[a]pyrenyl-dG adduct opposite dC in a DNA duplex: intercalation of the covalently attached BP ring into the helix with base displacement of the modified deoxyguanosine into the major groove. *Biochemistry* **1996,** *35,* 9850–9863.

97. Giri, I.; Stone, M. P. Wobble dC.dA pairing 5′ to the cationic guanine N7 8,9-dihydro-8-(N7-guanyl)-9-hydroxyaflatoxin B1 adduct: implications for nontargeted AFB1 mutagenesis. *Biochemistry* **2003,** *42,* 7023–7034.

98. Kim, M. S.; Guengerich, F. P. Synthesis of oligonucleotides containing the ethylene dibromide-derived DNA adducts S-[2-(N7-guanyl)ethyl]-glutathione, S-[2-(N2-guanyl)ethyl]glutathione, and S-[2-(O6-guanyl)ethyl]glutathione at a single site. *Chem. Res. Toxicol.* **1997,** *10,* 1133–1143.

99. Huang, Y.; Torres, M. C.; Iden, C. R.; Johnson, F. Regioselective synthesis of 1,N(2)-etheno-2′-deoxyguanosine and its generation in oligomeric DNA. *Chem. Res. Toxicol.* **2003,** *16,* 708–714.

100. Wang, H.; Kozekov, I. D.; Harris, T. M.; Rizzo, C. J. Site-specific synthesis and reactivity of oligonucleotides containing stereochemically defined 1,N2-deoxyguanosine adducts of the lipid peroxidation product trans-4-hydroxynonenal. *J. Am. Chem. Soc.* **2003,** *125,* 5687–5700.

101. Hsu, I. C.; Metcalf, R. A.; Sun, T.; Welsh, J. A.; Wang, N. J.; Harris, C. C. Mutational hotspot in the p53 gene in human hepatocellular carcinomas. *Nature* **1991,** *350,* 427–428.

102. Smela, M. E.; Hamm, M. L.; Henderson, P. T.; Harris, C. M.; Harris, T. M.; Essigmann, J. M. The aflatoxin B1 formamidopyrimidine adduct plays a major role in causing the types of mutations observed in human hepatocellular carcinoma. *Proc. Natl. Acad. Sci. USA* **2002**, *99*, 6655–6660.

103. Maki, H. Origins of spontaneous mutations: specificity and directionality of base-substitution, frameshift, and sequence-substitution mutageneses. *Annu. Rev. Genet.* **2002**, *36*, 279–303.

104. Morgan, A. R. Base mismatches and mutagenesis: how important is tautomerism? *Trends Biochem. Sci.* **1993**, *18*, 160–163.

105. Vogel, E. W.; Nivard, M. J. Model systems for studying germ cell mutagens: from flies to mammals. *Adv. Exp. Med. Biol.* **2003**, *518*, 99–114.

106. Lindee, M. S. Genetic disease since 1945. *Nat. Rev. Genet.* **2000**, *1*, 236–241.

107. Cardon, L. R.; Abecasis, G. R. Using haplotype blocks to map human complex trait loci. *Trends Genet.* **2003**, *19*, 135–140.

108. Stenson, P. D.; Ball, E. V.; Mort, M.; Phillips, A. D.; Shiel, J. A.; Thomas, N. S.; Abeysinghe, S.; Krawczak, M.; Cooper, D. N. Human Gene Mutation Database (HGMD): 2003 update. *Hum. Mutat.* **2003**, *21*, 577–581.

109. Sommer, S. S.; Scaringe, W. A.; Hill, K. A. Human germline mutation in the factor IX gene. *Mutat. Res.* **2001**, *487*, 1–17.

110. Mulvihill, J. J. Sentinel and other mutational effects in offspring of cancer survivors. *Prog. Clin. Biol. Res.* **1990**, *340C*, 179–186.

111. McAuley, D. F.; Elborn, J. S. Cystic fibrosis: basic science. *Paediatr. Respir. Rev.* **2000**, *1*, 93–100.

112. Frias, S.; Van, H. P.; Meistrich, M. L.; Lowe, X. R.; Hagemeister, F. B.; Shelby, M. D.; Bishop, J. B.; Wyrobek, A. J. NOVP chemotherapy for Hodgkin's disease transiently induces sperm aneuploidies associated with the major clinical aneuploidy syndromes involving chromosomes X, Y, 18, and 21. *Cancer Res.* **2003**, *63*, 44–51.

113. DeMarini, D. M.; Shelton, M. L.; Levine, J. G. Mutation spectrum of cigarette smoke condensate in *Salmonella*: comparison to mutations in smoking-associated tumors. *Carcinogenesis* **1995**, *16*, 2535–2542.

5

▷

Oncogenes,

Tumor

Suppressor

Genes,

and

Mutations

in

Cancer

Cells

HISTORICAL DEVELOPMENT OF THE LINK
BETWEEN CARCINOGENESIS AND MUTAGENESIS

The idea that cancer is a consequence of somatic mutations arose in the 19th century, when microscopic examination revealed that chromosome abnormalities were a frequent feature of cancer cells. Wilhelm Konrad Röntgen (Nobel Prize in Physics, 1901) discovered X-rays in 1895, and within weeks the new radiation was being used by surgeons to inspect bone fractures. The next year, in France, Henri Becquerel (Nobel Prize in Physics, 1903, shared with Pierre and Marie Curie) announced that uranium salts emitted high-energy rays, and physicists rushed to explore the phenomenon of radioactive decay. The damaging effects of ionizing radiation on cells and organisms were appreciated as soon as scientists and patients suffered radiation burns. Many early investigators of radio-activity, such as Marie Curie, later developed cancers induced by radiation exposure.

Hermann J. Müller discovered the mutagenic action of X-rays on *Drosophila melanogaster* in 1927 (Nobel Prize in Physiology or Medicine, 1946). This breakthrough had an immediate impact on fruit-fly genetics, because it meant that scientists no longer needed to wait for spontaneous "natural" mutants to come along. Mutants, the raw material of genetic research, could now be generated at the behest of the researcher. In a few days, Müller could create as many *Drosophila* mutants as his mentor T. H. Morgan (Nobel Prize in Physiology or Medicine, 1933) had discovered in a decade. The jigsaw puzzle pieces of radiation mutagenesis and radiation carcinogenesis seemed to fit together, linked by the idea that cancer is a somatic genetic disease.

Nevertheless, many facts about carcinogenesis refused to conform to the somatic mutation paradigm. Dating back at least as far as the observations of Sir James Paget (1) in the 19th century, doctors appreciated that some cancers were familial, which seemed to be at odds with the idea that somatic mutations were responsible. In 1911 Peyton Rous (Nobel Prize in Physiology or Medicine, 1966; perhaps a record for length of time between a Nobel prize-winning discovery and its eventual recognition!) showed that a virus could transmit sarcoma between chickens. Viral etiology seemed to place cancer in the realm of infectious, rather than genetic, diseases. The science of experimental chemical carcinogenesis developed in the early 20th century (see other chapters in this book), but the active chemical carcinogens, such as polycyclic aromatic hydrocarbons, were completely inactive in tests for mutagenic activity. Working at the Institute of Animal Genetics, Edinburgh, UK, during World War II, Charlotte Auerbach (2) discovered that mustard gas (see chapter 15) was a mutagen. This was the first known chemical mutagen, but the compound seemed an unlikely carcinogen: it was an acutely toxic poison gas. The link between mutagenesis and carcinogenesis could be made in the case of radiation, but apparently not for viruses or chemicals. By the 1950s, many scientists doubted whether there existed any meaningful relationship between mutagenesis and carcinogenesis (*3*).

Scientific advances lifted the veil of confusion. As discussed elsewhere in this text, the development of the concept of metabolic activation, and the construction of sensitive short-term mutagenicity assays, revealed that all of the major classes of environmental chemical carcinogens were indeed mutagenic, when tested in appropriate systems. Alkylating agent chemical mutagens (see chapter 15) proved to be carcinogenic in animals (at least those compounds for which the toxicity was not so great as to prevent an adequate carcinogenicity bioassay). Tumor viruses were characterized as retroviruses that could integrate into, and thereby alter, the animal genome. In 1960 Peter Nowell and David Hungerford reported that a specific chromosome abnormality, which they named the "Philadelphia" chromosome, after the location of its discovery, was an almost invariable karyotypic marker of *chronic myelogenous leukemia* (*4*). The Philadelphia chromosome is an abnormally shortened chromosome (eventually identified as chromosome 22). In 1972 Janet Rowley discovered that the abnormality was not a simple deletion of part of chromosome 22, as had first been thought, but a *translocation* of genetic material between chromosomes 9 and 22 (*5*). (The functional significance of the Philadelphia chromosome is discussed later in this chapter.) The discovery of the Philadelphia chromosome meant that, for the first time, *a specific genetic change was linked to a specific malignancy.*

THE DISTINCTION BETWEEN ONCOGENES AND TUMOR SUPPRESSOR GENES

This scientific progress came to fruition when molecular biology made possible the molecular analysis of cancer genetics (*6a*). The few genes of oncogenic viruses such as SV40 and Rous sarcoma virus were identified. In 1976 Michael Bishop, Harold Varmus (Nobel Prize in Physiology or Medicine, 1989), and their colleagues discovered that *src*, the transforming gene of Rous sarcoma virus, hybridizes to a gene present in normal chicken cells (*6b, 7*). This highly conserved eukaryotic gene was named c-*src*, the cellular homologue of the viral *oncogene* v-*src*. The link between genetic change and malignancy was moving from the chromosome/karyotype scale to the molecular scale.

"Cancer genes" can be divided into two classes: *oncogenes* and *tumor suppressor genes* (*8–11*) (see table 5-1). In chapter 4, we distinguished between reversion assays, in which a few specific mutations restore function to an inactive gene, and forward mutation assays, in which any one of a wide spectrum of mutations inactivates a functional gene. The distinction between oncogenes and tumor suppressor genes echoes this idea. Oncogenes are cancer-related genes that become functionally *activated* by specific mutations, usually resulting in constitutive activity of a protein that transmits or transduces cellular growth signals. Tumor suppressor genes, in contrast, are genes that become functionally *in*activated by any

TABLE 5-1.

Representative Oncogenes/Oncoproteins

ONCOGENE	PROTEIN/ FUNCTION	REFERENCE
sis	Platelet-derived growth factor (B-chain)	*(15)*
PDGRF	Platelet-derived growth factor receptor tyrosine kinase	*(16)*
c-kit	Stem cell factor receptor tyrosine kinase	*(17)*
H-ras	G-protein	*(18, 19)*
src	Tyrosine kinase	*(20, 21)*
fos, jun	Components of AP-1 transcription factor	*(22)*
myc	Transcription factor component	*(23, 24)*

This table is far from exhaustive.

one of a wide spectrum of mutations, usually resulting in the loss of a cellular function that restrains cell proliferation.

FAMILIAL CANCERS

Mutations in oncogenes and tumor suppressor genes may be either inherited (familial cancers (*8*)) or acquired somatically (sporadic cancers). Many tumor suppressor genes were identified through the study of hereditary predispositions to specific cancers. In these conditions, one copy of the gene is already inactivated in the germ line and the second copy becomes inactivated by somatic mutation. At a cellular level, tumor suppressor genes are *recessive*: cancer is associated with inactivation or loss of both cellular copies; oncogenes are *dominant*: activation of a single copy of the gene causes its carcinogenic effect. In terms of Mendelian inheritance, however, cancer-prone diseases due to mutations in tumor suppressor genes are usually autosomal *dominant* traits (e.g., hereditary non-polyposis colorectal carcinoma (HNPCC), retinoblastoma). In individuals who have inherited a germline mutation in one allele, the probability of a second, somatic mutation—inactivating the other allele and leading to a cancer—is very high. (Also, some alleles may act as dominant-negatives, whereby the protein product of the negative allele inactivates the product of the positive allele. Vogelstein et al. have shown that this can occur in HNPCC (*9*)). Some germline tumor suppressor gene mutations are dominant, but incompletely penetrant, for example BRCA1 and BRCA2 (*10*), so that the cancer risk of carriers is substantially less than 100%. In contrast, activating mutations of oncogenes are not often inherited, presumably because most such mutations in the germline are lethal early in development. A few examples are known, presumably in situations where the activated oncogene is only expressed in specific cell types (*11–13*). In cancers that are *not* familial, somatic mutational events have activated one or more oncogenes, or inactivated one or more tumor suppressor genes (or both types of events have taken place) in the clonal evolution of the tumor cells. The great majority of cases of the common human carcinomas (lung, skin, breast, colon, bladder, liver) probably fall into this class.

From the standpoint of cancer induction/maintenance, oncogene action involves activation and tumor suppressor gene action involves inactivation. Consequently, the protein products of oncogenes present therapeutic targets: we can try to develop drugs to inhibit them (*12*). Gleevec (STI571) has been the first spectacularly successful example of this new approach to cancer therapy (*13*). Combating the consequences of tumor suppressor gene inactivation may be a fundamentally more difficult task.

The field of cancer genetics has mushroomed in recent years. The cellular roles of cancer genes encompass much of eukaryotic cell biology, including signal transduction and cell–cell communication; cell cycle control; regulation of transcription; DNA repair; and apoptosis. It would be impossible to cover so much ground in one chapter, and, in any case, these topics are more appropriate for a textbook on cell biology. However, certain aspects of cancer gene biology are essential to modern molecular toxicology. The present discussion focuses on two aspects. First, tumor suppressor gene products are essential to the maintenance of genomic stability (discussed also in chapter 3). Second, analysis of the mutational spectra of oncogenes and tumor suppressor genes in human cancers provides fundamental insight into environmental carcinogenesis and molecular epidemiology.

Before proceeding to the discussions of specific genes and tumors, we need to pause and consider the complexity of carcinogenesis and cancer, as a precaution against oversimplifications. Cancer is not one disease but more than 100 diseases sharing the biological features of uncontrolled cell division and (in most cases) metastasis (spread through the circulation to reach new sites). We have drawn a distinction between oncogenes and tumor suppressor genes, but, as already noted, most human cancers probably involve both types of genetic change. These two classes of cancer genes coexist within the cell, and the pathways that they mediate are interconnected. Mutations in these genes can be described as "activating" or "inactivating," but the protein products are complicated molecular machines, and the consequences of a particular mutation may be subtle.

The diversity of cancer biology is vast. Cancers can arise in epithelial tissues (carcinomas), mesenchymal cells, such as fibroblasts or endothelial cells (sarcomas), or elements of the blood (leukemias). Most cancers are diseases of old age, but a few occur mainly, or even exclusively, in children. Some forms of cancer are strongly associated with environmental exposures, others apparently not at all. It would be naive to expect any single mechanism to explain the origins of all forms of cancer, or any single therapy to be effective against all forms. We will look for general principles but must expect many exceptions and special cases.

ONCOGENES

Let us recapitulate the logic of the identification of oncogenes carried by tumor viruses. These viruses can *transform* cultured cells, conferring properties, such as loss of contact inhibition, which resemble those of tumor cells. Genetic analysis of one class of tumor viruses, the retroviruses (which carry RNA genomes), revealed that the presence of specific genes (*oncogenes*) was required for tumor induction. Hybridization analysis then showed that these viral oncogenes were related to—indeed, derived from—normal cellular genes (*protooncogenes*); apparently, the viruses captured certain cellular genes and modified them, to produce active oncogenes (*14*).

Although many oncogenes were identified on the basis of their role in viral carcinogenesis, the significance of cellular oncogenes is much more general. Independent of viral infection, protooncogenes can be activated by mutation to become active oncogenes, which push cells towards malignancy. The products of protooncogenes perform a variety of cellular functions, leading to cell growth when appropriate biochemical signals are received. Activation of oncogenes overrides these signals and invokes uncontrolled cell division. Oncogenes encode proteins that act as growth factors (e.g., *sis*), growth factor receptors (e.g., *PDGFR*, *c-kit*), components of signal transduction pathways (e.g., *ras*), and transcription factors (e.g., *fos, jun*).

CHRONIC MYELOGENOUS LEUKEMIA; THE *BCR–ABL* FUSION GENE

As mentioned earlier, chronic myelogenous leukemia (CML) cells almost always show a characteristic chromosomal rearrangement: a portion of chromosome 9 has become attached to part of chromosome 22, to create the *Philadelphia chromosome* (*25*). The *ABL* gene, which encodes a tyrosine kinase, is located at the chromosome 9 breakpoint. When the Philadelphia chromosome is formed, the 3′-end of *ABL* becomes fused to the 5′-end of *BCR* (on chromosome 22). The result of this reciprocal translocation is the production of Bcr–Abl fusion protein, which has constitutive tyrosine kinase activity (*26*) and contributes to the development of leukemia.

One of the great success stories in cancer therapy has been the recent development of selective small-molecule inhibitors of the Bcr–Abl tyrosine kinase. These agents, notably STI571 (also called Gleevec or imatinib mesylate), have produced dramatic results in the treatment of CML and certain solid tumors (*27, 28*).

RAS

Members of the *ras* family were the first cellular oncogenes cloned (*29*). Mouse embryonic cells (NIH-3T3) were transfected with genomic DNA from a transformed *human* cell line. Foci of transformed cells that grew in the transfected culture were isolated and DNA libraries were prepared from these transformed cell lines. Human DNA contains characteristic repetitive (*alu*) sequences, and, by isolating the transfected DNA bearing these signature sequences, the (human) gene responsible for transformation could be identified.

The *ras* protooncogenes encode small guanine nucleotide-binding proteins (G-proteins) (*30*). *G-proteins* are guanyl nucleotide-binding signal transduction proteins; Alfred G. Gilman and Martin Rodbell received the Nobel Prize in Physiology or Medicine (1994) for the discovery of this class of proteins. Ras is posttranslationally processed by (among other events) the covalent addition of an isoprenyl group required for its binding to the plasma membrane (*31*). There are three distinct human *ras* genes, encoding four Ras proteins (see below). Ras proteins (*32*, p. 415) are among the many mediators of the complex signal transduction pathways leading from membrane-bound receptor protein-tyrosine kinases (which receive and respond to extracellular messenger molecules) to nuclear transcription factors (*33*). Ultimately, these transcriptional activation processes result in cell proliferation. When Ras is activated by specific mutations (see below), or overexpressed, control of cell proliferation is lost, because Ras activity becomes constitutive: its growth-promoting signal is transmitted continuously to its downstream effectors, including Raf and MEK protein serine-threonine kinases and phosphoinositide 3-kinase lipid kinases. These pathways are not considered in this chapter; see (*34*) for further discussion. Many other oncogenes (e.g., *c-kit*, *PTEN*, *myc*, *jun*, *fos*) also act by up-regulating protein-kinase-mediated signal transduction pathways (*35*).

Active Ras protein is GTP-bound (*36*). Upon interaction with *GTPase activating protein* (GAP), the intrinsic GTPase activity of Ras hydrolyses the bound GTP to GDP, leaving Ras in its inactive form (*37*). Activating mutations in *ras* often correspond to amino acid changes at specific residues involved in catalysis of GTP hydrolysis (*38*). These mutant forms of Ras can still interact with GAP, but lack GTPase activity, and therefore remain in the active, GTP-bound form (*39*). Transgenic mice bearing activated alleles of K-*ras* develop lung adenocarcinomas and other tumors at a high rate and within only a few weeks after birth (*40*).

RAS MUTATIONS IN HUMAN CANCER

Four human Ras proteins are known: Ha-Ras,[1] N-Ras, Ki-Ras A, and Ki-Ras B (*41, 42*). Both Ki-Ras proteins are encoded by a single gene; the Ki-*ras* mRNA undergoes alternative splicing of two fourth exons. These four proteins have very high sequence identity (figure 5-1), aside from the poorly conserved C-terminal score of residues. Why should four proteins

```
1         11         21         31         41
MTEYKLVVVG AGGVGKSALT IQLIQNHFVD EYDPTIEDSY RKQVVIDGET CLLDILDTAG
MTEYKLVVVG AGGVGKSALT IQLIQNHFVD EYDPTIEDSY RKQVVIDGET CLLDILDTAG
MTEYKLVVVG AGGVGKSALT IQLIQNHFVD EYDPTIEDSY RKQVVIDGET CLLDILDTAG
MTEYKLVVVG AGGVGKSALT IQLIQNHFVD EYDPTIEDSY RKQVVIDGET CLLDILDTAG


61         71         81         91         101
QEEYSAMRDQ YMRTGEGFLC VFAINNTKSF EDIHQYREQI KRVKDSDDVP MVLVGNKCDL
QEEYSAMRDQ YMRTGEGFLC VFAINNTKSF EDIHHYREQI KRVKDSEDVP MVLVGNKCDL
QEEYSAMRDQ YMRTGEGFLC VFAINNTKSF EDIHHYREQI KRVKDSEDVP MVLVGNKCDL
QEEYSAMRDQ YMRTGEGFLC VFAINNSKSF ADINLYREQI KRVKDSDDVP MVLVGNKCDL


121        131        141        151        161
AARTVESRQA QDLARSYGIP YIETSAKTRQ GVEDAFYTLV REIRQHKLRK LNPPDESGPG
PSRTVDTKQA QDLARSYGIP FIETSAKTRQ RVEDAFYTLV REIRQYRLKK ISKEEKTPGC
PSRTVDTKQA QDLARSYGIP FIETSAKTRQ GVDDAFYTLV REIRKHKEKM SKDGKKKKKK
PTRTVDTKQA HELAKSYGIP FIETSAKTRQ GVEDAFYTLV REIRQYRMKK LNSSDDGTQG


181
CMSCKCVLS    H-ras
VKIKKCIIM    K-ras A
SKT-KCVIM    K-ras B
CMGLPCVVM    N-ras
```

FIGURE 5-1.
The sequences of the four human Ras proteins are aligned. Nonconserved residues are shown in bold type. Exons 1 and 3 are underlined. Note the high degree of sequence conservation across the protein, except for the last approximately 20 residues. The yellow highlighting represents the variant segment of the Ki-Ras A and Ki-Ras B products, which are generated by alternative splicing of a single primary transcript. *Note*: A full-color version of this figure appears on the website.

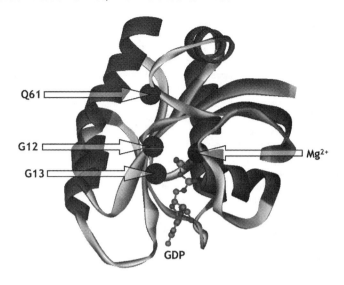

FIGURE 5-2.

Crystal structure of H-Ras protein–GDP complex; coordinates from file 4Q21.pdb. (*Milburn, M. V.; Tong, L.; deVos, A. M.; Brunger, A.; Yamaizumi, Z.; Nishimura, S.; Kim, S. H. Molecular switch for signal transduction: structural differences between active and inactive forms of protooncogenic Ras proteins.* Science **1990**, 247, 939–945.) The bound Mg^{2+} ion and the three amino acid residues at which activating mutations are found are indicated by arrows. *Note*: A full-color version of this figure appears on the website.

with such great similarity be required? Shields et al. (*34*) commented that "The high degree of sequence identity, coupled with the essentially identical ability of mutated forms of [the four Ras proteins] to cause transformation of NIH 3T3 and other cell types, have lulled us into a mindset that all Ras proteins were created equal." Knockout mouse studies, among other research, are revealing biological differences among the Ras proteins, but clear delineation of specific roles is not yet possible (*43*).

Almost all mutations activating ras affect one of three codons: 12, 13, and 61 (*44*). The corresponding amino acid residues, glycine 12, glycine 13, and glutamine 61, are all located near the GDP/GTP binding site (figure 5-2) (*39*) and are located within completely conserved regions of the amino acid sequence. These residues are either structurally or catalytically important, and substitutions result in loss of GTPase activity, as already mentioned. Highly destabilizing mutations (which will certainly occur at many sites on the *ras* genes/proteins) are not oncogenic, because they would result in complete loss of Ras function. In contrast, the oncogenic mutations result in *constitutively active* Ras. For example, at position 12, every possible amino acid substitution has been studied by site-directed mutagenesis, and all are oncogenic except for G12P. Of course, only certain amino acid substitutions can result from single-base substitution mutations within codons 12, 13, and 61. Common oncogenic mutations of human *ras* genes include G12V and Q61L (see below). Because the number of activating *ras* mutations is limited, the presence of such mutations in a tumor sample can be tested by PCR or hybridization with appropriate probes. Restriction fragment length polymorphism (RFLP) and single-strand conformational polymorphism (SSCP) analysis (see sidebar) are also used to detect *ras* mutations.

▶ Single-Strand Conformational Polymorphism (SSCP)

When we run mutagenesis assays on bacteria or on cultured cells, using selective growth conditions to obtain mutants, we can be confident that one or two sequencing runs on the target gene will identify the mutation. In studies of human mutations, we have no such guarantee. Even if we are confident that a tumor sample does carry a coding-sequence mutation in, say, the *p53* or *BRCA1* gene, many exons need to be examined. Sequencing the entire gene is a straightforward, but laborious, method for pinpointing the mutation. If possible, however, we would prefer to identify and sequence only the region of the gene that bears the mutation. The SSCP technique can be used to screen large numbers of similar samples (e.g., products of PCR amplification of a specific *p53* exon from many tumor samples (45)) for the presence of mutations (46).

Consider a single-stranded DNA oligonucleotide folding into a native conformation under nondenaturing conditions. If no complementary strand is present, standard duplex formation is impossible. Instead, short stretches of partially complementary internal sequence will anneal, twisting the molecule into a "knot." Even a single base difference between two oligonucleotide sequences can cause a substantial difference in the knotted conformation. This altered molecular shape will probably result in altered electrophoretic mobility on a gel. SSCP analysis exploits these differences. Strand length also affects mobility, of course, so we use SSCP to search for variant molecules (apparent as shifted bands) within a population of oligonucleotides of a given length. dsDNA samples, such as PCR products, are heat-denatured and then cooled rapidly, so that internal "knotting" is favored relative to duplex formation. The folded samples are run on a gel (figure 5-3, left). Mutant samples will usually show a mobility differing from that of control DNA, although there is no simple way to predict the change. In any case, the purpose of the SSCP run is to find a few mutants among many samples. The putative mutants are then sequenced, and we save the effort of repeatedly sequencing wild-type samples. ◀

In chapter 4, bacterial reversion mutation assays were presented. We saw that such assays consist of a genetic target that can be reverted ("activated") by a small number of specific mutational events (e.g., base substitutions at a particular nucleotide), giving rise to cells with altered phenotypic properties (e.g., the ability to catabolize lactose) that allow them to grow under selective conditions. *We can conceptualize mammalian carcinogenesis as a comparable system.* Each cell that might give rise to a cancer (e.g., an epithelial stem cell) contains a small number of genetic targets (e.g., *ras* genes) that can be activated by a few specific somatic mutational processes (e.g., base substitutions that yield nonsynonymous mutations in codons 12, 13, and 61, as discussed above). These rare events give rise to cells with enhanced proliferative potential that ultimately give rise to tumors. Just as we can analyze the mutational specificity of a mutagen by studying the DNA sequences of the target genes in the reversion mutants that it induces, *we should be able to analyze the mutational specificity of a carcinogen by studying the DNA sequences of the activated ras genes in the tumors that it induces.* We will examine such studies below. However, we must bear in mind that the three *ras* genes are not equal in their capacity to transform specific target cells, and some tumors do not contain activated *ras* genes at all.

MUTATIONAL SPECIFICITY OF *RAS* ACTIVATING MUTATIONS IN CHEMICALLY INDUCED RODENT TUMORS

Studies of activating mutations in *ras* genes of chemically induced tumors in laboratory animals are of mechanistic interest and can also serve as benchmarks for comparison with mutations in human cancers. However, as discussed in chapter 4, much more efficient experimental systems for analysis of mutational specificity are available, such as selectable endogenous genes or transgenic phage λ-based assays. In terms of experimental practicality, analysis of *ras* genes is considerably less attractive: it is necessary

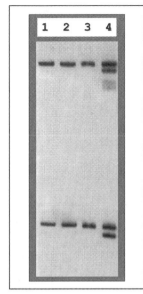

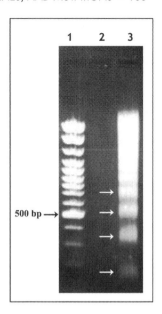

FIGURE 5-3.

Left: detection of mutations in the *p53* gene by single-strand conformation polymorphism analysis. DNA was prepared from primary human bronchial epithelial cells and transformed cell lines derived from these cells. Using PCR with intronic primers, a 290-nucleotide segment encompassing exon 5 of the *p53* gene was amplified. Samples (2 µL PCR product + 2 µL denaturing solution) were heated at 95°C for 5 min; placed on ice to prevent reannealing of the single-stranded DNA; electrophoresed at 600 V for 90 min at 10°C; and the gel was silver-stained to visualize the bands. Lanes represent: 1, primary cells; 2 and 3, cell lines with no mutations in exon 5; 4, a cell line with a mutation in exon 5; subsequent DNA sequencing of this mutant identified the altered codon, K139N. (*Piao, C. Q.; Willey, J. C.; Hei, T. K. Alterations of p53 in tumorigenic human bronchial epithelial cells correlate with metastatic potential.* Carcinogenesis **1999,** 20, 1529–1533. Copyright Oxford University Press.) Right (see p. 174): cultured cells undergoing apoptosis display DNA fragmentation visible as a "ladder" in ethidium bromide-stained agarose gels. Lane 1: molecular weight marker; lane 2: DNA extracted from epithelial cells treated under control conditions (DMSO vehicle only); lane 3: DNA from cells treated with cycloheximide, 10 µg/mL, for 48 hours. Note the extensive DNA fragmentation, visible as bands with masses corresponding to multiples of 180 base pairs (arrows).

to wait for tumor formation to provide material for analysis, and some tumors may prove not to harbor activated *ras* genes. (Similar considerations apply to studies of p53 mutations, discussed later.) Nevertheless, several studies of *ras* mutations in laboratory rodents have been reported.

In 1985 the first such study examined mammary carcinomas induced in rats by the alkylating agent MNU (*N*-methyl-*N*-nitrosourea). All of the activating mutations detected in the tumors were identical: a G:C → A:T transition[2] in the second base of Ha-*ras* codon 12 (*47*). As discussed in chapter 15, G:C → A:T transition is a characteristic mutational "fingerprint" of alkylating agents. In mice, the nitrosamines dimethylnitrosamine and 4-(*N*-methyl-*N*-nitrosamino)-1-(3-pyridyl)-1-butanone (NNK; see chapter 7) are lung carcinogens, and all tumors examined had Ki-*ras* mutations; these, too, were all G:C → A:T transition at the second base of codon 12 (*48*).

Polycyclic aromatic hydrocarbon-induced rodent tumors have been found to bear a variety of *ras* mutations (*49*). The potent carcinogen cyclopenta[*cd*]pyrene induces lung tumors in mice, and G:C → C:T transversions in the first base of Ki-*ras* codon 12 were the most common mutations found (*50*). 3-Methylcholanthrene-induced liver tumors in mice also showed a G:C → C:T transversion in Ki-*ras*, but it was located in the first base of codon 13 (*51*). In 7H-dibenzo[*c,g*]carbazole-induced mouse liver tumors (*52*), mutations in Ha-*ras* codons 12 and 13 were absent, but A:T → T:A transversions at the second base of codon 61 were common.

MUTATIONAL SPECIFICITY OF *RAS* ACTIVATING MUTATIONS IN HUMAN CANCER

Ki-Ras is the Ras form most often mutated in many human cancers (*53*), although N-*ras* mutations are common in acute myeloid leukemia (*54*). Point mutations in Ki-*ras* have been found in a majority of human colon (*55*) and pancreatic tumors (*56*) and they are also common in lung tumors (*57*).

In experimental studies in rodents, animals are exposed to a known carcinogen and the mutational consequences are characterized. In clinical/epidemiological studies with humans, the exposures are usually much less well defined, and we hope to identify (or confirm) the causative exposures by molecular analysis of the tumors. Lung cancers often have Ki-*ras* mutations, and tobacco smoke is the main carcinogenic exposure, so this is the most studied case. However, cigarette smoke contains almost every mutagen known (polycyclic aromatic hydrocarbons, aromatic amines, nitrosamines, etc.), so it is not at all easy to determine the most important chemical carcinogens in the mix. The most common *ras* mutations in human lung adenocarcinomas occur at Ki-*ras* codon 12. Lung cancer in nonsmokers is a rare disease. Remarkably, the *ras* mutation pattern is very different: Ki-*ras* mutations are much rarer in nonsmokers' lung cancers, which suggests that the etiology of the disease is different in nonsmokers (*58*).

The LMPCR method for mapping the distribution of DNA adducts along a gene (discussed later in this chapter) has been applied in a study of the three human *ras* genes (*59*). Damage sites caused by exposure to 7,8-benzo[*a*]pyrene dihydrodiol 9,10-epoxide (BPDE) in exons 1 (codons 1–37) and exon 2 (codons 38–97) of each of the three genes were mapped. Cultured human bronchial epithelial cells were treated with BPDE; also, purified genomic DNA from these cells was incubated with BPDE. In both systems, Ki-*ras* codon 12 was a hot-spot for BPDE damage, with little or no binding occurring at Ki-*ras* codons 13 or 61. In contrast, codon 12 was not a hot-spot for binding in either the Ha-*ras* or N-*ras* genes. These results are strikingly concordant with the patterns of *ras* mutations in human lung cancers. However, the mechanism by which BPDE targets Ki-*ras* codon 12 is unknown and, indeed, mysterious, since almost the same DNA sequence is present in the other two *ras* genes.

In summary, the human *ras* genes present an important target for carcinogen-induced mutations, and some information about chemical and mutational specificity can be garnered by studying these mutations. However, the chemical and biological factors influencing the relative susceptibilities of *ras* genes, and specific sites within those genes, remain to be delineated.

TUMOR SUPPRESSOR GENES

We now turn to a discussion of tumor suppressor genes. As our knowledge of these genes and their protein products has grown, appreciation of their importance in human cancer has also increased. Tumor suppressor genes are now being studied intensively as markers of human exposure to environmental mutagens. We begin by tracing the discovery of some important tumor suppressor genes and their biological roles.

KINETICS OF RETINOBLASTOMA INCIDENCE

Analysis of the rare cancer retinoblastoma has had a major influence on the development of our understanding of tumor suppressor genes. Retinoblastoma is a unique cancer. It occurs only in the eye and only in young children. The target cell type is believed to be the precursor of a photoreceptor cell of the retina. This target probably ceases to exist after early childhood, because, by then, all the cells have undergone terminal differentiation and ceased to divide. Roughly half of the cases of retinoblastoma are familial and half sporadic. Most (but not all) of the familial cases are bilateral, that is, both eyes develop tumors. Sporadic cases are invariably unilateral. Retinoblastoma is usually treated by surgical removal of the affected eye, an effective but devastating response to a potentially lethal cancer.

Alfred Knudson published an astute analysis of the incidence of retinoblastoma in 1971 (*60, 61*). He assembled data on about 50 cases of retinoblastoma, and sorted them into familial and sporadic cases, based on family histories and the unilateral/bilateral criterion. For each case in each group, he noted the age at diagnosis. He then analyzed each group of patients as though it were a population of cells, calculating, as a function of age, a "survival value," that is, the *fraction of the group in which no tumor had yet been diagnosed*. Plotting this fraction as a function of age produces a survival curve for each group (figure 5-4). Clearly, the familial cases have, on average, a much earlier onset than do the sporadic cases. The onset of the familial cases is a declining exponential function of age, reminiscent of a single-hit, single-target cell survival curve. Knudson hypothesized that the development of retinoblastoma required the *inactivation of both alleles* of a putative gene: a tumor suppressor gene. He predicted that the familial retinoblastoma patients inherited one inactive allele, with the exponential onset representing the kinetics of inactivation of the second allele. The later onset of the sporadic cases is explained by the requirement for two independent inactivation events. Indeed, 15 years later, the retinoblastoma susceptibility gene, *Rb*, was cloned, and it had the role in the disease that Knudson had predicted: both alleles of Rb are inactivated in the tumor cells, whether familial or sporadic in origin, and the familial cases inherit one germline inactive allele.

(Knudson's analysis is often described as "proving the two-hit model" of retinoblastoma induction. However, one cannot predict, from these

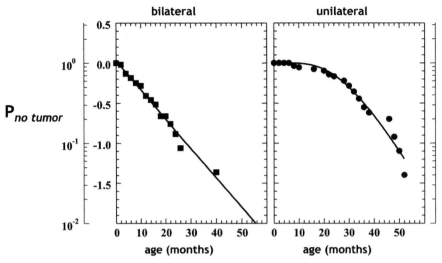

FIGURE 5-4.

Knudson's 1971 data on retinoblastoma incidence; left: bilateral cases; right: unilateral cases.

data, the integral number of genetic targets that must be mutated for retinoblastoma induction to occur. The age of retinoblastoma diagnosis curves do not represent true cell survival curves, and their shape is dictated not only by mutational events but also by the kinetics of growth of the target cells and the tumor cells. Indeed, recent evidence indicates that additional genetic changes beyond Rb gene inactivation are necessary for retinoblastoma to develop (*62*). We should also be very cautious about extrapolating from retinoblastoma to other cancers, most of which have a completely different age-of-onset behavior.)

GENETIC EVIDENCE FOR TUMOR SUPPRESSOR GENES

Whole cell fusion experiments between tumorigenic and nontumorigenic cell lines can produce hybrids that are nontumorigenic (*63*). This establishes that a dominant factor from the nontumorigenic cell line can confer its phenotype upon a tumorigenic one. Experimental results of this kind were the first clear evidence for *tumor suppressor* genes (or "antioncogenes"). Molecular analysis provided additional evidence that the loss of tumor suppressor genes is involved in the development of some tumors. While normal tissue from an affected individual is often heterozygous for a particular DNA sequence, tumor tissue sometimes shows loss of heterozygosity (LOH) for the same region (*64*). LOH is usually observed in patients who carry one (germline) wild-type allele and one mutant allele of a tumor suppressor gene. When the wild-type copy is lost through a deletion, the LOH can be observed in the resulting tumor tissue. In some cases, tumors that usually showed chromosomal abnormalities at specific locations had no such rearrangement. When these same tumors were examined at the molecular level, LOH was observed, even though, in these cases, the chromosomal change was cytogenetically undetectable.

Many tumor suppressor genes were cloned by the *positional cloning* strategy (*65*). This technique relies upon analysis of (cytogenetically observed) chromosomal abnormalities and LOH in a given tumor type. Once the chromosomal location of a putative tumor suppressor gene has been defined, the task of isolating the gene begins. In typical searches, DNA probes from the region of interest were isolated, and a "chromosome walk" was carried out, using these probes as starting point. Along the way, the isolated DNA sequences were checked for the hallmarks of expressed sequences (such as evolutionarily conserved sequences). Once an expressed sequence is found, DNA from many tumors was examined, to determine whether this sequence was altered or disrupted. Variations of this technique were used to clone the *Rb* (retinoblastoma), *DCC* (deleted in colorectal cancer), *WT-1* (Wilm's tumor), *NF1* (neurofibromatosis type I), and *BRCA1* and *BRCA2* (breast cancer) tumor suppressor genes. The completion of the human genome sequence has, of course, vastly simplified the task of positional cloning. Unfortunately, positional cloning tells us nothing about the biochemical/biological function of a gene. Even with the clone in hand, we may be unable to decipher what the sequence information is trying to tell us. Consequently, for many tumor suppressor genes, we still know frustratingly little about the functions of the encoded proteins.

The protein products of the tumor suppressor genes discovered so far (see table 5-2) have the common feature of retarding cell growth; the methods by which they perform this function vary. Tumor suppressors that resemble cell adhesion molecules (DCC), control the cell cycle (Rb and p53), interact with the Ras oncoprotein (rap1), and act in DNA repair (BRCA1) have been identified.

Earlier in this chapter, we drew an analogy between somatic oncogene-activating mutations and bacterial reversion assays. Extending this analogy, we can compare somatic tumor suppressor gene mutations to bacterial forward mutation assays. Each cell that might give rise to a cancer contains certain genetic targets (e.g., *p53*) that can be inactivated by a wide variety of mutational processes (e.g., almost any codon change that alters or eliminates the DNA-binding specificity of the core domain of p53 protein,

TABLE 5-2.

Some Tumor Suppressor Genes and Their Characteristics

GENE	INHERITED MALIGNANCY	FUNCTION	REFERENCE
p53	Li-Fraumeni syndrome	Transcription factor; cell cycle arrest; apoptosis	(*66*)
BRCA1	Breast and ovarian cancer	DNA double-strand break repair?	(*67*)
BRCA2	Breast cancer		(*68*)
Rb	Retinoblastoma	Regulates cell cycle progression?	(*69*)
hMSH2	HNPCC*	DNA mismatch repair	(*70*)
hMLH1	HNPCC		(*71*)
PTEN	Various tumors	Phosphatidylinositol phosphatase	(*72*)
APC	Familial adenomatous polyposis colorectal cancer	Multiple functions in adhesion, signaling?	(*73*)

HNPCC = hereditary nonpolyposis colorectal carcinoma.

as discussed below). These events give rise to cells that can evade apoptosis, or develop severe genetic instability, or possess other, as yet poorly characterized, properties that confer a survival advantage and a tendency to proliferation. These changes (perhaps combined with oncogene-activating mutations) ultimately give rise to tumors. *We should be able to analyze the mutational specificity of a carcinogen by studying the DNA sequences of the inactivated tumor suppressor genes in the tumors that it induces.* Because the spectrum of inactivating ("forward") mutations is so much broader than the spectrum of activating ("reversion") mutations, we might anticipate that tumor suppressor gene mutational spectra would be more informative than oncogene mutational spectra. We discuss such mutational spectra later in the chapter.

BREAST CANCER SUSCEPTIBILITY GENES *BRCA1* AND *BRCA2*

Germline mutations in the *BRCA1* gene result in familial predisposition to breast and ovarian cancers, with tumors often developing early in life (*74*). The susceptible individuals are heterozygous carriers of *BRCA1* mutations: germline homozygosity is unknown, presumably due to embryonic lethality. In the breast tumors that arise in these kindreds, LOH or other somatic mutational events inactivating the second *BRCA1* allele are observed (*75–77*).

Familial *BRCA1* mutations account for only a few percent of breast cancers. The role of the *BRCA1* gene in sporadic breast cancer remains unclear; somatic *BRCA1* mutations are very rarely observed in such cases (*78*).

The *BRCA1* gene was identified by positional cloning. Human BRCA1 protein is a polypeptide of 1863 amino acids, encoded by 24 exons. The biochemical functions of BRCA1 remain poorly understood, but it interacts with proteins involved in DNA double-strand break repair, cell cycle regulation, and transcriptional control (*79–82*). Murine *BRCA1* homozygous knockout mice die *in utero*. Using conditional knockout technology (*83*), Chu-Xia Deng and co-workers constructed a transgenic mouse line in which a specific recombinase, expressed from the mammary-specific *MMTV* promoter, inactivates *BRCA1* only in the mammary gland (*84*). These animals are viable but develop mammary tumors at a high frequency before the age of one year. The tumors are aneuploid and usually have *p53* mutations.

BRCA2 was also identified by positional cloning (*85, 86*). The very large (3418 amino acids) BRCA2 protein is believed to play a role in homologous recombination and DNA double-strand break repair, as mentioned in chapter 3 (*87–89*). Recent work by Ashok Venkitaraman and colleagues (University of Cambridge, UK) demonstrates that BRCA2 function is required for normal *cytokinesis*, the division of the cytoplasm into two daughter cells at mitosis (*90*).

THE RETINOBLASTOMA GENE, *RB*

The protein product of the retinoblastoma susceptibility gene *Rb* (*91*) blocks entry of cells into the S (DNA synthesis) phase of the cell cycle.

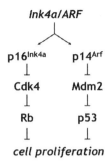

FIGURE 5-5.

p16^{Ink4a} and the regulatory network controlling the p53 and Rb proteins. This is a simplified schematic. Flat-headed arrows represent inhibitory actions. (*Adapted from Sherr, C. J. The INK4a/ARF network in tumour suppression. Nat. Rev. Mol. Cell Biol.* **2001,** *2, 731–737.*)

Cell division requires the inhibition of the Rb protein by phosphorylation, catalyzed by cyclin-dependent kinases. *Rb* is a tumor-suppressor gene and genes such as *CDK4*, which encode Rb-inactivating protein kinases, are oncogenes. In mice, *Rb* is required for viability; homozygous knockout mice die during embryonic development (*92*). While the deletion or mutation of *Rb* is characteristic of retinoblastoma, *Rb* is also altered in some breast and prostate carcinomas and osteosarcomas. Most frequently, in retinoblastoma, the *Rb* gene is inactivated by small deletions or duplications that result in a premature stop codon.

The *p16^{Ink4a}* (*93*) tumor-suppressor gene encodes a protein, p16, which inhibits the cyclin-dependent kinases and therefore activates Rb (figure 5-5). *p16^{Ink4a}* is deleted or mutated in many cancers, especially melanomas. Germline mutations in *p16* are associated with familial predisposition to malignant melanoma (*94*). Remarkably, the *p16^{Ink4a}* locus is the same as that of a second tumor-suppressor gene, *Arf*. Two proteins are expressed from the same gene through a complex alternative splicing arrangement; in fact, one exon encodes parts of both the p16^{Ink4a} and p14^{Arf} proteins, in two different reading frames (the name *Arf* stands for "alternate reading frame"). p14^{Arf} protein activates p53 (see next section) by blocking the action of its inhibitor Mdm2 (figure 5-5). Thus, the *p16^{Ink4a}* gene links the regulatory networks controlling the expression of two very important tumor suppressors, Rb and p53 (*95*).

p53

The p53 protein[3] was discovered in 1979 (*96–98*). Antisera against a mouse sarcoma, raised in syngeneic mice, were found to recognize a protein with Mr = 53 kDa in extracts of many different transformed mouse cells. p53 protein was purified (*99, 100*) and the *p53* gene was cloned (*101*). Germline missense mutations in the *p53* gene (in heterozygous individuals) cause *Li-Fraumeni syndrome* (*102–104*), a cancer-prone condition characterized by a spectrum of cancers including breast carcinomas; bone, brain, and soft tissue sarcomas; and leukemias. *p53* mutations are also frequently detected in sporadic cancers and indeed *p53 is now recognized as the most commonly altered gene in human cancers* (*105, 106*).

The cellular functions of p53 protein center on control of the cell cycle (*107*) and depend on the protein's DNA-binding properties. Homotetrameric p53 protein (*108, 109*) binds to DNA sequences containing two or more copies of a ten base-pair consensus half-site sequence (*110*) (figure 5-6). As with many other DNA-binding proteins, p53 contains distinct domains involved in DNA binding and oligomerization (*111–114*)

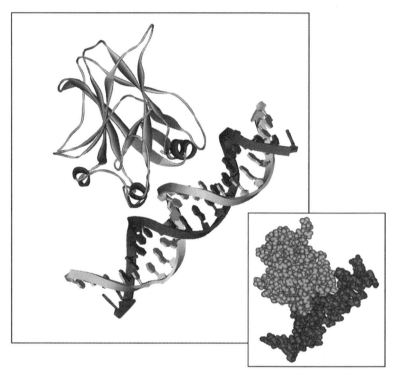

FIGURE 5-6.

Crystal structure of the core domain of p53 protein bound to a consensus binding-site duplex oligonucleotide. Left: space-filling model, with protein colored green. Right: schematic model, from the same angle. *Note*: A full-color version of this figure appears on the website. (*Cho, Y.; Gorina, S.; Jeffrey, P. D.; Pavletich, N. P. Crystal structure of a p53 tumor suppressor-DNA complex: understanding tumorigenic mutations.* Science **1994,** *265, 346–355.*)

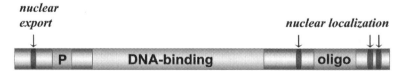

FIGURE 5-7.

Functional organization of the human p53 protein. The core region is a sequence-specific DNA-binding domain. Nuclear export signals are present near the amino and carboxyl (not shown) termini. The carboxy terminal region also contains the oligomerization domain and nuclear localization signals. *Note*: A full-color version of this figure appears on the website.

(figure 5-7). The DNA-binding property of p53 is lost in most tumorigenic *p53* mutants. p53 protein regulates a cell cycle "checkpoint." Cells that suffer severe DNA damage undergo a characteristic series of degradative processes, including proteolysis, degradation of chromosomal DNA, and dismantling of the cytoskeleton, culminating in cell disintegration. This process is called *apoptosis* or *programmed cell death* (see section on apoptosis). *Functional p53 protein is essential for induction of apoptosis in cells that have suffered extensive DNA damage (115).* In the absence of apoptosis, such cells can proliferate (*116*). Vousden (*117*) describes p53 as a "protein of many talents, including activation of cell cycle arrest, senescence, and differentiation . . . an apoptotic superhero, a protein that functions to selectively destroy stressed or abnormal cells, thereby protecting the organism from cancer development." Lane (*118*) described p53 protein as the "guardian of the genome," arresting the cell cycle in G1 in cells that have incurred DNA damage, thereby giving the cell time to effect DNA repair (*119*); and enforcing apoptosis in cells that suffered such extensive damage that they have "passed the point of no return."

Kinzler and Vogelstein (*120*) categorized tumor suppressor genes/proteins as either "caretakers" or "gatekeepers." *Caretakers*, such as DNA nucleotide excision repair and mismatch repair proteins, ATM, and probably BRCA1 and BRCA2, *maintain the stability of the genome*. Inactivation of these genes contributes to cancer development indirectly, by enhancing mutagenesis. The caretaker proteins play similar functional roles in all cell types, and germline inactivation usually leads to cancer development in many tissues and organs. *Gatekeepers*, such as Rb and APC, *regulate cell death*. Inactivation of these genes contributes to cancer development directly, by permitting abnormal cells to divide. Gatekeeper proteins may be expressed only in particular cell types, and germline mutations lead to specific tumors (e.g., retinoblastoma, polyposis colorectal carcinoma). p53 is the gatekeeper protein *par excellence* (*121*).

Cancer cells often exhibit chromosome instability (as noted at the start of this chapter) or microsatellite instability (chapter 3). "Mutators," that is, cancer cells with greatly elevated mutation rates, may result from early somatic mutations inactivating "caretaker" genes. These cells then accumulate mutations in "gatekeeper" tumor suppressor genes, and/or activating mutations in oncogenes, as the clones evolve towards greater malignancy. Some researchers have proposed that development of a "mutator phenotype" is a general phenomenon in carcinogenesis (*122*). Not all human cancers are genetically unstable mutators, however. The results of large-scale genomic sequencing analysis of colorectal cancer cell lines were not consistent with an elevated mutation rate in these cells (*123*), for example. The "mutator phenotype" may be a characteristic of certain tumors that have suffered loss of caretaker functions, and such tumors would be more likely to evolve rapidly towards greater malignancy and resistance to chemotherapy.

Knockout mouse technology has been used extensively to probe p53 biology (*124–128*). Targeted gene disruption (see sidebar on knockout mouse technology in chapter 8) was used to construct transgenic mice, either homozygous or heterozygous for a mutation that removes much of the *p53* gene coding region, eliminating biosynthesis of the p53 protein (*129*). Homozygous $p53^{\Delta}/p53^{\Delta}$ mice were viable and fertile, but had enormously enhanced susceptibility to cancer. Most animals die within six months, from lymphomas, osteosaracomas, teratomas, and other cancers (*127*). Heterozygotes (an animal model of the human Li-Fraumeni syndrome) had slightly reduced lifespans and increased cancer rates, compared to animals with wild-type p53. Since these mice display enhanced susceptibility to chemically induced tumors, in terms of both the magnitude and rapidity of carcinogenesis, they have been studied extensively as an alternative to the standard (two-year) carcinogenicity assays with wild-type mice (*128, 130, 131*).

APOPTOSIS

The term *apoptosis* (derived from the Greek for "a falling away, as leaves in autumn"; also known as *programmed cell death*) describes a particular type of cellular demise, which should be distinguished from cellular necrosis (*132, 133*). Necrosis is a tissue-based form of pathological cell death, mediated mainly by external factors such as traumatic injury, oxygen deficiency, and other gross cellular damage. Necrosis involves multiple cells (and often entire regions of organs) and induces an inflammatory response when the plasma membrane ruptures. In contrast, apoptosis is individualized in nature and is an energy-dependent internally scheduled process. Single cells undergo apoptosis independent of the fates of their neighbors. Undesirable cells are eliminated without leakage of the intracellular contents to the surrounding medium and no immune response is therefore triggered.

Apoptosis is an important response to toxicity, but also a pivotal process in differentiation and organogenesis in multicellular organisms. Factors inducing apoptosis can include genetic programming (e.g., loss of specific cells during development, as is well characterized in the nematode *C. elegans*); loss of trophic factors (e.g., for certain classes of lymphocytes); death-inducing signaling (e.g., through engagement of tumor necrosis factor (TNF)-α receptors); and intracellular events such as DNA damage and loss of mitochondrial integrity (*134*).

Regardless of how apoptosis is induced, the final common pathway involves cleavage of essential cellular elements (such as cytoskeletal and DNA repair proteins) and DNA fragmentation. A family of specific cysteine proteases known as *caspases* (EC 3.4.22) (*135, 136*) mediate the protein fragmentation and the activation of DNAses in apoptotic cells (*134, 137, 138*). Caspases catalyze the hydrolysis of proteins on the C-terminal side of aspartic acid residues. In the healthy cell, caspases exist as inactive procaspase molecules. They are divided into two groups: effector caspases, whose targets are essential cellular proteins, and initiator caspases, which activate the effector caspases via a cascade of proteolytic cleavage events (*139*).

As with other proteolytic cascades, such as the blood clotting pathway, the caspase cascade amplifies a small signal to produce a massive biochemical effect. The only way to activate procaspases is through hydrolysis by cysteine proteases, and caspases are the only known cysteine proteases in the mammalian cell. Apparently, then, active caspases are required to initiate caspase activation, a situation which seems to present a "chicken-and-egg" paradox. This paradox was resolved by the discovery of two mechanisms available to initiate procaspase-to-caspase activation. In the first characterized pathway, members of the TNF-α superfamily (membrane-bound receptor–ligand pairs, such as Fas and FasL) interact on adjacent cells, leading to receptor clustering and recruitment of adaptor proteins to the cytoplasmic domain (140). These adaptor proteins (such as FADD) bind via their so-called "death domain" motifs, and recruit a scaffold protein complex (death-induced signaling complex or DISC) that includes inactive procaspase 8 (or procaspase 10 in some cells). Proximity leads to conformational changes, auto- or cross-activation between closely apposed procaspase 8 molecules (141), and the subsequent release of activated caspase 8, which then initiates a cascade of caspase activation leading to activation of the effector caspases 3, 6, and 7 (139, 142).

Cells lacking TNF-α superfamily receptors can still undergo apoptosis (143) and apoptosis can also be triggered by ionizing radiation (144). An alternative pathway for caspase activation exists. This route requires the release of the small respiratory-chain heme protein cytochrome c from the mitochondrion, the organelle to which it is normally confined (145). Cytochrome c release activates cytoplasmic Apaf-1. Apaf-1 then forms an elaborate multimeric scaffold known as the apoptosome, which is able to recruit procaspase 9, resulting in its autoactivation to the effector caspase 9 (146, 147). DISC activity also leads to the generation of truncated Bid, a proapoptotic member of the Bcl-2 family (132). Truncated Bid induces release of cytochrome c from mitochondria (possibly by forming pore-like complexes with family member Bax). Thus, the two pathways (DISC and apoptosome) are interrelated. There is also growing evidence that release of cytochrome c from mitochondria may be triggered by caspase activity, suggesting that this component of the apoptotic machinery is more relevant for amplification, rather than initiation, of apoptosis (148, 149). Additional levels of control modulate the cellular response. Other members of the Bcl-2 family, such as Bcl-2 and Bcl-X, are antiapoptotic, protecting mito-chondrial integrity (132). The cytoplasm contains several members of the inhibitors of apoptosis protein (IAP) family, including XIAP and survivin, which inactivate caspases and also prevent the conversion of procaspases into their active forms (150, 151). Once mitochondrial integrity is lost, additional proteins, such as the DNAses endonuclease G and AIF, are released. Smac/Diablo and Omi are also released from mitochondria, and they interfere with the action of IAPs, thus allowing apoptosis to continue (152, 153). Further modulation is due to upstream events such as PI3K activation of the serine/threonine protein kinase AKT, leading to reduced expression of Bim (via phosphorylation of the transcription factor fork-head), and phosphorylation of other members of the apoptosis machinery (such as caspase 9 and Bad) resulting in their inactivation or sequestra-tion (154). AKT is also central to survival signals related to cell–cell and cell–substrate adhesion (155); loss of such adhesion and of subsequent AKT activity induces some cells types to undergo a form of apoptosis known as *anoikis* (from the Greek for "death due to homelessness") (156–158).

Apoptosis is frequently triggered as a response to cytotoxic and geno-toxic insult or stress (159), and has great relevance to our understanding of cancer (160). One of the central "guardians" of genome integrity is the p53 protein. The p53 protein responds to DNA damage by halting cell cycle progression, stimulating DNA repair mechanisms, and, in those cases where DNA damage cannot be repaired, inducing the cell to undergo apoptosis (*144, 161*). Over 70% of human cancers display loss or mutation of the gene encoding p53 protein. Such cells are able to avoid p53-mediated cell cycle arrest and apoptosis in response to DNA damage, thus giving rise to immortalized daughter cells with a mutated genome (*162*). Apoptosis is studied through several approaches, which rely on detection of characteristic nuclear and/or cytoplasmic events. The hallmark of apoptosis is fragmentation of DNA into nucleosomes, which can be detected by DNA ladder gel electrophoresis (figure 5-3), nucleosome ELISA, or the comet assay (see chapter 3) (*157, 163*). However, all of these techniques require that cells be dispersed from their tissues, and thus they cannot be used to verify that apoptosis has occurred in individual cells. Since cells undergoing necrosis may also display DNA fragmentation (*136*), in situ methods that preserve the tissue architecture are needed.

An extensively used and powerful technique for detecting apoptosis is the TdT-mediated dUTP nick-end labeling (TUNEL) assay (*157, 164*). This assay uses the enzyme TdT (terminal deoxyribonucleotidyl transferase; DNA nucleotidylexotransferase (EC 2.7.7.31)) to add modified nucleotides to the DNA double-strand breaks formed in apoptotic cells. Subsequent fluorescence or immunodetection methods, followed by microscopy, are used to visualize these incorporated bases and quantify apoptotic (TUNEL-positive) nuclei. Additional apoptotic assays involve evaluating caspase activation by western blotting to detect conversion of pro- to active caspases; proteolytic cleavage of known caspase substrates; and immunostaining cells and tissues with antibodies which detect activated caspase molecules (*157, 165*). Since the schedule of apoptotic events is cell- and tissue-dependent, and influenced by the nature of the signal or insult, it is prudent to evaluate this process using a combination of the above techniques.[4]

ANALYSIS OF *p53* MUTATIONS

Thousands of publications have reported studies of p53 protein expression or *p53* gene mutation in animal or human tumors. p53 protein down-regulates its own expression, in a feedback loop that depends on its sequence-specific binding to DNA (*166*). In normal cells, p53 protein expression is so low that it cannot be detected by standard immunoblotting protocols. Most *p53* mutations in tumors destroy the autoregulatory function of p53 protein by altering codons corresponding to the DNA-binding domain. As a result, p53 protein becomes highly overexpressed and visible by immunoblotting or immunohistochemical staining. This high-level expression can be used as an indicator (albeit indirect and imperfect) of the presence of *p53* mutations in tumors (*167, 168*).

A massive effort has gone into the characterization of *p53* mutations in human cancers and rodent tumors, and public databases of *p53* mutations are accessible on the Internet. The density of characterized human cancer mutations along the *p53* coding sequence is shown in figure 5-8. This near-saturation coverage is reminiscent of the analysis of *lacI* mutations discussed in chapter 4. About three-quarters of the *p53* mutations

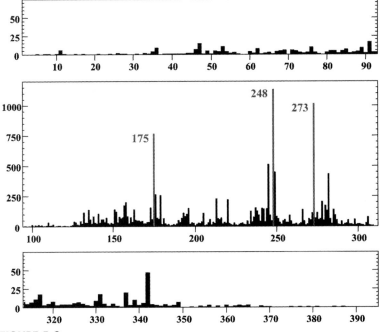

FIGURE 5-8.

The distribution of human tumor *p53* mutations across the coding sequence. A total of 15,208 base-substitution mutants from all tumor types are represented in this data set. The top, middle, and bottom panels represent the N-terminal, DNA-binding core, and C-terminal regions of the protein. Note the greatly reduced vertical scale for the center panel. The three strongest hot-spots are shown in red. *Note*: A full-color version of this figure appears on the website. (*Dataset kindly provided by Professor Thierry Soussi, Laboratoire de Génotoxicologie des tumeurs, Hôpital Tenon, Paris, France.*)

in human cancers are missense mutations. As in *lacI*, the DNA-binding domain is especially sensitive, that is, mutations affecting codons in that domain are especially likely to be functionally defective. Mutations are very strongly clustered in the central exons of *p53* encoding the DNA-binding domain. (About four-fifths of *p53* mutations are found in the corresponding exons 5–8.) A few very strong hot-spots are evident, but the diversity of affected sites is remarkable. Figure 5-9 shows the types of somatic and germline mutations found in the *p53* gene.

(How are *p53* mutations detected and identified? In contrast to the situation with *ras*, the number of possible *p53* mutations in tumors is very large, so hybridization methods are not applicable. As mentioned above, p53 protein overexpression is a good indicator of *p53* mutation. Most commonly, the SSCP method is used to screen for mutations in *p53* exons amplified by PCR. This narrows the search to a particular exon, and DNA sequencing can then be used to pinpoint the mutation.)

In our earlier discussion of *ras* mutations, we saw that patterns of oncogene-activating mutations in cancers can provide clues to the mutational specificity of known carcinogens, and may indict particular environmental mutagens in the etiology of human cancers: the mutagen leaves

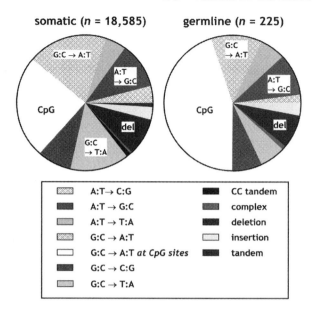

FIGURE 5-9.

The distribution of human tumor *p53* mutations among the classes of mutational events. The pie charts show the results of sequencing somatic (all tumor types combined) and germline (Li-Fraumeni) *p53* mutations. The legend lists the mutation types in order, proceeding counterclockwise from the stippled segment. CpG indicates G:C → A:T transitions occurring at CpG sites, which are likely to have arisen from 5-methylcytosine deamination events. *Note*: A full-color version of this figure appears on the website. (*Data obtained from the database maintained by the International Agency for Research on Cancer (http://www.iarc.fr/p53/).*)

its mutational "fingerprints" on the gene. This idea applies even more strongly to *p53* mutations, since (i) *p53* mutations are found so commonly in human cancers; and (ii) the diversity of *p53*-inactivating mutations is so great that very distinctive "fingerprints" may be anticipated (*169*).

p53 MUTATIONS IN HUMAN TUMORS

Possible associations between environmental mutagens and *p53* mutational spectra have been investigated for many human cancers (*170, 171*). The most intensively studied examples are those malignancies in which (i) the cancers are relatively common; (ii) *p53* mutations are frequent; and (iii) likely environmental mutagens have already been associated with the cancer, providing known "fingerprints" of mutational specificity.

In skin carcinomas (*172–174*), C → T transitions and CC → TT tandem transitions are common, consistent with sunlight-induced photoproducts as premutagenic lesions (*175*). Particular hot-spots are CCG and TCG codons, where a cytosine is present both in a Py-Py sequence that can give rise to a pyrimidine dimer, and in a CpG sequence where the cytosine is 5-methylated (*176*). This suggests mutational mechanisms involving both pyrimidine dimer formation and cytosine deamination; see (*177*) for further discussion.

Earlier in the chapter, we noted that *ras* mutations in lung cancers among cigarette smokers have a high frequency of Ki-*ras* codon 12 mutations. *p53* spectra show a relatively high frequency of $G \rightarrow T$ transversions in this group, which suggests that bulky adducts of polycyclic aromatic hydrocarbons are possible mutagens (*178–180*). Breast cancers show a wide range of *p53* mutations, and the spectra vary among different regions/countries (*181*), and this has been interpreted as evidence for contributions by diverse environmental mutagens to human breast cancer.

Liver cancers (hepatocellular carcinoma) have proved to be a particularly interesting case study. Liver cancer is rare in the industrialized world but common in many tropical regions. Contamination of stored grain by the fungal secondary metabolite aflatoxin is an endemic problem in many tropical regions, including sub-Saharan Africa and southern China.[5] In many of these areas, liver cancer rates are very high. *p53* mutations are detected in one-third to one-half of liver cancers, and a large number of these mutations have been mapped. *p53* codon 249 is only about the fifth most commonly altered codon in the complete *p53* mutation database. However, the *p53* spectra of liver cancers from tropical countries with high aflatoxin exposure are dominated, to a remarkable degree, by a single mutation, codon 249 AGG $\rightarrow$ AGT (R249S). This hot-spot transversion event is thought to be a marker of aflatoxin mutagenesis (*182, 183*) and may be caused primarily by the aflatoxin-Fapy adduct (*184*) (see chapter 4).

Figure 5-10 shows data on the incidence of liver cancer within the population, and the frequency of *p53* R249S in these cancers, for a variety of countries representing high, medium, and low liver cancer rates. The three variables liver cancer incidence, *p53* R249S, and estimated average

hepatocellular carcinoma, males; rate per 100,000 per year

	<20	20-40	>40
PRC, Mozambique (103)			95%
Taiwan (316)		37%	
Japan (483)		26%	
Europe, USA (152)	6%		

FIGURE 5-10.

Frequency of the *p53* hot-spot mutation R249S in liver cancer cases from various geographical regions. The columns indicate low, medium, and high rates of hepatocellular carcinoma. PRC designates data obtained in Qidong, southern China, an area with a very high rate of liver cancer. Numbers in each cell indicate the percentage of *p53* mutations occurring in the hot-spot; the total number of *p53* mutations characterized is given at left. (*Data from Montesano, R.; Hainaut, P.; Wild, C. P. Hepatocellular carcinoma: from gene to public health.* J. Natl. Cancer Inst. **1997**, 89, 1844–1851.)

dietary intake of aflatoxin (data not shown) are highly correlated. This does not prove a causative role for aflatoxin, but it is strongly suggestive that *different agents* (rather than different exposure levels of similar agents) are responsible for liver carcinogenesis in the low- vs. high-incidence regions.

p53 MUTATIONS IN RODENT TUMORS

Spectra of *p53* mutations in rodent tumors induced by chemical carcinogens would seem to offer useful benchmarks for analysis of human *p53* spectra. However, there are both practical and theoretical limits to such an extrapolation. (i) *p53* spectra are much more difficult to construct than spectra of mutations in *selectable* genes, such as the *lacI* transgene (chapter 4). (ii) A given carcinogen may induce tumors in different organs of the rat vs. mouse vs. human; even if the target organ is the same, the frequencies of *p53* (or other gene) mutations may be different. (iii) The *p53* genes and proteins themselves are different; there are multiple sequence differences, even within the core domain, and the rat *p53* gene contains only ten exons, rather than 11, as in the mouse and human genes (*185*).

The $G \rightarrow T$ transversion mutation R249S is believed to be an aflatoxin "signature," as just discussed. However, the mouse *p53* codon (R246, CGA) corresponding to the site of the human "signature" mutation (R249, AGG) cannot mutate to a serine codon by a single base substitution; a tandem change (CGA → TCA) would be required. The same is true for the rat, where the corresponding codon is R247, CGG. So, with respect to this particular mutational event, neither the rat nor the mouse is a good model for the human. In female mice, aflatoxin administration produced pulmonary adenomas and carcinomas. Four-fifths of the tumors had *p53* mutations, but these were mainly transitions rather than transversions (*186*).

▶ The Ligation-Mediated Polymerase Chain Reaction (LMPCR)

The ligation-mediated polymerase chain reaction (LMPCR) makes possible the mapping at nucleotide resolution of the positions of DNA adducts in a specific gene (*187, 188*). This approach can be applied to determine the relative susceptibility to damage of each base in a gene of interest, such as p53 or ras. The template for the LMPCR process (figure 5-11) is damaged DNA. For example, DNA could be isolated from cells that have been treated with a mutagen. Or, isolated chromosomal DNA can be exposed to a reactive intermediate, such as BPDE, in vitro. LMPCR makes use of the principle of the PCR for gene amplification, and can therefore be applied to very small samples of genomic DNA (typically 1 μg).

As in all DNA sequencing methods, the LMPCR encodes base-specific information as fragment length information, which can be read out on a sequencing gel. The critical step for converting adduct position information into fragment length information occurs at the beginning of the LMPCR process. The damaged DNA is treated to convert adducts into strand breaks. For example, the DNA can be incubated with the E. coli excinuclease enzyme UvrABC (see chapter 3), which recognizes bulky adducts and creates single-strand breaks at defined sites 3' and 5' to the adducts, or with T4 endonuclease V, which cuts at the sites of cyclobutane pyrimidine dimer photoproducts.

This treatment generates a manifold of DNA molecules bearing single-strand breaks, and the strategy is to amplify these broken DNA molecules, using the PCR. However, since we do not know where the breaks have occurred, we cannot use primers complementary to each end of the gene of interest for the PCR reaction. Instead, we proceed as follows.

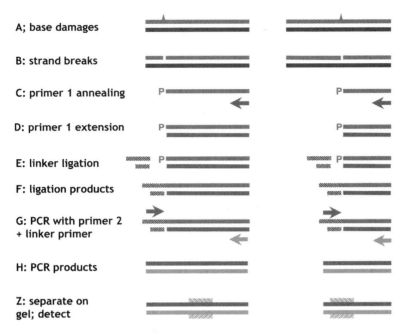

FIGURE 5-11.

Mapping DNA damage by the ligation-mediated polymerase chain reaction (LMPCR). See text for details. *Note*: A full-color version of this figure appears on the website.

First, a gene-specific primer is added and extended by DNA polymerase for one cycle only. The primer will extend from the site to which it anneals until the polymerase reaches the strand break. The product of this first extension reaction is a set of DNA molecules terminating in blunt ends. In the next step, a specially designed double-stranded oligonucleotide *linker* is added. This primer has two strands of unequal length (so that it is less likely to self-ligate). The blunt-end ligation is carried out using T4 DNA ligase enzyme. However, in contrast to standard ligation procedures, *ATP is not added*. Consequently, ligation can only occur by virtue of the 5′ phosphates present at the ends of the broken DNA strands. (This modification also reduces the possibility of self-ligation of the linkers or primers.) The product molecules result from the blunt-ended ligation of the linkers to the blunt-ended double-stranded DNA molecules generated in the previous primer-extension step. Most of the genomic DNA in the sample does not terminate in blunt double-stranded ends. Therefore, linker ligation occurs preferentially at the gene of interest.

At this point, the fragments of the gene of interest are bracketed by, at one end, a known sequence specified by the first primer, and, at the other end, by the known linker sequence. Consequently, we can now carry out PCR amplification of the gene of interest, as shown. Two primers are used, one complementary to the gene of interest and one complementary to the linker. After multiple rounds of the PCR, we obtain amplified products corresponding to the fragments of the gene of interest. The lengths of these fragments are determined by the positions of the original adducts on the genomic DNA.

The amplified DNA is now run out on the sequencing polyacrylamide gel (figure 5-12) and the molecules are separated based on their length. The DNA is transferred to a nylon membrane, as for a Southern blot. The blotted DNA is then hybridized with a radiolabeled probe specific for the gene of interest. (This visualization step provides additional specificity.) The final plot shows a pattern of bands whose intensities correspond to the extent of adduct formation at each site in the gene of interest.

To orient the bands on the gel, a second sample of (untreated) genomic DNA is sequenced by the Maxam–Gilbert procedure. This method produces strand breaks at specific bases. The Maxam–Gilbert cleavage products are treated by LMPCR in the same manner as the mutagen-treated DNA and run on the same gel, providing a benchmark sequencing ladder. ◀

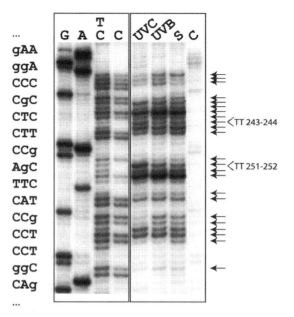

FIGURE 5-12.

The induction of cyclobutane pyrimidine dimers (CPDs) by ultraviolet or visible radiation in Chinese hamster ovary cells was mapped across exon 2 of the adenine phosphoribosyltransferase (aprt) locus. Aprt is a selectable locus often used in mammalian cell mutagenesis studies. CPD formation was analyzed by LMPCR of T4 endonuclease V-treated genomic DNA. Left half of gel: the four lanes correspond to LMPCR of DNA cleaved according to the standard Maxam–Gilbert DNA-sequencing chemical cleavage reactions for G, A, (T+C), and C, as indicated. Each arrow (right) indicates a Py-Py site; the arrow is positioned between the adjacent pyrimidines. Right half of gel: LMPCR of DNA isolated from cells irradiated with UVC (254 nm), UVB (295–320 nm), broad-spectrum simulated sunlight (S), or control (no irradiation, C), as indicated. Note that strand cleavage has occurred almost exclusively at Py-Py sites. The three radiations induce very similar site-specific patterns of CPDs. UVA radiation gave a distinct pattern of damages (data not shown here). (Only part of the full-length gel is shown here). (*From Rochette, P. J.; Therrien, J. P.; Drouin, R.; Perdiz, D.; Bastien, N.; Drobetsky, E. A.; Sage, E. UVA-induced cyclobutane pyrimidine dimers form predominantly at thymine–thymine dipyrimidines and correlate with the mutation spectrum in rodent cells.* Nucleic Acids Res. **2003**, 31, 2786–2794. *Copyright Oxford University Press.*)

Notes

1. The nomenclature derives from the presence of corresponding viral oncogenes on the Harvey and Kirsten sarcoma retroviruses; N-ras was cloned from neuroblastoma cells; Ha-ras and Ki-ras are often written as H-ras and K-ras. Ras protein is also referred to as p21 or p21^{ras}, based on its 21 kDa molecular mass.

2. In the rat, H-*ras* codon 12 (glycine) is GGA; MNU-induced mutation changes this codon to GAA (glutamate). In the human H-*ras* gene, the synonymous GGC is found at this position.

3. p53 is also referred to as TP53.

4. This section written by Brenda L. Coomber, Department of Biomedical Sciences, University of Guelph, Canada.

5. Efforts to ameliorate aflatoxin-induced liver cancer, by a chemo-prevention strategy, are mentioned in chapter 11.

References

1. Coppes-Zantinga, A. R.; Coppes, M. J. Sir James Paget (1814–1889): a great academic Victorian. *J. Am. Coll. Surg.* **2000,** *191,* 70–74.

2. Kilbey, B. J. In memoriam Charlotte Auerbach, FRS (1899–1994). *Mutat. Res.* **1995,** *327,* 1–4.

3. Burdette, W. J. The significance of mutation in relation to the origin of tumors: a review. *Cancer Res.* **1955,** *15,* 201–226.

4. Tjio, J. H.; Carbone, P. P.; Whang, J.; Frei, E., III. The Philadelphia chromosome and chronic myelogenous leukemia. *J. Natl. Cancer Inst.* **1966,** *36,* 567–584.

5. Rowley, J. D. Chromosome translocations: dangerous liaisons revisited. *Nat. Rev. Cancer* **2001,** *1,* 245–250.

6. (a) Pecorino, L. *Molecular Biology of Cancer;* Oxford University Press: New York, 2005. (b) Stehelin, D.; Varmus, H. E.; Bishop, J. M.; Vogt, P. K. DNA related to the transforming gene(s) of avian sarcoma viruses is present in normal avian DNA. *Nature* **1976,** *260,* 170–173.

7. Martin, G. S. The road to Src. *Oncogene* **2004,** *23,* 7910–7917.

8. Weinberg, R. A. How cancer arises. *Sci. Am.* **1996,** *275,* 62–70.

9. Varmus, H. E.; Weinberg, R. A. *Genes and the Biology of Cancer;* Scientific American Books, WH Freeman: New York, 1992.

10. Weir, B.; Zhao, X.; Meyerson, M. Somatic alterations in the human cancer genome. *Cancer Cell* **2004,** *6,* 433–438.

11. Vogelstein, B.; Kinzler, K. W. Cancer genes and the pathways they control. *Nat. Med.* **2004,** *10,* 789–799.

12. Cox, A. D.; Der, C. J. Ras family signaling: therapeutic targeting. *Cancer Biol. Ther.* **2002,** *1,* 599–606.

13. Roskoski, R., Jr. STI-571: an anticancer protein-tyrosine kinase inhibitor. *Biochem. Biophys. Res. Commun.* **2003,** *309,* 709–717.

14. Sugden, B. How some retroviruses got their oncogenes. *Trends Biochem. Sci.* **1993,** *18,* 233–235.

15. Heldin, C.-H.; Westermark, B. Mechanism of action and in vivo role of platelet-derived growth factor. *Physiol Rev.* **1999,** *79,* 1283–1316.

16. Claesson-Welsh, L. Platelet-derived growth factor receptor signals. *J. Biol. Chem.* **1994,** *269,* 32023–32026.

17. Mol, C. D.; Lim, K. B.; Sridhar, V.; Zou, H.; Chien, E. Y.; Sang, B. C.; Nowakowski, J.; Kassel, D. B.; Cronin, C. N.; McRee, D. E. Structure of a c-kit product complex reveals the basis for kinase transactivation. *J. Biol. Chem.* **2003,** *278,* 31461–31464.

18. Ayllon, V.; Rebollo, A. Ras-induced cellular events (review). *Mol. Membr. Biol.* **2000,** *17,* 65–73.

19. Malumbres, M.; Pellicer, A. RAS pathways to cell cycle control and cell transformation. *Front Biosci.* **1998,** *3,* d887–d912.

20. Russello, S. V.; Shore, S. K. Src in human carcinogenesis. *Front Biosci.* **2003,** *8,* s1068–s1073.

21. Warmuth, M.; Damoiseaux, R.; Liu, Y.; Fabbro, D.; Gray, N. SRC family kinases: potential targets for the treatment of human cancer and leukemia. *Curr. Pharm. Des.* **2003,** *9,* 2043–2059.

22. Jochum, W.; Passegue, E.; Wagner, E. F. AP-1 in mouse development and tumorigenesis. *Oncogene* **2001**, *20*, 2401–2412.
23. Pelengaris, S.; Khan, M.; Evan, G. c-MYC: more than just a matter of life and death. *Nat. Rev. Cancer* **2002**, *2*, 764–776.
24. Pelengaris, S.; Khan, M. The many faces of c-MYC. *Arch. Biochem. Biophys.* **2003**, *416*, 129–136.
25. Groffen, J.; Stephenson, J. R.; Heisterkamp, N.; de Klein, A.; Bartram, C. R.; Grosveld, G. Philadelphia chromosomal breakpoints are clustered within a limited region, bcr, on chromosome 22. *Cell* **1984**, *36*, 93–99.
26. Konopka, J. B.; Watanabe, S. M.; Witte, O. N. An alteration of the human c-abl protein in K562 leukemia cells unmasks associated tyrosine kinase activity. *Cell* **1984**, *37*, 1035–1042.
27. Mauro, M. J.; O'Dwyer, M.; Heinrich, M. C.; Druker, B. J. STI571: a paradigm of new agents for cancer therapeutics. *J. Clin. Oncol.* **2002**, *20*, 325–334.
28. Dancey, J.; Sausville, E. A. Issues and progress with protein kinase inhibitors for cancer treatment. *Nat. Rev. Drug Discov.* **2003**, *2*, 296–313.
29. Parada, L. F.; Tabin, C. J.; Shih, C.; Weinberg, R. A. Human EJ bladder carcinoma oncogene is homologue of Harvey sarcoma virus ras gene. *Nature* **1982**, *297*, 474–478.
30. Linder, M. E.; Gilman, A. G. G proteins. *Sci. Am.* **1992**, *267*, 56–5.
31. Seabra, M. C. Membrane association and targeting of prenylated Ras-like GTPases. *Cell Signal.* **1998**, *10*, 167–172.
32. Berg, J. M.; Tymoczko, J. L.; Stryer, L. *Biochemistry;* WH Freeman: New York, 2001.
33. Hall, A. Ras-related proteins. *Curr. Opin. Cell Biol.* **1993**, *5*, 265–268.
34. Shields, J. M.; Pruitt, K.; McFall, A.; Shaub, A.; Der, C. J. Understanding Ras: "it ain't over 'til it's over." *Trends Cell Biol.* **2000**, *10*, 147–154.
35. Sulis, M. L.; Parsons, R. PTEN: from pathology to biology. *Trends Cell Biol.* **2003**, *13*, 478–483.
36. McCormick, F. Signal transduction. How receptors turn Ras on. *Nature* **1993**, *363*, 15–16.
37. Hall, B. E.; Bar-Sagi, D.; Nassar, N. The structural basis for the transition from Ras-GTP to Ras-GDP. *Proc. Natl. Acad. Sci. USA* **2002**, *99*, 12138–12142.
38. Maegley, K. A.; Admiraal, S. J.; Herschlag, D. Ras-catalyzed hydrolysis of GTP: a new perspective from model studies. *Proc. Natl. Acad. Sci. USA* **1996**, *93*, 8160–8166.
39. Krengel, U.; Schlichting, L.; Scherer, A.; Schumann, R.; Frech, M.; John, J.; Kabsch, W.; Pai, E. F.; Wittinghofer, A. Three-dimensional structures of H-ras p21 mutants: molecular basis for their inability to function as signal switch molecules. *Cell* **1990**, *62*, 539–548.
40. Johnson, L.; Mercer, K.; Greenbaum, D.; Bronson, R. T.; Crowley, D.; Tuveson, D. A.; Jacks, T. Somatic activation of the K-ras oncogene causes early onset lung cancer in mice. *Nature* **2001**, *410*, 1111–1116.
41. Ehrhardt, A.; Ehrhardt, G. R.; Guo, X.; Schrader, J. W. Ras and relatives: job sharing and networking keep an old family together. *Exp. Hematol.* **2002**, *30*, 1089–1106.
42. Voice, J. K.; Klemke, R. L.; Le, A.; Jackson, J. H. Four human ras homologs differ in their abilities to activate Raf-1, induce transformation, and stimulate cell motility. *J. Biol. Chem.* **1999**, *274*, 17164–17170.
43. Matallanas, D.; Arozarena, I.; Berciano, M. T.; Aaronson, D. S.; Pellicer, A.; Lafarga, M.; Crespo, P. Differences on the inhibitory specificities of

H-Ras, K-Ras, and N-Ras (N17) dominant negative mutants are related to their membrane microlocalization. *J. Biol. Chem.* **2003,** *278,* 4572–4581.

44. Lowy, D. R.; Willumsen, B. M. Function and regulation of ras. *Annu. Rev. Biochem.* **1993,** *62,* 851–891.

45. Conway, K.; Edmiston, S. N.; Cui, L.; Drouin, S. S.; Pang, J.; He, M.; Tse, C. K.; Geradts, J.; Dressler, L.; Liu, E. T.; Millikan, R.; Newman, B. Prevalence and spectrum of p53 mutations associated with smoking in breast cancer. *Cancer Res.* **2002,** *62,* 1987–1995.

46. Orita, M.; Iwahana, H.; Kanazawa, H.; Hayashi, K.; Sekiya, T. Detection of polymorphisms of human DNA by gel electrophoresis as single-strand conformation polymorphisms. *Proc. Natl. Acad. Sci. USA* **1989,** *86,* 2766–2770.

47. Zarbl, H.; Sukumar, S.; Arthur, A. V.; Martin-Zanca, D.; Barbacid, M. Direct mutagenesis of Ha-ras-1 oncogenes by N-nitroso-N-methylurea during initiation of mammary carcinogenesis in rats. *Nature* **1985,** *315,* 382–385.

48. Devereux, T. R.; Anderson, M. W.; Belinsky, S. A. Role of ras proto-oncogene activation in the formation of spontaneous and nitrosamine-induced lung tumors in the resistant C3H mouse. *Carcinogenesis* **1991,** *12,* 299–303.

49. Ross, J. A.; Nesnow, S. Polycyclic aromatic hydrocarbons: correlations between DNA adducts and ras oncogene mutations. *Mutat. Res.* **1999,** *424,* 155–166.

50. Nesnow, S.; Ross, J. A.; Nelson, G.; Wilson, K.; Roop, B. C.; Jeffers, A. J.; Galati, A. J.; Stoner, G. D.; Sangaiah, R.; Gold, A. Cyclopenta[*cd*]pyrene-induced tumorigenicity, *Ki-ras* codon 12 mutations and DNA adducts in strain A/J mouse lung. *Carcinogenesis* **1994,** *15,* 601–606.

51. Gressani, K. M.; Rollins, L. A.; Leone-Kabler, S.; Cline, J. M.; Miller, M. S. Induction of mutations in Ki-ras and INK4a in liver tumors of mice exposed in utero to 3-methylcholanthrene. *Carcinogenesis* **1998,** *19,* 1045–1052.

52. Mitchell, K. R.; Warshawsky, D. Frequent Ha-ras mutations in murine skin and liver tumors induced by 7H-dibenzo[*c,g*]carbazole. *Mol. Carcinog.* **1999,** *25,* 107–112.

53. Ellis, C. A.; Clark, G. The importance of being K-Ras. *Cell Signal.* **2000,** *12,* 425–434.

54. Kiyoi, H.; Naoe, T.; Nakano, Y.; Yokota, S.; Minami, S.; Miyawaki, S.; Asou, N.; Kuriyama, K.; Jinnai, I.; Shimazaki, C.; Akiyama, H.; Saito, K.; Oh, H.; Motoji, T.; Omoto, E.; Saito, H.; Ohno, R.; Ueda, R. Prognostic implication of FLT3 and N-RAS gene mutations in acute myeloid leukemia. *Blood* **1999,** *93,* 3074–3080.

55. Kressner, U.; Bjørheim, J.; Westring, S.; Wahlberg, S. S.; Påhlman, L.; Glimelius, B.; Lindmark, G.; Lindblom, A.; Børresen-Dale, A. L. Ki-ras mutations and prognosis in colorectal cancer. *Eur. J. Cancer* **1998,** *34,* 518–521.

56. Flanders, T. Y.; Foulkes, W. D. Pancreatic adenocarcinoma: epidemiology and genetics. *J. Med. Genet.* **1996,** *33,* 889–898.

57. Minamoto, T.; Mai, M.; Ronai, Z. K-*ras* mutation: early detection in molecular diagnosis and risk assessment of colorectal, pancreas, and lung cancers: a review. *Cancer Detect. Prev.* **2000,** *24,* 1–12.

58. Ahrendt, S. A.; Decker, P. A.; Alawi, E. A.; Zhu Yr, Y. R.; Sanchez-Cespedes, M.; Yang, S. C.; Haasler, G. B.; Kajdacsy-Balla, A.; Demeure, M. J.; Sidransky, D. Cigarette smoking is strongly associated

with mutation of the K-ras gene in patients with primary adenocarcinoma of the lung. *Cancer* **2001**, *92*, 1525–1530.

59. Feng, Z.; Hu, W.; Chen, J. X.; Pao, A.; Li, H.; Rom, W.; Hung, M. C.; Tang, M. S. Preferential DNA damage and poor repair determine ras gene mutational hotspot in human cancer. *J. Natl. Cancer Inst.* **2002**, *94*, 1527–1536.

60. Knudson, A. G., Jr. Mutation and cancer: statistical study of retino-blastoma. *Proc. Natl. Acad. Sci. USA* **1971**, *68*, 820–823.

61. Knudson, A. G., Jr. Two genetic hits (more or less) to cancer. *Nat. Rev. Cancer* **2001**, *1*, 157–162.

62. Chen, D.; Pajovic, S.; Duckett, A.; Brown, V. D.; Squire, J. A.; Gallie, B. L. Genomic amplification in retinoblastoma narrowed to 0.6 megabase on chromosome 6p containing a kinesin-like gene, RBKIN. *Cancer Res.* **2002**, *62*, 967–971.

63. Sager, R. Genetic suppression of tumor formation. *Adv. Cancer Res.* **1985**, *44*, 43–68.

64. Lasko, D.; Cavenee, W.; Nordenskjöld, M. Loss of constitutional heterozygosity in human cancer. *Annu. Rev. Genet.* **1991**, *25*, 281–314.

65. Collins, F. S. Positional cloning moves from perditional to traditional. *Nat. Genet.* **1995**, *9*, 347–350.

66. Bourdon, J. C.; Laurenzi, V. D.; Melino, G.; Lane, D. p53: 25 years of research and more questions to answer. *Cell Death. Differ.* **2003**, *10*, 397–399.

67. Jhanwar-Uniyal, M. BRCA1 in cancer, cell cycle and genomic stability. *Front Biosci.* **2003**, *8*, s1107–s1117.

68. Welcsh, P. L.; Owens, K. N.; King, M. C. Insights into the functions of BRCA1 and BRCA2. *Trends Genet.* **2000**, *16*, 69–74.

69. DiCiommo, D.; Gallie, B. L.; Bremner, R. Retinoblastoma: the disease, gene and protein provide critical leads to understand cancer. *Semin. Cancer Biol.* **2000**, *10*, 255–269.

70. Drotschmann, K.; Clark, A. B.; Kunkel, T. A. Mutator phenotypes of common polymorphisms and missense mutations in MSH2. *Curr. Biol.* **1999**, *9*, 907–910.

71. Meyers, M.; Wagner, M. W.; Hwang, H. S.; Kinsella, T. J.; Boothman, D. A. Role of the hMLH1 DNA mismatch repair protein in fluoro-pyrimidine-mediated cell death and cell cycle responses. *Cancer Res.* **2001**, *61*, 5193–5201.

72. Eng, C. PTEN: one gene, many syndromes. *Hum. Mutat.* **2003**, *22*, 183–198.

73. Fodde, R.; Smits, R.; Clevers, H. APC, signal transduction and genetic instability in colorectal cancer. *Nat. Rev. Cancer* **2001**, *1*, 55–67.

74. King, M. C.; Marks, J. H.; Mandell, J. B. Breast and ovarian cancer risks due to inherited mutations in BRCA1 and BRCA2. *Science* **2003**, *302*, 643–646.

75. Smith, S. A.; Easton, D. F.; Evans, D. G.; Ponder, B. A. Allele losses in the region 17q12-21 in familial breast and ovarian cancer involve the wild-type chromosome. *Nat. Genet.* **1992**, *2*, 128–131.

76. Neuhausen, S. L.; Marshall, C. J. Loss of heterozygosity in familial tumors from three BRCA1-linked kindreds. *Cancer Res.* **1994**, *54*, 6069–6072.

77. Osorio, A.; de la Hoya, M.; Rodriguez-Lopez, R.; Martinez-Ramirez, A.; Cazorla, A.; Granizo, J. J.; Esteller, M.; Rivas, C.; Caldes, T.; Benitez, J. Loss of heterozygosity analysis at the BRCA loci in tumor samples from patients with familial breast cancer. *Int. J. Cancer* **2002**, *99*, 305–309.

78. Staff, S.; Isola, J.; Tanner, M. Haplo-insufficiency of BRCA1 in sporadic breast cancer. *Cancer Res.* **2003**, *63*, 4978–4983.

79. Deng, C. X.; Brodie, S. G. Roles of BRCA1 and its interacting proteins. *Bioessays* **2000**, *22*, 728–737.

80. Deng, C. X.; Brodie, S. G. Knockout mouse models and mammary tumorigenesis. *Semin. Cancer Biol.* **2001**, *11*, 387–394.

81. Venkitaraman, A. R. Tracing the network connecting Brca and Fanconi anaemia proteins. *Nat. Rev. Cancer* **2004**, *4*, 266–276.

82. Venkitaraman, A. R. Cancer susceptibility and the functions of BRCA1 and BRCA2. *Cell* **2002**, *108*, 171–182.

83. Feil, R.; Brocard, J.; Mascrez, B.; LeMeur, M.; Metzger, D.; Chambon, P. Ligand-activated site-specific recombination in mice. *Proc. Natl. Acad. Sci. USA* **1996**, *93*, 10887–10890.

84. Xu, X.; Wagner, K. U.; Larson, D.; Weaver, Z.; Li, C.; Ried, T.; Hennighausen, L.; Wynshaw-Boris, A.; Deng, C. X. Conditional mutation of Brca1 in mammary epithelial cells results in blunted ductal morphogenesis and tumour formation. *Nat. Genet.* **1999**, *22*, 37–43.

85. Wooster, R.; Bignell, G.; Lancaster, J.; Swift, S.; Seal, S.; Mangion, J.; Collins, N.; Gregory, S.; Gumbs, C.; Micklem, G. Identification of the breast cancer susceptibility gene BRCA2. *Nature* **1995**, *378*, 789–792.

86. Lancaster, J. M.; Wooster, R.; Mangion, J.; Phelan, C. M.; Cochran, C.; Gumbs, C.; Seal, S.; Barfoot, R.; Collins, N.; Bignell, G.; Patel, S.; Hamoudi, R.; Larsson, C.; Wiseman, R. W.; Berchuck, A.; Iglehart, J. D.; Marks, J. R.; Ashworth, A.; Stratton, M. R.; Futreal, P. A. BRCA2 mutations in primary breast and ovarian cancers. *Nat. Genet.* **1996**, *13*, 238–240.

87. Thompson, L. H.; Schild, D. Recombinational DNA repair and human disease. *Mutat. Res.* **2002**, *509*, 49–78.

88. Powell, S. N.; Kachnic, L. A. Roles of BRCA1 and BRCA2 in homologous recombination, DNA replication fidelity and the cellular response to ionizing radiation. *Oncogene* **2003**, *22*, 5784–5791.

89. Narod, S. A.; Foulkes, W. D. BRCA1 and BRCA2: 1994 and beyond. *Nat. Rev. Cancer* **2004**, *4*, 665–676.

90. Daniels, M. J.; Wang, Y.; Lee, M.; Venkitaraman, A. R. Abnormal cytokinesis in cells deficient in the breast cancer susceptibility protein BRCA2. *Science* **2004**, *306*, 876–879.

91. Goodrich, D. W.; Lee, W. H. Molecular characterization of the retinoblastoma susceptibility gene. *Biochim. Biophys. Acta* **1993**, *1155*, 43–61.

92. Lee, E. Y.; Chang, C. Y.; Hu, N.; Wang, Y. C.; Lai, C. C.; Herrup, K.; Lee, W. H.; Bradley, A. Mice deficient for Rb are nonviable and show defects in neurogenesis and haematopoiesis. *Nature* **1992**, *359*, 288–294.

93. Sharpless, N. E.; Alson, S.; Chan, S.; Silver, D. P.; Castrillon, D. H.; DePinho, R. A. p16(INK4a) and p53 deficiency cooperate in tumorigenesis. *Cancer Res.* **2002**, *62*, 2761–2765.

94. Hussussian, C. J.; Struewing, J. P.; Goldstein, A. M.; Higgins, P. A.; Ally, D. S.; Sheahan, M. D.; Clark, W. H., Jr.; Tucker, M. A.; Dracopoli, N. C. Germline p16 mutations in familial melanoma. *Nat. Genet.* **1994**, *8*, 15–21.

95. Sherr, C. J.; McCormick, F. The RB and p53 pathways in cancer. *Cancer Cell* **2002**, *2*, 103–112.

96. DeLeo, A. B.; Jay, G.; Appella, E.; DuBois, G. C.; Law, L. W.; Old, L. J. Detection of a transformation-related antigen in chemically induced sarcomas and other transformed cells of the mouse. *Proc. Natl. Acad. Sci. USA* **1979**, *76*, 2420–2424.

97. Linzer, D. I.; Levine, A. J. Characterization of a 54K dalton cellular SV40 tumor antigen present in SV40-transformed cells and uninfected embryonal carcinoma cells. *Cell* **1979**, *17*, 43–52.

98. Hofseth, L. J.; Hussain, S. P.; Harris, C. C. p53: 25 years after its discovery. *Trends Pharmacol. Sci.* **2004**, *25*, 177–181.

99. Crawford, L. The 53,000-dalton cellular protein and its role in transformation. *Int. Rev. Exp. Pathol.* **1983**, *25*, 1–50.

100. Leppard, K.; Totty, N.; Waterfield, M.; Harlow, E.; Jenkins, J.; Crawford, L. Purification and partial amino acid sequence analysis of the cellular tumour antigen, p53, from mouse SV40-transformed cells. *EMBO J.* **1983**, *2*, 1993–1999.

101. Oren, M.; Levine, A. J. Molecular cloning of a cDNA specific for the murine p53 cellular tumor antigen. *Proc. Natl. Acad. Sci. USA* **1983**, *80*, 56–59.

102. Li, F. P.; Fraumeni, J. F., Jr.; Mulvihill, J. J.; Blattner, W. A.; Dreyfus, M. G.; Tucker, M. A.; Miller, R. W. A cancer family syndrome in twenty-four kindreds. *Cancer Res.* **1988**, *48*, 5358–5362.

103. Srivastava, S.; Zou, Z. Q.; Pirollo, K.; Blattner, W.; Chang, E. H. Germ-line transmission of a mutated p53 gene in a cancer-prone family with Li-Fraumeni syndrome. *Nature* **1990**, *348*, 747–749.

104. Chompret, A. The Li-Fraumeni syndrome. *Biochimie* **2002**, *84*, 75–82.

105. Hollstein, M.; Sidransky, D.; Vogelstein, B.; Harris, C. C. p53 mutations in human cancers. *Science* **1991**, *253*, 49–53.

106. Sigal, A.; Rotter, V. Oncogenic mutations of the p53 tumor suppressor: the demons of the guardian of the genome. *Cancer Res.* **2000**, *60*, 6788–6793.

107. Prives, C.; Manfreid, J. J. The p53 tumor suppressor protein: meeting review. *Genes Dev.* **1993**, *7*, 529–534.

108. Jeffrey, P. D.; Gorina, S.; Pavletich, N. P. Crystal structure of the tetramerization domain of the p53 tumor suppressor at 1.7 angstroms. *Science* **1995**, *267*, 1498–1502.

109. May, P.; May, E. Twenty years of p53 research: structural and functional aspects of the p53 protein. *Oncogene* **1999**, *18*, 7621–7636.

110. Liu, Y.; Kulesz-Martin, M. p53 protein at the hub of cellular DNA damage response pathways through sequence-specific and non-sequence-specific DNA binding. *Carcinogenesis* **2001**, *22*, 851–860.

111. Kato, S.; Han, S. Y.; Liu, W.; Otsuka, K.; Shibata, H.; Kanamaru, R.; Ishioka, C. Understanding the function–structure and function–mutation relationships of p53 tumor suppressor protein by high-resolution missense mutation analysis. *Proc. Natl. Acad. Sci. USA* **2003**, *100*, 8424–8429.

112. Lee, W.; Harvey, T. S.; Yin, Y.; Yau, P.; Litchfield, D.; Arrowsmith, C. H. Solution structure of the tetrameric minimum transforming domain of p53. *Nat. Struct. Biol.* **1994**, *1*, 877–890.

113. Arrowsmith, C. H.; Morin, P. New insights into p53 function from structural studies. *Oncogene* **1996**, *12*, 1379–1385.

114. Arrowsmith, C. H. Structure and function in the p53 family. *Cell Death. Differ.* **1999**, *6*, 1169–1173.

115. Haupt, S.; Berger, M.; Goldberg, Z.; Haupt, Y. Apoptosis: the p53 network. *J. Cell Sci.* **2003**, *116*, 4077–4085.

116. Thompson, C. B. Apoptosis in the pathogenesis and treatment of disease. *Science* **1995**, *267*, 1456–1462.

117. Vousden, K. H. p53: death star. *Cell* **2000**, *103*, 691–694.

118. Lane, D. P. Cancer. p53, guardian of the genome. *Nature* **1992**, *358*, 15–16.

119. Schwartz, D.; Rotter, V. p53-dependent cell cycle control: response to genotoxic stress. *Semin. Cancer Biol.* **1998**, *8*, 325–336.

120. Kinzler, K. W.; Vogelstein, B. Cancer-susceptibility genes. Gatekeepers and caretakers. *Nature* **1997**, *386*, 761, 763.

121. Levine, A. J. p53, the cellular gatekeeper for growth and division. *Cell* **1997**, *88*, 323–331.

122. Loeb, L. A.; Loeb, K. R.; Anderson, J. P. Multiple mutations and cancer. *Proc. Natl. Acad. Sci. USA* **2003**, *100*, 776–781.

123. Wang, T. L.; Rago, C.; Silliman, N.; Ptak, J.; Markowitz, S.; Willson, J. K.; Parmigiani, G.; Kinzler, K. W.; Vogelstein, B.; Velculescu, V. E. Prevalence of somatic alterations in the colorectal cancer cell genome. *Proc. Natl. Acad. Sci. USA* **2002**, *99*, 3076–3080.

124. Donehower, L. A.; Harvey, M.; Slagle, B. L.; McArthur, M. J.; Montgomery, C. A., Jr.; Butel, J. S.; Bradley, A. Mice deficient for p53 are developmentally normal but susceptible to spontaneous tumours. *Nature* **1992**, *356*, 215–221.

125. Donehower, L. A. The p53-deficient mouse: a model for basic and applied cancer studies. *Semin. Cancer Biol.* **1996**, *7*, 269–278.

126. French, J.; Storer, R. D.; Donehower, L. A. The nature of the heterozygous Trp53 knockout model for identification of mutagenic carcinogens. *Toxicol. Pathol.* **2001**, *29* (Suppl.), 24–29.

127. Dumble, M. L.; Donehower, L. A.; Lu, X. Generation and characterization of p53 mutant mice. *Methods Mol. Biol.* **2003**, *234*, 29–49.

128. Storer, R. D.; French, J. E.; Donehower, L. A.; Gulezian, D.; Mitsumori, K.; Recio, L.; Schiestl, R. H.; Sistare, F. D.; Tamaoki, N.; Usui, T.; van Steeg, H. Transgenic tumor models for carcinogen identification: the heterozygous Trp53-deficient and RasH2 mouse lines. *Mutat. Res.* **2003**, *540*, 165–176.

129. Jacks, T.; Remington, L.; Williams, B. O.; Schmitt, E. M.; Halachmi, S.; Bronson, R. T.; Weinberg, R. A. Tumor spectrum analysis in p53-mutant mice. *Curr. Biol.* **1994**, *4*, 1–7.

130. Storer, R. D.; French, J. E.; Haseman, J.; Hajian, G.; LeGrand, E. K.; Long, G. G.; Mixson, L. A.; Ochoa, R.; Sagartz, J. E.; Soper, K. A. P53+/− hemizygous knockout mouse: overview of available data. *Toxicol. Pathol.* **2001**, *29* (Suppl.), 30–50.

131. Wijnhoven, S. W.; van Steeg, H. Transgenic and knockout mice for DNA repair functions in carcinogenesis and mutagenesis. *Toxicology* **2003**, *193*, 171–187.

132. Cory, S.; Adams, J. M. The Bcl2 family: regulators of the cellular life-or-death switch. *Nat. Rev. Cancer* **2002**, *2*, 647–656.

133. Raffray, M.; Cohen, G. M. Apoptosis and necrosis in toxicology: a continuum or distinct modes of cell death? *Pharmacol. Ther.* **1997**, *75*, 153–177.

134. Vaux, D. L.; Strasser, A. The molecular biology of apoptosis. *Proc. Natl. Acad. Sci. USA* **1996**, *93*, 2239–2244.

135. Degterev, A.; Boyce, M.; Yuan, J. A decade of caspases. *Oncogene* **2003**, *22*, 8543–8567.

136. Boyce, M.; Degterev, A.; Yuan, J. Caspases: an ancient cellular sword of Damocles. *Cell Death. Differ.* **2004**, *11*, 29–37.

137. Greidinger, E. L.; Miller, D. K.; Yamin, T. T.; Casciola-Rosen, L.; Rosen, A. Sequential activation of three distinct ICE-like activities in Fas-ligated Jurkat cells. *FEBS Lett.* **1996**, *390*, 299–303.

138. Thornberry, N. A.; Bull, H. G.; Calaycay, J. R.; Chapman, K. T.; Howard, A. D.; Kostura, M. J.; Miller, D. K.; Molineaux, S. M.; Weidner, J. R.; Aunins, J. A novel heterodimeric cysteine protease is required for interleukin-1 beta processing in monocytes. *Nature* **1992**, *356*, 768–774.

139. Curtin, J. F.; Cotter, T. G. Live and let die: regulatory mechanisms in Fas-mediated apoptosis. *Cell Signal.* **2003**, *15*, 983–992.

140. Muzio, M.; Chinnaiyan, A. M.; Kischkel, F. C.; O'Rourke, K.; Shevchenko, A.; Ni, J.; Scaffidi, C.; Bretz, J. D.; Zhang, M.; Gentz, R.; Mann, M.; Krammer, P. H.; Peter, M. E.; Dixit, V. M. FLICE, a novel FADD-homologous ICE/CED-3-like protease, is recruited to the CD95 (Fas/APO-1) death-inducing signaling complex. *Cell* **1996**, *85*, 817–827.

141. Medema, J. P.; Scaffidi, C.; Kischkel, F. C.; Shevchenko, A.; Mann, M.; Krammer, P. H.; Peter, M. E. FLICE is activated by association with the CD95 death-inducing signaling complex (DISC). *EMBO J.* **1997**, *16*, 2794–2804.

142. Ohta, T.; Kinoshita, T.; Naito, M.; Nozaki, T.; Masutani, M.; Tsuruo, T.; Miyajima, A. Requirement of the caspase-3/CPP32 protease cascade for apoptotic death following cytokine deprivation in hematopoietic cells. *J. Biol. Chem.* **1997**, *272*, 23111–23116.

143. Eischen, C. M.; Kottke, T. J.; Martins, L. M.; Basi, G. S.; Tung, J. S.; Earnshaw, W. C.; Leibson, P. J.; Kaufmann, S. H. Comparison of apoptosis in wild-type and Fas-resistant cells: chemotherapy-induced apoptosis is not dependent on Fas/Fas ligand interactions. *Blood* **1997**, *90*, 935–943.

144. Kaina, B. DNA damage-triggered apoptosis: critical role of DNA repair, double-strand breaks, cell proliferation and signaling. *Biochem. Pharmacol.* **2003**, *66*, 1547–1554.

145. Jiang, X.; Wang, X. Cytochrome c-mediated apoptosis. *Annu. Rev. Biochem.* **2004**, *73*, 87–106.

146. Acehan, D.; Jiang, X.; Morgan, D. G.; Heuser, J. E.; Wang, X.; Akey, C. W. Three-dimensional structure of the apoptosome: implications for assembly, procaspase-9 binding, and activation. *Mol. Cell* **2002**, *9*, 423–432.

147. Renatus, M.; Stennicke, H. R.; Scott, F. L.; Liddington, R. C.; Salvesen, G. S. Dimer formation drives the activation of the cell death protease caspase 9. *Proc. Natl. Acad. Sci. USA* **2001**, *98*, 14250–14255.

148. Lassus, P.; Opitz-Araya, X.; Lazebnik, Y. Requirement for caspase-2 in stress-induced apoptosis before mitochondrial permeabilization. *Science* **2002**, *297*, 1352–1354.

149. Marsden, V. S.; O'Connor, L.; O'Reilly, L. A.; Silke, J.; Metcalf, D.; Ekert, P. G.; Huang, D. C.; Cecconi, F.; Kuida, K.; Tomaselli, K. J.; Roy, S.; Nicholson, D. W.; Vaux, D. L.; Bouillet, P.; Adams, J. M.; Strasser, A. Apoptosis initiated by Bcl-2-regulated caspase activation independently of the cytochrome c/Apaf-1/caspase-9 apoptosome. *Nature* **2002**, *419*, 634–637.

150. Deveraux, Q. L.; Takahashi, R.; Salvesen, G. S.; Reed, J. C. X-linked IAP is a direct inhibitor of cell-death proteases. *Nature* **1997**, *388*, 300–304.

151. Li, F. Survivin study: what is the next wave? *J. Cell Physiol.* **2003**, *197*, 8–29.

152. Deng, Y.; Lin, Y.; Wu, X. TRAIL-induced apoptosis requires Bax-dependent mitochondrial release of Smac/DIABLO. *Genes Dev.* **2002**, *16*, 33–45.

153. Vaux, D. L.; Silke, J. Mammalian mitochondrial IAP binding proteins. *Biochem. Biophys. Res. Commun.* **2003**, *304*, 499–504.

154. Brunet, A.; Bonni, A.; Zigmond, M. J.; Lin, M. Z.; Juo, P.; Hu, L. S.; Anderson, M. J.; Arden, K. C.; Blenis, J.; Greenberg, M. E. Akt promotes cell survival by phosphorylating and inhibiting a Forkhead transcription factor. *Cell* **1999**, *96*, 857–868.

155. Scheid, M. P.; Woodgett, J. R. Unravelling the activation mechanisms of protein kinase B/Akt. *FEBS Lett.* **2003**, *546*, 108–112.

156. Frisch, S. M.; Screaton, R. A. Anoikis mechanisms. *Curr. Opin. Cell Biol.* **2001**, *13*, 555–562.

157. Mirakian, R.; Nye, K.; Palazzo, F. F.; Goode, A. W.; Hammond, L. J. Methods for detecting apoptosis in thyroid diseases. *J. Immunol. Methods* **2002**, *265*, 161–175.

158. Valentijn, A. J.; Zouq, N.; Gilmore, A. P. Anoikis. *Biochem. Soc. Trans.* **2004**, *32*, 421–425.

159. Vaux, D. L. Apoptosis and toxicology: what relevance? *Toxicology* **2002**, *181–182*, 3–7.

160. Yu, J.; Zhang, L. Apoptosis in human cancer cells. *Curr. Opin. Oncol.* **2004**, *16*, 19–24.

161. Fridman, J. S.; Lowe, S. W. Control of apoptosis by p53. *Oncogene* **2003**, *22*, 9030–9040. Appella, E.; Anderson, C. W. Post-translational modifications and activation of p53 by genotoxic stresses. *Eur. J. Biochem.* **2001**, *268*, 2764–2772.

162. Polyak, K.; Xia, Y.; Zweier, J. L.; Kinzler, K. W.; Vogelstein, B. A model for p53-induced apoptosis. *Nature* **1997**, *389*, 300–305.

163. Olive, P. L.; Johnston, P. J.; Banath, J. P.; Durand, R. E. The comet assay: a new method to examine heterogeneity associated with solid tumors. *Nat. Med.* **1998**, *4*, 103–105.

164. Itoh, G.; Tamura, J.; Suzuki, M.; Suzuki, Y.; Ikeda, H.; Koike, M.; Nomura, M.; Jie, T.; Ito, K. DNA fragmentation of human infarcted myocardial cells demonstrated by the nick end labeling method and DNA agarose gel electrophoresis. *Am. J. Pathol.* **1995**, *146*, 1325–1331.

165. Kohler, C.; Orrenius, S.; Zhivotovsky, B. Evaluation of caspase activity in apoptotic cells. *J. Immunol. Methods* **2002**, *265*, 97–110.

166. Hudson, J. M.; Frade, R.; Bar-Eli, M. Wild-type p53 regulates its own transcription in a cell-type specific manner. *DNA Cell Biol.* **1995**, *14*, 759–766.

167. Marks, J. R.; Davidoff, A. M.; Kerns, B. J.; Humphrey, P. A.; Pence, J. C.; Dodge, R. K.; Clarke-Pearson, D. L.; Iglehart, J. D.; Bast, R. C., Jr.; Berchuck, A. Overexpression and mutation of p53 in epithelial ovarian cancer. *Cancer Res.* **1991**, *51*, 2979–2984.

168. Bartek, J.; Bartkova, J.; Vojtesek, B.; Staskova, Z.; Rejthar, A.; Kovarik, J.; Lane, D. P. Patterns of expression of the p53 tumour suppressor in human breast tissues and tumours in situ and in vitro. *Int. J. Cancer* **1990**, *46*, 839–844.

169. Hernandez-Boussard, T.; Montesano, R.; Hainaut, P. Analysis of somatic mutations of the p53 gene in human cancers: a tool to generate hypotheses about the natural history of cancer. *IARC Sci. Publ.* **1999**, 43–53.

170. Hussain, S. P.; Harris, C. C. Molecular epidemiology and carcinogenesis: endogenous and exogenous carcinogens. *Mutat. Res.* **2000**, *462*, 311–322.

171. Hollstein, M.; Hergenhahn, M.; Yang, Q.; Bartsch, H.; Wang, Z. Q.; Hainaut, P. New approaches to understanding p53 gene tumor mutation spectra. *Mutat. Res.* **1999**, *431*, 199–209.

172. Brash, D. E.; Rudolph, J. A.; Simon, J. A.; Lin, A.; McKenna, G. J.; Baden, H. P.; Halperin, A. J.; Pontén, J. A role for sunlight in skin cancer: UV-induced p53 mutations in squamous cell carcinoma. *Proc. Natl. Acad. Sci. USA* **1991**, *88*, 10124–10128.

173. Ziegler, A.; Leffell, D. J.; Kunala, S.; Sharma, H. W.; Gailani, M.; Simon, J. A.; Halperin, A. J.; Baden, H. P.; Shapiro, P. E.; Bale, A. E. Mutation hotspots due to sunlight in the p53 gene of nonmelanoma skin cancers. *Proc. Natl. Acad. Sci. USA* **1993**, *90*, 4216–4220.

174. Giglia-Mari, G.; Sarasin, A. TP53 mutations in human skin cancers. *Hum. Mutat.* **2003**, *21*, 217–228.

175. Ziegler, A.; Jonason, A. S.; Leffell, D. J.; Simon, J. A.; Sharma, H. W.; Kimmelman, J.; Remington, L.; Jacks, T.; Brash, D. E. Sunburn and p53 in the onset of skin cancer. *Nature* **1994**, *372*, 773–776.

176. Tornaletti, S.; Pfeifer, G. P. Complete and tissue-independent methylation of CpG sites in the p53 gene: implications for mutations in human cancers. *Oncogene* **1995**, *10*, 1493–1499.

177. You, Y. H.; Pfeifer, G. P. Similarities in sunlight-induced mutational spectra of CpG-methylated transgenes and the p53 gene in skin cancer point to an important role of 5-methylcytosine residues in solar UV mutagenesis. *J. Mol. Biol.* **2001**, *305*, 389–399.

178. Pfeifer, G. P.; Denissenko, M. F.; Olivier, M.; Tretyakova, N.; Hecht, S. S.; Hainaut, P. Tobacco smoke carcinogens, DNA damage and p53 mutations in smoking-associated cancers. *Oncogene* **2002**, *21*, 7435–7451.

179. Pfeifer, G. P.; Hainaut, P. On the origin of G-T transversions in lung cancer. *Mutat. Res.* **2003**, *526*, 39–43.

180. Hainaut, P.; Pfeifer, G. P. Patterns of p53 G-T transversions in lung cancers reflect the primary mutagenic signature of DNA-damage by tobacco smoke. *Carcinogenesis* **2001**, *22*, 367–374.

181. Hill, K. A.; Sommer, S. S. p53 as a mutagen test in breast cancer. *Environ. Mol. Mutagen.* **2002**, *39*, 216–227.

182. Shen, H. M.; Ong, C. N. Mutations of the p53 tumor suppressor gene and ras oncogenes in aflatoxin hepatocarcinogenesis. *Mutat. Res.* **1996**, *366*, 23–44.

183. Montesano, R.; Hainaut, P.; Wild, C. P. Hepatocellular carcinoma: from gene to public health. *J. Natl. Cancer Inst.* **1997**, *89*, 1844–1851.

184. Smela, M. E.; Hamm, M. L.; Henderson, P. T.; Harris, C. M.; Harris, T. M.; Essigmann, J. M. The aflatoxin B1 formamidopyrimidine adduct plays a major role in causing the types of mutations observed in human hepatocellular carcinoma. *Proc. Natl. Acad. Sci. USA* **2002**, *99*, 6655–6660.

185. Hulla, J. E.; Schneider, R. P. Structure of the rat p53 tumor suppressor gene. *Nucleic Acids Res.* **1993**, *21*, 713–717.

186. Tam, A. S.; Foley, J. F.; Devereux, T. R.; Maronpot, R. R.; Massey, T. E. High frequency and heterogeneous distribution of p53 mutations in aflatoxin B1-induced mouse lung tumors. *Cancer Res.* **1999**, *59*, 3634–3640.

187. Pfeifer, G. P.; Steigerwald, S. D.; Mueller, P. R.; Wold, B.; Riggs, A. D. Genomic sequencing and methylation analysis by ligation mediated PCR. *Science* **1989**, *246*, 810–813.

188. Pfeifer, G. P.; Drouin, R.; Holmquist, G. P. Detection of DNA adducts at the DNA sequence level by ligation-mediated PCR. *Mutat. Res.* **1993**, *288*, 39–46.

SURVIVAL ASSAYS

Toxicology studies often involve the quantitative measurement of cell death. Consider, for example, the requirements of cancer therapy. A solid tumor weighing 1 g (which might easily escape clinical detection) already contains as many as 10^9 cells. Any single surviving cell may have the potential to regrow into a tumor, so, to be curative, radiotherapy or chemotherapy might require better than 99.999999% killing. Similar considerations apply to the problem of disinfection: to ensure the effective sterilization of contaminated medical instruments, we want to prevent the survival of any bacteria—even a few cells might transfer a disease.

A variety of techniques are available for measuring cytotoxicity/cell survival. Intact mammalian cells will exclude a "vital dye" such as trypan blue. Cells that have disrupted plasma membranes (and are presumably dead) become stained by the dye (e.g., (*1*)) and can be counted under the microscope. Another rapid cytotoxicity assay measures the reduction of the indicator 3-(4,5-dimethylthiazol-2-yl)-2,5-diphenyltetrazolium (MTT); living cells reduce this compound to blue formazan crystals (*2*). This assay is readily adapted to the 96-well plate format (*3*) for high-throughput screening applications.

Clonogenic survival assays (e.g., (*4*)) are often regarded as the "gold standard" of cytotoxicity measurements. A population of cells is exposed to a lethal agent and then plated in Petri dishes so that surviving cells can proliferate. After a suitable growth period (typically a week, for mammalian cells), survivors have formed colonies large enough to be counted by eye (after staining). Although this assay requires much more time than the "acute toxicity" assays mentioned previously, it has several important advantages. First, it measures the ability of cells to *reproduce* and form colonies. A cell with severely damaged DNA and unable to proliferate might still have an intact cell membrane and appear viable in a dye-exclusion assay. Second, the clonogenic assay principle is applicable to any type of cell that can be grown in culture, whether it be an animal, plant, yeast, or bacterial cell. Even viruses can be studied this way, for example by counting plaques on a lawn of bacteria. Third, clonogenic assays have a very large "dynamic range." This is a topic we need to explore in more detail.

Dynamic Range of Survival Assays

Both the high survival/low killing and low survival/high killing regimes are of scientific interest. We already noted situations, such as cancer therapy, in which it is critically important to achieve extremely low survival levels. The other end of the dynamic range is significant when we want to evaluate the toxicological consequences of low-level exposures, such as to natural background radiation or trace environmental chemicals. Frustratingly, these high-dose and low-dose effects are usually the hardest to quantify.

Consider the dye-exclusion assay, for example. At very low doses, almost all cells survive. To measure killing, we would have to search for a few stained cells among a very large number of viable cells. But any cell preparation is bound to contain a few dead cells, independent of exposure. So how can we reliably measure the presence of a few additional dead cells that may have been killed by the experimental treatment? At the other extreme, very high doses, almost all of the cells are dead, so we would have to search for a few *un*stained cells among a very large number of stained cells. These will be hard to find, and to measure a survival level of 10^{-6}, we would need to examine at least one million cells under the microscope. Similar limitations apply to the MTT assay.

Clonogenic assays perform better than rapid cytotoxicity tests at the low-survival extreme. Suppose survival has been reduced to, say, 10^{-4}; if we can plate 10^5 cells into a Petri dish (which is realistic, even with mammalian cells), then approximately 10 of them should be able to form colonies, and this is sufficient to give a reasonably accurate measurement of survival. With bacteria, one can readily measure survival even at the 10^{-8} level. At the high-survival end of the range, however, we encounter the familiar difficulty of measuring a small difference between two large numbers. The *plating efficiency* (i.e., the percentage of plated cells that grow into colonies) is never 100%, whether because of spontaneous lethal mutations, physical damage to cells during manipulation and plating, or other ill-defined factors. With mammalian cells, 75% plating efficiency may be considered good. Suppose we wish to measure killing at the 1% level (i.e., 99% survival). We plate 100 cells into a control dish and another 100 cells into the experimental dish. Seventy-five colonies grow in the former and 74 in the latter; but the statistical error in either of the values is much more than the difference between them.

In fact, the situation is usually worse than this. Rather than plating 100 cells, counted out one at a time, we simply dilute the preparation of cells to a density of, say, 1000 cells per mL, and then plate 0.1 mL aliquots into each dish. This aliquoting procedure, in itself, incurs a statistical variability of magnitude approximately equal to the square root of the number of cells plated; with 100 cells per dish, this amounts to ±10% error. To overcome this limitation, several research groups (5–7) have introduced computer-automated microscopy image analysis systems, which scan the Petri dishes electronically, detecting each cell plated. At time intervals during the incubation period, the dishes are re-scanned, and the fate (growth or death/disintegration) of each cell is recorded. These systems have improved the accuracy of low-dose survival curve measurements.

TARGET THEORY

His little bureau is dominated now by a glimmering map . . . written names and spidering streets, an ink ghost of London, ruled off into 576 squares, a quarter square kilometer each. Rocket strikes are represented by red circles. The Poisson equation will tell, for a number of total hits arbitrarily chosen, how many squares will get none, how many 1, 2, 3, and so on ... When it does happen, we are content to call it "chance". Or we have been persuaded. But to the likes of employees such as Roger Mexico it is music, not without its majesty, this power series $Ne^{-m}(1 + m + m^2/2! + m^3/3! + ... + m^{n-1}/(n-1)!)$, terms numbered according to rocket-falls per square, the Poisson dispensation ruling not only these annihilations no man can run from, but also cavalry accidents, blood counts, radioactive decay, number of wars per year ...

Thomas Pynchon, *Gravity's Rainbow*, 1973 (pp. 63 and 163)

Pynchon's great novel is set in London during World War II. On a gridded map of the city, Mr. Roger Mexico, a War Department bureaucrat, plots the impact sites of German flying bombs and observes that they follow a Poisson statistical distribution (8). The formula for the Poisson distribution is:

$$P(n) = \frac{e^{-x}x^n}{n!}$$

where $P(n)$ is the probability of n events, and x is the average number of events.

Pynchon's fiction is based on historical fact; figure 6-1 compares the actual data set[1] (number of grid squares, N, suffering number of bomb hits, k, in south[2] London, during the Blitz) with the results of a calculation using the Poisson distribution (8, p. 150). Note how closely the bars line up: this agreement proves that the widespread impression that the bomb strikes tended to "cluster" in certain areas was incorrect; their local distribution was completely random.

Pynchon observes that the same law applies to phenomena as disparate as road accidents and blood cell counts.[3] The factor that all these situations have in common is *statistical independence*. The fact that a rocket bomb landed in Piccadilly Circus last week neither increases nor decreases the chance that one will land there this week. (Gamblers believe that each losing throw of the dice makes the next roll more likely to win, but this is pure delusion.)

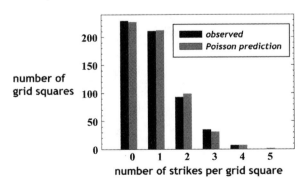

FIGURE 6-1.
The Poisson distribution. Black bars: number of grid squares, N, suffering number of bomb hits, k, in south London during the Blitz of World War II. Red bars: values predicted by the Poisson distribution. *Note*: A full-color version of this figure appears on the website.

Notice that, for any value of x (the average number of events), the value of $P(0)$ is simply e^{-x}. That is, the number of grid squares in which no bomb has landed ("survivors") *declines exponentially with the total number of bombs dropped.*

Now we will make the transition from a discussion of flying bombs and road accidents to cellular toxicology. Consider, then, a population of cells—say, mammalian fibroblasts in a Petri dish—exposed to a dose of a toxic agent. (We will make the simplifying assumption that the cells are clonal and all have identical sensitivity.) *We will assume that the fate (life or death) of an individual cell is dictated by the same statistical rules as those that describe the impact of flying bombs.* Instead of grid squares on a map, we have individual cells in the population. Instead of bomb strikes, we have biological "hits," which might be mutations, DNA strand breaks, or membrane ruptures. *The analysis of the kinetics of lethality is called "target theory" because of this close analogy.* Target theory was developed around the time of World War II, notably by D.E. Lea (9). Typically, we do not have direct information about the number of "hits" (damaging events of an unspecified nature) that have occurred in each cell in the population. Rather, we perform a *survival assay* on the population, as discussed above. Instead of counting the number of grid squares (cells) that have been hit, we will simply measure S, the surviving fraction of the population, in a clonogenic assay.

The Single-Hit, Single-Target Model

Let us analyze this situation mathematically (*10*, ch. 4). We will assume that *one "hit" will kill one cell.* (This may seem to be an unsophisticated model for the phenomenon of cell death, and we will construct a more complex model later, but the simplest theory is the best place to start.)

An increment of dose will inactivate an increment of targets:

$$-\frac{dN}{dD} = \lambda N$$

where N is the initial number of targets, D is the dose, and λ is a proportionality constant.

$$\int_{N_0}^{N} \frac{dN}{N} = -\lambda \int_{0}^{D} dD$$

Integrating this equation gives a formula for the surviving fraction, S:

$$\ln \frac{N}{N_0} = -\lambda D$$

$$S = \frac{N}{N_0} = e^{-\lambda D} = e^{-D/D_0}$$

where $D_0 = 1/\lambda$. What is the interpretation of the term D_0? When $D = D_0$, $S = e^{-1} = 0.37$ (37% survival). We call D_0 the "inactivation dose"; it is *the dose that causes, on average, one lethal event per cell* and reduces survival to $1/e$.

This "one-hit, one-target" equation predicts that survival of the population of cells will decrease exponentially with dose (i.e., *a plot of log S versus dose will give a straight line*) as one would have expected from the form of the Poisson distribution. This pure exponential model works remarkably well as a description of certain lethal processes. We will look at a couple of examples.

The inactivation of macromolecules by radiation is the clearest case of one-hit kinetics. When high-energy radiation (such as β-particles or γ-rays) interacts with the electrons of an atom in a protein, a large amount of energy is released by electronic excitations and ionizations. Each primary interaction releases enough energy to break many covalent bonds, almost certainly fragmenting the polypeptide chain and many amino acid side chains. We would expect that even one such "hit" would inactivate a protein molecule, for example destroy the catalytic activity of an enzyme molecule (figure 6-2). Indeed, an activity assay of an irradiated enzyme sample shows that V_{max} decreases exponentially with dose, while K_M is unchanged. Enzyme activity V_{max} as a function of radiation dose (measured in energy units such as rads or grays) follows exponential kinetics *and the slope of the plot is proportional to the mass of the holoenzyme.* This linear relationship between mass and inactivation rate is the same for all macromolecules (proteins, DNA, even viruses) because they are all composed of the same sorts of atoms (C, N, O). Indeed, measurement of radiation inactivation

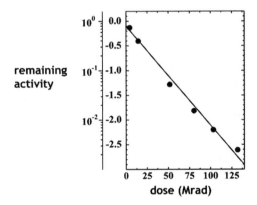

FIGURE 6-2.

Radiation inactivation of an enzyme. Recombinant human hepatic lipase was expressed in Chinese hamster ovary cells and purified. Aliquots of enzyme were frozen on dry ice and irradiated at −135°C with 13 MeV electrons. The aliquots were subsequently thawed and assayed for enzyme activity. From the slope of the inactivation curve, the molecular weight of the enzyme was calculated to be 109 kDa, closely matching the value of 106.8 kDa for a homodimer calculated from the sequence. (*Hill, J. S. et al. Human hepatic lipase subunit structure determination.* J. Biol. Chem. **1996**, 271, 22931–22936.) The radiation inactivation method measures the size of the functional enzyme unit, so it is valuable for determining whether an enzyme protein's activity is associated with a monomer or multimer. (Note that the radiation doses used to inactivate enzyme samples are vastly higher than the doses required to kill cells; doses this high would destroy almost every macromolecule within a cell.) For this and subsequent inactivation/survival curves, the data are plotted semi-logarithmically (linear abscissa and logarithmic ordinate); vertical scales show both the *S* and log *S* values.

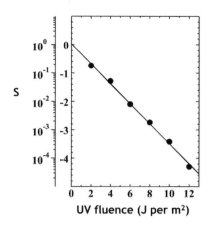

FIGURE 6-3.

UV survival curve for *E. coli* cells bearing the *uvrA*6 (UV-sensitivity) mutation. Cultures were grown to log phase, resuspended in phosphate buffer, treated with 254 nm radiation, and then plated on nutrient agar. (*Data from Song, Y.; Sargentini, N. J. Escherichia coli DNA repair genes radA and sms are the same gene.* J. Bacteriol. **1996**, 178, 5045–5048.)

kinetics provides a very accurate technique for measuring the molecular weight of a macromolecule (*11–13*).

Turning to cells, we find that many survival curves follow exponential kinetics remarkably closely. For example, figure 6-3 shows the results of an ultraviolet (UV) survival curve for a strain of *E. coli* (*14*). The cells were grown in rich medium, resuspended in buffer, treated with various doses of UV radiation (254 nm), and then plated on nutrient agar to determine survival. The plotted line represents a regression fit of the one-hit/one-target model to the data, and clearly fits the data very well.

The Multitarget Model

Although some experimental survival curves appear to be purely exponential, as we have just seen, many survival curves show a distinct "shoulder." That is, S remains close to 100% until a certain "threshold" dose range is reached, and only then begins to drop steeply. This behavior is inconsistent with the simple Poisson model we have developed, and we need to generalize our model to account for it.

Inactivating one target may not be sufficient to kill a cell. Let us assume that each cell contains a certain small number, n, of "targets," *all of which* must be inactivated to kill the cell. This is referred to as the "single-hit, multitarget" model, and it is analyzed as follows.

For each target, the probability that the target has *survived* (not been hit) at dose D is

$$S = e^{-D/D_0}$$

So, the probability that the target *has* been hit is

$$P = 1 - e^{-D/D_0}$$

And the probability that n (identically sensitive) independent targets have all been hit, that is, the probability that the cell has been *killed*, is the product of these n terms:

$$P = \left(1 - e^{-D/D_0}\right)^n$$

Finally, the probability that the cell has *survived* is $1 - P$:

$$S = 1 - \left(1 - e^{-D/D_0}\right)^n \tag{6-1}$$

This well-known equation for the "single-hit, multitarget" model describes many dose–response curves remarkably well. Other models of survival curves have been constructed (*10*), but this equation works satisfactorily for most situations involving a homogeneous cell population. Figure 6-4 (left) shows the calculated shape of the curve for values of n from 1 to 5. (Of course, n does not need to be integral.) For $n = 1$, the equation reduces to the straight-line, single-target equation.

At the high-dose limit, equation (6-1) approximates[4] to

$$S \approx n e^{-D/D_0}$$

This equation describes a straight line on the plot of $\log S$ versus D, resembling the single-target case discussed previously. *The value of n is simply the intercept, on the S axis, of the straight line drawn tangent to the survival curve at high doses.* This is illustrated in figure 6-4 (right) for the case $n = 4$. We can easily see why the equation has this limit. At high doses, almost all of the targets have already been hit, so most of the surviving cells have only one remaining target.

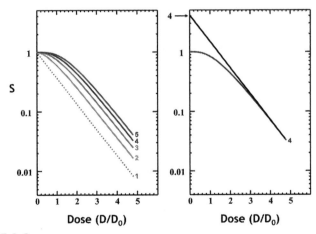

FIGURE 6-4.
The multitarget theory equation (see text) describes survival (*S*) as a function of dose, represented here as the (dimensionless) ratio D/D_0. Survival is plotted on a logarithmic scale. Left: predicted dose–response curves for integral values of n (target number) 1, 2, 3, 4, and 5. Note how the width of the "shoulder" increases with n. Right: multitarget theory equation, $n = 4$, illustrating that the value of n represents the y-intercept of the tangent to the curve at high doses. *Note*: A full-color version of this figure appears on the website.

At low doses ($D \rightarrow 0$), the first derivative of equation (6-1) is zero (for $n > 1$).[5] This means that, in the low-dose limit, no cell killing occurs if the number of targets is greater than one, then the first increment of dose cannot kill a cell. Experimental studies of radiation survival curves tend *not* to support this model; some lethality is detected even at very low doses (*15*); however, as we have noted, survival measurements at low dose are fraught with difficulty. Alternative models, such as the linear-quadratic model

$$S = e^{-\alpha D - \beta D^2}$$

allow for a nonzero initial slope, although the mechanistic validity of this model is debatable (*16–18*). In practice, other than at very low doses, both models tend to fit experimental data reasonably well.

Let us look at some real in vitro survival curve data. Figure 6-5 shows a data set for the survival of rat mammary epithelial cells exposed to the alkylating agent *N*-ethyl-*N*-nitrosourea (ENU). The data are fit very well by the multitarget equation with $n = 2.0$. Figure 6-6 shows an X-ray survival curve for the human fibroblast cell line AG1522 (*4*). In this case, the "shoulder" is wider ($n = 3.2$). (Determining the target theory equation parameters accurately requires nonlinear regression analysis of the log S vs. dose data set. This can now be done rather easily with commercially available computer software. In the older literature, the usual approach was to estimate n graphically, by drawing a tangent to the high-dose data points.)

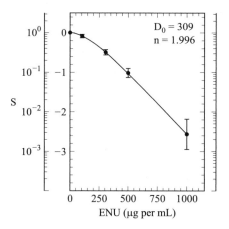

FIGURE 6-5.

Rat mammary epithelial cells were grown to 70–90% confluency in culture dishes and then treated with *N*-ethyl-*N*-nitrosourea (ENU) in serum-free medium. After treatment for 3 h, the cells were rinsed and allowed to recover in fresh medium. After 24 h, cells were harvested by trypsinization and counted. Plates containing either 200 or 1000 cells were prepared and incubated for about two weeks. Colonies were stained with crystal violet and counted. Survival indicates the percentage of cells that formed colonies, relative to the untreated control cells. (*Data from: McDiarmid, H. M.; Douglas, G. R.; Coomber, B. L.; Josephy, P. D. Epithelial and fibroblast cell lines cultured from the transgenic BigBlue rat: an in vitro mutagenesis assay. Mutat. Res.* **2001**, *497, 39–47.*)

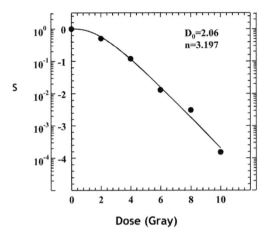

FIGURE 6-6.

Survival curve for AG1522 human fibroblast cells exposed to 250 kV X-rays at a dose rate of 1.42 Gy per min. Data were fit to the multitarget equation. (*Data from Niedbala, M.; Alsbeih, G.; Ng, C. E.; Raaphorst, G. P. Equivalence of pulsed-dose-rate to low-dose-rate irradiation in tumor and normal cell lines.* Radiat. Res. ***2001***, *155, 297–303.*)

INTERPRETATION OF TARGET THEORY PARAMETERS

The target theory equation provides an excellent fit to survival curves obtained for agents as diverse as chemical alkylating agents, ionizing radiation, nonionizing radiation, and hyperthermia. One should not be too surprised when the equation fails to fit a data set, because the assumptions made to derive the equation were drastic. For example, in a real population of cells, biological variation means that some cells may be substantially more resistant or more sensitive. Such subpopulations manifest as high-dose "tails" or other substructure on the survival curve.

The greater surprise, perhaps, is that the target theory model works so well for so many agents. In the case of radiation damage, DNA is certainly the most critical target for cell killing, but some chemical agents might act primarily against proteins, membranes, or other targets. How should we interpret the parameters in the target theory equation? D_0 is a parameter reflecting the sensitivity of the target—smaller values indicate more sensitive cells/more toxic agents. But what biological property does the "number of targets" n, which is a measure of the "width of the shoulder" of the survival curve, measure? This question has been much debated.

Perhaps, for any agent, each cell's survival is determined by a specific set of critical targets. For example, perhaps a cell has six genes encoding DNA polymerase enzymes. Any one of these genes is sufficient to produce enzyme and to permit replication; however, once all six genes have been damaged, the cell cannot divide: $n = 6$. But it seems unlikely that a minuscule number of specific genes could determine life or death of a cell, and, in fact, the sensitivity of mammalian cells to radiation is far higher than could be accounted for by such small targets. A looser interpretation is that a small number of chromosome-damaging events is required to kill a cell, and these damages can occur in any of a large number of different genes. DNA double-strand breaks have most often been put forward as the lesions most likely to cause cell death (*19, 20*).

An alternative analysis of target theory ascribes the "shoulder" not to the presence of multiple targets in each cell, but instead to the capacity of cells to repair damage. In this interpretation, the "shoulder" effect indicates that a certain level of sublethal damage can be tolerated by the cell, but beyond a threshold value, repair systems are overwhelmed and cell death ensues (*21*). Regardless of the interpretation, the target theory provides a useful empirical framework for modeling survival curves, and the distinction between factors (chemical or genetic) that modify D_0 and those that modify n can be helpful.

Notes

1. Indeed, there were 576 quarter-square-kilometer grid squares, just as Pynchon wrote.

2. Of course, analyzed over a larger geographical scale, the distribution was not at all random, since the bombs, although highly inaccurate in their trajectories, were all aimed in the general direction of London.

3. That is, spreading a drop of blood onto a gridded microscope slide, and then counting the number of cells in each grid square.

4. The reader should prove this.

5. The reader should prove this.

References

1. Parran, D. K.; Mundy, W. R.; Barone S., Jr. Effects of methylmercury and mercuric chloride on differentiation and cell viability in PC12 cells. *Toxicol. Sci.* **2001**, *59*, 278–290.

2. Morgan, D. M. Tetrazolium (MTT) assay for cellular viability and activity. *Methods Mol. Biol.* **1998**, *79*, 179–183.

3. Campling, B. G.; Pym, J.; Galbraith, P. R.; Cole, S. P. Use of the MTT assay for rapid determination of chemosensitivity of human leukemic blast cells. *Leuk. Res.* **1988**, *12*, 823–831.

4. Niedbala, M.; Alsbeih, G.; Ng, C. E.; Raaphorst, G. P. Equivalence of pulsed-dose-rate to low-dose-rate irradiation in tumor and normal cell lines. *Radiat. Res.* **2001**, *155*, 297–303.

5. Spadinger, I.; Palcic, B. Cell survival measurements at low doses using an automated image cytometry device. *Int. J. Radiat. Biol.* **1993**, *63*, 183–189.

6. Barber, P. R.; Vojnovic, B.; Kelly, J.; Mayes, C. R.; Boulton, P.; Woodcock, M.; Joiner, M. C. Automated counting of mammalian cell colonies. *Phys. Med. Biol.* **2001**, *46*, 63–76.

7. Bohrnsen, G.; Weber, K. J.; Scholz, M. Measurement of biological effects of high-energy carbon ions at low doses using a semi-automated cell detection system. *Int. J. Radiat. Biol.* **2002**, *78*, 259–266.

8. Feller, W. *An Introduction to Probability Theory and Its Applications*; John Wiley: New York, 1957.

9. Lea, D. E. *Actions of Radiations on Living Cells*; Cambridge University Press: Cambridge, 1946.

10. Alper, T. *Cellular Radiobiology*; Cambridge University Press: Cambridge, 1979.

11. Kempner, E. S. Advances in radiation target analysis. *Anal. Biochem.* **1999,** *276*, 113–123.

12. Hill, J. S.; Davis, R. C.; Yang, D.; Wen, J.; Philo, J. S.; Poon, P. H.; Phillips, M. L.; Kempner, E. S.; Wong, H. Human hepatic lipase subunit structure determination. *J. Biol. Chem.* **1996,** *271*, 22931–22936.

13. Kempner, E. S. Novel predictions from radiation target analysis. *Trends Biochem. Sci.* **1993,** *18*, 236–239.

14. Song, Y.; Sargentini, N. J. *Escherichia coli* DNA repair genes *radA* and *sms* are the same gene. *J. Bacteriol.* **1996,** *178*, 5045–5048.

15. Malaise, E. P.; Fertil, B.; Deschavanne, P. J.; Chavaudra, N.; Brock, W. A. Initial slope of radiation survival curves is characteristic of the origin of primary and established cultures of human tumor cells and fibroblasts. *Radiat. Res.* **1987,** *111*, 319–333.

16. Brenner, D. J.; Hall, E. J. The origins and basis of the linear-quadratic model. *Int. J. Radiat. Oncol. Biol. Phys.* **1992,** *23*, 252–253.

17. Brenner, D. J.; Herbert, D. E. The use of the linear-quadratic model in clinical radiation oncology can be defended on the basis of empirical evidence and theoretical argument. *Med. Phys.* **1997,** *24*, 1245–1248.

18. Herbert, D. Comment on "Point/counterpoint: the use of the linear-quadratic model in clinical radiation oncology can be defended on the basis of empirical evidence and theoretical argument" [*Med. Phys.* **1997,** *24*, 1245–1248]. *Med. Phys.* **1997,** *24*, 1329.

19. Stewart, R. D. Two-lesion kinetic model of double-strand break rejoining and cell killing. *Radiat. Res.* **2001,** *156*, 365–378.

20. Frankenberg-Schwager, M.; Frankenberg, D. Survival curves with shoulders: damage interaction, unsaturated but dose-dependent rejoining kinetics or inducible repair of DNA double-strand breaks? *Radiat. Res.* **1994,** *138*, S97–S100.

21. Bos, C. J.; Stam, P.; van der Veen, J. H. Interpretation of UV-survival curves of *Aspergillus* conidiospores. *Mutat. Res.* **1988,** *197*, 67–75.

Part Two

Enzymology
of
Biotransformation

Cytochrome P450: Chemical and Biochemical Aspects

INTRODUCTION

The significance of P450 enzymes in modern pharmacology and toxicology can hardly be overstated. The activities of these enzymes determine the pharmacokinetics of many drugs and toxicants. Furthermore, explanation of the unusual catalytic activities of P450s presents a fascinating challenge to chemists and biochemists. Although P450 enzymes are now among the most intensively studied protein families, cytochrome P450 was only discovered relatively recently, in the mid-1960s. This chapter begins with a discussion of the historical developments in biochemistry and pharmacology that led to the discovery of P450. We then consider the elements of P450 biochemistry, such as enzyme assays, protein structure, and reaction mechanisms. P450 enzymes are widely distributed throughout nature, but we focus on human P450s, particularly the human liver P450 enzymes that carry out the biotransformation of drugs. In chapter 8, we consider biological aspects of P450, including regulation of protein expression and P450 genetics.

▶ A Guide to the Usage of the Term "P450"

We shall refer to these enzymes as "P450," written in just this manner, with no dashes or subscripts, and often omitting the word "cytochrome": it is redundant, since all P450s are cytochromes. The synonymous terms "P-450" or "P$_{450}$" are used in older literature. As discussed below, the name "P450," assigned to the enzyme by its discoverers, refers to the enzyme's characteristic optical absorption spectrum. Much later, it was recognized that P450 enzymes share certain structural features and, on this basis, they are sometimes referred to as "heme-thiolate proteins."

P450 enzymes are often identified by their catalytic activities. The common feature to P450 catalysis is insertion of a single oxygen atom into an organic substrate, hence the name "monooxygenase" (preferred to the archaic terminology, "mixed-function oxidase"). Specific P450 catalytic activities are denoted as, for example, "mephenytoin hydroxylase" or "benzphetamine N-demethylase." This is the usual practice in biochemistry: enzymes are designated either on the basis of their protein structure or their catalytic activities. The abbreviation "CYP," designating the genes encoding P450s, is also widely used to describe specific enzymes, for example, "CYP1A2." We will return to P450 nomenclature issues later in this chapter. ◀

OXYGEN AND ENZYMATIC OXIDATIONS

The surprisingly late (1964) discovery of P450 monooxygenases was the culmination of independent lines of investigation in enzymology and protein chemistry. Since the discovery of oxygen in the 18th century, its importance to life processes was recognized: a mouse or bird deprived of oxygen soon died. But how did oxygen participate in metabolism? By the 1930s, a vigorous scientific controversy about the nature of tissue respiration had developed. Otto Warburg (Nobel Prize, 1931) demonstrated that an iron-containing respiratory enzyme ("Atmungsferment," now known as cytochrome c oxidase) could activate molecular oxygen. Warburg believed that this enzyme constituted a direct link between oxygen and intermediary metabolism. The contrasting opinion, advocated by Wieland, and others, was that the enzymatic oxidation–reduction reactions of intermediary metabolism take place by "trans-hydrogenation," that is, the transfer of hydride (H^-) equivalents between organic donors and acceptors. The cofactors NAD^+, $NADP^+$, FMN, and FAD were isolated and recognized as the most important biochemical oxidizing agents. The student of biochemistry quickly appreciates that the redox reactions of the citric acid cycle, fatty acid oxidation, and other central aerobic catabolic processes generate the reduced forms of these cofactors, in reactions catalyzed by dehydrogenases:

$$\text{Reduced substrate} + \text{oxidized cofactor}$$
$$\rightarrow \text{oxidized substrate} + \text{reduced cofactor}$$

The views of Warburg and Wieland were reconciled with the realization that reoxidation of reduced cofactors is carried out by the respiratory electron transport chain (in the mitochondria). The mitochondrial chain passes reducing equivalents from NADH and other reduced cofactors, via coenzyme Q and cytochrome c, to cytochrome oxidase. Electron transport is dependent on the supply of molecular oxygen, because the ultimate process in the transport chain is the oxidation of cytochrome oxidase by O_2. (We apply the term *oxidase* to an enzyme that catalyzes the reduction of molecular oxygen to water or, in certain cases, superoxide or hydrogen peroxide.) Under anoxic conditions, respiration halts and reduced cofactors accumulate.

The involvement of oxygen in intermediary metabolism is limited, then, to a single critical reaction: the reduction of oxygen to water, at the final stage of the respiratory electron transport chain. Oxygen atoms incorporated into substrates are derived from water, not from O_2. Consider, for example, the first steps of fatty acid ω-oxidation, in which an acyl CoA is oxidized to a hydroxyacyl CoA. This is accomplished in two reactions: oxidation of the fatty acid by FAD to give an alkene; and subsequent hydration of the alkene to give an alcohol. The delineation of the electron transport chain explained the ability of intermediary metabolic processes to oxidize carbohydrates and fats to CO_2 and H_2O, despite the apparent absence of enzymes catalyzing the direct reaction of O_2 with organic substrates.

The reduction of oxygen to water by almost any biochemical reductant is thermodynamically favorable. Nevertheless, there is a kinetic barrier to the reaction of oxygen with organic compounds, accounting for the commonplace observation that most organic materials do not oxidize rapidly at room temperature. The ground-state O_2 molecule has net electron spin = 1, a *ground-state triplet*: oxygen is paramagnetic. The two highest-energy electrons in molecular oxygen occupy degenerate molecular orbitals (antibonding π^* orbitals) and have parallel spins. Consequently, the reaction of O_2 with most (diamagnetic) organic molecules is hindered by spin restriction. *Molecular oxygen combines two characteristics that are often incompatible: thermodynamic potency and kinetic stability.* The energy available from the reduction of O_2 can only be released if the spin restriction on its reduction is overcome. This can be accomplished by very high temperatures (combustion) or by interaction with transition metal ions, as in P450 and other metalloenzymes.

This picture of oxidative metabolism, in which oxygen acts only as the terminal oxidant in the electron transport chain, was upset in 1955 by the discovery of enzymatic processes in which oxygen atoms derived from O_2 are incorporated directly into organic substrates (1). Tracing the fate of the oxygen atoms was achieved by use of O_2 labeled with the stable heavy isotope ^{18}O: mass spectrometry revealed the incorporation of the labeled atoms in the product. In the USA, Howard Mason et al. (2) discovered the prototype *monooxygenase* reaction (incorporation of one atom of oxygen from molecular oxygen into an organic substrate): the hydroxylation of a phenol derivative to give the corresponding catechol (*ortho*-dihydroxybenzene). Osamu Hayaishi and colleagues (3) observed the incorporation of both atoms of O_2 into an organic substrate (*dioxygenase* reaction) in the oxidation of catechol to pyrocatechuic acid.

Simultaneously, researchers at the Laboratory for Clinical Pharmacology, National Institutes of Health (NIH), Bethesda, Maryland, USA, led by Bernard B. Brodie, were pioneering the in vitro study of drug metabolism reactions (4). Hepatic microsomes were found to carry out the aromatic hydroxylation of, for example, acetanilide to give *p*-acetylaminophenol (acetaminophen). The source of the phenolic oxygen atom was determined to be O_2, and the stoichiometry of the reaction was established as:

$$NADPH + H^+ + RH + O_2 \rightarrow NADP^+ + ROH + H_2O$$

The hepatic microsomal drug oxidation system was recognized as a monooxygenase; this is one strand of the history of the discovery of P450. We now recognize this stoichiometry as the general formulation of a P450-dependent drug oxidation.

▶ R.T. Williams and the "Two Phases" of Drug Metabolism

Richard Tecwyn Williams (1909–1979) was one of the founders of the study of drug metabolism at the molecular level (5, 6). R.T. Williams is perhaps best remembered for introducing the idea of "Phase 1" versus "Phase 2" drug metabolism, a classification that has greatly influenced subsequent thinking in pharmacology and toxicology. Williams was born in the town of Abertillery, South Wales. In school, he developed an early interest in chemistry, excelling both in academics and sports (especially rugby). After earning his B.Sc. degree from University College, Cardiff, Williams began Ph.D. research at the Physiology Institute. His focus was on glucuronic acid. The structure of this compound was not yet fully characterized, although it was known to be metabolically conjugated to some xenobiotics. The preferred method for preparing glucuronic acid, at that time, was to isolate bornyl glucuronide from the urine of dogs fed borneol ("Sumatra camphor"):

> The first dog that had been fed with borneol had probably been house-trained, and although kept in a metabolic cage for four days, it failed to pass a single drop of urine. Tecwyn became sorry for the captive dog and let him out of the cage. The dog wagged his tail and then comfortably proceeded to urinate all over the floor ... The only course of action left to Tecwyn was to pursue the dog and suck up the urine with a large pipet. About 100 mL ... was recovered, and from this bornyl glucuronide was ... isolated (6a).

Williams established the structure of glucuronic acid in 1931. Later, he pursued the characterization of metabolites of terpenes, phenols, and drugs, including amphetamine and thalidomide.

Williams' influential textbook *Detoxication Mechanisms: The Metabolism of Drugs and Allied Organic Compounds* was published in 1947; a second edition appeared in 1959. In the second edition of his book,

William distinguished between two classes of drug metabolism, which he called "Phase 1" and "Phase 2." "Phase 1" included oxidation, reduction, and hydrolysis reactions, which can be regarded as "functionalization" processes, introducing hydroxyl groups or other functions into the substrate. (Note that this insight was achieved long before the discovery of monooxygenase reactions or P450 proteins.) "Phase 2" encompassed conjugation reactions, such as glucuronidation and sulfation, which typically yield water-soluble urinary metabolites. Williams also recognized (long before bioactivation became an established paradigm in toxicology) that metabolism could result in either detoxication or increased toxicity.

Williams' categorization of drug metabolism into two distinct "phases" helped to systematize the science and has been adhered to rather rigidly in many later presentations of the subject. However, we have avoided using the designations "Phase 1" and "Phase 2" in this book. In the era when Williams introduced these terms, the enzymes of xenobiotic metabolism had not yet been characterized and their roles in metabolic processes could only be inferred indirectly. The "Phase 1" versus "Phase 2" distinction is much too crude to provide a mechanistic basis for categorizing the diverse enzymatic reactions of xenobiotic metabolism (6b). For those who demand classification systems, we can distinguish at least the following groups of reactions:

1. *Oxidations*, catalyzed mainly by P450 enzymes but also by peroxidases, flavin-containing monooxygenase, alcohol dehydrogenase, and so on; these reactions encompass most of the so-called "Phase 1" processes. Within the realm of P450-mediated reactions, we can distinguish many alternative chemical transformations leading to different end products.

2. *Reductions*; these are much less numerous than oxidations because few functional groups are readily reduced. Relevant substrates include aldehydes, quinones, and compounds containing nitro or azo groups. Reductions have usually been considered as "Phase 1" processes, like oxidations. However, unlike oxidations (e.g., hydroxylations), reductions do not introduce functional groups at previously nonfunctionalized sites.

3. Reactions between electrophilic groups of xenobiotic substrates and the most important cellular nucleophiles, namely water and glutathione. These processes include the hydrolysis of esters, amides, epoxides, and so on, and the many and varied reactions catalyzed by glutathione transferases. (The tradition, following Williams, has been to classify hydrolysis, along with oxidation and reduction, as a "Phase 1" process, and to place glutathione conjugation, along with glucuronidation, sulfation, etc., in the "Phase 2" group. But there is no mechanistic basis, and little, if any, pharmacological basis, for doing so.)

4. Reactions of nucleophilic functional groups (alcohols, amines, thiols, etc.) in xenobiotics with endogenous electrophilic conjugating agents (UDPGA, acetyl CoA, PAPS, etc.). This class encompasses the traditional "Phase 2" drug metabolism processes, such as glucuronidation, sulfation, acetylation, and amino acid conjugation.

5. Membrane transport processes, such as the ATP-dependent export of glutathione conjugates and glucuronides across cell membranes, catalyzed by transporters such as MRP (see chapter 9). Membrane transport processes were little studied at the time of Williams, when drug metabolism was still examined almost exclusively in living animals. Cellular transport processes have been described as "Phase 3" drug metabolism, to emphasize that the substrates are often the products of prior conjugation reactions.

Even this five-fold classification is far from comprehensive. For example, the downstream biotransformation of glutathione conjugates into mercapturic acids (chapter 9) does not fit cleanly into any of these categories, nor do the formation, metabolism, and repair of covalent adducts to DNA or protein. ◀

▶ B.B. Brodie and the NIH Laboratory for Clinical Pharmacology

Bernard B. Brodie[1] (1909–1989) was one of the founders of modern pharmacology and toxicology (7). Brodie was raised in Ottawa, Canada, where his father ran a clothing store. He had a "slow start" to his academic career: he dropped out of high school and joined the Canadian army. He enrolled at McGill University in Montreal, supposedly after winning the money he needed to pay his tuition fees in a poker game. In his final undergraduate year, he had an opportunity to do laboratory work for a chemistry professor, W.H. Hatcher, and this experience set him on a research career. He earned a Ph.D. in organic chemistry at New York University and joined their Pharmacology Department. During World War II he worked on antimalarial drugs, which were desperately needed for the war effort in the Pacific. Brodie's studies of the metabolism of atabrine (quinacrine) assisted the development of a dosing regimen that minimized toxic side effects of the drug. Later, as head of the Laboratory for Clinical Pharmacology at the US National Institutes of Health (1950–1970), Brodie put

continues next page

continued from previous page
together a group of researchers who made pioneering contributions to the study of drug metabolism. His studies with Julius Axelrod of methemoglobinemia induced by the pain remedy acetanilide led to the discovery of enzymatic deacetylation (to give aniline) and aromatic hydroxylation (to give acetylaminophenol, which became an even more important pain relief medication: acetaminophen). These studies laid the foundation of P450 biochemistry. Brodie published almost 400 scientific papers in his career. ASPET, the American Society for Pharmacology and Experimental Therapeutics, presents a biennial Bernard B. Brodie Award to recognize outstanding research contributions in drug metabolism. ◀

Despite the characterization of microsomal monooxygenase enzyme activity, the hepatic protein responsible for drug oxidation was still mysterious. A second line of research, starting with studies of respiratory electron transport proteins, led to the discovery of P450 protein.

The mitochondrial electron transport chain is a complex assembly of protein and nonprotein carriers. Britton Chance and colleagues, at the Johnson Foundation, University of Pennsylvania, were investigating the components of the respiratory chain (*8*). To understand the operation of the chain, one needs to know the order in which electrons pass through it. Chance recognized that respiratory inhibitors, such as antimycin, block the electron transport chain at specific points. As discussed earlier, carriers that are "higher" (closer to $NADH/FADH_2$) than such a block become fully reduced; carriers that are "lower" (closer to O_2) than the block become fully oxidized. By using a variety of respiratory inhibitors, the order of electron transport could be deduced—but only if the redox state of the various carriers could be determined in intact mitochondria. Many of the electron transport chain components (NADH, coenzyme Q, cytochrome c, etc.) have optical absorption spectra that shift in characteristic ways upon reduction. Therefore, in principle, optical spectroscopy of mitochondria can be used to examine the redox state of these components. In practice, the spectral shifts are rather small, and must be measured against a large background of light absorbance by other components of the mitochondrion. To put this strategy into practice, Chance constructed double-beam spectrophotometers that could record accurate spectra from highly turbid (light-scattering) preparations, such as mitochondria. These spectra could be recorded in "difference mode": the light beam is rapidly chopped (i.e., passed alternately through two parallel light paths) between a sample and a reference cuvette. If the transmitted intensities differ between the two paths (that is, between the reference and sample cuvettes), chopping generates an alternating current (square wave signal) proportional to this difference. Such a signal can be measured electronically with high accuracy. This instrument design allows small shifts in a spectrum (say, following addition of a respirable substrate) to be detected.

THE DISCOVERY OF P450

Most of the Chance group's studies were performed with mitochondria (known to be the site of aerobic energy generation). In late 1954 Martin Klingenberg set out to study microsomal heme proteins by the same methods. In a recent recollection (*9*), he describes what happened next:

> Britton Chance proposed to study the redox kinetics of cytochrome b_5 in microsomes from rat liver. With the "split-beam

spectrophotometer," I recorded difference spectra in microsomes using dithionite and "DPNH" to reduce cytochrome b_5. [DPNH is the old name for NADH.] To prevent the autoxidation of cytochrome b_5 I applied CO. Unexpectedly, a strong band at 450 nm appeared ... These studies were performed from November 1954 to May 1955. David Garfinkel joined the Johnson Foundation in summer 1955 and we tried to isolate cytochrome b_5 as well as the new pigment ... with mixed success ... Due to various circumstances, my work on the CO-induced 450-nm pigment was published only in 1958 ... Ryo Sato joined the Johnson Foundation late in 1955 but did not participate in this research. In Osaka in a systematic study he and Tsuneo Omura associated the P450 pigment ... with the CO-420-nm compound [and] the nature of P450 as a hemoprotein was established.

Let us recapitulate these studies. Knowing that many ferrous heme proteins form characteristic carbon monoxide (CO) complexes, Klingenberg treated rat liver microsomes with *sodium dithionite*, to reduce any heme proteins to the ferrous state. This preparation was pipetted into both the sample and the reference cuvettes of a double-beam spectrophotometer, and then CO gas was bubbled into the sample cuvette only. The *reduced-CO difference spectrum* (figure 7-1) showed a strong absorption peak at $\lambda_{max} = 450$ nm; this was a surprising result (*10*), because no previously characterized cytochrome had displayed a Soret band[2] at such a long wavelength.[3] In 1962 Omura and Sato purified the protein responsible for the strange 450 nm chromophore. They confirmed that the absorption was due to a previously unknown class of heme proteins (*11*) which they named *cytochrome P450*. They measured the reduced-CO difference spectrum of purified P450; comparing the 450 nm peak to the baseline at a longer wavelength (490 nm), they calculated $\varepsilon_{450-490} = 91$ mM^{-1}. This value is still used to quantitate the total amount of P450 protein in a sample.[4] Omura and Sato also appreciated that P450 was susceptible to irreversible denaturation, converting the enzyme into an inactive form, with a ferrous–CO complex absorption at 420 nm ("cytochrome P420").

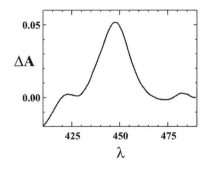

FIGURE 7-1.
The optical difference spectrum of a P450 enzyme, measured by the procedure of Omura and Sato. This spectrum was obtained using a membrane preparation from an *E. coli* strain engineered to express recombinant human P450 1A2. The sample and reference cuvettes contained dithionite-reduced P450; the sample cuvette only was bubbled with CO gas. (The negative deflection seen below about 420 nm is due to endogenous *E. coli* cytochromes.)

▶ **Dithionite and Carbon Monoxide**

Sodium dithionite (or sodium hydrosulfite) is $Na_2S_2O_4$. (This compound should not be confused with single-sulfur species such as sodium sulfite, Na_2SO_3.) We can regard the dithionite anion, $S_2O_4^{2-}$, as a dimer of SO_2^- (compare sulfur dioxide, SO_2). Sodium dithionite is a strong one-electron reducing agent; this is the rationale for the use of dithionite to reduce heme proteins. (It is also widely used as a reducing agent in industrial applications.) Since aqueous solutions of sodium dithionite are unstable, the compound is added directly to protein preparations as a solid.

Carbon monoxide, CO, is a powerful Lewis base (electron pair donor) that binds tightly to many transition metals to give characteristic coordination complexes. The Lewis (electron-dot) structure of CO may be represented as $^-C\equiv O^+$; CO binds to transition metal ions by a carbon-to-metal bond. Note that the ferrous–CO form of P450 is not a normal participant in the enzyme's catalytic cycle (discussed below); indeed, CO is a potent inhibitor of P450 activity. The reduced-CO form is simply a stable form of the protein with a characteristic absorption spectrum, useful for identifying and distinguishing various heme proteins. Typical heme proteins other than P450 (myoglobin, cytochrome c) have $\lambda_{max} \sim 420$ nm for the reduced-CO difference spectrum. ◀

These two independent paths to the discovery of P450—the characterization of microsomal drug hydroxylation activity and the purification of a new kind of heme protein from liver microsomes—converged with the demonstration that P450 protein is the monooxygenase enzyme. Ronald Estabrook showed that the inhibition of microsomal hydroxylation by CO could be reversed by photoirradiation, which dissociates the CO complex; 450 nm radiation was most effective. (These experiments recalled much earlier work by Warburg, who had shown that cellular respiration could also be inhibited by CO and photo-reactivated in a wavelength-specific manner.) The final proof of the identity of P450 and the microsomal hydroxylase was the reconstitution of monooxygenase enzyme activity with purified P450, as discussed later.

THE DISTRIBUTION OF P450 ENZYMES

P450 is an ancient superfamily of proteins, probably having arisen soon after green plants began to liberate oxygen into the atmosphere. Today, P450 enzymes are found throughout the major divisions of life, including archaea, eubacteria, plants, and animals. P450 apoproteins are single polypeptide chains of about 500 amino acids in length. Human genes encode about 66 functional P450 proteins as well as 30 pseudogenes[5] (evolutionary relics of once functional genes). Eukaryotic P450 genes are encoded by multiple exons. The human gene encoding P450 1A2, for example, is about 8 kbp in length and comprises seven exons/six introns (12).

A dozen or so P450 enzymes dominate the metabolism of drugs and xenobiotics; these enzymes (from families 1, 2, 3, and 4) are the focus of our attention. Microsomal P450 enzymes are classified as EC 1.14.14.1 (unspecific monooxygenase). Many other P450s catalyze specific steps in secondary metabolism, particularly steroid synthesis (13, 14, p. 734). Most multicellular animals seem to have similar numbers of P450 genes, for example, about 90 functional P450 genes in the mouse, about 90 in the fruit-fly *Drosophila melanogaster*, and about 80 in the nematode worm *Caenorhabditis elegans*. Flowering plants seem to be particularly rich in P450s; the *Arabidopsis thaliana* (thale cress) genome encodes nearly 300 P450s, comprising about 1% of its total complement of genes! This abundance probably reflects the requirement for multiple P450s for the synthesis of plant secondary metabolites, such as pigments (15), alkaloids, and terpenoids (16). Sequence-based analysis of P450 evolution indicates that the number of animal P450 genes increased suddenly about 400 million years ago, at about the time when animals moved from the sea to the land. Frank Gonzalez and Daniel Nebert have speculated that the selective pressure resulting from fierce molecular struggles between plants (evolving biosynthetic pathways for elaboration of natural product toxins, to deter foraging animals) and animals (evolving detoxication enzymes to metabolize these toxins, thereby allowing the animals to eat the plants) drove this expansion of the P450 superfamily (17).

Although there are no P450 genes in *E. coli*, many bacteria do express P450 enzymes, notably those species that assimilate unusual carbon sources. P450$_{cam}$ (P450 101; EC 1.14.15.1) from *Pseudomonas putida* (414 amino acids) catalyzes the first step in the catabolism of camphor (figure 7-2), which this organism can use as its sole carbon source.[6] Bacterial P450

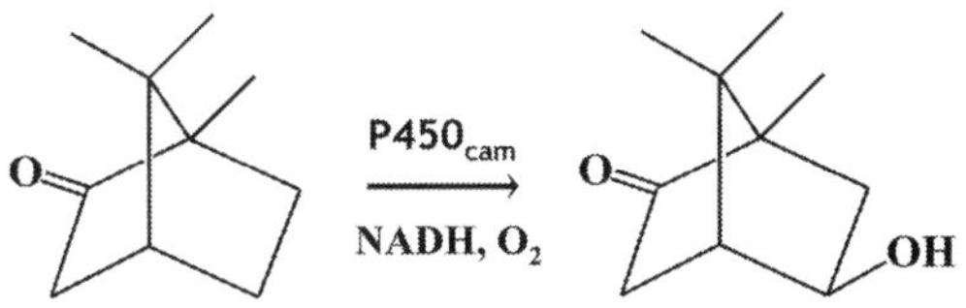

FIGURE 7-2.
The regiospecific hydroxylation of camphor catalyzed by cytochrome P450$_{cam}$.

enzymes are soluble proteins, smaller than their eukaryotic counterparts and more easily purified and crystallized. They have been used in many important studies of P450 structure and function.

Mammalian P450 enzymes are membrane-bound. The P450 enzymes involved in the biosynthesis of sterols are found mainly in steroidogenic organs, such as the adrenals, testis, ovaries, and placenta. P450 enzymes involved in the oxidation of drugs and xenobiotics are widely distributed, with highest concentrations in the endoplasmic reticulum of liver, kidney, lung (*18*), nasal passages (*19*), gut, and skin (*20*)—organs that must cope with exposure to diverse foreign compounds.

THE P450 GENE SUPERFAMILY

Studies of hepatic P450 enzyme induction (see chapter 8) and purification revealed the existence of multiple P450 enzymes with differing catalytic activities and distinct, if similar, physical properties. Some of the better-expressed forms were successfully purified to homogeneity, but the difficulty of separating closely related forms impeded progress. Cloning and expression of P450 cDNAs shattered this barrier.

P450 ENZYME CLASSIFICATION

The different forms of P450 found in a given organism were once referred to as P450 *isoenzyme*s (or isozymes). Strictly speaking, isozymes are enzymes that catalyze the same reaction. In most cases, however, different P450s catalyze different reactions. For this reason, the term *isoform* has been introduced, in preference to isozyme. However, the most straightforward terminology is to refer simply to specific P450 *enzymes*, as we will do here.

Before the advent of molecular cloning, P450 enzymes were identified in ad hoc fashion according to electrophoretic mobility, chromophore λ_{max}, substrate specificity, and so on, resulting in considerable confusion. The contemporary classification is based on sequence homology, giving a systematic (if somewhat arbitrary) taxonomy. Enzymes sharing > 40% amino acid sequence identity are assigned to the same *family*. Generally, family numbers 1–50 are used for animal P450s; 50–65, fungal P450s; 70–100 plant P450s; 100 and above, bacterial P450s. (This scheme may break down as additional families are discovered.) P450 proteins that share >55% identity are classified as members of the same *subfamily*.[7] Individual enzymes are identified by a family number, subfamily letter, and finally another number. For example, P450 3A4[8] (a major human hepatic enzyme) is the fourth member of family 3, subfamily A. "CYP3A4" is equivalent to "P450 3A4." Italicized (*CYP3A4*), this notation designates the corresponding gene. Trivial nonsystematic names are still widely used to identify the function of the enzyme under discussion. For example, *aromatase* (systematically, CYP19A) removes the 19-methyl carbon and aromatizes the A-ring of the steroid androstene-3,17-dione.

Enzymatic function usually correlates, at least in a general fashion, with sequence similarity. For example, all P450 4A enzymes catalyze the ω-hydroxylation of fatty acids. However, one must be very cautious about inferring activity on the basis of sequence homology.

P450 ENZYME ASSAYS

Since P450 monooxygenases catalyze a vast and diverse range of chemical transformations, many different methods can be (and are) used to assay P450 enzyme activity (*21*). Ideally, we would like to have both "universal" P450 substrates (oxidized by any enzyme) and completely enzyme-specific substrates, but such substances do not exist. A variety of sensitive and convenient P450 assays have been developed; each provides some clues about the kinds and amounts of P450 present in a sample. A few of these assays are discussed here (figure 7-3). As we look at these substrates, we will also begin to explore the diverse chemical reactions catalyzed by P450s. The mechanisms of these reactions are considered in more detail later in this chapter.

Many P450 substrates bear N- or O-alkyl substituents. Hydroxylation of the methylene carbon adjacent to the heteroatom gives an unstable product that decomposes to an aldehyde plus the dealkylated substrate (as discussed in the section on hydroxylation mechanisms later in this chapter). In the case of an N- or O-methyl substrate, the resulting aldehyde is formaldehyde ($CH_2=O$). Formaldehyde formation can be assayed easily by means of the *Nash assay* (*22*), which is based on the chemistry of the Hantzsch pyridine synthesis (1882) (figure 7-4). Formaldehyde reacts

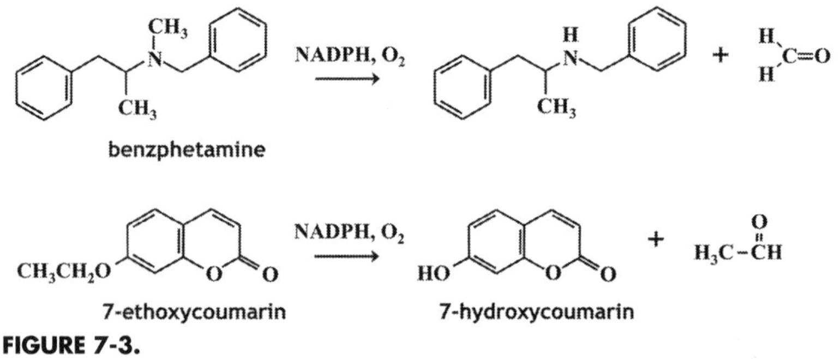

benzphetamine

7-ethoxycoumarin   7-hydroxycoumarin

FIGURE 7-3.
Typical P450 assays.

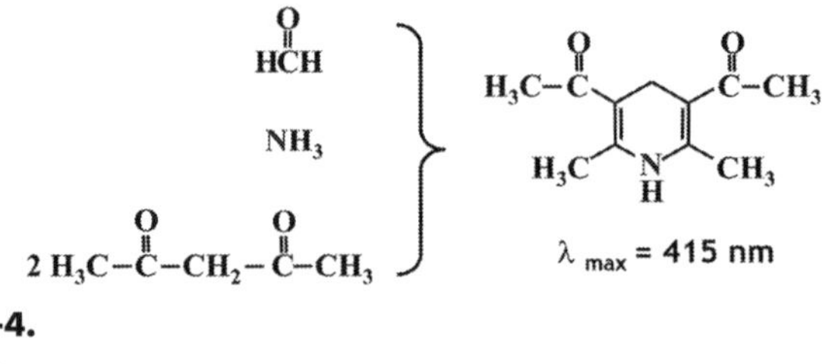

$\lambda_{max} = 415$ nm

FIGURE 7-4.
Nash assay.

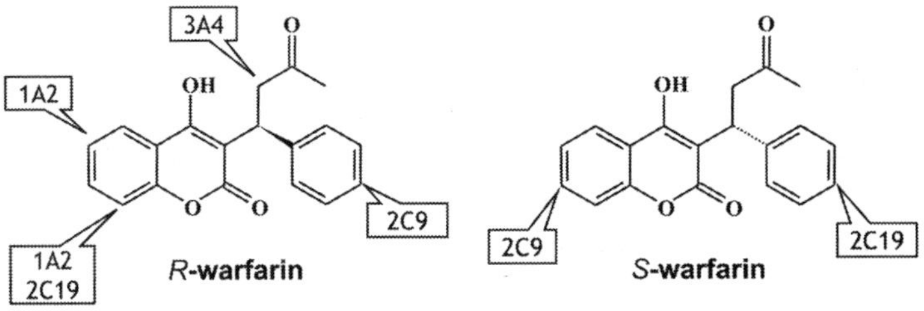

FIGURE 7-5.
Warfarin can be used as a probe drug in microsomal incubations; different P450 enzymes oxidize the drug at characteristic positions. The two enantiomeric forms of warfarin are metabolized differently. At low concentrations, warfarin metabolism in humans is dominated by hepatic P450 2C9. (*Adapted from Kaminsky, L. S.; Zhang, Z. Y. Human P450 metabolism of warfarin. Pharmacol. Ther. 1997, 73, 67–74.*)

with ammonia and acetylacetone (2,4-pentanedione) to give the yellow product diacetyldihydrolutidine, $\lambda_{max} = 412$ nm, which is measured by spectrophotometry, fluorescence, HPLC with fluorescence detection (*23*), and so on. A commonly used substrate that generates formaldehyde is benzphetamine.

Another routine P450 enzyme assay measures the O-deethylation of 7-ethoxycoumarin to give 7-hydroxycoumarin (and acetaldehyde). After incubation, the product and substrate are coextracted with chloroform; the phenolic product is back-extracted into aqueous base and quantitated by fluorescence (*21*).

Many substrates are metabolized to multiple isomeric products in P450-catalyzed reactions; the rodenticide warfarin is an example (figure 7-5). Chromatographic methods such as HPLC are used to separate the isomers. Typically, different P450 enzymes will yield different products. Analysis of the metabolites formed from such substrates can provide information about the P450 enzymes present in a microsomal sample (*24*).

PURIFICATION OF MICROSOMAL P450

Although P450 activity can be studied in crude microsomal preparations, it is preferable to reconstitute P450 activity from purified proteins, so that interference from other enzymes is absent. Purification of active membrane-bound P450 enzymes depends on solubilization of the enzyme. This can be accomplished with nonionic detergents, such as Nonoxynol or octyl glucoside. P450 is usually stabilized by the presence of 20% glycerol. P450 protein is purified by column chromatography on media such as hydroxyapatite, *n*-octylaminosepharose, and DEAE-sepharose. Complete separation of individual enzymes from native sources may be difficult to achieve by column chromatography; isoelectric focusing has been successfully applied (*25*). Purification of specific P450 enzymes from natural sources has largely been replaced, since the 1980s, by the expression of recombinant enzymes in bacterial or eukaryotic host cells (*26*).

As we discuss later, P450 activity requires the presence not only of P450 itself, but also of the accessory flavoprotein *P450 reductase* (EC 1.6.2.4), which transfers electrons from NADPH to P450. Sterol 11-hydroxylase, a biosynthetic enzyme from adrenal mitochondria, was the first P450 system (P450 + reductase) to be solubilized and separated into its components (27). The purification and reconstitution of active microsomal P450 enzyme were accomplished by A.Y.H. Lu and M.J. Coon at the University of Michigan (28–30). This achievement was crucial for the biochemical analysis of P450 function, but the difficulty of separating the multiple enzymes of P450 found in natural sources such as mammalian liver remained an obstacle to defining the activities of specific P450s.

HUMAN HEPATIC P450 ENZYMES: NOMENCLATURE AND CHARACTERISTICS

With the completion of several mammalian genome projects, including human, mouse, and rat, the enumeration of mammalian P450 families is nearly complete. The P450-dependent metabolism of xenobiotics and drugs is primarily catalyzed by enzymes of the CYP1, CYP2, CYP3, and CYP4 families. In this section, we briefly consider the features of the major human hepatic P450 enzymes from these four families. Table 7-1 summarizes the properties of these enzymes and table 7-2 lists some important drug and toxicant substrates.

Human hepatic microsomes contain about 0.5 nmol (25 µg) P450 per mg protein, as assayed spectrally (31), although interindividual variation is large. Immunoassay analysis, combined with knowledge of the expression patterns of specific human P450 enzymes, indicates that most of

TABLE 7-1.

Some Human Hepatic P450 Enzymes of Toxicological and Pharmacological Importance

ENZYME	TYPICAL SUBSTRATES OR ACTIVITIES	REMARKS	
1A1	Polycyclic aromatic hydrocarbons	All P450 1 family enzymes	Extrahepatic; e.g., lung
1A2	Aromatic and heterocyclic amines (N-hydroxylation)	are inducible by ligands of the Ah receptor, e.g., TCDD,	Hepatic
1B1	Activity overlaps with 1A1, 1A2	β-Naphthoflavone	Extrahepatic; expressed in lung; mutated in congenital glaucoma
2A6	Nicotine oxidation, coumarin 7-hydroxylation	Hepatic; probably non-inducible	
2B6	Phenobarbital, efavirenz	Hepatic (minor) and extrahepatic	
2C9	(S)-Warfarin 7-hydroxylation	Hepatic	
2C19	(S)-Mephenytoin 4′-hydroxylation	Hepatic; highly polymorphic	
2D6	Debrisoquine, dextromethorphan	Hepatic; most substrates are bases; highly polymorphic	
2E1	Dimethylnitrosamine, ethanol	Hepatic (abundant); inducible by ethanol, isoniazid	
3A4	Nifedipine and many other drugs	Much the most abundant hepatic P450	
4A11	Fatty acid ω-hydroxylase	Rat orthologue (4A1) is inducible by hypolipidemic drugs (e.g., clofibrate)	

TABLE 7-2.

Typical Substrates of Selected Human Hepatic P450 Enzymes

1A2	2C19	3A4	4A
Acetaminophen	Mephenytoin	Aldrin	Arachidonic acid
Aflatoxin B_1	Omeprazole	Alfentanil	Lauric acid
Caffeine		Cortisol	
Clozapine	2D6	Cyclosporin	
Ethoxyresorufin	Bufuralol	Dapsone	
Phenacetin	Debrisoquine	Diltiazem	
	Desipramine	Erythromycin	
2A6	Dextromethorphan	17-estradiol	
Coumarin	Propranolol	Lidocaine	
Nicotine	Sparteine	Lovastatin	
Methyl *t*-butyl ether		Nifedipine	
	2E1	Quinidine	
2B6	Acetaminophen	Taxol	
Aflatoxin B_1	Acetone		
Cyclophosphamide	Aflatoxin B_1		
Diazepam	Aniline		
Tamoxifen	Caffeine		
	Chlorzoxazone		
2C9	Ethanol		
Aminopyrene	Halothane		
Celecoxib			
Hexobarbital			
Tienilic acid			
Tolbutamide			

the hepatic P450 content can be accounted for by enzymes 1A2, the 2C subfamily (2C8, 2C9, 2C18, and 2C19, which are difficult to distinguish by immunoassay), 2E1, and the most abundant P450 enzyme, 3A4. It should be borne in mind, however, that even a P450 expressed at a low level may control the metabolism of a substance for which it has high specificity. For example, P450 2A6 is probably not one of the highly expressed hepatic forms, but it accounts for most of the nicotine detoxication activity.

In this section, we examine some of the major human hepatic P450 enzymes of importance in toxicology and pharmacology. Biological aspects of these enzymes are discussed in more detail in chapter 8.

P450 1 Family

Administration of agents such as 3-methylcholanthrene or TCDD to rodents leads to the *induction* (see chapter 8) of hepatic P450 enzymes that are almost undetectable in noninduced animals. These enzymes have characteristic absorption peaks around 447–448 nm, rather than the typical 450 nm. *They catalyze several reactions associated with carcinogen activation, including the hydroxylation of polycyclic aromatic hydrocarbons and the N-oxidation of aromatic amines (32).* Once described as "cytochrome P448," the induced enzymes are 1A1, 1A2, and 1B1, the three members of the mammalian P450 1 family. (P450 enzymes 1A1 and 1A2 were characterized in the 1970s and referred to as rat liver forms "c" and "d," respectively; P450 1B1 (*33*) was not discovered until the 1990s (*34*).) There is considerable overlap among all three enzymes, in terms of catalytic activity. Two of the most intensively studied activities of P450 family 1 enzymes are the oxidation of aromatic amines and polycyclic aromatic hydrocarbons (PAH), processes that are central to the metabolic activation of these prevalent environmental carcinogens. (We return to these bioactivation reactions in chapters 17 and 18, respectively.) PAH are oxidized to epoxides, which give rise to phenols and dihydrodiols. This enzyme activity was referred to as AHH ("aryl hydrocarbon hydroxylase") before the characterization of the relevant P450 enzymes. P450 1A2, especially, catalyzes the N-oxidation of aromatic amines to give arylhydroxylamines (*32*). In humans, P450 1A1 is exclusively extrahepatic while 1A2 is a major hepatic P450.

The human *CYP1B1* gene is a locus[9] of the autosomal recessive disorder *primary congenital glaucoma* (buphthalmos or "ox-eye," because of the distended appearance of the eye, due to increased intraocular pressure) (*35, 36*). This is the first known instance in which a mutation of a human P450 gene from families 1–4 cold be associated with an inherited disease.[10] Knockout mice lacking the gene for P450 1B1 do not show obvious symptoms of ocular pathology. However, careful studies revealed abnormal development of the anatomical structures (Schlemm's canal and trabecular meshwork) that regulate drainage of intraocular fluid. The effect of the CYP1B1 knockout is much more severe in albino (tyrosinase-deficient) mice (*37*). P450 1B1 activity may be required for metabolism of retinoids which control the development of these ocular structures.

All three enzymes of the P450 1 family are induced by compounds such as 3-methylcholanthrene, as mentioned above. Analysis of this regulatory mechanism led to the discovery of the AH receptor protein, which is discussed in detail in chapter 8. As we will see, the induction of P450 1 enzymes is distinctly different from the regulation of other P450s.

P450 2A6

The *CYP2A6* gene is one member of a complex cluster of 2A, 2B, and 2F subfamily P450 genes on human chromosome 19. This group of genes presumably arose by duplication and subsequent divergent evolution (*38*). P450 2A6 is probably the only member of the group expressed at substantial levels in the liver. 7-Hydroxylation of coumarin, a widely distributed lactone natural product, is a characteristic activity of 2A6. Nicotine metabolism (*39*) is also strongly dependent on P450 2A6 (see sidebar). The high-resolution structure of human P450 2A6 has recently been published (*40*).

▶ **Tobacco, Nicotine, and P450**

Nicotine (figure 7-6) is the addictive alkaloid constituent of tobacco; the compound is named for the French diplomat Jean Nicot (1530–1600), who brought tobacco to Europe. Orally ingested nicotine is very rapidly metabolized by hepatic P450 ("first-pass" effect), so that the substance is only pharmacologically active when it is absorbed directly into the bloodstream, via the lungs (smoking), nasal epithelium (snuff), oral epithelium (chewing tobacco), or skin (nicotine "patch"). Smokers are addicted to nicotine and adjust their smoking habits so as to maintain their blood nicotine levels above a threshold level, to avoid the unpleasant effects of nicotine withdrawal. Rachel Tyndale (*41*) and her colleagues have found that the activity of P450 2A6, which is highly variable in the population, is a major determinant of smoking behavior. Individuals with high activity metabolize nicotine quickly, and smoke frequently—in some cases, waking with nicotine cravings and smoking at night. The metabolic activity level does not affect the likelihood of addiction or the ability to quit; these factors are probably influenced more by the physiology and genetics of the receptors for nicotine (42).

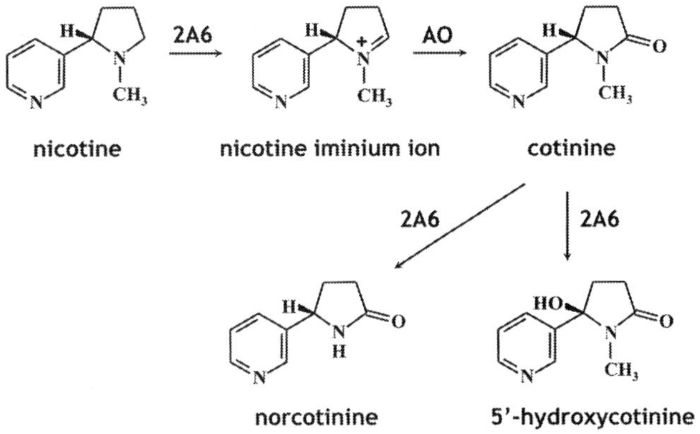

FIGURE 7-6.

Nicotine. (*Adapted from Oscarson, M. Genetic polymorphisms in the cytochrome P450 2A6 (CYP2A6) gene: implications for interindividual differences in nicotine metabolism.* Drug Metab. Dispos. ***2001***, 29, 91–95.)

P450 2B6

The rat enzymes P450 2B1 (rat form "b") and 2B2 have long been recognized as major phenobarbital-inducible hepatic enzymes; 2B6 is the only member of this subfamily in humans.

Although 2B6 was once thought to be only a minor hepatic form in humans, recent studies indicate that it may account for about 5% of hepatic P450 (43). It is also expressed in kidney and lung. This enzyme has received increasing attention as its role in metabolism of some important drugs, including tamoxifen and the HIV reverse transcriptase inhibitor efavirenz, has been recognized (44).

P450 2C Subfamily

There are four members in the 2C subfamily; the corresponding genes are arranged in a cluster on chromosome 10, in the order 2C18–2C19–2C9–2C8 (45). P450 2C9 and 2C19 are the more important hepatic drug-metabolizing forms. Many important drugs are metabolized by the 2C enzymes, including omeprazole (a proton pump inhibitor for the treatment of acid reflux from the stomach) and diclofenac (an antiinflammatory agent). The clinically consequential polymorphism of P450 2C19 (46) was revealed by large differences in the metabolism of the anticonvulsant drug mephenytoin.

P450 2D6

This enzyme is expressed in human liver at relatively low levels (a few percent of total P450), but its substrates include a large number of drugs, typically compounds bearing a basic nitrogen (amines, substituted amines, pyridines, etc.) (47). Fluoxetine (Prozac^{TM}) and tricyclic antidepressants used in psychiatry are important examples. Basic substrates are believed to bind to the enzyme with the assistance of an electrostatic interaction between the protonated, positively charged substrate and one or more acidic residues on the protein (48). The P450 2D6 polymorphism was discovered in May 1977 during studies of the pharmacokinetics of the antihypertensive agent *debrisoquine*. The director of the laboratory performing the research used himself as one of the experimental subjects (*49*). Not long after taking the first pill, he collapsed onto the floor, due to a drastic drop in blood pressure! As soon as he regained consciousness, he began drafting a report on the debrisoquine poor-metabolizer phenotype.

P450 2E1

Ethanol is the xenobiotic that humans consume in the largest quantities: grams rather than milligrams. Because fermentation is a natural process occurring in fruits and other food sources, humans have always been exposed to ethanol. The major pathway of ethanol metabolism is catalyzed by the cytosolic enzyme alcohol dehydrogenase, which catalyzes its NAD-dependent oxidation to acetaldehyde. However, alcohol oxidation activity was also discovered in microsomal fraction (*50*) and found to be P450-dependent. This "microsomal ethanol oxidation system" (MEOS) can be thought of as a backup to the alcohol dehydrogenase system. MEOS activity is associated with P450 2E1[11] (*51*), which catalyzes both the oxidation of ethanol to acetaldehyde and the further oxidation of acetaldehyde to acetic acid (*52*). The preferred substrates for P450 2E1 are typically small molecules, including solvents such as ethanol, acetone, chloroform (*53*), and *N,N*-dimethylacetamide. Ethanol and acetone are also inducers of 2E1. (The regulation of P450 2E1 gene expression differs markedly from that of other hepatic forms, as is discussed in chapter 8.) This form is also associated with the metabolic activation of carcinogenic nitrosamines (see sidebar) and the hepatotoxic analgesic drug acetaminophen.

▶ **Nitrosamines**

Dialkylnitrosamines (R_1R_2–N–N=O; nitrosodialkylamines) are synthesized by treating dialkylamines (secondary amines) with nitrous acid, HNO_2. The same synthetic reaction can potentially occur in the stomach: secondary amines are present in the diet, and nitrous acid can be formed from dietary nitrite, at the acid pH of the stomach.

Many nitrosamines are mutagenic and carcinogenic in animals. Like the nitrosoureas, nitrosamines are alkylating agents (see chapter 15) and cause covalent modification of DNA bases. Dialkylnitrosamines are chemically unreactive. Hydroxylation of the carbon atom adjacent to the amine nitrogen atom (α-hydroxylation), catalyzed principally by P450 2E1, yields highly reactive α-hydroxynitrosamines (figure 7-7). α-Hydroxynitrosamines can be prepared chemically (e.g., by the reduction of α-hydroperoxynitrosamine precursors). They decompose very rapidly to yield reactive electrophiles (diazonium ions and alkyl cations) (*54*).

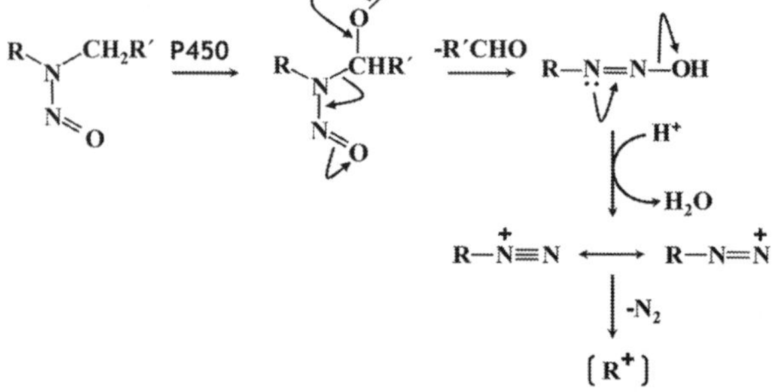

FIGURE 7-7.
Nitrosamines.

Tobacco contains several nicotine-related nitrosamines (55). These "tobacco-specific nitrosamines" (an example is shown in figure 7-8) are found in both tobacco and tobacco smoke, at levels up to hundreds of nanograms per cigarette. The processes of tobacco curing and combustion during smoking generate these compounds by nitrosation of precursor alkaloids. Tobacco-specific nitrosamines are mutagens and carcinogens, and they are probably important contributors to the carcinogenic action of tobacco and smoking.

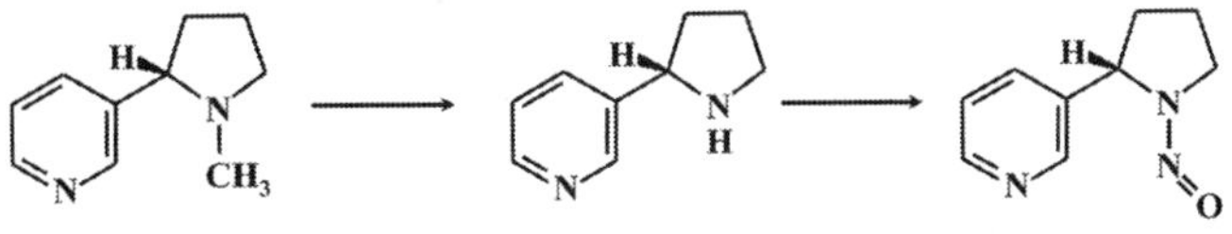

nicotine   nornicotine   NNN

FIGURE 7-8.
Formation of a tobacco-specific nitrosamine, NNN.

P450 3A4

This enzyme is the most highly expressed human hepatic P450. P450 3A4[12] has extremely wide substrate specificity (substrate *promiscuity* would be a more apt description) (56). As many as half of all commonly used drugs are metabolized, at least in part, in 3A4-catalyzed reactions. In contrast to 2E1, which is a specialist in small substrates, 3A4 can accommodate very large substrates, such as cyclosporin A (cyclosporine) (57), which has a molar mass greater than 1000. Indeed, the active site of 3A4 is apparently spacious enough to bind multiple substrates simultaneously, as manifested by its unusual kinetic behavior (58).

P450 4A11

Enzymes of P450 family 4 are inducible in the rat by hypolipidemic drugs such as clofibrate, which cause the proliferation of peroxisome organelles in the liver (see chapter 8). P450 4A11 is the human hepatic member of this family; in the rat, the corresponding hepatic form is 4A1.[13] Both enzymes are active as fatty acid ω-hydroxylases (see below).

Until recently, it had been thought that the mode of binding of the heme prosthetic group to apoprotein, in P450 enzymes, was always noncovalent. However, Paul Ortiz de Montellano and colleagues have discovered that P450 family 4 enzymes are an exception: a covalently linkage (ester bond) links a conserved glutamic acid residue in the I-helix to modified 5-hydroxymethylheme (59, 60).

WHY ARE SO MANY P450 ENZYMES NEEDED?

Why should humans express so many different P450 enzymes? The enzymes of intermediary metabolism are usually both highly efficient (high turnover numbers and enormous rate enhancements relative to the uncatalyzed reactions) and highly substrate-specific. High catalytic efficiency demands a precise chemical fit between the substrate and enzyme, and this fit, in turn, dictates stringent substrate specificity. In contrast, *many of the enzymes of xenobiotic metabolism are characterized by broad substrate specificity and relatively low catalytic efficiency.* These enzymes represent a metabolic compromise: the ability to metabolize diverse substances is achieved at the cost of reduced precision of substrate binding to the enzyme. *Many of the enzymes are present in very large amounts.* In the liver, P450 enzymes are the predominant proteins of the endoplasmic reticulum. A large amount of versatile (but low-efficiency) catalyst substitutes for a small amount of highly efficient catalyst. Many of the enzymes of biotransformation have diverged evolutionarily into *large families of catalysts with overlapping substrate specificities.* Each enzyme carries out the same general reaction (oxygen insertion, in the case of P450) but handles slightly different groups of substrates.

P450 STRUCTURE

As recently as the mid-1980s, some doubt remained with regard to the identification of the proximal ligand to the heme iron atom in P450s. Much spectroscopic evidence indicated that this ligand was a cysteine thiolate ($-CH_2S^-$), but direct proof was lacking until the first P450 X-ray crystal structure, that of P450$_{cam}$ (*61*), was determined in 1987. Structures of other bacterial P450 enzymes soon followed, including the terpineol-oxidizing enzyme P450$_{terp}$ (CYP108) (*62*) and the heme-containing domain of P450BM-3 (CYP102) (*63*). (P450BM-3 shares higher sequence similarity with mammalian enzymes of the 4A family than with P450$_{cam}$ or other bacterial enzymes.) The first structure of a mammalian P450 (rabbit 2C5) was published in 2000 (*64*) and Schlichting et al. determined the structures of oxygenated P450 intermediates by application of low-temperature X-ray crystallography techniques (*65*). The first structures of human P450s were published in 2003 (2C9) (*66, 67*) and 2004 (3A4) (*68–70*). These developments are swiftly expanding our understanding of P450 biochemistry.

The Structure of a Bacterial P450, P450$_{cam}$

All published P450s (*71*) show many similar structural features, so analysis of a single P450 should provide insight into the entire super-family. We will focus on P450$_{cam}$ before briefly considering the distinctive features of rabbit 2C5. P450$_{cam}$ (figures 7-9 and 7-10) is a globular

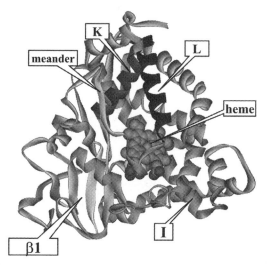

FIGURE 7-9.

Proximal view of the tertiary structure of P450$_{cam}$. Structure file 2cpp.pdb was used. *Note*: A full-color version of this figure appears on the website.

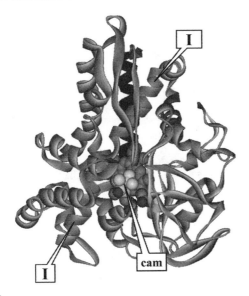

FIGURE 7-10.
Distal view of the tertiary structure of P450$_{cam}$. Structure file 2cpp.pdb was used. *Note*: A full-color version of this figure appears on the website.

protein with the approximate shape of a triangular prism, enfolding a single heme prosthetic group. Twelve α-helical segments (lettered A–L in primary structure order, starting from the amino terminus) encompass almost half of the amino acid residues and dominate the secondary structure. We distinguish between two "faces" of the prism: on the *proximal* face, we see the cysteine thiolate ligand to the heme iron; on the *distal* face, we see the substrate-binding site. When P450$_{cam}$ is crystallized in the presence of camphor, the bound substrate is clearly seen in the structure, proving that it is held in a fixed orientation in the active site.

The heme prosthetic group is "sandwiched" between two α-helices, the L-helix (on the proximal side) and the I-helix (on the distal side) (figure 7-11). The proximal L-helix forms part of the outer surface of the protein; the distal I-helix extends across the hydrophobic interior. Indeed, the very long I-helix, which traverses the entire protein, is a striking feature of P450 structure. The heme group is held in place (noncovalently) by hydrophobic contacts with the two helices, hydrogen bonds between the negatively charged propionic acid substituents of the heme and basic residues Arg-299 and His-355, and by the thiolate ligand to the iron, which is provided by Cys-357. This cysteine residue is located just before the N-terminus of the proximal (L) helix. The liganded cysteine is absolutely conserved in all P450 enzyme sequences, and many of the residues in its vicinity are also strongly conserved. Replacement of this cysteine by any other residue, in site-directed mutagenesis experiments, destroys the P450 chromophore and eliminates catalytic activity (*72*). The amide groups of several residues close to this cysteine residue stabilize the thiolate anion by electrostatic or hydrogen bonding interactions (figure 7-12) (*73*). Figure 7-13 shows a gallery of heme protein active

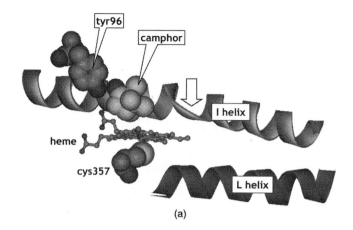

(a)

1A2	LFGMGKRRCIGEVLAKW
2C5	PFSAGKRMCVGEGLARM
86	AFNAGPRTCLGKDLAYN
101	TFGHGSHLCLGQHLARR
61	VFGCGPHVCLGQTYVMI
79	SFSTGRRGCIAASLGTA

(b)

FIGURE 7-11.

(a) The active site of the camphor–P450$_{cam}$ complex. The heme ring is shown as a ball-and-stick model. The camphor substrate, proximal cysteine residue 357, and tyrosine residue 96, which forms a hydrogen bond to the substrate, are shown space-filling. The I and L helices are shown as ribbons. Note the "kink" in the middle of the I-helix (arrow). Structure file 2cpp.pdb was used. (b) Amino acid sequences in the conserved cysteine (proximal ligand) region of cytochrome P450; strongly conserved residues are shown in red. The P450 enzymes aligned here are: human 1A2, rabbit 2C5, *Arabidopsis thaliana* 86, *Pseudomonas putida* P450$_{cam}$ (CYP101), *Saccharomyces cerevisiae* (yeast) P450 61, and *Sorghum bicolor* P450 79. The plant CYP 79 family is the only instance in which the residue two residues past the conserved cysteine is not glycine (*74*). *Note*: A full-color version of this figure appears on the website.

sites and allows a comparison of the iron/ligand environments in these proteins.

The crystal structure of P450$_{cam}$ with camphor bound in the active site reveals a hydrogen bond between the camphor carbonyl group and the phenolic hydroxyl group of Tyr-96 (figure 7-14). In addition to this important hydrogen bond, camphor has several other contacts with the enzyme, notably with residues Phe-87, Leu-244, Val-247, and Val-295. These interactions position the camphor group approximately 4 Å above the heme plane, directly adjacent to the oxygen binding site. Site-specific mutagenesis studies, and the use of camphor analogues from which the carbonyl or methyl groups have been deleted, show that the hydrogen bond and the hydrophobic interactions of the methyl groups with the protein are not essential for catalytic turnover. In the absence of these interactions, however, the oxidation of camphor no longer exclusively yields 5-*exo*-hydroxycamphor (*75*). (We will return to the issue of the

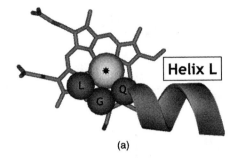

(a)

1A2	KIVNLVNDIFGAGFDTVTTAISWSLMYLVTKP
2C5	SLVIAVSDLFGAGTETTSTTLRYSLLLLLKHP
86	VLQRIALNFVLAGRDTSSVALSWFFWLVMNNR
101	EAKRMCGLLLVGGLDTVVNFLSFSMEFLAKSP
61	EISEAVFTFLFASQDASSSLACWLFQIVADRP
79	TVKAQSQDITFAAVDNPSNAVEWALAEMVNNP

(b)

FIGURE 7-12.

(a) The proximal side of the P450$_{cam}$ active site. The heme ring is shown as sticks. The beginning of helix L is shown as a ribbon, and atoms from the four residues closest to the heme iron are shown as balls. The sulfur atom of cysteine residue 357, coordinated to the heme iron, is shown as a light ball. The amide N atoms of residues 358–360 are shown as darker balls, labeled L, G, and Q. These amide NH groups contribute partial positive charges that stabilize the cysteine thiolate anion. Structure file 2cpp.pdb was used. (*Yoshioka, S.; Takahashi, S.; Ishimori, K.; Morishima, I. Roles of the axial push effect in cytochrome P450cam studied with the site-directed mutagenesis at the heme proximal site.* J. Inorg. Biochem. **2000**, *81, 141–151.*) (b) Amino acid sequences in the vicinity of the strongly conserved I-helix threonine (shown in red) of cytochrome P450; atypically, an alanine residue is found at this position in P450 61 and an asparagine in P450 79. The P450 enzymes are the same as in the preceding figure. *Note:* A full-color version of this figure appears on the website.

regiospecificity of alkane hydroxylation later in this chapter.) Another effect is also seen. In the oxidation of camphor by wild-type P450$_{cam}$, the consumption of oxygen and NADH is tightly coupled to substrate oxidation. But this coupling weakens when the interactions between the enzyme and the substrate are weakened, either by supplying the enzyme with a nonnatural substrate or when the enzyme structure is altered by site-directed mutagenesis. Under such uncoupled conditions, reducing equivalents from NAD(P)H drive the reduction of oxygen to hydrogen peroxide without achieving substrate oxidation.

Examination of the crystal structure shows that the heme and the substrate are almost completely buried within the core of the globular P450 protein (figure 7-15). How, then, does the substrate reach the active site? As with many enzymes, entry of the substrate requires conformational changes in the protein structure, opening a channel into the active site. These conformational changes can be thought of as a "breathing" motion of the protein, opening and closing the channel. Crystallization of the protein "traps" the structure in one of its conformations and prevents

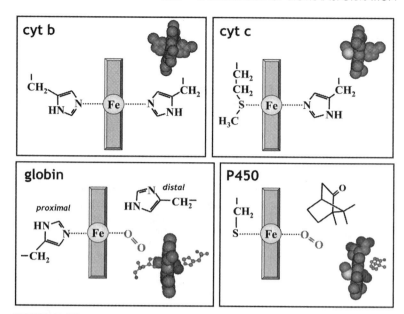

FIGURE 7-13.

The heme environments of four classes of heme proteins are illustrated both schematically and with crystal structure representations (small insets). In each case, the heme ring is viewed edge on. The protein classes are cytochrome b; cytochrome c; oxygen-binding globins such as myoglobin; and P450 enzymes. In the cases of globins and P450s, bound molecular oxygen is also shown. *Note*: A full-color version of this figure appears on the website.

observation of the entry channel, but analysis of the structure suggests that the channel is opened by movement of residues Phe-87, Phe-193, and Ile-395.

Sequence comparisons of $P450_{cam}$ with other P450 enzymes show that a threonine residue analogous to Thr-252 in the I-helix of $P450_{cam}$ is highly conserved, although a few enzymes are known in which it is replaced by Ser or Asn. Thr-252 in the $P450_{cam}$ structure forms a hydrogen bond to the peptide carbonyl of Gly-248 and thereby forces a distinct disruption in the middle of the otherwise-regular I-helix (figure 7-11). Site-directed mutation of Thr-252 in $P450_{cam}$ causes increased uncoupling (reduction of oxygen to hydrogen peroxide), although the enzyme retains some catalytic activity. In mammalian P450 enzymes, however, mutations of the corresponding residue do not always interfere with catalytic activity. In rat P450 1A2, for example, the mutation Thr-319 → Ala suppresses the enzyme's ability to oxidize benzphetamine, but does not alter its ability to oxidize 7-ethoxycoumarin (*76*).

Additional features of P450 active site structure are discussed in the later section on the P450 catalytic cycle.

Structures of Mammalian P450 Enzymes

Sequence alignments suggest that the main structural features of the membrane-bound mammalian enzymes are similar to those of bacterial P450 enzymes. The overall structural similarity of P450BM-3 to $P450_{cam}$ is also reassuring, in this regard, because P450BM-3 shows higher

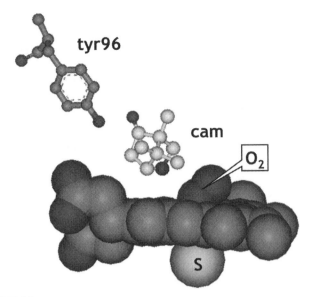

FIGURE 7-14.

The active site of the P450$_{cam}$ ferrous oxy complex, showing the heme ring (edge on), the sulfur atom of proximal cysteine 357, camphor substrate, tyrosine 96, and molecular oxygen bound to the heme iron. The C-5 position of camphor, which is the site of hydroxylation, is highlighted in a darker color. H atoms not shown. Coordinates: 1DZ8.pdb. *Note*: A full-color version of this figure appears on the website. *(Schlichting, I.; Berendzen, J.; Chu, K.; Stock, A. M.; Maves, S. A.; Benson, D. E.; Sweet, R. M.; Ringe, D.; Petsko, G. A.; Sligar, S. G. The catalytic pathway of cytochrome P450$_{cam}$ at atomic resolution. Science **2000**, 287, 1615–1622.)*

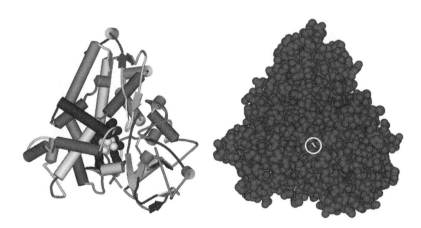

FIGURE 7-15.

Two views of the camphor-P450$_{cam}$ complex. Left: schematic view of the protein; the camphor substrate is shown as a space-filling model near the center of the protein. Right: the same view of the protein is shown as a space-filling model. The circle highlights the barely visible camphor substrate. *Note*: A full-color version of this figure appears on the website.

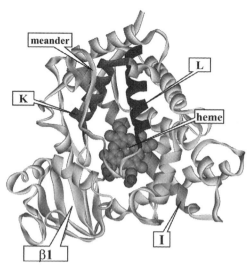

FIGURE 7-16.

The overall tertiary structure of recombinant rabbit P450 2C5. Coordinates: 1DT6.pdb. *Note*: A full-color version of this figure appears on the website. (*Williams, P. A.; Cosme, J.; Sridhar, V.; Johnson, E. F.; McRee, D. E. Mammalian microsomal cytochrome P450 monooxygenase: structural adaptations for membrane binding and functional diversity.* Mol. Cell **2000**, 5, *121–131*.)

sequence identity with the mammalian P450 4A1 family than with P450$_{cam}$. The first mammalian microsomal P450 structure solved is a modified form of recombinant rabbit 2C5; the amino-terminal hydrophobic residues were deleted and several internal residues were replaced by the corresponding residues of rabbit 2C3 in a successful attempt to increase solubility and ease of crystallization. The structure of 2C5 (figure 7-16) did indeed prove to have a great deal in common with the bacterial enzymes, including the overall shape of the protein and the major secondary structure elements. When compared to the bacterial P450 structures, the geometry of the 2C5 heme "sandwich" formed by the I- and L-helices is closely similar. The β-sheet region near the amino-terminal end of 2C5 is positioned somewhat differently relative to the heme, however, and a shift in the position of the F-helix gives the active site a distinct shape. Although the crystal structure is of substrate-free protein, computer "docking" methods were able to identify the binding geometry for progesterone, an endogenous substrate for this P450. By analysis of P450 sequence alignments, six "substrate recognition sequences" (SRSs), stretches of primary structure that may account for the substrate specificities of P450 enzymes, have been inferred (77). Indeed, the postulated SRS regions contain the residues that contact the "docked" progesterone molecule in the 2C5 structure.

The first high-resolution structure of a human P450—a modified form of P450 2C9—was published in 2003 (*66*), and two independent reports of the structure of human P450 3A4 appeared in 2004 (*68, 69*). In view of its important role in the metabolism of a wide variety of drugs, researchers had anticipated that P450 3A4 would have an unusually large active site cavity. Surprisingly, this proved to be incorrect; the accessible volume of the active site was rather smaller than that of P450 2C9. A distinctive feature of P450 3A4 is the cluster of phenylalanine residues in

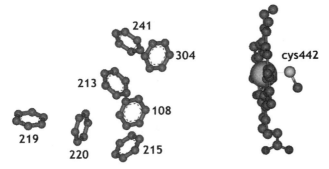

FIGURE 7-17.

The "Phe-cluster" of recombinant human P450 3A4. The sulfur atom of cysteine 442 is shown to the right of the heme group and the cluster of phenylalanine residues (numbered) in the active site is shown to the left. Coordinates: 1W0E.pdb. *Note*: A full-color version of this figure appears on the website.

the active site (figure 7-17). Previous site-directed mutagenesis studies had identified some of these Phe residues as participating in substrate binding.

Membrane Topology of Microsomal P450

The orientation of microsomal P450 enzymes in the endoplasmic reticulum is still not well understood. Amino acid sequences of microsomal P450 forms always contain a section of about 25 very hydrophobic residues at the amino terminus. This hydrophobic region is recognized by a signal recognition particle (SRP), which directs insertion of the enzyme into the endoplasmic reticulum membrane, and also functions as a stop-transfer sequence (see chapter 12). The consensus view is that microsomal P450s are exposed on the cytosolic side of the endoplasmic reticulum and anchored into the ER membrane by the amino-terminal hydrophobic "tail," although additional hydrophobic regions of the protein assist membrane association (*78, 79*).

SPECTROSCOPIC PROPERTIES OF P450 ENZYMES

The heme group is a very strong chromophore and its spectroscopic properties are sensitive to the *nature of the ligands* bound to the heme iron, to the iron *oxidation state*, and to the *protein environment* in which the heme is located. The unique feature of P450 enzymes, which led to their discovery and accounts for their name, is the 450 nm absorption maximum of the reduced (ferrous, Fe^{2+}) carbon monoxide complex of the protein. Among different P450 enzymes, λ_{max} ranges from 447 to 452 nm. The analogous $Fe^{2+}CO$ complex of a spectroscopically typical heme protein is near 420 nm; myoglobin, for example, has $\lambda_{max} = 423$ nm. The position of λ_{max} for the $Fe^{2+}CO$ complex of a hemoprotein is strongly influenced by the identity of the ligand coordinated to the iron on the side opposite to that occupied by CO. This axial ligand, in myoglobin and most other hemoproteins, is a nitrogen atom of a histidine imidazole ring. The unusual P450 chromophore suggested the presence of an unusual ligand: evidence from chemical model systems, spectroscopy, and crystallography showed that the *P450 axial ligand is the deprotonated sulfur of a cysteine* (*thiolate*). Only proteins with a thiolate ligand have reduced CO complexes with λ_{max}

near 450 nm (*80*). The thiolate ligand causes the Soret absorption band to split into the band at about 450 nm and a second band, of comparable intensity, at about 370 nm. (A few other proteins, notably nitric oxide synthase (*81*) and chloroperoxidase, also have a thiolate ligand and, therefore, an $Fe^{2+}CO$ complex λ_{max} near 450 nm. These proteins may be regarded as close "cousins" to P450, although their tertiary structures and activities may differ.) From the original work of Omura and Sato, it was already clear that denaturation of P450 caused a shift in λ_{max} from 450 nm to about 420 nm. *The unique spectroscopic signature of P450 is due to a structural feature—the thiolate ligand—that is required for P450 mono-oxygenase enzyme activity.*

THE CATALYTIC CYCLE OF P450

Substrate hydroxylation by P450 is represented by the following stoichiometric equation:[14]

$$NADPH + H^+ + RH + O_2 \rightarrow NADP^+ + ROH + H_2O$$

From this equation, we can deduce that several distinct chemical events must occur during the catalytic cycle. The enzyme must bind substrate and oxygen; accept two reducing equivalents and two protons; split the bond between the oxygen atoms of O_2; insert an oxygen atom into the substrate; and release products, water and oxygenated substrate. In what order do these molecular events occur, and what intermediate states of the enzyme exist? Much effort has been devoted to answering these questions. The tools that have been applied to studying the P450 reaction cycle include enzyme kinetics, X-ray diffraction structural analysis, many forms of spectroscopy, and theoretical calculations. The catalytic cycle of P450 has been best defined for the bacterial enzyme $P450_{cam}$ (*82*), but the essential features appear to apply to the mitochondrial and microsomal P450 enzymes as well. Our present understanding of the P450 catalytic cycle is outlined here (figure 7-18).

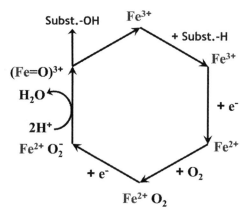

FIGURE 7-18.

The catalytic cycle of P450 enzymes. The oxidation states of the heme iron and oxygen are indicated. Note that other representations are also possible for the redox states of the intermediates, as described in the text. All intermediates between the substrate-binding and product-release steps include bound substrate, but this is not shown, for simplicity.

P450 Spin States

Optical spectroscopy of heme proteins provides us with insight into the chemical environment of the active site. To understand heme protein chemistry and spectroscopy, we need to review the elementary "crystal field" model of the electronic structure of transition metal ions (83). The valence electrons in transition metals occupy d orbitals, and ligands coordinated to the metals (Lewis bases) influence the energies of these five orbitals. In field-free space, all five d orbitals (figure 7-19) are degenerate, that is, they have identical energies. In Fe^{3+}, which has five d electrons, each of the orbitals is occupied by a single electron; this configuration satisfies Hund's rule, which is a consequence of the energy cost of putting two electrons with paired spins into the same orbital. Let us now consider what happens if, as occurs in an octahedral complex, we bring negative charges (in the form of free electron pairs on ligand donor atoms) close to the d_{x2-y2} and d_{z2} orbitals, but not close to the d_{xy}, d_{xz}, or d_{yz} orbitals. Because of the electrostatic charge repulsion between the electrons in the d orbitals and those of the free electron pairs in the ligands approaching along the x, y, and z axes, the five d orbitals are no longer degenerate, but split into two sets of orbitals separated by an energy gap (figure 7-19). Energetically, it is more expensive to place an electron into one of the first two orbitals (d_{x2-y2}, d_{z2}) than the latter three (d_{xy}, d_{xz}, d_{yz}), that is, the energies of

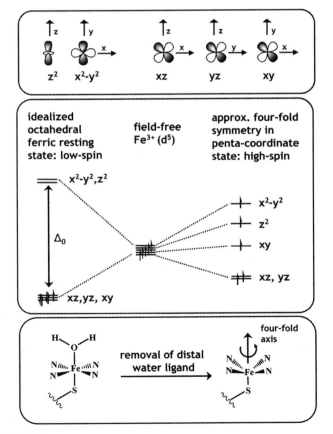

FIGURE 7-19.

P450 spin states; see text for further details.

the two orbitals closest in space to the negative charges on the ligands are increased. Note that in an idealized octahedron, with all ligands being identical, the orbitals within a given set will again be energetically degenerate, that is, d_{x2-y2} and d_{z2} will have the same energy as d_{xy}, d_{xz}, and d_{yz}. While the iron center in P450 does not quite fulfill the criterion of perfect octahedral symmetry, we can adopt this simplified orbital splitting pattern as a good approximation. The energy gap between the two sets of orbitals is referred to as the *crystal field splitting energy* and denoted $\triangle_0$. Typically, $\triangle_0 \sim 300\,kJ/mol$. If this energy gap separating the higher and lower energy orbitals is greater than the spin-pairing energy, the five Fe^{3+} d electrons will occupy the lower three orbitals, giving rise to a net unpaired electron spin of ½. This orbital occupancy is known as the "low-spin state" and is shown on the left-hand side of figure 7-19.

In a heme group, the iron atom is bonded to the four nitrogen atoms of the porphyrin; to the proximal axial ligand provided by the protein (cysteine thiolate in P450); and, in some circumstances, to a distal sixth ligand such as H_2O, O_2, or CO. In the Fe^{3+} (ferric) "resting-state" $P450_{cam}$, the distal ligand is a water molecule. (This probably also holds for membrane-bound P450 enzymes.) The hexacoordinated iron lies almost exactly in the plane of the porphyrin ring with the proximal and distal ligands occupying the axial positions, that is, the coordination sphere of the iron does indeed approximate the ideal octahedral environment and should have a d orbital splitting pattern very similar to the one shown on the left-hand side of figure 7-19. Two of the d orbitals in the hexaco-ordinated heme group are, therefore, at higher energies than the other three, favoring the low-spin state for the ferric resting state.

Removal of the distal ligand (induced by the binding of certain ligands or substrates in proximity to, but not on, the iron center) breaks the symmetry of the octahedron and gives a pentacoordinated species of approximate four-fold symmetry, in which the iron experiences an overall weaker crystal field. As a consequence, the iron atom moves out of the plane of the heme, towards the fifth (proximal) ligand. The d_{x2-y2} orbital then points less directly at the porphyrin nitrogens and the d_{z2} orbital interaction with the distal ligand is reduced. At the same time, the inter-action between the d_{xy} orbital and the four porphyrin nitrogens increases slightly, leading to an additional splitting of the energies of the three lower energy orbitals, d_{xy}, d_{xz}, and d_{yz}, as shown on the right-hand side of figure 7-19. The differences between the energy levels of d_{xz}/d_{yz} and the d_{xy} and the d_{xy} and d_{z2} orbitals, respectively, are now less than the spin pairing energy, resulting in an electron configuration in which each orbital is occupied by one electron. This is called the "high-spin state."

Thus, the spin state of a heme protein can tell us whether the iron is coordinated to a sixth ligand. The low-spin and high-spin states of "resting" (ferric, Fe^{3+}) P450 are characterized by $\lambda_{max} = 416–419\,nm$ and $\lambda_{max} = 390–416\,nm$, respectively. Spin state can also be probed by electron paramagnetic resonance spectroscopy.

Substrate Binding to P450

Ferric P450 is stable (at least, in the absence of reducing equivalents and oxygen), and the distal ligand in this state is usually a water molecule, as noted above. Diverse compounds bind to ferric P450 enzymes (*84*) and cause a characteristic shift in the protein's ultraviolet–visible absorbance spectrum. Binding of a small organic molecule to the P450 active site can displace the bound water, causing a shift from the hexacoordinate to the pentacoordinate state and consequently from the low-spin to the high-spin state. To measure this shift, a difference spectrum is recorded: ferric enzyme versus ferric enzyme + compound of interest (e.g., (85)). This spectral blue-shift, showing a maximum at 385–390 nm and a trough at about 420 nm, is known as a "type I difference spectrum" (figure 7-20). Many compounds induce the type I difference spectrum, including toluene, DDT, phenobarbital, chlorpromazine, and so on. Some, but not all, of these compounds are P450 substrates. In the case of P450$_{cam}$, the shift in spin state accompanying camphor binding changes the protein's redox potential from −300 to −170 mV. The substrate-bound enzyme is thus much more easily reduced.

A distinct type of difference spectrum is observed when certain compounds, particularly those containing nitrogen heterocycles or other nitrogen functions (e.g., aniline, imidazole, pyridine, nicotine), are added to P450 enzymes. This spectrum displays a trough at 390–405 nm and a maximum at 425–435 nm—roughly the opposite of the type I spectrum. This "type II difference spectrum" (e.g., (86)) is associated with the binding of compounds that coordinate to the iron even more strongly than

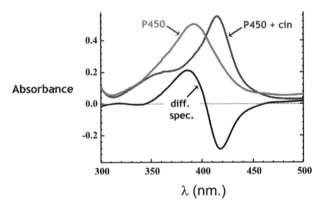

FIGURE 7-20.

The P450 type I optical difference spectrum. Three traces are shown: the absolute spectra of the (ferric) P450 enzyme in the absence and presence of ligand, and the resulting difference spectrum. Note the characteristic "differential" shape of the difference spectrum, which is centered at $\triangle A = 0$. (These spectra of the ferric enzyme should not be confused with the 450 nm chromophore of the ferrous-CO complex.) In this example, the P450 enzyme is P450$_{cin}$ and the ligand is its substrate cineole. The reader should consult the published paper (*Hawkes, D. B.; Adams, G. W.; Burlingame, A. L.; Ortiz de Montellano, P. R.; De Voss, J. J. Cytochrome P450(cin) (CYP176A), isolation, expression, and characterization*. J. Biol. Chem. **2002**, *277, 27725–27732*) and note how a plot of the magnitude of the spectral shift ($\triangle A_{392-415\,nm}$) versus cineole concentration allows calculation of K_D for the enzyme–ligand (enzyme–substrate) complex. *Note*: A full-color version of this figure appears on the website. (*Data graciously provided by James De Voss, Department of Chemistry, University of Queensland, Australia.*)

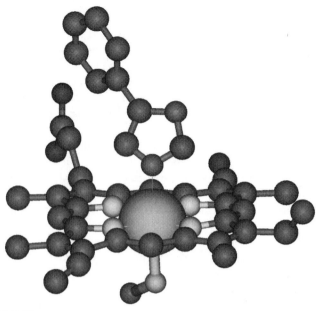

FIGURE 7-21.

Crystal structure of the complex of P450$_{cam}$ and a typical type II binding compound, phenylimidazole; heme environment. The view is slightly out of the plane of the heme ring. The central iron atom is shown as a space-filling ball, surrounded by the four heme N atoms coordinating to the iron. The sulfur atom of cysteine residue 357, the protein's proximal ligand to the heme iron, is shown below the heme plane, and the liganding phenylimidazole is shown above. Coordinates: 1phd.pdb. *Note*: A full-color version of this figure appears on the website.

does water. Figure 7-21 shows the structure of the heme environment of a P450 enzyme complexed with phenylimidazole, a type II binder.

Some compounds resemble water in their coordination to the iron, and produce a variant of the type II spectrum, known as a reverse type I spectrum. In this spectrum, the maximum occurs at approximately 420 nm and the trough at 388–390 nm. The mixture of P450 states present in a sample is shifted from the pentacoordinate, high-spin state toward the hexacoordinated, low-spin state by compounds that give either type II or reverse type I spectra.

Electron Transport to P450

P450 heme iron accepts electrons one at a time, whereas NADPH and NADH are two-electron donors. The electrons provided by the pyridine nucleotides to the heme group must, therefore, pass through a "transformer," which accepts paired electrons (in the form of hydride anion, H$^-$, or equivalent) but delivers single electrons to the iron atom. These functions are satisfied either by a flavoprotein plus an iron–sulfur protein, or by a single protein with two flavin prosthetic groups.

Electron transfer from reduced pyridine nucleotides to microsomal P450s, including the enzymes involved in mammalian xenobiotic metabolism, is mediated by the enzyme *NADPH-cytochrome P450 reductase*. P450 reductase[15] was, in fact, discovered long before P450 itself! B.L. Horecker, in 1950, identified a hepatic microsomal enzyme that catalyzed the reduction of cytochrome c (Fe^{3+} to Fe^{2+}) by NADPH (*87*). The activity was detected by monitoring the shift in the absorbance spectrum of cytochrome c accompanying reduction. Cytochrome c, of course, is a mitochondrial, not a microsomal, protein; it was used simply as a convenient protein electron acceptor. Consequently, Horecker named the new enzyme "NADPH-cytochrome c reductase." After the discovery of P450, it became clear that the true physiological substrate for the reductase is P450, and the enzyme was renamed as NADPH-cytochrome P450 reductase (NADPH-ferrihemoprotein reductase; EC 1.6.2.4). Nevertheless, cytochrome c reduction is still used as the standard assay substrate for quantitation of reductase activity.

Lu and Coon, in their original work on reconstitution of P450 activity from purified microsomal components (*28*), demonstrated that the necessary and sufficient constituents required for P450 enzyme activity are P450 hemeprotein, NADPH-cytochrome P450 reductase, and phospholipid. (The phospholipid presumably provides a suitable milieu for association of P450 and reductase, and is not required with soluble forms of P450.)

The reductase (MW ~78 kDa) consists of a large cytosolic domain, which binds one molecule each of FMN and FAD, and an N-terminal hydrophobic peptide that anchors the protein to the membrane (*88*). Electron flow is believed to occur sequentially from NADPH to reductase-bound FAD, then to bound FMN, and finally to P450 heme.

Cytochrome b_5

Although NADPH-cytochrome P450 reductase is the only accessory protein absolutely required for reconstitution of P450 activity in a purified system, other microsomal proteins might facilitate P450 activity in vivo. Hepatic microsomes also contain the heme enzyme, cytochrome b_5 and the flavoprotein, cytochrome b_5 reductase. (Microsomal cytochrome b_5 is a membrane-bound form of the cytosolic enzyme cytochrome b_5 found in red blood cells.) The principal enzymatic activity of the b_5/b_5 reductase system is desaturation of fatty acids (*14*, p. 627). However, the P450-catalyzed turnover of some substrates can be increased synergistically by electron transfer from cytochrome b_5 (*89, 90*). NADH alone will not support microsomal P450 activity, but the addition of NADH results in a several-fold increase in product formation, above the rate obtained with NADPH alone. Similar stimulation of product formation is observed, in some instances, when cytochrome b_5 is included in a system reconstituted from purified P450 and P450 reductase. (Cytochrome b_5 reductase is not required in such reconstitution studies, because cytochrome b_5 can be reduced directly by NADPH-cytochrome P450 reductase.) The physiological significance (if any) of such "crosstalk" electron flow between the microsomal b_5 and P450 systems remains unclear (*91, 92*).

Electron supply to P450 enzymes can occur by several different pathways (*93*). In adrenal mitochondria, where P450 activity is important for the biosynthesis of steroid hormones, a flavoprotein known as *adrenodoxin reductase* supplies electrons to P450. Adrenodoxin reductase has a single FAD prosthetic group. The companion protein *adrenodoxin* has an active site with two iron atoms, each coordinated to two cysteinyl sulfurs and bridged by two inorganic sulfur atoms ([2Fe–2S] cluster (*14*, p. 500)).

Transfer of H^- from NADPH to FAD yields a two-electron reduced form of the reductase, which is reoxidized in two discrete, one-electron transfers by the iron–sulfur protein. The iron–sulfur proteins subsequently transfer the electron to the P450 heme iron atom. The corresponding proteins that supply electrons to bacterial $P450_{cam}$ are known as *putidaredoxin reductase* (reduced by NADH rather than NADPH) and *putidaredoxin*, respectively. Putidaredoxin has a redox potential of $-196\,mV$ when bound to $P450_{cam}$. As we noted earlier, the shift in spin state upon substrate binding changes the P450 protein's redox potential from -300 to $-170\,mV$. Thus, reduction of $P450_{cam}$ by putidaredoxin becomes thermodynamically accessible once substrate binds to P450. Consequently, the P450 enzyme is quiescent, in the absence of substrate, but becomes catalytically activated when a substrate is available.[16]

Oxygen Binding and the First Reduction Step

The ferrous substrate-bound form of the enzyme rapidly reacts with oxygen to give the ferrous dioxygen-bound complex. Binding of oxygen to the ferrous form of P450 is formally analogous to the binding of oxygen to hemoglobin or myoglobin, which function as reversible oxygen carriers in the ferrous state. Oxygen binding is also reversible in the P450 enzymes. The ferrous dioxygen-bound form of the enzyme can be observed spectroscopically (*94*) and by low-temperature X-ray crystallography (*65*) (figure 7-14). However, the P450 dioxygen complex is much less stable with respect to autooxidation (generating superoxide) than is the case with hemoglobin or myoglobin:

$$P450\ (Fe^{2+})\ O_2\ SH \leftrightarrow P450\ (Fe^{3+})\ O_2^{\bullet-}\ SH$$

Under physiological conditions, transfer of the second electron usually occurs before autoxidation takes place, so superoxide generation is only a trace side reaction.

The Second Reduction Step: Formation of the Reactive Species

Transfer of the second electron completes the assembly of the P450 reactive intermediate and triggers the remaining rapid steps of the catalytic cycle: dioxygen cleavage, proton uptake, and substrate hydroxylation. The second reduction step generates a complex that (in formal "electron-bookkeeping" terms, at least) is electronically equivalent to coordination of hydrogen peroxide (dianion) with the ferric enzyme:

$$Fe^{2+}\ O_2 + e^- \leftrightarrow Fe^{1+}O_2 \leftrightarrow Fe^{2+}\ O_2^{\bullet-} \leftrightarrow Fe^{3+}\ O_2^{2-}$$

The P450 intermediate reached at this stage of the catalytic cycle is formally at the same oxidation state as an intermediate formed in the catalytic cycle of heme *peroxidases*, enzymes that catalyze the decomposition of hydrogen peroxide. The initial step in the peroxidase catalytic cycle is reaction of the ferric enzyme with hydrogen peroxide to give an intermediate that is readily detected by optical spectroscopy,[17] peroxidase "compound I". For this reason, some scientists refer to the P450 reactive intermediate as "P450 compound I." Indeed, in some instances, *hydrogen peroxide can replace enzymatically reduced molecular oxygen in the P450 catalytic cycle*; that is, P450 plus hydrogen peroxide can carry out hydroxylation reactions even in the absence of NADPH and P450 reductase (96). However, this analogy between P450 and peroxidases is limited. Peroxidases are not heme thiolate proteins[18] (the peroxidase proximal heme ligand is histidine); they do not catalyze hydroxylation of alkanes; and P450 compound I is much less stable than peroxidase compound I (98).

In principle, dioxygen cleavage might occur either before or after substrate hydroxylation. That is to say, the active hydroxylating enzyme intermediate might contain either one or two oxygen atoms. The ability of iodosylbenzene (C_6H_5–I=O) to drive P450-catalyzed hydroxylations (99) lends support to the idea of a one-oxygen-atom hydroxylating species, but direct evidence concerning the structure of the short-lived P450 compound I intermediate has proven elusive. Uptake of two protons, followed by heterolytic cleavage of the O–O bond, with loss of a molecule of water, would give a P450 compound I heme species that could be written as:

$$Fe^{3+} O_2^{2-} + 2H^+ \rightarrow H_2O + Fe^{3+}O^0$$

This representation, which is usually written $(Fe=O)^{3+}$, shows a ferric iron species (Fe^{3+}) coupled to a neutral oxygen atom (O^0) which is formally a six-electron species. In 1964 Gordon Hamilton pointed out the analogy between P450-mediated chemistry and the behavior of *carbenes*, reactive species in which a carbon atom bears six electrons (100). Carbenes add to olefins, to produce cyclopropyl derivatives, just as P450 inserts an oxygen atom into an olefin to generate an epoxide. Hamilton called the P450 intermediate an "oxenoid" species. (He originally suggested the term "oxene," which would designate a free neutral oxygen atom, but a referee of his manuscript suggested that "oxenoid" is a better description, since the single oxygen atom is bound to the enzyme, rather than free.) The term "oxenoid intermediate" has gained wide currency in the description of P450 chemistry.

Another designation for the oxenoid intermediate is $[Fe^V=O]$, representing a highly oxidized iron atom (Fe^V, so-called "perferryl iron") coupled to an oxygen atom at the redox state of water (O^{2-}). The high oxidation state of the oxenoid intermediate is certainly shared among the heme iron, oxygen, and porphyrin (101). The porphyrin ring (102) is probably oxidized to a π cation radical ($P^{•+}$), leaving the iron at the oxidation state Fe^{IV} (ferryl) (103). We would then represent the oxenoid intermediate as $(Fe=O)^{+3} P^{•+}$. Undoubtedly, interaction with the cysteine thiolate ligand also helps to stabilize this species (104, 105).

In the final step of the catalytic process, the oxygen atom of the ferryl species reacts with, and is usually transferred to, the substrate. The substrate, presumably, remains bound to the enzyme throughout the electron transfer and oxygen activation sequence, and is released after reaction with the ferryl oxygen. In the case of substrates that are relatively difficult to oxidize, the ferryl oxygen can apparently be reduced to water by additional electrons, provided by the accessory reductase or reductase/iron–sulfur protein pair. To the extent that superoxide, hydrogen peroxide, and water are produced during the catalytic turnover of P450, the reaction is said to be *uncoupled*, and deviates from the ideal monooxygenase stoichiometry.

Next, we consider the chemical events that take place when the $(Fe=O)^{3+}$ enzyme species interacts with substrate. Of course, the outcome differs for each of the major chemical classes of P450 substrate.

P450-CATALYZED REACTIONS

The diversity of P450-catalyzed chemistry is impressive. However, many of these metabolites arise by secondary, nonenzyme-catalyzed decompositions of the products initially formed by the enzymes, and most of the reactions directly catalyzed by P450 enzymes are variations on a limited set of chemical processes:

- *hydroxylation*: replacement of hydrogen by hydroxyl
- *epoxidation*: addition of oxygen to a carbon–carbon π-bond
- *heteroatom oxidation*: addition of oxygen to an electron lone pair on a heteroatom such as nitrogen, sulfur, or halogen.

In the following sections, we discuss the chemical mechanisms of some of these transformations. We have seen that the P450 catalytic cycle splits the O_2 molecule and generates a potent heme-bound oxidant species, formally $[Fe^V=O]$. Here, we focus on the substrates, considering the mechanisms of oxygenation and the subsequent chemical events that it triggers.

Hydroxylation of Alkanes

P450 activates molecular oxygen to a reactive species that can attack relatively inert chemical sites, such as unactivated carbon–hydrogen bonds and aromatic rings. Oxidation of alkanes is the quintessential P450-catalyzed reaction and has been the primary focus of mechanistic investigations (*106*). Some P450 enzymes, such as P450$_{cam}$ or P450 4A (which catalyzes fatty acid ω-oxidation), seem to have "specialized" in the oxidation of alkyl groups. Although recent advances in inorganic catalysis have provided some synthetic tools for alkane oxidation (*107*), any synthetic organic chemist would refrain from trying to oxidize a compound at an unactivated hydrocarbon site—the harsh conditions required (such as lighting a match!) are indiscriminate (*108*, page 747). The ability of P450 enzymes to catalyze the selective oxidation of specific C–H bonds in hydrocarbons is astonishing. Nevertheless, the efficiency of alkane hydroxylation, as measured by enzyme turnover numbers, is low; one molecule of P450$_{cam}$ can oxidize, at best, a few molecules of camphor per second (*109*). Chemists and biochemists have been studying (and arguing about) the mechanism of these reactions for about 50 years, but our understanding remains incomplete. A key issue is the characterization of the reactive oxygen species that is formed during the enzyme's reaction cycle, and much progress has been made in this regard. We will return to this issue in the subsequent discussion of the P450 catalytic cycle.

Typical substrates for P450-catalyzed alkane hydroxylation, such as camphor or fatty acids, have multiple alkyl groups that are potential sites of reaction. Nevertheless, P450-catalyzed oxidations invariably discriminate among these sites. Thermodynamic factors intrinsic to the substrate, especially the energy required to break the C–H bond, can be major determinants of the site of hydroxylation (regiospecificity). However, we must remember the overriding principle that the enzyme is a participant in the transition state: the enzyme positions the substrate with respect to the reactive oxygen and thus restricts the sites on the substrate at which oxygen can react. The catalytic outcome is thus governed both by the *geometry of the enzyme–substrate complex* and by the *relative reactivities of the accessible positions on the substrate.*

The hydroxylation of camphor elegantly illustrates the ability of the enzyme to direct hydroxylation by orienting a substrate in the active site. Camphor has 17 hydrogen atoms, any of which, in principle, could be converted to a hydroxy group. Nevertheless, the reaction is regiospecific and stereospecific: the exclusive product is 5-*exo*-hydroxycamphor. A tyrosine residue (tyr-96) of P450$_{cam}$ forms a hydrogen bond to the ketone oxygen atom of camphor (its only functional group), locking the substrate into position with its C5 carbon proximate to the heme iron (figure 7-14); the hydrogen atom closest to the iron is the site of camphor hydroxylation.

Some P450 enzymes can catalyze the hydroxylation of simple hydrocarbons, devoid of functional groups. For example, the yeast *Candida maltosa* assimilates *n*-alkanes via P450-dependent hydroxylation (*110*). P450$_{cam}$ also hydroxylates hydrocarbons. A small simple hydrocarbon substrate is like a coffee mug with no handle: the enzyme can grab the molecule, but cannot hold it firmly in a fixed orientation. In such cases, it is reasonable to predict that chemical factors intrinsic to the substrate will determine the regiospecificity of hydroxylation. Let us look at such a case, the hydroxylation of the small branched hydrocarbon 2-methylpentane catalyzed by P450$_{cam}$ (figure 7-22). This reaction was examined, catalyzed either by the wild-type enzyme or by a modified enzyme (P450$_{cam}$ Y96F) in which tyr-96 was replaced by phenylalanine via site-directed mutagenesis (*111*). The Y96F modification greatly increased the enzyme's affinity for hydrocarbons. The substrate has three primary, two secondary, and one

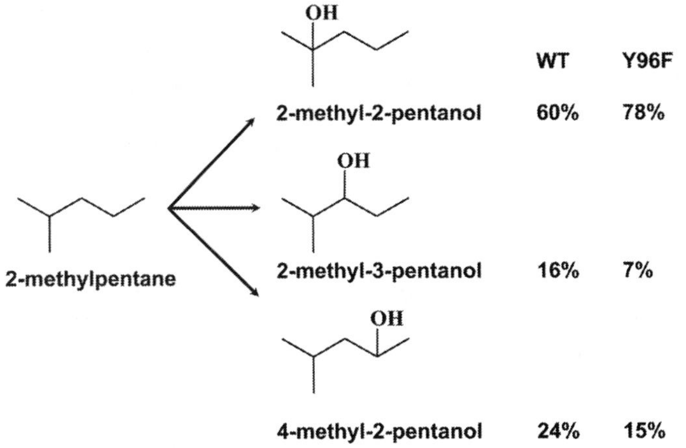

	WT	Y96F
2-methyl-2-pentanol	60%	78%
2-methyl-3-pentanol	16%	7%
4-methyl-2-pentanol	24%	15%

FIGURE 7-22.
Regiospecific products of hydroxylation of a hydrocarbon by P450$_{cam}$. Percentages indicate yield (% of total) for the wild-type enzyme (WT) and for the Y96F mutant. 4-Methyl-1-pentanol was not detected. (*Data from Stevenson, J.-A.; Westlake, A. C. G.; Whittock, C.; Wong, L. L. The catalytic oxidation of linear and branched alkanes by cytochrome P450cam.* J. Am. Chem. Soc. **1996**, 118, 12846–12847.)

tertiary carbon, so there are nine primary, four secondary, and one tertiary hydrogen atoms that could be converted to −OH groups. Nevertheless, the major product was the tertiary alcohol 2-methyl-2-pentanol and no primary alcohol products were formed. This result has been seen with a variety of P450 enzymes and substrates (112, 113). The bond dissociation energies (kJ/mol) for homolytic cleavage of C−H bonds in hydrocarbons $(RH \rightarrow R^{\bullet} + H^{\bullet})$ are typically: primary, CH_3CH_2−H, 410; secondary, $(CH_3)_2CH$−H, 400; tertiary, $(CH_3)_3C$−H, 380. Thus, the intrinsic reactivities of carbon−hydrogen bonds in alkane substrates follow the order of the ease of C−H bond breakage: tertiary > secondary > primary.

Of course, for certain substrates, the enzyme may disregard these intrinsic chemical effects and "steer" a reaction into a pathway that, in the uncatalyzed process, is disfavored. (We have seen this effect already, in the case of camphor hydroxylation by $P450_{cam}$.) Such control is possible because the enzyme itself participates in the transition state of the catalyzed reaction. Another striking example where enzyme-directed regiospecificity contradicts the expected "chemical" selectivity order is seen with P450 4A enzymes, which catalyze ω-hydroxylation of the fatty acid lauric acid (C12:0): the carbon atom that becomes oxidized is that of the terminal primary methyl group, exactly the position *disfavored* on chemical reactivity grounds (114, 115). A polar site on the P450 4A protein binds the fatty acid's carboxylic acid group, and the alkyl chain binds in a confined hydrophobic "tunnel" leading towards the heme iron. Decanoic acid (C10:0), just two carbons shorter than lauric acid, is a very poor substrate, presumably because it is not long enough to stretch between the polar carboxylic acid binding site and the heme iron (116).

Hydroxylation reactions are highly favored when the C−H bond is *weakened* by the presence of an adjacent heteroatom or π-bond. Hydroxylation of a methyl substituent on an aromatic ring is a common P450-catalyzed reaction. However, oxidation of C−H bonds stronger than those of a terminal −CH$_3$ group (e.g., vinylic or aromatic C−H bonds) rarely, if ever, occurs; such bonds are so strong that hydroxylation does not compete effectively with other possible reactions. In the case of *aromatic* rings, hydroxylation proceeds by a route that does not involve oxygen insertion into the C−H bond. Aromatic hydroxylation is considered later in this chapter.

▶ Isotopes of Hydrogen

Three isotopes of hydrogen exist: the common isotope ^{1}H ("protium"), D (^{2}H; deuterium, stable), and T (^{3}H; tritium, radioactive). Isotope labeling makes it possible to distinguish the fates of specific hydrogen atoms in a molecule. We will see an example of this application of isotopic labeling in the discussion of the NIH shift mechanism later in this chapter. Furthermore, the large mass differences among hydrogen isotopes result in substantial chemical kinetic isotope effects, that is, *isotopic differences in the rates of chemical reactions*, effects that are much larger than those observed with heavier atoms. Isotope effects can yield valuable information about the mechanisms of reactions involving hydrogen atoms (117). The quantum mechanical zero-point vibrational energies of C−H bonds are in the order C−H > C−D > C−T, due to the different masses (figure 7-23). As a result, *the C−H bond is significantly weaker than the C−D (or C−T) bond*. If a C−H bond is broken in the transition state of a reaction, then the rate of that step will be faster for a C−H bond than for a C−D bond. The maximum possible kinetic isotope effect (which can be calculated on simple theoretical grounds) is $k_H/k_D = 7$. The magnitude of the isotope effect can be much *lower*, if C−H bond breaking is only partially rate limiting, or much *higher*, if tunneling and other quantum mechanical effects are taken into consideration.

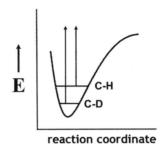

reaction coordinate

FIGURE 7-23.

The energy curve of a hypothetical C–H bond is shown, illustrating the greater depth of the potential energy well for a C–D bond, due to the lower quantum mechanical zero-point energy of the heavier isotope. ◀

Kinetic Isotope Effects in P450-Catalyzed Alkane Hydroxylation

As we will see later in this chapter, the P450 reaction cycle is comprised of a sequence of many discrete chemical steps. In this overall cycle, steps other than the oxygen insertion event (e.g., electron transfer to the P450 heme) are usually rate limiting. Therefore, when we compare the overall rates of product formation between substrates with H versus D atoms at the site of the reaction (e.g., comparing the overall rates of hydroxylation of the methyl groups of xylene, H_3C–phenyl–CH_3, and methyl-deuterated xylene, D_3C–phenyl–CD_3), the differences are usually small. However, suppose we prepare a substrate with equivalent C–H and C–D bonds *within the same substrate molecule*, such as H_3C–phenyl–CD_3. If the enzyme's active site is sufficiently flexible to allow the catalytic group of the enzyme to "choose" between the equivalent methyl substituents, then substantial *isotopic discrimination* between the C–H and C–D bonds may be observed. This *intramolecular isotope effect* can be calculated from the change in the ratio of H to D substitution in the substrate and product. Substitution of D at one of two equivalent alkyl C–H bonds shifts P450-dependent oxidation from the deuterated to the nondeuterated site and gives rise to large intramolecular isotope effects (figure 7-24) (*118*). This result indicates that C–H bond breakage occurs during the P450 catalytic cycle, and lends support to the so-called "oxygen rebound" mechanism of alkyl hydroxylation, discussed below.

Oxygen Rebound

Regiospecific alkyl hydroxylation is, as we have noted, the quintessential P450-catalyzed reaction and a process with little chemical precedent. Much research effort has gone into the study of the mechanism of this reaction and lively controversies have arisen. Hydroxylation mechanisms may be classed as either *stepwise*, proceeding via discrete (albeit short-lived) activated-carbon intermediates (e.g., radicals or carbocations), or *concerted*, that is, mechanisms in which the oxygen atom is inserted directly into the C–H bond, without intermediates. If discrete intermediates, such as carbon-centered radicals, are formed during the reaction, then they might

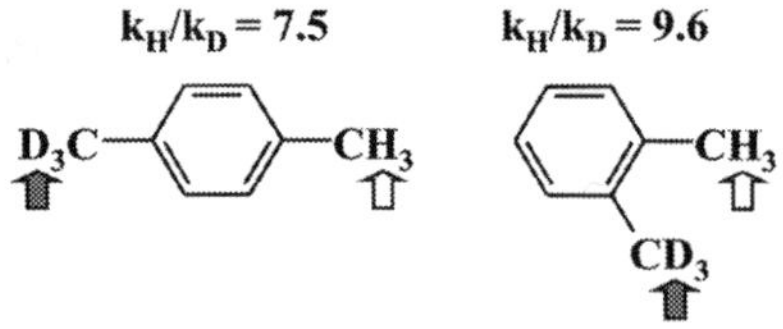

$$k_H/k_D = 7.5 \qquad\qquad k_H/k_D = 9.6$$

FIGURE 7-24.

The intramolecular isotope ratios for hydroxylation of the methyl substituents in *ortho*- and *para*-xylene. (*Data from Hanzlik, R. P.; Ling, K. H. Active site dynamics of xylene hydroxylation by cytochrome P-450 as revealed by kinetic deuterium isotope effects.* J. Am. Chem. Soc. **1993**, 115, 9363–9370.)

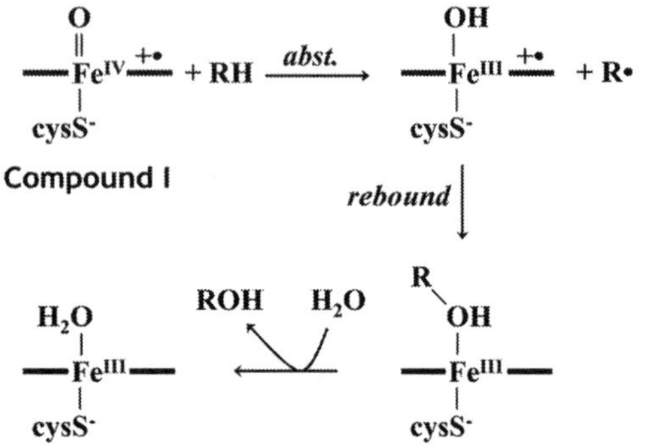

FIGURE 7-25.

Oxygen rebound mechanism of alkane hydroxylation. The thick horizontal line represents the heme ring. The steps shown are: (1) H-atom abstraction by compound I; (2) oxygen rebound; (3) product release. (*Adapted from Shaik, S.; De Visser, S. P.; Ogliaro, F.; Schwarz, H.; Schröder, D. Two-state reactivity mechanisms of hydroxylation and epoxidation by cytochrome P-450 revealed by theory.* Curr. Opin. Chem. Biol. **2002**, 6, 556–567.)

have the opportunity to undergo rearrangements, leading to "scrambled" products, for example products with altered stereochemistry. However, if the reaction mechanism is concerted, stereochemistry should remain intact.[19] There is evidence for both possibilities. Stereochemistry is usually, but not always, preserved, as expected for concerted mechanisms. But the correlation between C–H bond strength and reactivity, discussed earlier, suggests C–H bond breakage and a stepwise mechanism.

The so-called oxygen rebound mechanism of alkane hydroxylation (*119*) postulates that the enzyme abstracts a H atom from the substrate, generating a transient carbon radical on the substrate and forming an iron-bound hydroxyl radical (or equivalent) on the enzyme. These radicals then recombine to form the product (figure 7-25).

Evidence for such a stepwise oxygen insertion mechanism was obtained in a study of the hydroxylation of *exo*-tetradeuterated norbornane, which yields (in part) products in which D is retained in the *endo* configuration on the hydroxylated C atom (figure 7-26) (*119*). This inversion of D stereochemistry requires the formation of a discrete intermediate, in which the geometry of the tetrahedral carbon can undergo inversion. Several examples are now known of reactions that occur with loss of stereo- or regiochemistry and that, therefore, must proceed via an intermediate.

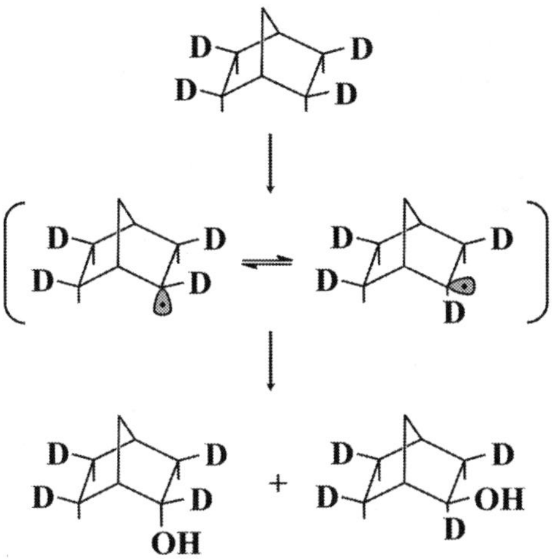

FIGURE 7-26.
The loss of stereochemistry observed during the hydroxylation of *exo*-tetradeuterated norbornane by rabbit liver microsomal P450 implies that the reaction proceeds via an intermediate in which the reaction site can undergo stereochemical inversion.

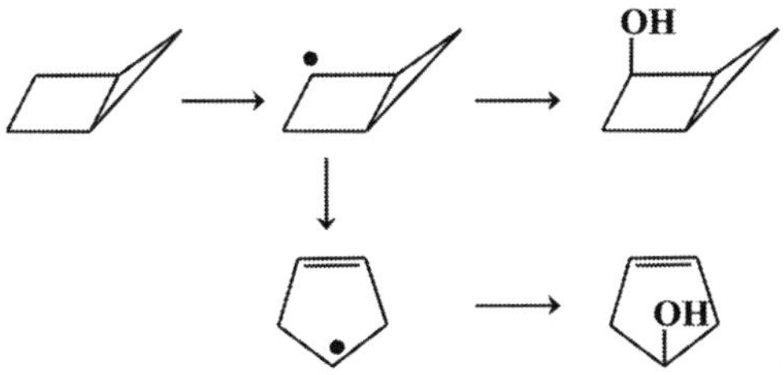

FIGURE 7-27.
Bicyclo[2.1.0]pentane is oxidized to a radical that rearranges on an ultrafast (picosecond) timescale. (*See Bowry, V. W.; Ingold, K. U. A radical clock investigation of microsomal cytochrome P-450 hydroxylation of hydrocarbons. Rate of oxygen rebound.* J. Am. Chem. Soc. *1991*, 113, 5699–5707.)

The rate of the recombination reaction has been measured by the use of "radical clock" probes. A "radical clock" is a radical that rearranges to a different radical, at a known rate (figure 7-27). Such rearrangements have been observed with several hydrocarbon substrates, and experiments indicate that the lifetime of the carbon-centered radical in the P450 active site is of the order of 50 ps (*120*). Theoretical studies suggest that both low-spin and high-spin states of compound I participate in substrate hydroxylation (two-state reactivity model) (*121*) and give predictions consistent with the oxygen rebound mechanism (*122*).

Oxidation of Alkyl Groups Adjacent to Heteroatoms or Halogens

Hydroxylation of a methyl group attached to an O or N atom is facile, and such reactions are common P450-catalyzed biotransformations. In the O-alkyl case, hydroxylation yields a *hemiacetal*, which usually fragments to give an aldehyde plus an alcohol product. In the N-alkyl case, hydroxylation

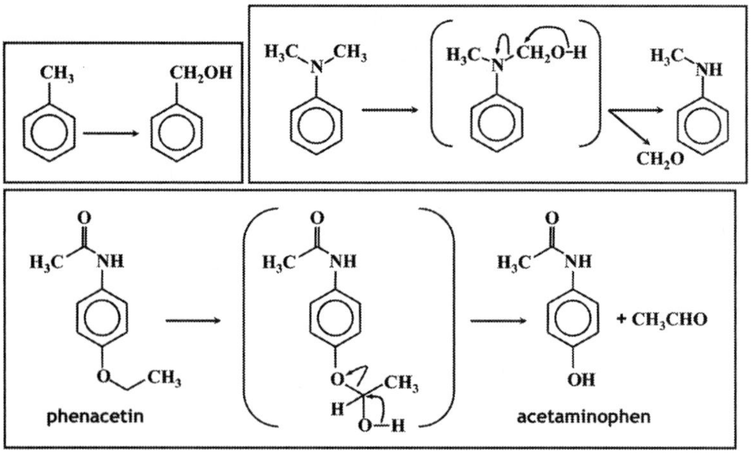

FIGURE 7-28.

Hydroxylations of benzylic carbons and carbons adjacent to oxygen and nitrogen atoms are generally favored, because the corresponding C–H bonds are relatively reactive. Hydroxylation adjacent to a heteroatom produces an alcohol, which usually eliminates the heteroatom, yielding a carbonyl compound and an alcohol or amine product.

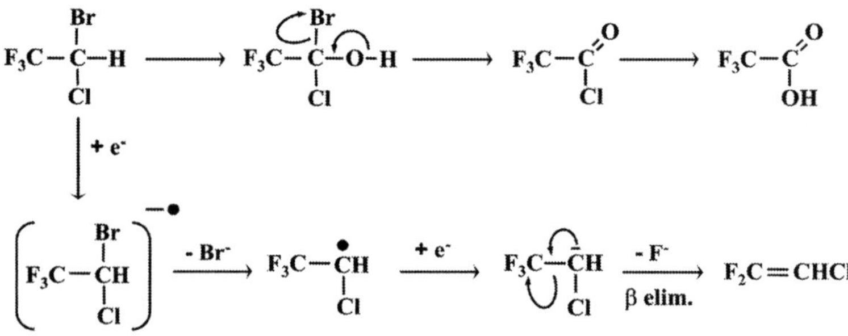

FIGURE 7-29.

Oxidative (upper scheme) and reductive (lower scheme) metabolism of halothane. In each case, only one product is shown, for simplicity. In the reductive route, the substrate receives a single electron from ferrous P450. Loss of bromide anion (the most weakly bound halogen) generates a neutral carbon-centered radical. The radical may abstract another reducing equivalent from P450 (or membrane lipid) to form an anion; β-elimination generates the indicated alkene.

yields an *aminal*, which fragments to give an aldehyde plus an amine (figure 7-28). *The outcome of hydroxylation adjacent to a N or O is therefore N- or O-dealkylation.* The same sort of fragmentation is observed after hydroxylation adjacent to halogens or other heteroatoms.

Hydroxylation of a carbon bearing more than one halogen atom gives rise to reactive species that can acylate protein residues, perturbing protein structure and function. Halothane (1-bromo-1-chloro-2,2,2-trifluoroethane) is a widely used inhalation anesthetic (figure 7-29). Oxidation of halothane catalyzed by P450 2E1 generates reactive intermediates that acylate liver proteins (*123*), including P450 2E1 itself;

the covalently modified proteins can trigger autoimmune reactions and severe liver damage, in rare cases.

Epoxidation

Olefins are oxidized by P450 to the corresponding epoxides. (The formal similarity of this reaction to the reaction of carbenes with olefins, to give cyclopropyl groups, prompted Hamilton to suggest the "oxenoid" character of activated P450, as discussed earlier in this chapter.) Olefin stereochemistry is retained (figure 7-30, upper panel). The epoxidation reaction, therefore, does not proceed via an intermediate that allows free rotation about the C–C bond. The simplest explanation for this finding is that the reaction, like nonenzymatic epoxidation by peracids, involves *simultaneous formation of both carbon–oxygen bonds of the epoxide*. The enzymatic reaction, like the peracid reaction, occurs more readily with electron-rich than with electron-poor olefins, consistent with such a mechanism. The occasional formation of carbonyl derivatives as minor reaction products, however, requires either the existence of a second mechanism in addition to a concerted addition, or formulation of a more complex mechanism that can account for all the reactions. A concerted mechanism does not explain, for example, the formation of trichloroacetaldehyde from 1,1,2-trichloroethylene, under conditions where it can be shown that the carbonyl products are not formed by rearrangement of the epoxide (figure 7-30, lower panel) (*124*). The 1,2-migration of a hydrogen or halide, required for the formation of such products, indicates that a cationic intermediate is formed, at least in the pathway that leads to the rearranged products.

Inactivation of P450 accompanies the oxidation of terminal olefins such as ethylene and octene (*125*). Although each of these olefins is primarily converted to its epoxide, the epoxidation reaction occasionally results in *alkylation of a pyrrole nitrogen of the enzyme's heme group by the terminal carbon of the olefin*. The heme alkylation reaction (figure 7-31) is triggered

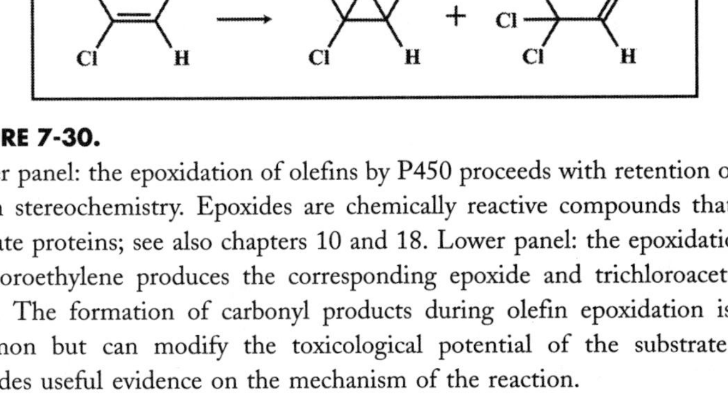

FIGURE 7-30.
Upper panel: the epoxidation of olefins by P450 proceeds with retention of the olefin stereochemistry. Epoxides are chemically reactive compounds that can alkylate proteins; see also chapters 10 and 18. Lower panel: the epoxidation of trichloroethylene produces the corresponding epoxide and trichloroacetaldehyde. The formation of carbonyl products during olefin epoxidation is not common but can modify the toxicological potential of the substrate and provides useful evidence on the mechanism of the reaction.

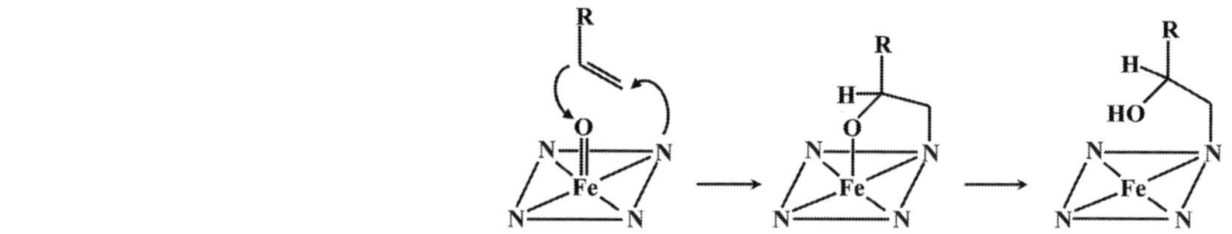

FIGURE 7-31.

Alkylation of the prosthetic heme group of a P450 enzyme, inactivating the enzyme, during catalytic oxidation of a terminal olefin.

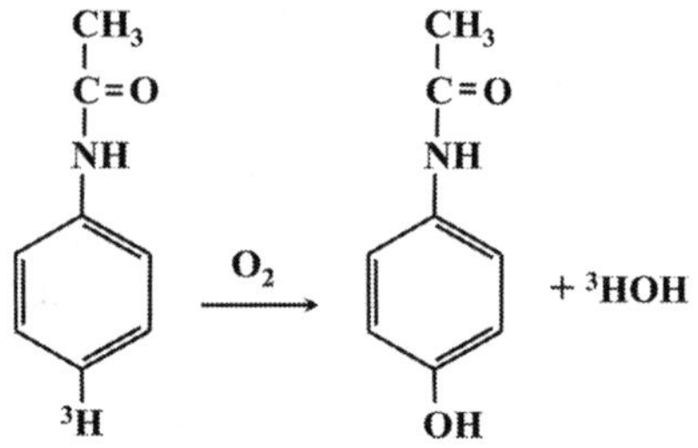

FIGURE 7-32.

Acetanilide hydroxylation.

by transfer of the activated oxygen to the internal carbon of the double bond. The N-alkylated prosthetic heme groups obtained with several olefins have been extracted from the protein. Removal of the iron gives an N-alkylated porphyrin; these have been characterized by NMR and other techniques. Because the inactivation requires catalytic oxidation of the inhibitor and involves inactivation of the very same enzyme molecule that catalyzes the oxidation, it is known as a *mechanism-based* or "suicide" inactivation.

Oxidation of Aromatic Rings; The NIH Shift

P450 hydroxylates aromatic substrates. Indeed, the formation of phenolic metabolites incorporating ^{18}O derived from $^{18}O_2$ was the first evidence for monooxygenation reactions in biochemistry, as discussed earlier. Even before the discovery of P450 protein, Bernard Brodie's group at NIH was studying the hydroxylation of acetanilide by hepatic microsomes (4). These investigations first highlighted the pharmacological significance of microsomal drug metabolism and established the existence of a microsomal hydroxylase enzyme. Because of the pharmacological and toxicological significance of aromatic hydroxylation, this biotransformation has been the focus of research in many laboratories.

The NIH group made a surprising discovery during their investigation of acetanilide hydroxylation (*126*). Acetanilide is hydroxylated to *para*-hydroxyacetanilide, in what is now known to be a typical P450-catalyzed monooxygenase reaction. Udenfriend and colleagues reasoned that a simple enzyme assay for this activity could be devised: they synthesized [4-^{3}H]-acetanilide, and expected that the amount of tritium radioactivity released as tritiated water (HTO) would equal the amount of product *para*-hydroxyacetanilide formed (figure 7-32). They were perplexed to discover that the amount of tritium released was variable, and much less than the amount of organic product formed (as measured by a colorimetric assay). Perhaps the radiolabel had been misincorporated into another position on the ring? But the same phenomenon was observed in the enzymatic conversion of [4-^{3}H]-phenylalanine into tyrosine. Deuterated [4-^{2}H] substrates were then synthesized; this allowed the position of incorporation, and subsequent fate, of the substituent at the *para* position to be monitored by NMR spectroscopy. This approach proved that the *para* hydrogen could either be released as water or migrate to the adjacent ring position. This "NIH shift" was subsequently observed for many different aromatic hydroxylation reactions. Not only hydrogen, but also halogen and alkyl substituents can migrate (*127*).

What is the mechanism of the NIH shift? The analogous migration of hydrogen, alkyl, or aryl substituents from a carbon to an adjacent electron-deficient carbon is known as a 1,2-shift, and is exemplified by the pinacol rearrangement, discovered by Fittig in 1860 (figure 7-33). The rearrangement occurs with diols, such as pinacol, and also with epoxides (figure 7-34). A carbenium ion is formed by the rupture of the epoxide ring, and the migrating substituent moves to this site, with its electron pair. In the case of the pinacol rearrangement, the reaction is driven by the

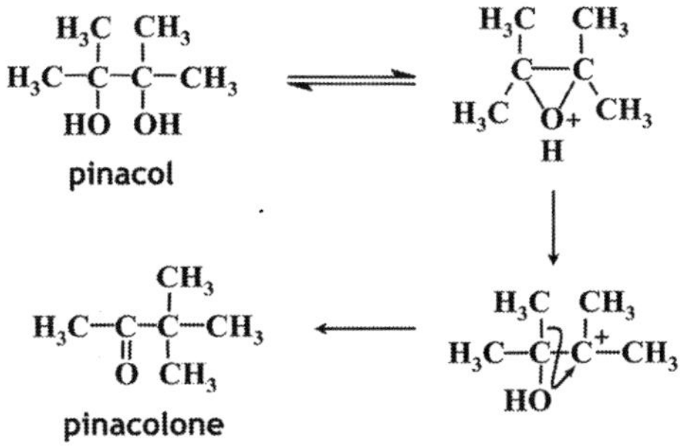

FIGURE 7-33.
Pinacol rearrangement.

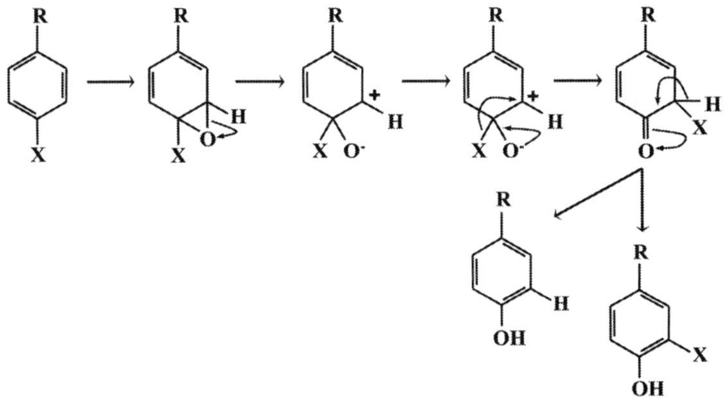

FIGURE 7-34.
Mechanism of the NIH shift in P450-catalyzed aromatic hydroxylation.

favorable formation of the ketone product. Jerina and colleagues suggested that the NIH shift proceeded via an arene oxide intermediate, which ruptures to form a carbenium ion. The validity of this model was demonstrated by the direct observation of isotope migration during the isomerization of synthetic arene oxides. For example, [1-^{2}H]-4-methylbenzene 1,2-oxide rearranges to 4-methylphenol and most of the deuterium is retained. *The NIH shift is indirect evidence for the intermediacy of arene oxides (epoxides formed on aromatic rings) in the enzymatic oxidation of aromatic hydrocarbons to phenols.* Direct proof was obtained when Jerina and colleagues isolated naphthalene 1,2-oxide as a microsomal metabolite of naphthalene (*128*).

Arene Oxides

The first arene oxide, the 9,10-oxide ("K-region" epoxide[20]) of phenanthrene, was synthesized in 1964 and, in the following years, arene oxide chemistry has been explored thoroughly (*129*). Arene oxides can, in principle, rearrange to the isomeric *oxepins* (figure 7-35), in which the carbon–carbon bond of the epoxide ring has broken to form a seven-membered ring incorporating the oxygen atom. The equilibrium between the arene oxide and oxepin forms depends on their relative thermodynamic stabilities. The colorless benzene oxide rapidly interconverts with the isomeric, conjugated, yellow oxepin valence bond tautomer. In the case of the naphthalene 1,2- and 2,3-oxides, the forms with aromatic benzene rings predominate: that is, the epoxide form of the former compound, and the oxepin form of the latter (figure 7-36). The epoxide ring can exist in two optically enantiomeric forms ("above" and "below" the plane of the aromatic rings) (figure 7-37). Reversible equilibration with the oxirane form, of course, results in racemization (loss of optical activity) of an initially pure enantiomer, and can be used as a probe of oxepin formation. All K-region epoxides that have been studied exist only in the epoxide form, as would be expected from a consideration of aromaticity. Again, this behavior reflects the alkene-like properties of the K-region double bond. However, the epoxides derived from aromatic rings (arene oxides) are much less stable than olefinic epoxides: cleavage of one of the carbon–oxygen bonds yields a cation that is stabilized by conjugation to the remaining double bonds of the aromatic ring. Formation of this cation initiates the NIH shift rearrangement, which leads to a hydroxylated product. The product is identical to that which would have been formed by direct insertion of oxygen into the C–H bond (*130*) but a direct mechanism could not account for the NIH shift.

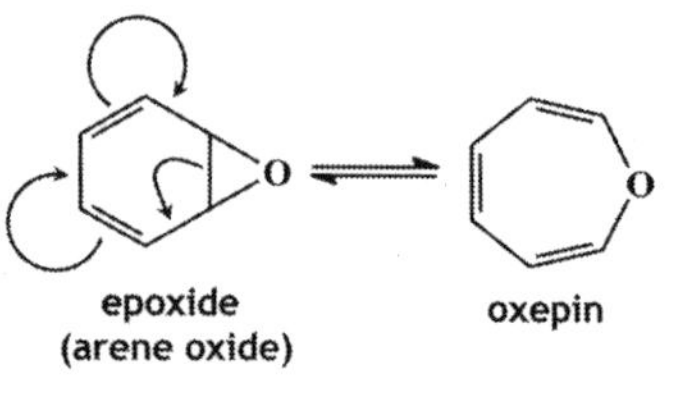

epoxide
(arene oxide)   oxepin

FIGURE 7-35.

Valence bond tautomerism interconverts an oxepin with an arene oxide.

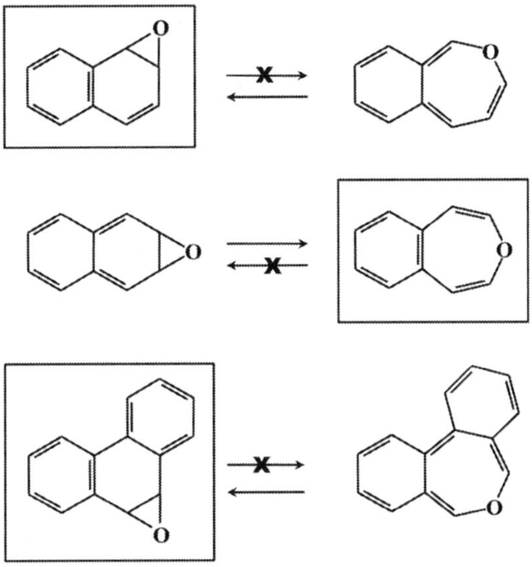

FIGURE 7-36.
Equilibrium strongly favors the arene oxide forms of the K-region epoxides formed from naphthalene (top) and anthracene (bottom). In the case of the naphthalene non-K-region epoxide (middle), the oxepin form is favored.

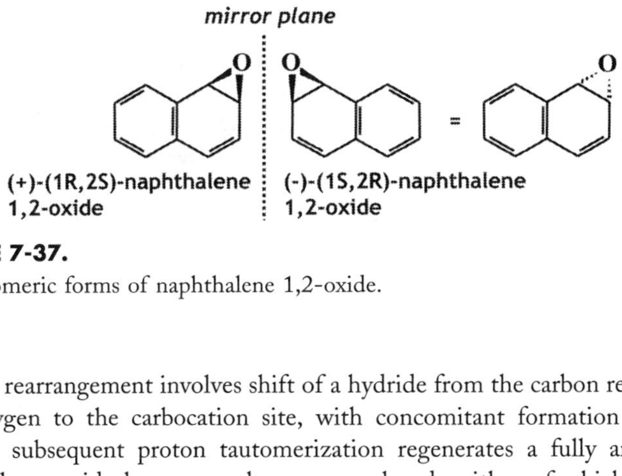

FIGURE 7-37.
Enantiomeric forms of naphthalene 1,2-oxide.

The rearrangement involves shift of a hydride from the carbon retaining the oxygen to the carbocation site, with concomitant formation of the ketone; subsequent proton tautomerization regenerates a fully aromatic ring. The epoxide has two carbon–oxygen bonds, either of which could, in principle, be broken, so the reaction can give rise to two different phenolic products. If cleavage of one of the carbon–oxygen bonds yields a cation that is significantly more stable than that obtained by cleavage of the other, then one product will predominate. For example, if the aromatic ring is substituted with an electron-donating methoxy group, formation of the *para*-hydroxy product is favored; formation of the *meta*-hydroxy product is favored if the substituent is an electron-withdrawing nitro group (figure 7-38).

The oxidation of aromatic π-bonds is subject to mechanistic ambiguities comparable to those that beset the oxidation of simple olefins. For example, although the epoxides of some aromatic substrates can

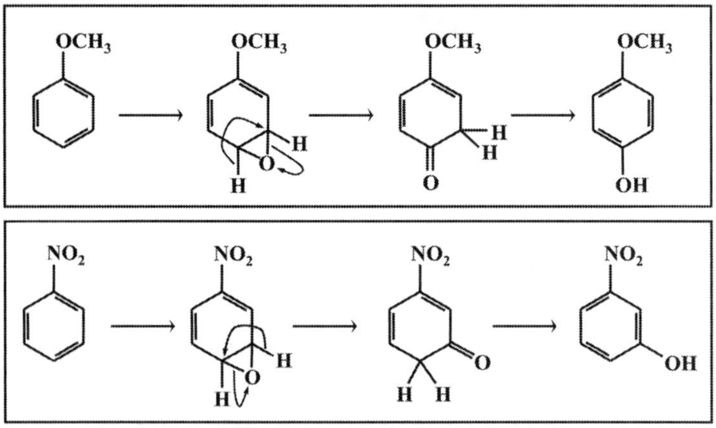

FIGURE 7-38.
Electron-donating (e.g., methoxy) and electron-withdrawing (e.g., nitro) substituents have opposite effects on the regiospecificity of the NIH shift.

actually be isolated and shown to undergo the NIH shift, aromatic substrates that have strong electron-donating substituents could possibly proceed to the NIH shift (or other reactions) without actually forming a discrete epoxide intermediate.

Oxidation of N and S Centers

Until this point, we have considered only the hydroxylation of C–H bonds in a variety of chemical contexts. P450 can also catalyze the hydroxylation of nitrogen (figure 7-39) and sulfur (figure 7-40) functionalities. The reactions of molecules bearing nitrogen or sulfur atoms with P450 are dominated by the availability of free electron pairs on the heteroatoms. In general, the more electronegative the atom, the more tightly it holds its electron pairs, and the less reactive it is towards oxidation by P450. Nitrogen and sulfur are readily oxidized, but oxygen is not.

The simplest reaction of P450 with a heteroatom involves transfer of the electron-deficient ferryl oxygen from the iron to one of the electron pairs of the heteroatom: nitrogen is oxidized to the N-oxide[21] ($R_3N\rightarrow O \leftrightarrow R_3N^+-O^-$) and sulfur to the sulfoxide ($R_2S=O \leftrightarrow R_2S^+-O^-$). The oxidations of arylamines (to hydroxylamines) and arylamides (to hydroxamic acids) (figure 7-41) are toxicologically important examples of P450-catalyzed nitrogen oxidation and are discussed further in chapter 17. Sulfoxides can be further oxidized to the sulfones (R_2SO_2). However, the free electron pair is more difficult to oxidize in the sulfoxide than in the sulfide, because of the partial positive charge on the sulfur. Oxidation of a sulfoxide to a sulfone is, therefore, more difficult than that of a sulfide to a sulfoxide. The sulfhydryl group can be oxidized to a sulfenic acid ($RSH \rightarrow RSOH$); the high electronegativity of oxygen, however, makes the O–H bond very strong and rules out the analogous hydroxylation of alcohols to peroxides ($ROH \rightarrow ROOH$).

Acetaminophen (4-hydroxyacetanilide, Tylenol®) is a widely used non-prescription analgesic and antipyretic. Although safe at therapeutic doses, acetaminophen overdose is potentially life-threatening; acetaminophen

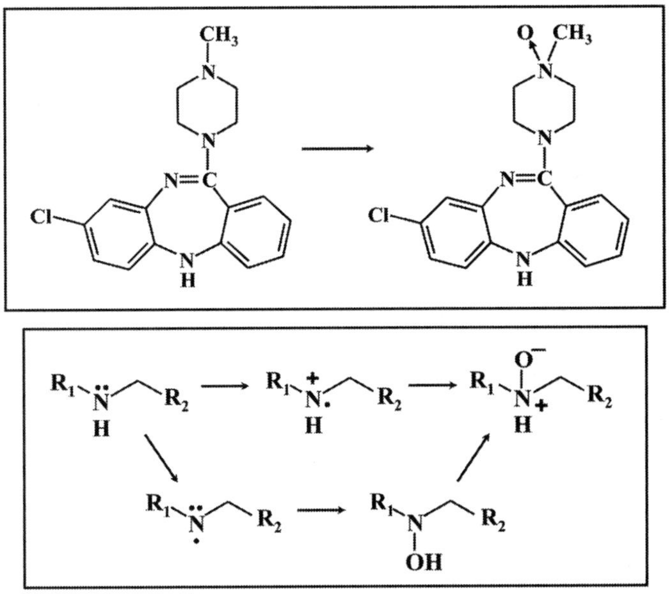

FIGURE 7-39.

Oxidation of a nitrogen bearing a hydrogen to the N-hydroxy product could involve either hydrogen abstraction followed by oxygen recombination or formation of an N-oxide that tautomerizes to the N-hydroxy product. An aliphatic amine, the antipsychotic drug clozapine, is converted to an N-oxide. (*Tugnait, M.; Hawes, E. M.; McKay, G.; Eichelbaum, M.; Midha, K. K. Characterization of the human hepatic cytochromes P450 involved in the in vitro oxidation of clozapine.* Chem. Biol. Interact. ***1999***, *118, 171–189.*)

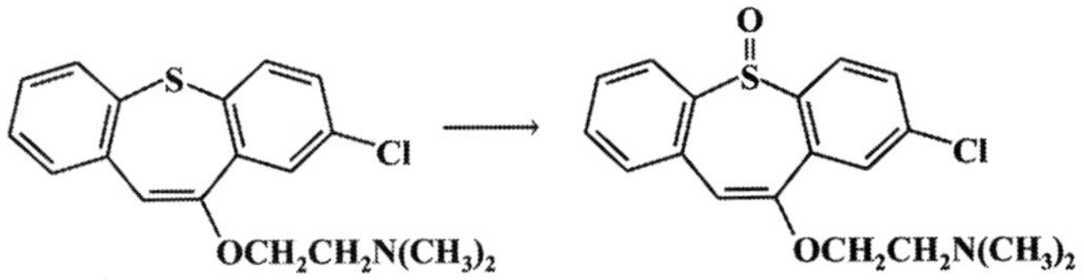

FIGURE 7-40.

An example of P450-catalyzed oxidation of a sulfide to a sulfoxide; the substrate is the antipsychotic agent zotepine. (*Shiraga, T.; Kaneko, H.; Iwasaki, K.; Tozuka, Z.; Suzuki, A.; Hata, T. Identification of cytochrome P450 enzymes involved in the metabolism of zotepine, an antipsychotic drug, in human liver microsomes.* Xenobiotica ***1999***, *29, 217–229.*)

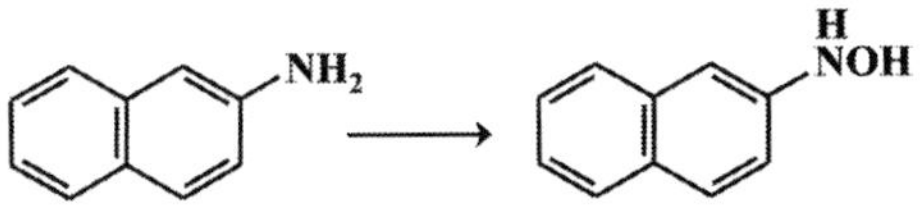

FIGURE 7-41.

N-hydroxylation of 2-naphthylamine, followed by sulfate or acetate conjugation of the hydroxyl group, is believed to be responsible for the potent carcinogenic properties of the arylamine (see chapter 17).

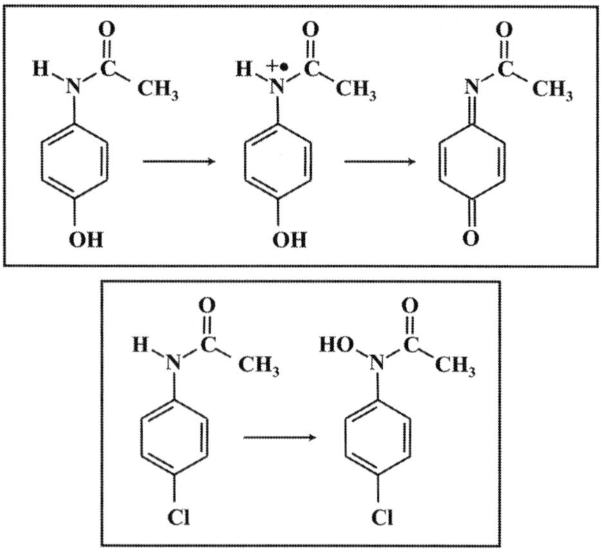

FIGURE 7-42.
P450-catalyzed oxidation of acetaminophen (chapter 19) generates reactive
N-acetyl-p-benzoquinone imine (NAPQI). Oxidation of p-chloroacetanilide,
in contrast, gives a stable N-hydroxylated product.

is a frequent cause of accidental poisoning in children and attempted suicide
in adults (see chapters 9 and 19). Acetaminophen metabolism by P450
produces a reactive iminoquinone (*132*) that is responsible for the hepatotoxic effects of the drug (*133*). The oxidation of acetaminophen illustrates
some of the mechanistic complications involved in nitrogen oxidation
reactions. The demonstration that the iminoquinone is the reactive species
(figure 7-42) was initially thought to be consistent with N-hydroxylation
of the amide function, followed by chemical elimination of a molecule
of water. Related compounds, such as p-chloroacetanilide, give isolable
amounts of the N-hydroxy derivatives. Synthesis of the proposed
N-hydroxy derivative of acetaminophen, however, clearly showed that
the water elimination step was too slow to account for the observed rate
of formation of the iminoquinone. It is now believed that the N-hydroxy
intermediate is never formed; one-electron removal from the substrate
by P450 gives a radical intermediate; deprotonation and transfer of a
second electron to the heme group occurs more rapidly than collapse to
give the N-hydroxy derivative. Although the detailed sequence of hydrogen
and electron transfer steps remains a matter of debate, the evidence
strongly suggests that the iminoquinone is formed without the formation
of an intermediate, other than a transient radical.

Reductions

It seems odd that P450, the oxidizing enzyme of unequalled potency,
should be able to carry out reductions. However, molecular oxygen is
reduced during the catalytic cycle, and if the supply of molecular oxygen
is limited, some substrates may act as alternative electron acceptors (*134*).
Another possible scenario is that a substrate may block oxygen binding

and be reduced even under aerobic conditions. As discussed above, the anesthetic gas halothane is metabolized primarily by oxidative routes, but a small percentage of an administered dose undergoes reductive metabolism (*135*) (figure 7-29).

P450 INHIBITORS

Several nonspecific chemical inhibitors of P450 activity are available, such as metyrapone and SKF 5252A. CO itself is an inhibitor, since it binds almost irreversibly to the ferrous form of P450. However, CO gas is not applicable in whole animal studies, for obvious reasons. Many researchers have sought enzyme-selective inhibitors of P450 activity (*136*). Such agents can be used experimentally to test the involvement of particular enzyme forms in bioactivation or detoxication processes. Among the available inhibitors with reasonably good specificity for human P450 enzymes are furafylline (1A2) (*137*), quinidine (2D6), diethyldithiocarbamic acid (2A6 and 2E1), and ketoconazole (3A4) (*138*). Since some forms of P450 (such as 1A1 and 1A2) bioactivate environmental carcinogens, enzyme-specific inhibitors might also have potential as chemopreventive agents (*139, 140*).

P450 inhibition can also have important pharmacological consequences: one drug or environmental chemical may inhibit the metabolism of another, leading to overdose toxicity. The antihistamine (allergy) medication terfenadine (marketed as Seldane™) was found to induce ventricular arrhythmia as a rare, and sometimes fatal, adverse reaction. This side effect was mainly associated with an interaction in which a second drug (particularly the antifungal agent ketoconazole) reduced terfenadine metabolism by inhibition of P450 3A4, resulting in dangerously elevated plasma levels of terfenadine (*141*). This drug interaction led to the withdrawal of terfenadine from the market.

P450 inhibition can be exploited to improve drug pharmacokinetics. Oral bioavailability of many drugs is limited by first-pass metabolism in the gastrointestinal tract, and P450 3A4 is usually a major contributor. Ritonavir, an HIV protease inhibitor, is also a very potent inhibitor of P450 3A4 (*142*). The use of ritonavir greatly prolongs the metabolic half-life of another HIV protease inhibitor, saquinavir; combination therapy with a cocktail including the two drugs actually *reduces* the number of pills that a patient needs to take daily, making therapy more effective. Another HIV protease inhibitor combination, Kaletra™, is a coformulation of ritonavir and lopinavir. The role of ritonavir in this combination is simply to improve the pharmacokinetics of lopinavir by inhibiting its P450 3A4-dependent metabolism.

The inhibition of P450 enzymes by components of grapefruit juice was discovered by accident. Volunteers in a study of felodipine, an antihypertensive agent, were routinely given orange juice to wash down their pills; one day, grapefruit juice was used as a substitute, and, suddenly, the metabolism of the drug was much slower than usual (*143*)! It is now recognized that components of grapefruit juice—not found in other citrus fruit juices—inhibit P450 3A4, with possible alterations to the pharmacokinetics of numerous drugs (*144*). One active constituent of grapefruit is *bergamottin* (figure 7-43), but the derivative referred to as the

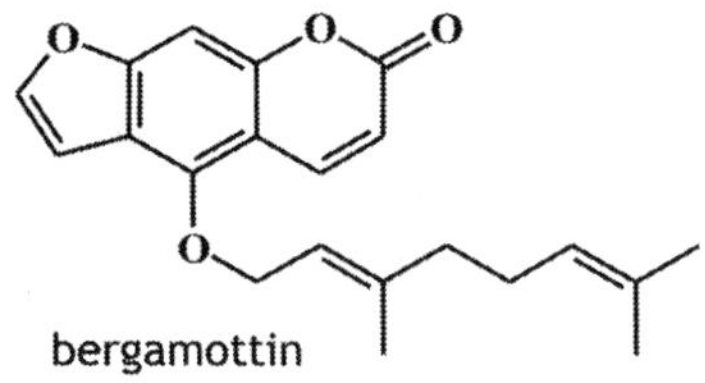

bergamottin

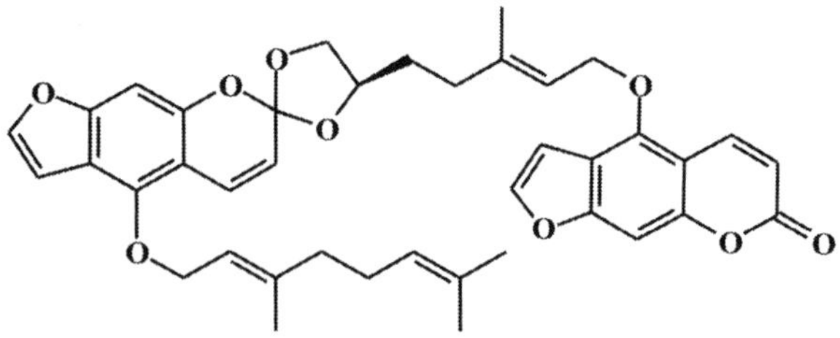

spiro ortho ester

FIGURE 7-43.

Structure of bergamottin and the spiro ortho ester P450 inhibitor.

"spiro ortho ester" is an even more potent P450 3A4 inhibitor, and might be applicable as an agent for improving the pharmacokinetics of poorly bioavailable drugs.

IDENTIFYING THE P450 ENZYME RESPONSIBLE FOR A SPECIFIC BIOTRANSFORMATION

As we have seen, many forms of P450 contribute to monooxygenase activity in human liver and additional forms are expressed extrahepatically. The catalytic activities of these forms often overlap. It is often desired to identify the specific P450 enzymes that catalyze a specific biotransformation. For example, when a new chemical entity is evaluated as a drug candidate, we want to know which P450 enzymes are responsible for its metabolism, so that we can be alerted to its potential interactions with other drugs. Several types of in vitro experiment can help to answer this question. It is now routine for pharmaceutical companies to assemble tissue banks of human liver samples (obtained from cadavers or from surgical removal of liver material, e.g., in hepatic cancer patients) for use in such studies. These liver samples are then characterized for various P450 enzymes by assaying the metabolism of specific substrates or by immunoassays (*145*).

We can test the ability of specific P450 forms (e.g., recombinant enzymes expressed in *E. coli*) to catalyze oxidation of the test substrate. This can rule out candidate enzymes, if they prove to be inactive. However, if several enzymes display activity (as is often the case), it may be hard to gauge their relative importance in vivo: this will depend on their levels of expression in various tissues, their kinetic parameters (V_{max} and K_M), and so on.

We can measure the rate of oxidation of the substrate by each of the individual liver samples in the tissue bank. These samples will previously have been characterized for the level of activity of each of the major human P450s, by assays with diagnostic substrates. Scatter-plots are constructed to measure the correlation between the activity with the substrate of interest and the activities with each of the diagnostic substrates. A high correlation indicates that the same P450 enzyme is responsible for metabolism of the test compound and the diagnostic substrate.

If inhibitory antibodies, specific for particular P450 enzymes, are available, we can test whether they inhibit metabolism of the test compound. This approach may be limited by the degree of specificity of the antibodies, which typically cross-react, at least with members of a given P450 family. (The corresponding approach can be taken with chemical inhibitors rather than antibodies.)

Recent studies of this kind have identified the principal human P450 enzymes that carry out the metabolism of the cyclooxygenase-2 inhibitor celecoxib (2C9 (*146*)), the vinca alkaloid vinorelbine (3A4 (*147*)), the antimalarial agent amodiaquine (2C8 (*148*)), and so on.

Finally, the use of transgenic animals should be noted. The mouse gene "knockout" technology is a powerful tool for determining the role of a given P450 enzyme in metabolism or toxicology of a specific agent, and results of such studies can provide guidance to analysis of orthologous human enzymes.

Some P450 Internet Resources

1. Directory of P450-containing systems: http://p450.abc.hu/

2. David Nelson's P450 pages at the Department of Molecular Sciences, University of Tennessee: http://drnelson.utmem.edu/Cytochrome P450.html

3. Home page of the human cytochrome P450 allele nomenclature committee: http://www.imm.ki.se/CYPalleles/

4. Todd D. Porter's "Biology of P450 reductase" page at the University of Kentucky: http://www.uky.edu/Pharmacy/ps/porter/CPR_biology.htm

5. PROMISE: The Prosthetic groups and Metal Ions in Protein Active Sites database: http://metallo.scripps.edu/PROMISE/

Notes

1. Additional sources: NIH: http://history.nih.gov/exhibits/bowman/BioBrodie.htm; International Society for the Study of Xenobiotics: http://www.issx.org/hissept.html.

2. The Soret band (named after its discoverer) is the very strong optical absorbance band (chromophore) above 400 nm displayed by heme proteins; it corresponds to a $\pi-\pi^*$ transition of the conjugated porphyrin ring.

3. P450 enzymes have characteristic reduced-CO peaks λ_{max} values, which range from about 447.5 to 452 nm.

4. This assay measures total P450 holoenzyme but does not assay catalytic activity; P450 enzyme assays are discussed later in this chapter.

5. Interindividual genetic variations and other genomic ambiguities make this number less than definitive.

6. The ability of certain bacteria to effect the biodegradation of hydrophobic natural products via P450-catalyzed oxidation suggests the idea of using these organisms or their enzymes for the bioremediation of persistent organic pollutants. However, this goal has been difficult to implement; one of the obstacles is the low catalytic efficiency of these oxidation reactions.

7. Genes encoding multiple members of a given subfamily are always found on the same chromosome, at least in humans.

8. Originally, a Roman numeral was used for the family number, e.g., IIIA4, but this convention has been replaced by the use of standard Arabic numbers (3A4).

9. *CYP1B1* is one of several loci; multiple genes are involved.

10. Many inherited disorders are associated with P450 enzymes responsible for steroid metabolism. For example, the lipid storage disease *cerebrotendinous xanthomatosis*, in which cholesterol deposits accumulate in the brain, is due to mutations in the CYP27A1 gene, which encodes the sterol 27-hydroxylase enzyme.

11. Originally referred to as rat P450j.

12. In rats, two members of the 3A family are expressed in the liver, designated 3A1 (previously P450p) and 3A2 (previously P450l).

13. Ideally, orthologues (enzymes of related sequence and activity in different species) would receive the same designation, but this may not be possible when a particular subfamily has multiple members in a given species.

14. NADH rather than NADPH is used by some bacterial enzymes.

15. The enzyme is sometimes abbreviated as "CPR," "RED," or "fp" (flavoprotein).

16. It remains unclear whether this is a general control mechanism for all P450 enzymes.

17. Peroxidase compound I was discovered by Britton Chance, in one of the earliest experimental demonstrations of the existence of the enzyme–substrate complex (*95*).

18. *Chloroperoxidase*, EC 1.11.1.10, a heme thiolate protein from the marine filamentous fungus *Caldariomyces fumago*, is an unusual enzyme that combines the properties of peroxidases and P450s. Chloroperoxidase catalyzes a chlorination reaction required for biosynthesis of the secondary metabolite caldariomycin (2,2-dichloro-1,3-cyclopentanediol). The enzyme behaves as a peroxidase, using hydrogen peroxide to drive one-electron oxidations of organic substrates, but it also catalyzes typical P450 reactions, such as alkene epoxidation (*97*).

19. However, this simple analysis may be misleading, since the reactivity of a "discrete" intermediate could be restrained by strong interactions with the enzyme. Much of the debate over alkyl hydroxylation mechanisms hinges on this question.

20. The "K-region" of a polycyclic aromatic hydrocarbon is a region of high π-electron density that is particularly "alkene-like" in its reactivity. See chapter 18 for further discussion.

21. N-Oxide and sulfoxide metabolites are not only formed by the P450 system: these reactions are also catalyzed by the *flavin monooxygenase* enzyme (*131*).

References

1. Hamilton, G. A. Mechanisms of biological oxidation reactions involving oxygen and reduced oxygen derivatives. In *Biological Oxidation Systems*; Reddy, C. C., Hamilton, G. A., Madyastha, K. M., Eds.; Academic Press: San Diego, 1990; pp. 3–15.

2. Mason, H. S.; Fowlks, W. L.; Peterson, E. Oxygen transfer and electron transport by the phenolase complex. *J. Am. Chem. Soc.* **1955,** *77*, 2914–2915.

3. Hayaishi, O.; Katagiri, M.; Rothberg, S. Mechanism of the pyrocatechase reaction. *J. Am. Chem. Soc.* **1955,** *77*, 5450–5451.

4. Brodie, B. B.; Axelrod, J.; Cooper, J. R.; Gaudette, L.; La Du, B. N.; Mitoma, C.; Udenfriend, S. Detoxification of drugs and other foreign compounds by liver microsomes. *Science* **1955,** *121*, 603–604.

5. Parke, D. V. Richard Tecwyn Williams. **1977,** *Xenobiotica 7*, 1.

6. (a) Neuberger, A.; Smith, R. L. Richard Tecwyn Williams: the man, his work, his impact. **1983,** *Drug Metab. Rev. 14*, 559–607. (b) Josephy, P. D.; Guengerich, F. P.; Miners, J. O. "Phase I" and "phase II" drug metabolism: terminology that we should phase out? *Drug Metab. Rev.* **2006,** in press.

7. Costa, E.; Karczmar, A. G.; Vesell, E. S. Bernard B. Brodie and the rise of chemical pharmacology. *Annu. Rev. Pharmacol. Toxicol.* **1989,** *29*, 1–21.

8. Estabrook, R. W. A passion for P450s (remembrances of the early history of research on cytochrome P450). *Drug Metab. Dispos.* **2003,** *31*, 1461–1473.

9. Klingenberg, M. The dragging emergence of the P450 cytochrome. *Arch. Biochem. Biophys.* **2003,** *412*, 2.

10. Klingenberg, M. Pigments of rat liver microsomes. *Arch. Biochem. Biophys.* **1958,** *75*, 376–386.

11. Omura, T.; Sato, R. The carbon monoxide-binding pigment of liver microsomes. *J. Biol. Chem.* **1964,** *239*, 2370, 2379–2378, 2385.

12. Ikeya, K.; Jaiswal, A. K.; Owens, R. A.; Jones, J. E.; Nebert, D. W.; Kimura, S. Human CYP1A2: sequence, gene structure, comparison with the mouse and rat orthologous gene, and differences in liver 1A2 mRNA expression. *Mol. Endocrinol.* **1989,** *3*, 1399–1408.

13. Pikuleva, I.; Waterman, M. Cytochromes P450 in synthesis of steroid hormones, bile acids, vitamin D_3 and cholesterol. *Mol. Aspects Med.* **1999,** *20*, 33–37.

14. Berg, J. M.; Tymoczko, J. L.; Stryer, L. *Biochemistry*; WH Freeman: New York, 2001.

15. Holton, T. A.; Brugliera, F.; Lester, D. R.; Tanaka, Y.; Hyland, C. D.; Menting, J. G.; Lu, C. Y.; Farcy, E.; Stevenson, T. W.; Cornish, E. C. Cloning and expression of cytochrome P450 genes controlling flower colour. *Nature* **1993,** *366*, 276–279.

16. Arabidopsis Initiative. Analysis of the genome sequence of the flowering plant *Arabidopsis thaliana*. *Nature* **2000,** *408*, 796–815.

17. Gonzalez, F. J.; Nebert, D. W. Evolution of the P450 gene superfamily: animal–plant "warfare", molecular drive and human genetic differences in drug oxidation. *Trends Genet.* **1990,** *6*, 182–186.

18. Hukkanen, J.; Pelkonen, O.; Hakkola, J.; Raunio, H. Expression and regulation of xenobiotic-metabolizing cytochrome P450 (CYP) enzymes in human lung. *Crit. Rev. Toxicol.* **2002,** *32*, 391–411.

19. Ling, G.; Gu, J.; Genter, M. B.; Zhuo, X.; Ding, X. Regulation of cytochrome P450 gene expression in the olfactory mucosa. *Chem. Biol. Interact.* **2004,** *147*, 247–258.

20. Du, L.; Hoffman, S. M.; Keeney, D. S. Epidermal CYP2 family cytochromes P450. *Toxicol. Appl. Pharmacol.* **2004,** *195*, 278–287.

21. Guengerich, F. P. Analysis and characterization of enzymes and nucleic acids. In *Principles and Methods of Toxicology*; Hayes, A. W., Ed.; Taylor & Francis: Philadelphia, 2001; pp. 1625–1687.

22. Nash, T. The colorimetric estimation of formaldehyde by means of the Hantzsch reaction. *Biochem. J.* **1953**, *55*, 416–421.

23. Kobayashi, K.; Yamamoto, T.; Taguchi, M.; Chiba, K. High-performance liquid chromatography determination of N- and O-demethylase activities of chemicals in human liver microsomes: application of postcolumn fluorescence derivatization using Nash reagent. *Anal. Biochem.* **2000**, *284*, 342–347.

24. Kaminsky, L. S.; de Morais, S. M.; Faletto, M. B.; Dunbar, D. A.; Goldstein, J. A. Correlation of human cytochrome P4502C substrate specificities with primary structure: warfarin as a probe. *Mol. Pharmacol.* **1993**, *43*, 234–239.

25. Kuwada, M.; Maki, J.; Hasumi, H.; Furudate, S.; Takahasi, K. A simplified procedure for purification of cytochrome P-450 by preparative ampholine gel for isoelectric focusing. *Prep. Biochem. Biotechnol.* **2000**, *30*, 125–132.

26. Guengerich, F. P.; Hosea, N. A.; Parikh, A.; Bell-Parikh, L. C.; Johnson, W. W.; Gillam, E. M.; Shimada, T. Twenty years of biochemistry of human P450s: purification, expression, mechanism, and relevance to drugs. *Drug Metab. Dispos.* **1998**, *26*, 1175–1178.

27. Omura, T.; Sanders, E.; Estabrook, R. W.; Cooper, D. Y.; Rosenthal, O. Isolation from adrenal cortex of a nonheme iron protein and a flavoprotein functional as a reduced triphosphopyridine nucleotide-cytochrome P-450 reductase. *Arch. Biochem. Biophys.* **1966**, *117*, 660–673.

28. Lu, A. Y. H.; Coon, M. J. Role of hemoprotein P450 in fatty acid ω-hydroxylation in a soluble enzyme from liver microsomes. *J. Biol. Chem.* **1968**, *243*, 1331–1332.

29. Porter, T. D. Jud Coon: 35 years of P450 research, a synopsis of P450 history. *Drug Metab. Dispos.* **2004**, *32*, 1–6.

30. Coon, M. J. Cytochrome P450: nature's most versatile biological catalyst. *Annu. Rev. Pharmacol. Toxicol.* **2005**, *45*, 1–25.

31. Snawder, J. E.; Lipscomb, J. C. Interindividual variance of cytochrome P450 forms in human hepatic microsomes: correlation of individual forms with xenobiotic metabolism and implications in risk assessment. *Regul. Toxicol. Pharmacol.* **2000**, *32*, 200–209.

32. Kim, D.; Guengerich, F. P. Cytochrome P450 activation of arylamines and heterocyclic amines. *Annu. Rev. Pharmacol. Toxicol.* **2005**, *45*, 27–49.

33. Murray, G. I.; Melvin, W. T.; Greenlee, W. F.; Burke, M. D. Regulation, function, and tissue-specific expression of cytochrome P450 CYP1B1. *Annu. Rev. Pharmacol. Toxicol.* **2001**, *41*, 297–316.

34. Savas, U.; Bhattacharyya, K. K.; Christou, M.; Alexander, D. L.; Jefcoate, C. R. Mouse cytochrome P-450EF, representative of a new 1B subfamily of cytochrome P-450s. Cloning, sequence determination, and tissue expression. *J. Biol. Chem.* **1994**, *269*, 14905–14911.

35. Belmouden, A.; Melki, R.; Hamdani, M.; Zaghloul, K.; Amraoui, A.; Nadifi, S.; Akhayat, O.; Garchon, J. A novel frameshift founder mutation in the cytochrome P450 1B1 (CYP1B1) gene is associated with primary congenital glaucoma in Morocco. *Clin. Genet.* **2002**, *62*, 334–339.

36. Sarfarazi, M.; Stoilov, I. Molecular genetics of primary congenital glaucoma. *Eye* **2000**, *14* (3B), 422–428.

37. Libby, R. T.; Smith, R. S.; Savinova, O. V.; Zabaleta, A.; Martin, J. E.; Gonzalez, F. J.; John, S. W. Modification of ocular defects in mouse developmental glaucoma models by tyrosinase. *Science* **2003**, *299*, 1578–1581.

38. Hoffman, S. M.; Nelson, D. R.; Keeney, D. S. Organization, structure and evolution of the CYP2 gene cluster on human chromosome 19. *Pharmacogenetics* **2001,** *11,* 687–698.

39. Oscarson, M. Genetic polymorphisms in the cytochrome P450 2A6 (CYP2A6) gene: implications for interindividual differences in nicotine metabolism. *Drug Metab. Dispos.* **2001,** *29,* 91–95.

40. Yano, J. K.; Hsu, M.-H.; Griffin, K. J.; Stout, C. D.; Johnson, E. F. Structures of human microsomal cytochrome P450 2A6 complexed with coumarin and methoxsalen. *Nature Struct. Molec. Biol.* **2005,** *12,* 822–823.

41. Tyndale, R. F.; Sellers, E. M. Genetic variation in CYP2A6-mediated nicotine metabolism alters smoking behavior. *Ther. Drug Monit.* **2002,** *24,* 163–171.

42. Batra, V.; Patkar, A. A.; Berrettini, W. H.; Weinstein, S. P.; Leone, F. T. The genetic determinants of smoking. *Chest* **2003,** *123,* 1730–1739.

43. Stresser, D. M.; Kupfer, D. Monospecific antipeptide antibody to cytochrome P-450 2B6. *Drug Metab. Dispos.* **1999,** *27,* 517–525.

44. Ekins, S.; Wrighton, S. A. The role of CYP2B6 in human xenobiotic metabolism. *Drug Metab. Rev.* **1999,** *31,* 719–754.

45. Warner, S. C.; Finta, C.; Zaphiropoulos, P. G. Intergenic transcripts containing a novel human cytochrome P450 2C exon 1 spliced to sequences from the CYP2C9 gene. *Mol. Biol. Evol.* **2001,** *18,* 1841–1848.

46. Desta, Z.; Zhao, X.; Shin, J. G.; Flockhart, D. A. Clinical significance of the cytochrome P450 2C19 genetic polymorphism. *Clin. Pharmacokinet.* **2002,** *41,* 913–958.

47. Zanger, U. M.; Raimundo, S.; Eichelbaum, M. Cytochrome P450 2D6: overview and update on pharmacology, genetics, biochemistry. *Naunyn Schmiedebergs Arch. Pharmacol.* **2004,** *369,* 23–37.

48. Guengerich, F. P.; Hanna, I. H.; Martin, M. V.; Gillam, E. M. Role of glutamic acid 216 in cytochrome P450 2D6 substrate binding and catalysis. *Biochemistry* **2003,** *42,* 1245–1253.

49. Goldstein, D. B.; Tate, S. K.; Sisodiya, S. M. Pharmacogenetics goes genomic. *Nat. Rev. Genet.* **2003,** *4,* 937–947.

50. Lieber, C. S.; DeCarli, L. M. Role of hepatic microsomal ethanol metabolism. *Chem. Biol. Interact.* **1971,** *3,* 292–293.

51. Tanaka, E.; Terada, M.; Misawa, S. Cytochrome P450 2E1: its clinical and toxicological role. *J. Clin Pharm. Ther.* **2000,** *25,* 165–175.

52. Bell-Parikh, L. C.; Guengerich, F. P. Kinetics of cytochrome P450 2E1-catalyzed oxidation of ethanol to acetic acid via acetaldehyde. *J. Biol. Chem.* **1999,** *274,* 23833–23840.

53. Constan, A. A.; Sprankle, C. S.; Peters, J. M.; Kedderis, G. L.; Everitt, J. I.; Wong, B. A.; Gonzalez, F. L.; Butterworth, B. E. Metabolism of chloroform by cytochrome P450 2E1 is required for induction of toxicity in the liver, kidney, and nose of male mice. *Toxicol. Appl. Pharmacol.* **1999,** *160,* 120–126.

54. Mesic, M.; Peuralahti, J.; Blans, P.; Fishbein, J. C. Mechanisms of decomposition of α-hydroxydialkylnitrosamines in aqueous solution. *Chem. Res. Toxicol.* **2000,** *13,* 983–992.

55. Hecht, S. S. Tobacco carcinogens, their biomarkers and tobacco-induced cancer. *Nat. Rev. Cancer* **2003,** *3,* 733–744.

56. Guengerich, F. P. Cytochrome P-450 3A4: regulation and role in drug metabolism. *Annu. Rev. Pharmacol. Toxicol.* **1999,** *39,* 1–17.

57. Kelly, P. A.; Wang, H.; Napoli, K. L.; Kahan, B. D.; Strobel, H. W. Metabolism of cyclosporine by cytochromes P450 3A9 and 3A4. *Eur. J. Drug Metab. Pharmacokinet.* **1999**, *24*, 321–328.

58. Shou, M.; Dai, R.; Cui, D.; Korzekwa, K. R.; Baillie, T. A.; Rushmore, T. H. A kinetic model for the metabolic interaction of two substrates at the active site of cytochrome P450 3A4. *J. Biol. Chem.* **2001**, *276*, 2256–2262.

59. LeBrun, L. A.; Hoch, U.; Ortiz de Montellano, P. R. Autocatalytic mechanism and consequences of covalent heme attachment in the cytochrome P4504A family. *J. Biol. Chem.* **2002**, *277*, 12755–12761.

60. Colas, C.; Ortiz de Montellano, P. R. Autocatalytic radical reactions in physiological prosthetic heme modification. *Chem. Rev.* **2003**, *103*, 2305–2332.

61. Poulos, T. L.; Finzel, B. C.; Howard, A. J. High-resolution crystal structure of cytochrome P450$_{cam}$. *J. Mol. Biol.* **1987**, *195*, 687–700.

62. Boddupalli, S. S.; Hasemann, C. A.; Ravichandran, K. G.; Lu, J. Y.; Goldsmith, E. J.; Deisenhofer, J.; Peterson, J. A. Crystallization and preliminary x-ray diffraction analysis of P450$_{terp}$ and the hemoprotein domain of P450BM-3, enzymes belonging to two distinct classes of the cytochrome P450 superfamily. *Proc. Natl. Acad. Sci. USA* **1992**, *89*, 5567–5571.

63. Ravichandran, K. G.; Boddupalli, S. S.; Hasermann, C. A.; Peterson, J. A.; Deisenhofer, J. Crystal structure of hemoprotein domain of P450BM-3, a prototype for microsomal P450's. *Science* **1993**, *261*, 731–736.

64. Williams, P. A.; Cosme, J.; Sridhar, V.; Johnson, E. F.; McRee, D. E. Microsomal cytochrome P450 2C5: comparison to microbial P450s and unique features. *J. Inorg. Biochem.* **2000**, *81*, 183–190.

65. Schlichting, I.; Berendzen, J.; Chu, K.; Stock, A. M.; Maves, S. A.; Benson, D. E.; Sweet, R. M.; Ringe, D.; Petsko, G. A.; Sligar, S. G. The catalytic pathway of cytochrome P450$_{cam}$ at atomic resolution. *Science* **2000**, *287*, 1615–1622.

66. Williams, P. A.; Cosme, J.; Ward, A.; Angove, H. C.; Matak, V. D.; Jhoti, H. Crystal structure of human cytochrome P450 2C9 with bound warfarin. *Nature* **2003**, *424*, 464–468.

67. Wester, M. R.; Yano, J. K.; Schoch, G. A.; Yang, C.; Griffin, K. J.; Stout, C. D.; Johnson, E. F. The structure of human cytochrome P450 2C9 complexed with flurbiprofen at 2.0-Å resolution. *J. Biol. Chem.* **2004**, *279*, 35630–35637.

68. Williams, P. A.; Cosme, J.; Vinkovic, D. M.; Ward, A.; Angove, H. C.; Day, P. J.; Vonrhein, C.; Tickle, I. J.; Jhoti, H. Crystal structures of human cytochrome P450 3A4 bound to metyrapone and progesterone. *Science* **2004**, *305*, 683–686.

69. Yano, J. K.; Wester, M. R.; Schoch, G. A.; Griffin, K. J.; Stout, C. D.; Johnson, E. F. The structure of human microsomal cytochrome P450 3A4 determined by X-ray crystallography to 2.05-Å resolution. *J. Biol. Chem.* **2004**, *279*, 38091–38094.

70. Scott, E. E.; Halpert, J. R. Structures of cytochrome P450 3A4. *Trends Biochem. Sci.* **2005**, *30*, 5–7.

71. Hasemann, C. A.; Kurumbail, R. G.; Boddupalli, S. S.; Peterson, J. A.; Deisenhofer, J. Structure and function of cytochromes P450: a comparative analysis of three crystal structures. *Structure* **1995**, *3*, 41–62.

72. Yoshioka, S.; Takahashi, S.; Hori, H.; Ishimori, K.; Morishima, I. Proximal cysteine residue is essential for the enzymatic activities of cytochrome P450$_{cam}$. *Eur. J. Biochem.* **2001**, *268*, 252–259.

73. Yoshioka, S.; Takahashi, S.; Ishimori, K.; Morishima, I. Roles of the axial push effect in cytochrome P450$_{cam}$ studied with the site-directed mutagenesis at the heme proximal site. *J. Inorg. Biochem.* **2000,** *81,* 141–151.

74. Koch, B. M.; Sibbesen, O.; Halkier, B. A.; Svendsen, I.; Moller, B. L. The primary sequence of cytochrome P450$_{tyr}$, the multifunctional N-hydroxylase catalyzing the conversion of L-tyrosine to *p*-hydroxyphenylacetaldehyde oxime in the biosynthesis of the cyanogenic glucoside dhurrin in *Sorghum bicolor* (L.) Moench. *Arch. Biochem. Biophys.* **1995,** *323,* 177–186.

75. Atkins, W. M.; Sligar, S. G. Molecular recognition in cytochrome P450: alteration of regioselective alkane hydroxylation via protein engineering. *J. Am. Chem. Soc.* **1989,** *111,* 2715–2717.

76. Furuya, H.; Shimizu, T.; Hirano, K.; Hatano, M.; Fujii-Kuriyama, Y.; Raag, R.; Poulos, T. L. Site-directed mutageneses of rat liver cytochrome P-450d: catalytic activities toward benzphetamine and 7-ethoxycoumarin. *Biochemistry* **1989,** *28,* 6848–6857.

77. Gotoh, O. Substrate recognition sites in cytochrome P450 family 2 (CYP2) proteins inferred from comparative analyses of amino acid and coding nucleotide sequences. *J. Biol. Chem.* **1992,** *267,* 83–90.

78. Black, S. D. Membrane topology of the mammalian P450 cytochromes. *FASEB J.* **1992,** *6,* 680–685.

79. Urban, P.; Truan, G.; Gautier, J. C.; Pompon, D. Xenobiotic metabolism in humanized yeast: engineered yeast cells producing human NADPH-cytochrome P-450 reductase, cytochrome b$_5$, epoxide hydrolase and P-450s. *Biochem. Soc. Trans.* **1993,** *21,* 1028–1034.

80. Dawson, J. H.; Sono, M. Cytochrome P450 and chloroperoxidase: thiolate-ligated heme enzymes. Spectroscopic determination of their active site structures and mechanistic implications of thiolate ligation. *Chem. Rev.* **1987,** *87,* 1255–1276.

81. McMillan, K.; Masters, B. S. Prokaryotic expression of the heme- and flavin-binding domains of rat neuronal nitric oxide synthase as distinct polypeptides: identification of the heme-binding proximal thiolate ligand as cysteine-415. *Biochemistry* **1995,** *34,* 3686–3693.

82. Mueller, E. J.; Loida, P. J.; Sligar, S. G. Twenty-five years of P450$_{cam}$ research: mechanistic insights into oxygenase catalysis. In *Cytochrome P450: Structure, Mechanism and Biochemistry*; Ortiz de Montellano, P. R., Ed.; Plenum Press: New York, 1995; pp. 83–124.

83. Krishnamurthy, R. and Schaap, W. B. Computing ligand field potentials and relative energies of d orbitals. *J. Chem. Ed.* **1969,** *46,* 799–810.

84. Pylypenko, O.; Schlichting, I. Structural aspects of ligand binding to and electron transfer in bacterial and fungal P450s. *Annu. Rev. Biochem.* **2004,** *73,* 991–1018.

85. Luykx, D. M.; Prenafeta-Boldu, F. X.; de Bont, J. A. Toluene monooxygenase from the fungus *Cladosporium sphaerospermum. Biochem. Biophys. Res. Commun.* **2003,** *312,* 373–379.

86. Imai, Y.; Okamoto, N.; Nakahara, K.; Shoun, H. Absorption spectral studies on heme ligand interactions of P-450$_{nor}$. *Biochim. Biophys. Acta* **1997,** *1337,* 66–74.

87. Horecker, B. L. Triphosphopyridine nucleotide cytochrome c reductase in liver. *J. Biol. Chem.* **1950,** *183,* 593–605.

88. Wang, M.; Roberts, D. L.; Paschke, R.; Shea, T. M.; Masters, B. S.; Kim, J. J. Three-dimensional structure of NADPH-cytochrome P450

reductase: prototype for FMN- and FAD-containing enzymes. *Proc. Natl. Acad. Sci. USA* **1997,** *94,* 8411–8416.

89. Bonfils, C.; Balny, C.; Maurel, P. Direct evidence for electron transfer from ferrous cytochrome b_5 to the oxyferrous intermediate of liver microsomal cytochrome P-450 LM2. *J. Biol. Chem.* **1981,** *256,* 9457–9465.

90. Guryev, O. L.; Gilep, A. A.; Usanov, S. A.; Estabrook, R. W. Interaction of apo-cytochrome b_5 with cytochromes P4503A4 and P45017A: relevance of heme transfer reactions. *Biochemistry* **2001,** *40,* 5018–5031.

91. Yamazaki, H.; Shimada, T.; Martin, M. V.; Guengerich, F. P. Stimulation of cytochrome P450 reactions by apo-cytochrome b_5: evidence against transfer of heme from cytochrome P450 3A4 to apo-cytochrome b_5 or heme oxygenase. *J. Biol. Chem.* **2001,** *276,* 30885–30891.

92. Porter, T. D. The roles of cytochrome b_5 in cytochrome P450 reactions. *J. Biochem. Mol. Toxicol.* **2002,** *16,* 311–316.

93. Lambeth, J. D.; Seybert, D. W.; Lancaster, J. R.; Jr.; Salerno, J. C.; Kamin, H. Steroidogenic electron transport in adrenal cortex mito-chondria. *Mol. Cell Biochem.* **1982,** *45,* 13–31.

94. Bec, N.; Anzenbacher, P.; Anzenbacherova, E.; Gorren, A. C.; Munro, A. W.; Lange, R. Spectral properties of the oxyferrous complex of the heme domain of cytochrome P450 BM-3 (CYP102). *Biochem. Biophys. Res. Commun.* **1999,** *266,* 187–189.

95. Chance, B. Kinetics of the enzyme-substrate compound of peroxidase. *J. Biol. Chem.* **1943,** *151,* 553–577.

96. Rahimtula, A. D.; O'Brien, P. J.; Hrycay, E. G.; Peterson, J. A.; Estabrook, R. W. Possible higher valence states of cytochrome P-450 during oxidative reactions. *Biochem. Biophys. Res. Commun.* **1974,** *60,* 695–702.

97. Yi, X.; Mroczko, M.; Manoj, K. M.; Wang, X.; Hager, L. P. Replacement of the proximal heme thiolate ligand in chloroperoxidase with a histidine residue. *Proc. Natl. Acad. Sci. USA* **1999,** *96,* 12412–12417.

98. Bonagura, C. A.; Bhaskar, B.; Shimizu, H.; Li, H.; Sundaramoorthy, M.; McRee, D. E.; Goodin, D. B.; Poulos, T. L. High-resolution crystal structures and spectroscopy of native and compound I cytochrome c peroxidase. *Biochemistry* **2003,** *42,* 5600–5608.

99. Gelb, M. H.; Heimbrook, D. C.; Malkonen, P.; Sligar, S. G. Stereochemistry and deuterium isotope effects in camphor hydroxylation by the cytochrome $P450_{cam}$ monooxygenase system. *Biochemistry* **1982,** *21,* 370–377.

100. Hamilton, G. A. Oxidation by molecular oxygen. 11. The oxygen atom transfer mechanism for mixed-function oxidases and the model for mixed-function oxidases. *J. Am. Chem. Soc.* **1964,** *86,* 3391–3392.

101. Boche, G.; Lohrenz, J. C. The electrophilic nature of carbenoids, nitrenoids, and oxenoids. *Chem. Rev.* **2001,** *101,* 697–756.

102. Dolphin, D. Cytochrome P450: substrate and prosthetic-group free radicals generated during the enzymatic cycle. *Philos. Trans. R. Soc. Lond. B Biol. Sci.* **1985,** *311,* 579–591.

103. Weiss, R.; Bulach, V.; Gold, A.; Terner, J.; Trautwein, A. X. Valence-tautomerism in high-valent iron and manganese porphyrins. *J. Biol. Inorg. Chem.* **2001,** *6,* 831–845.

104. Ullrich, V. Thoughts on thiolate tethering. Tribute and thanks to a teacher. *Arch. Biochem. Biophys.* **2003,** *409,* 45–51.

105. Schoneboom, J. C.; Lin, H.; Reuter, N.; Thiel, W.; Cohen, S.; Ogliaro, F.; Shaik, S. The elusive oxidant species of cytochrome P450 enzymes: characterization by combined quantum mechanical/molecular mechanical (QM/MM) calculations. *J. Am. Chem. Soc.* **2002**, *124*, 8142–8151.

106. Ortiz de Montellano, P. R.; De Voss, J. J. Oxidizing species in the mechanism of cytochrome P450. *Nat. Prod. Rep.* **2002**, *19*, 477–493.

107. Hartmann, M.; Ernst, S. Selective oxidations of linear alkanes with molecular oxygen on molecular sieve catalysts: a breakthrough? *Angew. Chem. Int. Ed Engl.* **2000**, *39*, 888–890.

108. Hendrickson, J. B.; Cram, D. J.; Hammond, G. S. *Organic Chemistry*; McGraw-Hill: New York, 1970.

109. Sibbesen, O.; De Voss, J. J.; Montellano, P. R. Putidaredoxin reductase-putidaredoxin-cytochrome p450cam triple fusion protein. Construction of a self-sufficient *Escherichia coli* catalytic system. *J. Biol. Chem.* **1996**, *271*, 22462–22469.

110. Zimmer, T.; Ohkuma, M.; Ohta, A.; Takagi, M.; Schunck, W. H. The CYP52 multigene family of *Candida maltosa* encodes functionally diverse *n*-alkane-inducible cytochromes P450. *Biochem. Biophys. Res. Commun.* **1996**, *224*, 784–789.

111. Stevenson, J.-A.; Westlake, A. C. G.; Whittock, C.; Wong, L. L. The catalytic oxidation of linear and branched alkanes by cytochrome P450$_{cam}$. *J. Am. Chem. Soc.* **1996**, *118*, 12846–12847.

112. Frommer, U.; Ullrich, V.; Staudinger, H. Hydroxylation of aliphatic compounds by liver microsomes: I. The distribution pattern of isomeric alcohols. *Hoppe Seyler's Z. Physiol. Chem.* **1970**, *351*, 903–912.

113. White, R. E.; McCarthy, M. B.; Egeberg, K. D.; Sligar, S. G. Regioselectivity in the cytochromes P-450: control by protein constraints and by chemical reactivities. *Arch. Biochem. Biophys.* **1984**, *228*, 493–502.

114. Bambal, R. B.; Hanzlik, R. P. Active site structure and substrate specificity of cytochrome P450 4A1: steric control of ligand approach perpendicular to heme plane. *Biochem. Biophys. Res. Commun.* **1996**, *219*, 445–449.

115. Hoch, U.; Zhang, Z.; Kroetz, D. L.; Ortiz de Montellano, P. R. Structural determination of the substrate specificities and regioselectivities of the rat and human fatty acid omega-hydroxylases. *Arch. Biochem. Biophys.* **2000**, *373*, 63–71.

116. Chang, Y. T.; Loew, G. H. Homology modeling and substrate binding study of human CYP4A11 enzyme. *Proteins* **1999**, *34*, 403–415.

117. Kohen, A.; Limbach, H.-H., Eds. *Isotope Effects in Chemistry and Biology*; CRC Press: Boca Raton, FL, 2005.

118. Hjelmeland, L. M.; Aronow, L.; Trudell, J. R. Intramolecular determination of primary kinetic isotope effects in hydroxylations catalyzed by cytochrome P-450. *Biochem. Biophys. Res. Commun.* **1976**, *76*, 541–549.

119. Groves, J. T.; McClusky, G. A.; White, R. E.; Coon, M. J. Aliphatic hydroxylation by highly purified liver microsomal cytochrome P-450: evidence for a carbon radical intermediate. *Biochem. Biophys. Res. Commun.* **1978**, *81*, 160.

120. Auclair, K.; Hu, Z.; Little, D. M.; Ortiz de Montellano, P. R.; Groves, J. T. Revisiting the mechanism of P450 enzymes with the radical clocks norcarane and spiro[2,5]octane. *J. Am. Chem. Soc.* **2002**, *124*, 6020–6027.

121. Shaik, S.; De Visser, S. P.; Ogliaro, F.; Schwarz, H.; Schroder, D. Two-state reactivity mechanisms of hydroxylation and epoxidation by

cytochrome P-450 revealed by theory. *Curr. Opin. Chem. Biol.* **2002**, *6*, 556–567.

122. Kumar, D.; De Visser, S. P.; Sharma, P. K.; Cohen, S.; Shaik, S. Radical clock substrates, their C–H hydroxylation mechanism by cytochrome P450, and other reactivity patterns: what does theory reveal about the clocks' behavior? *J. Am. Chem. Soc.* **2004**, *126*, 1907–1920.

123. Njoku, D.; Laster, M. J.; Gong, D. H.; Eger, E. I.; Reed, G. F.; Martin, J. L. Biotransformation of halothane, enflurane, isoflurane, and desflurane to trifluoroacetylated liver proteins: association between protein acylation and hepatic injury. *Anesth. Analg.* **1997**, *84*, 173–178.

124. Miller, R. E.; Guengerich, F. P. Oxidation of trichloroethylene by liver microsomal cytochrome P-450: evidence for chlorine migration in a transition state not involving trichloroethylene oxide. *Biochemistry* **1982**, *21*, 1090–1097.

125. Ortiz de Montellano, P. R.; Reich, N. O. Inhibition of cytochrome P450 enzymes. In *Cytochrome P450: Structure, Mechanism and Biochemistry*; Ortiz de Montellano, P. R., Ed.; Plenum Press: New York, 1986; pp. 273–314.

126. Guroff, G.; Daly, J. W.; Jerina, D. M.; Renson, J.; Witkop, B.; Udenfriend, S. Hydroxylation-induced migration: the NIH shift. Recent experiments reveal an unexpected and general result of enzymatic hydroxylation of aromatic compounds. *Science* **1967**, *157*, 1524–1530.

127. Daly, J. W.; Jerina, D. M.; Witkop, B. Arene oxides and the NIH shift: the metabolism, toxicity and carcinogenicity of aromatic compounds. *Experientia* **1972**, *28*, 1129–1149.

128. Jerina, D. M.; Daly, J. W.; Witkop, B.; Zaltzman-Nirenberg, P.; Udenfriend, S. 1,2-Naphthalene oxide as an intermediate in the microsomal hydroxylation of naphthalene. *Biochemistry* **1970**, *9*, 147–156.

129. Boyd, D. R.; Jerina, D. M. Arene oxides-oxepins. In *Small Ring Heterocycles, Part 3: Oxiranes, Arene Oxides, Oxaziridines, Dioxetanes, Thietanes, Thietes, Thiazetes*; John Wiley: New York, 1985; pp. 197–282.

130. Jerina, D. M.; Daly, J. W. Arene oxides: a new aspect of drug metabolism. *Science* **1974**, *185*, 573–582.

131. Cashman, J. R. Human flavin-containing monooxygenase: substrate specificity and role in drug metabolism. *Curr. Drug Metab.* **2000**, *1*, 181–191.

132. Dahlin, D. C.; Miwa, G. T.; Lu, A. Y.; Nelson, S. D. N-Acetyl-*p*-benzoquinone imine: a cytochrome P-450-mediated oxidation product of acetaminophen. *Proc. Natl. Acad. Sci. USA* **1984**, *81*, 1327–1331.

133. Bessems, J. G.; Vermeulen, N. P. Paracetamol (acetaminophen)-induced toxicity: molecular and biochemical mechanisms, analogues and protective approaches. *Crit. Rev. Toxicol.* **2001**, *31*, 55–138.

134. Goeptar, A. R.; Scheerens, H.; Vermeulen, N. P. Oxygen and xenobiotic reductase activities of cytochrome P450. *Crit. Rev. Toxicol.* **1995**, *25*, 25–65.

135. Spracklin, D. K.; Kharasch, E. D. Human halothane reduction in vitro by cytochrome P450 2A6 and 3A4: identification of low and high KM isoforms. *Drug Metab. Dispos.* **1998**, *26*, 605–607.

136. Newton, D. J.; Wang, R. W.; Lu, A. Y. Cytochrome P450 inhibitors. Evaluation of specificities in the in vitro metabolism of therapeutic agents by human liver microsomes. *Drug Metab. Dispos.* **1995**, *23*, 154–158.

137. Clarke, S. E.; Ayrton, A. D.; Chenery, R. J. Characterization of the inhibition of P4501A2 by furafylline. *Xenobiotica* **1994**, *24*, 517–526.
138. Wojcikowski, J.; Pichard-Garcia, L.; Maurel, P.; Daniel, W. A. Contribution of human cytochrome p-450 isoforms to the metabolism of the simplest phenothiazine neuroleptic promazine. *Br. J. Pharmacol.* **2003**, *138*, 1465–1474.
139. Halpert, J. R.; Guengerich, F. P.; Bend, J. R.; Correia, M. A. Selective inhibitors of cytochromes P450. *Toxicol. Appl. Pharmacol.* **1994**, *125*, 163–175.
140. Hecht, S. S. Inhibition of carcinogenesis by isothiocyanates. *Drug Metab. Rev.* **2000**, *32*, 395–411.
141. von Moltke, L. L.; Greenblatt, D. J.; Duan, S. X.; Harmatz, J. S.; Shader, R. I. In vitro prediction of the terfenadine-ketoconazole pharmacokinetic interaction. *J. Clin. Pharmacol.* **1994**, *34*, 1222–1227.
142. Cooper, C. L.; van Heeswijk, R. P.; Gallicano, K.; Cameron, D. W. A review of low-dose ritonavir in protease inhibitor combination therapy. *Clin. Infect. Dis.* **2003**, *36*, 1585–1592.
143. Bailey, D. G.; Spence, J. D.; Munoz, C.; Arnold, J. M. Interaction of citrus juices with felodipine and nifedipine. *Lancet* **1991**, *337*, 268–269.
144. Kane, G. C.; Lipsky, J. J. Drug-grapefruit juice interactions. *Mayo Clin. Proc.* **2000**, *75*, 933–942.
145. Bourrie, M.; Meunier, V.; Berger, Y.; Fabre, G. Role of cytochrome P-4502C9 in irbesartan oxidation by human liver microsomes. *Drug Metab. Dispos.* **1999**, *27*, 288–296.
146. Tang, C.; Shou, M.; Mei, Q.; Rushmore, T. H.; Rodrigues, A. D. Major role of human liver microsomal cytochrome P450 2C9 (CYP2C9) in the oxidative metabolism of celecoxib, a novel cyclooxygenase-II inhibitor. *J. Pharmacol. Exp. Ther.* **2000**, *293*, 453–459.
147. Kajita, J.; Kuwabara, T.; Kobayashi, H.; Kobayashi, S. CYP3A4 is mainly responsible for the metabolism of a new vinca alkaloid, vinorelbine, in human liver microsomes. *Drug Metab. Dispos.* **2000**, *28*, 1121–1127.
148. Li, X.-Q.; Björkman, A.; Andersson, T. B.; Ridderström, M.; Masimi-rembwa, C. M. Amodiaquine clearance and its metabolism to N-desethylamodiaquine is mediated by CYP2C8: a new high affinity and turnover enzyme-specific probe substrate. *J. Pharmacol. Exp. Ther.* **2002**, *300*, 399–407.

8

P450:

Biological

Aspects,

Regulation,

and

Genetics

INTRODUCTION

Long before P450 protein was discovered, pharmacologists and toxicologists recognized that individuals varied greatly in their response to, and metabolism of, drugs and other xenobiotics. Both environmental and genetic factors contribute to this variation. Increased activity of an enzyme following exposure to an environmental factor (such as a dietary constituent, drug, or toxicant) is referred to as *induction*. The rise in enzyme activities, following administration of an inducing agent, usually takes several days to reach a maximum. Sustained elevation depends on the continued presence of the inducing agent: if the inducing agent is withdrawn, enzyme activities slowly return to baseline, due to normal messenger RNA and protein degradation and turnover. The level of induction depends on the concentration of the inducing agent and is saturable.

As the science of molecular toxicology developed, induction became an increasingly important field of research. But, for a long time, studies remained empirical rather than mechanistic. The main impediment to progress was the difficulty of identifying and characterizing the protein receptors that mediate the induction response and to which xenobiotics bind. Advances in biochemistry and molecular biology swept these obstacles away, beginning with the cloning of the AH (aryl hydrocarbon) receptor in the early 1990s. In the few years since the publication of the first edition of this text, understanding of the regulation of P450 expression has advanced enormously. This chapter focuses on P450 induction, with some extension to the wider field of biological regulation. We will also discuss genetic polymorphism of human P450s as a factor contributing to interindividual variation in metabolism of drugs and toxicants.

THE SIGNIFICANCE OF P450 INDUCTION

Why has induction been studied so intensively, since its discovery in the late 1950s? First, P450 induction is a phenomenon with significant implications for clinical pharmacology and toxicology. Humans are usually exposed not to single agents but to complex mixtures of chemicals in the environment; multiple drugs are often prescribed simultaneously ("polypharmacy"). The P450 induction effect of one agent may alter the pharmacological/toxicological actions of another. Induction can greatly change the rate of elimination of a xenobiotic from the body; alter the fraction of an oral dose of a drug that reaches a target organ; and shift the proportions of the various metabolites formed from a xenobiotic. Such changes occasionally increase the clinical effectiveness of a drug, but the more common outcome is to reduce it, because the pharmacologically active parent compound is metabolized more quickly to inactive products. For example, carbamazepine, a widely prescribed antiepileptic and antidepressant drug, induces P450 3A4 and can accelerate the metabolism of coadministered drugs, such as the anticonvulsant valproic acid (1). St. John's wort (*Hypericum perforatum*), a common herbal remedy, is also a potent 3A4 inducer (2); the major active ingredient is hyperforin. St. John's wort reduces the effectiveness of the chemotherapeutic drug irinotecan (3) and, in transplant patients, it can decrease the plasma levels of the immunosupressant drug cyclosporin A so significantly that tissue rejection occurs (4). The toxicity of acetaminophen, which is triggered by its oxidation to the iminoquinone (see chapters 7 and 19), is increased by exposure to agents that elevate the activities of P450 1A2 and P450 2E1, which catalyze this oxidation.

The levels of some P450 enzymes (notably 3-methylcholanthrene-inducible rat hepatic P450 1A1) are increased by orders of magnitude following administration of an inducing agent. Therefore, induction was an essential tool for the purification and characterization of many P450 enzymes. (Before the introduction of systematic nomenclature, some P450 enzymes were actually named for their chemical inducers.) Induction effects can be used to test the involvement of a given P450 enzyme in a metabolic process or toxic effect, as discussed at the end of chapter 7. P450 induction has been an important model experimental system for studying the regulation of gene expression in animals and, from a wider perspective, the nature of gene–environment interactions.

The increased metabolic activities following induction reflect an increase in the amounts of specific forms of P450 present in the tissue. *The amount of a given P450 can be increased by up to two orders of magnitude* by exposure to xenobiotics, although there is usually no more than a 2- to 3-fold increase in the *total* content of P450 in the tissue. Significant elevations in conjugating enzymes, such as glucuronosyl transferases and glutathione transferases (see chapters 10 and 12), also occur in response to xenobiotic exposures.

THE DISCOVERY OF THE INDUCTION OF P450 BY XENOBIOTICS

The concept that prior exposure to a small dose of a poison protects against a subsequent, larger dose goes back to antiquity. In the 1950s, as the scientific study of drug metabolism matured, several researchers independently discovered systems in which administration of one xenobiotic greatly altered a rodent's response to a subsequent exposure to another agent. Many different classes of chemical can act as inducers. Before examining the molecular mechanisms of induction, we will introduce some of these inducing agents and note how their effects were discovered. Structures of some P450 inducers are shown in figure 8-1. Aside from hydrophobicity, no single chemical theme typifies all of these agents.

Polycyclic Aromatic Hydrocarbons

In 1952 Richardson and colleagues discovered that feeding the polycyclic aromatic hydrocarbon (PAH) 3-methylcholanthrene to rats greatly

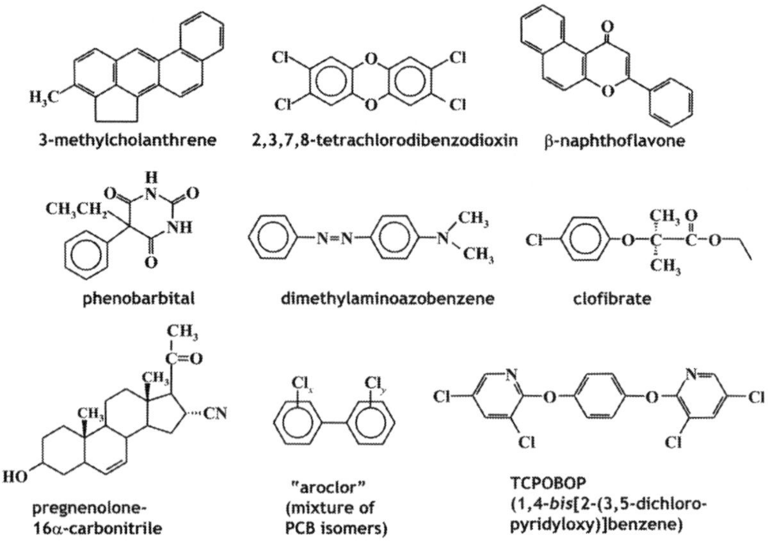

3-methylcholanthrene   2,3,7,8-tetrachlorodibenzodioxin   β-naphthoflavone

phenobarbital   dimethylaminoazobenzene   clofibrate

pregnenolone-
16α-carbonitrile

"aroclor"
(mixture of
PCB isomers)

TCPOBOP
(1,4-*bis*[2-(3,5-dichloro-
pyridyloxy)]benzene)

FIGURE 8-1.
Chemical structures of selected P450 inducers.

decreased the carcinogenic activity of a subsequently administered amino-azo dye (5). Allan Conney learned of this finding when he joined the University of Wisconsin's McArdle Laboratory for Cancer Research as a new graduate student (6):

> I wanted to enter the oncology Ph.D. program at McArdle, and [the director] introduced me to Drs. James and Elizabeth Miller ... I joined the Miller laboratory in September, 1952, and my first project was to synthesize 1-hydroxy-2-aminonaphthalene, a suspected carcinogenic metabolite of 2-naphthylamine (a bladder carcinogen). After many attempts to synthesize and purify the 2-naphthylamine derivative ... failed to yield pure product and also resulted in two explosions, the Millers realized that I did not have much future as a synthetic chemist; I believe they were also worried about the destruction of their laboratory. These concerns led to a change in my research project ... The Millers and I discussed earlier research ... indicating that administration of 3-methylcholanthrene inhibited the hepatocarcinogenic activity of 3'-methyl-4-dimethylaminoazo-benzene in rats. We discussed the possibility that treatment of rats with the protective hydrocarbon might alter the metabolism of carcinogenic aminoazo dyes, and ... I started studies on the effects of treating rats with 3-methylcholanthrene and other polycyclic aromatic hydrocarbons on the hepatic N-demethylation and azo-link reduction of aminoazo dyes—metabolic pathways that resulted in noncarcinogenic products. Almost immediately, I experienced the joys of discovery by finding that treatment of rats with a single i.p. injection of 3-methylcholanthrene caused a rapid and many-fold increase in azo dye N-demethylase activity... These studies... were early examples of enzyme induction in mammals.

3-Methylcholanthrene (3-MC) and many other PAHs were found to induce P450. As noted in chapter 7, the main 3-MC-inducible enzymes are the members of the mammalian P450 1 family, once described as "cytochrome P448."

TCDD and Other Chlorinated Aromatic Compounds

2,3,7,8-Tetrachlorodibenzo-p-dioxin (TCDD) is a potent toxicant in animals and humans. One of the serious and characteristic consequences of human exposure to TCDD is chloracne, a persistent cystic skin eruption. In animals, toxic effects include loss of body weight ("wasting syndrome") and liver damage (7). The toxicity of TCDD (measured as oral LD_{50}) varies greatly among species. In the guinea pig, the LD_{50} is about 1 µg per kg; in the rat and hamster, it is ten- to several thousand-fold higher, depending on the sex and strain. TCDD is an even more potent P450 inducer than are PAHs (8).

TCDD is a parts-per-million contaminant in the herbicide 2,4,5-trichlorophenoxyacetic acid (2,4,5-T), which was an ingredient in the defoliant *Agent Orange*.[1] Tens of millions of liters of Agent Orange—an environmental weapon of mass destruction—was sprayed from airplanes over Vietnam in the late 1960s, as part of the "Operation Ranch Hand" defoliation campaign by the US military. It is estimated that several hundred kilograms of TCDD was deposited in Vietnam during the war (9). Another serious human TCDD exposure occurred following the explosion of a reaction chamber for the industrial synthesis of 2,4,5-trichlorophenol in Seveso, Italy, on July 10, 1976 (10).

Polychlorinated biphenyls (PCBs) were used on a very large scale as (among other applications) electrical transformer fluids and plasticizers, until concern over their environmental persistence and toxicity led to a phase-out after 1974. "Aroclor 1254," a commercial preparation containing various PCB congeners (i.e., biphenyl derivatives bearing one or more chlorine substituents), is a powerful inducer of hepatic P450 enzymes (11). Aroclor is a complex chemical mixture and its spectrum of inducing activities is broad. Aroclor-induced rat liver S9 has been widely used as an activation system in mutagenicity tests (12) such as the Ames test (13). However, with the phase-out of PCB use, alternatives are needed. An induction protocol using phenobarbital plus β-naphthoflavone provides a better-defined replacement for the use of aroclor in S9 preparation (14).

Barbiturates

After completing his Ph.D. studies, Allan Conney continued exploring the induction of drug metabolism:

> I met with Dr. Bernard Brodie, whose Laboratory of Chemical Pharmacology in the Heart Institute at the National Institutes of Health was at the forefront of drug metabolism research ... and I discussed with him the possibility that drugs may induce increased levels of microsomal drug-metabolizing enzymes. In 1957, I ... started working with John Burns at the National Institutes of Health ... We then found that treatment of rats with phenobarbital, barbital, aminopyrine, phenylbutazone, orphenadrine, or benzo[a]-pyrene caused a marked increase in the activity of liver microsomal enzymes that metabolized several drugs.

The inducing activity of barbiturates and other sedative drugs was discovered independently by Herbert Remmer in Germany (15) and Ryuichi Kato in Japan.

P450 2 family enzymes are the most characteristically phenobarbital-inducible P450s (16). In addition to its induction of microsomal P450, phenobarbital administration also causes dramatic structural and biochemical changes in rat liver (17, 16). The entire organ becomes enlarged and the synthesis of protein and phospholipid increases. At the ultrastructural level, the smooth endoplasmic reticulum (in which P450 resides) proliferates within the hepatocyte. These effects occur much less, or not at all, with PAHs (18).

TCPOBOP (1,4-bis[2-(3,5-dichloropyridyloxy)]benzene)

This compound has a spectrum of activity similar to that of phenobarbital, but it is at least a thousand times more potent. Its inducing effect was discovered by Alan Poland and colleagues at the University of Wisconsin in 1980 (19). "A foreign company had entered into a deal with a US chemical company to test and manufacture an agricultural chemical ... TCPOBOP was a contaminant ... The company knew of my interest in chemicals that induce monooxygenase activities ... they informed me of the structure and provided a small amount of the chemical ... They let us publish, as long as ... we never mentioned its source."[2] Because of its potency, TCPOBOP has been used in many subsequent experimental protocols.

Steroids

Hans Selye (1907–1982), professor of medicine at the University of Montreal, was a leading authority on the medical effects of stress (figure 8-2). One of his major interests was the role of steroid hormones in stress and disease. Selye discovered that certain steroids, notably the synthetic agent *pregnenolone 16-α-carbonitrile* (PCN), acted to protect rats against subsequent exposure to toxicants (20). He referred to these agents as "catatoxic" steroids. Allan Conney picks up the story:

> In 1970, I visited Hans Selye in Montreal ... and we discussed [his] observation that treatment of rats with certain steroids inhibited the toxicity of a large number of foreign chemicals. PCN was one of Selye's most active compounds, and I suggested the possibility that this steroid was an inducer of microsomal detoxifying enzymes. In 1972, we identified PCN as a new type of inducer ... Treatment of rats with PCN induced a different profile of xenobiotic-metabolizing enzymes than occurred after treatment of rats with either phenobarbital or 3-methylcholanthrene.

Ethanol

Ethanol was recognized as an inducer of P450 in the 1960s (21, 22), following the development of liquid diet formulations that can be used to administer chronic high-dose ethanol to rats. Rubin and Lieber fed rats a diet in which ethanol made up 36% of total calories, for two weeks. Aniline hydroxylase activity (oxidation of aniline to aminophenol) increased more than two-fold after induction, while benzo[a]pyrene hydroxylase

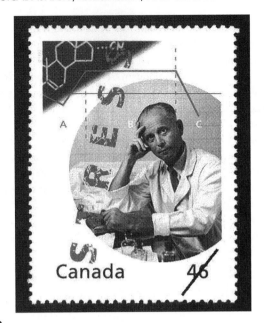

FIGURE 8-2.

Dr. Hans Selye (1907–1982) featured on a Canadian postage stamp (2000); note structure of the P450 inducer PCN in the top left corner. *Note*: A full-color version of this figure appears on the website.

(which we now recognize as a P450 1 activity) was little affected (*22*). Induction was also observed in human volunteers. Volunteers were administered a diet containing 42% calories as ethanol, for 12 days. Liver biopsies were performed before and after ethanol administration, and hydroxylase activity towards the barbiturate pentobarbital was found to have increased more than two-fold.

The major ethanol-inducible P450 enzyme is P450 2E1. The magnitude of induction of P450 2E1 by dietary ethanol in rats is typically less than ten-fold, although higher induction has been achieved by using alcohol intubation to maintain very high levels of blood alcohol (*23*). One of the biochemical activities induced by ethanol is ethanol oxidation, the "microsomal ethanol oxidizing system" (MEOS) associated with P450 2E1.

Peroxisome Proliferators

Clofibrate and related drugs have been used in the treatment of hyper-lipidemia. These drugs, and certain other compounds, such as the phthalate ester plasticizers, are *peroxisome proliferators* in rodents. They induce the production of peroxisomes, organelles responsible for β-oxidation of long-chain fatty acids and certain other pathways of lipid metabolism (see chapter 1). Other hepatic changes due to peroxisome proliferators include hypertrophy (increased liver size), increased cell proliferation, and tumorigenesis[3] (*24*). Rat P450 4A1, the enzyme that catalyzes fatty acid ω-hydroxylation, is induced by these agents (*25*).

P450 INDUCTION: EARLY MISCONCEPTIONS

As the above survey illustrates, very many xenobiotics, and some endo-genous agents, such as steroids, can act as P450 inducers. The structural diversity of P450 inducers is reminiscent of the diversity of P450 substrates. Many P450 inducers are indeed also P450 substrates. An early, but incorrect, idea was that each P450 substrate would induce the P450 activity responsible for its metabolism. This is occasionally true, but it is not a general rule. Another attractive, but false, hypothesis was that the P450 enzymes are themselves the receptors that mediate the induction process, perhaps by a single general mechanism. We now understand that induction is a complex biological response that may involve regulation at the transcriptional, translational, and posttranslational levels, and that no single mechanism can explain all aspects of induction. Nevertheless, transcriptional control is usually the most significant process in P450 regulation. Most inducers act by *binding to specific regulatory proteins that mediate signal transduction pathways leading to increased transcription* of the genes encoding one or more P450 enzymes. These regulatory proteins are the main focus of this chapter.

P450 INDUCTION: AN EXAMPLE

Let us look at a typical experiment on the induction of P450 activities by a drug, the anesthetic midazolam (*26*). Rats were treated for three consecutive days with either midazolam (50 mg/kg) or saline (controls), sacrificed, and hepatic microsomes were isolated. Enzyme activities in these microsomal fractions were determined by standard P450 assays, choosing substrates and assays with good specificity for several major hepatic P450 enzymes. The data in table 8-1 illustrate some typical features of P450 induction. One family of enzymes, P450 2B, is induced with marked, but not complete, specificity. Note the high level of induction: in this case, almost 100-fold increase in P450 2B activity. Closely related enzymes tend to share induction behavior; here, P450 2E1 is induced more than two-fold, but there is little or no induction of P450 1 enzymes.

The most important mechanism of P450 induction is enhanced transcription, although other mechanisms, such as mRNA and protein stabilization, can also contribute to increased enzyme activity. Therefore, to study the mechanisms of P450 induction, we need to start by reviewing the regulation of eukaryotic transcription and some of the experimental tools for studying this process.

TABLE 8-1.

Results of an Experiment on the Induction of P450 Activities

		ACTIVITY (pmol per min per mg protein)		
ASSAY	P450 (MAJOR)	CONTROL	MIDAZOLAM	FOLD INDUCTION
EROD	1A1	12.3	13.8	1.1
PHOD	1A2	829	1058	1.3
T16α	2B	4.4	416	95
*p*NP	2E1	67.2	168	2.5

EROD, ethoxyresorufin O-deethylation; PHOD, phenacetin O-deethylation; T16α, testosterone 16α hydroxylation; pNP, para-nitrophenol hydroxylation.

TOOLS FOR STUDYING TRANSCRIPTIONAL REGULATION

The major experimental strategies for studying transcription are briefly summarized here.

Northern blots[4] are gel electrophoretic assays in which mRNA molecules are separated on the basis of size and then detected by nucleic acid hybridization. Eukaryotic mRNA molecules undergo posttranscriptional processing reactions that add a polyA "tail" up to 200 nucleotides long to the 3′ end. Therefore, total mRNA can be conveniently isolated from eukaryotic cells by binding to oligo-dT affinity columns. When mRNA pools are run on an agarose gel, the mRNA species separate on the basis of size. mRNA molecules transcribed from a specific gene can be detected by hybridization to specific cDNA or oligonucleotide probes that have been labeled (e.g., with radioactive or fluorescent tags). The intensity of hybridization is a semiquantitative measure of the abundance of a particular transcript. Note that, even for a specific gene, the length of the corresponding transcript is variable, because the lengths of poly(A) tails are variable and mRNA is rapidly turned over in the cell. So, in any preparation, some of the transcripts will be partially degraded. As a result, northern blots usually show "fuzzy" bands (in contrast to the sharp bands of DNA restriction digests and Southern blots).

The use of northern blots to detect transcripts has largely been superseded by the development of the more sensitive *reverse transcriptase/ polymerase chain reaction (RT-PCR)* method (*27*). RT-PCR begins, like a northern blot, with an mRNA pool. The enzyme reverse transcriptase is used to make DNA copies of the mRNA (by extension of random oligonucleotide primers) and these DNA copies are then amplified by the PCR, using primers specific to the gene of interest. The PCR products can be visualized on an agarose gel. The information given by RT-PCR is similar to that of a northern blot, but with advantages of greater sensitivity and speed.

Microarray technology (*28*) extends the RT-PCR approach to examination of the transcription of large numbers (e.g., thousands) of genes simultaneously. Robotic technology is used to transfer gene-specific DNA probes (oligonucleotides or cDNA) onto a glass slide, forming an immobilized array. The microarray is then hybridized to fluorescently labeled mRNA pools and the extent of hybridization to specific probes is read by scanning the microarray. A typical experimental design is to compare two samples (e.g., cells before and after induction); each sample is labeled by incorporation of a distinct fluorescent dye (red vs. green) and the two samples are pooled before hybridization to the microarray. Genes expressed at higher levels in one of the samples will show up as red spots, and those expressed at higher levels in the other sample will show up as green spots. This technique can be used in a screening approach to identify genes induced in response to particular agents, for example xenobiotics (*29*).

Northern blots, RT-PCR, and microarrays evaluate the steady-state level of specific mRNAs, but a stronger band on a northern blot could reflect enhanced transcription of a gene, reduced degradation of the resulting message, or both. *Nuclear run-on assays* can distinguish between these possibilities, by measuring the relative rates at which different genes are being transcribed. Intact nuclei are isolated from cells. Deprived of the (cytosolic) supply of NTP building blocks, mRNA synthesis stops, leaving RNA polymerases stalled on the genes that they were transcribing. The isolated nuclei are then incubated with NTPs, including radiolabeled UTP, generating a pool of newly transcribed labeled mRNA molecules as the RNA polymerases "run on" along the actively transcribed genes. Specific transcripts are then isolated by hybridization to corresponding cDNAs.

Reporter Assays

The transcription assays described above generally require cell disruption and isolation of mRNA, followed by specific detection, using hybridization to oligonucleotide probes. These steps are laborious and technically demanding. (RNAse enzymes, which are ubiquitous and remarkably persistent, can degrade RNA molecules during isolation, so researchers working with RNA need to be scrupulous about avoiding contamination.) A recombinant *reporter assay* provides a simple, sensitive, and specific— albeit indirect—assay that allows the researcher to monitor expression of any gene of interest (*30, 31*). Many specific reporter assay systems have been commercialized, but the general principles are the same. A reporter gene is simply a gene whose protein product is easily measured in transfected cells. (It is also desirable that the gene not be expressed endogenously in the cells of interest, so that there is no background interference with the assay of the reporter gene.) Some commonly used reporter genes are listed in table 8-2, which indicates how the corresponding protein product (usually an enzyme) is detected.

The regulatory sequences upstream of a gene of interest (as much as several kilobases) are cloned into a site in a plasmid, such that they control not the endogenous gene (say, a P450 gene) but, instead, a reporter gene. The plasmid is transfected into the cells of interest. The cells are then treated as desired (e.g., exposed to an inducing agent) and expression of the reporter gene is assayed. Induction can be observed as an increase in reporter activity following exposure of the transfected cells to the inducer.

TABLE 8-2.
Reporter Genes

REPORTER GENE	PROTEIN PRODUCT/ACTIVITY	TYPICAL DETECTION METHOD
Bacterial CAT	Chloramphenicol acetyltransferase; catalyzes acetylation of the antibiotic chloramphenicol	Separation of ^{14}C-labeled acetyl-chloramphenicol from chloramphenicol (thin-layer chromatography) followed by autoradiography
E. coli β-gal	β-Galactosidase; hydrolyzes lactose and other galactosides	Hydrolysis of *o*-nitrophenyl-β-D-galactoside (OPNG) to give yellow product
Firefly luciferase	Catalyzes oxidative carboxylation of luciferin	Luminometer detects photons (chemiluminescence)

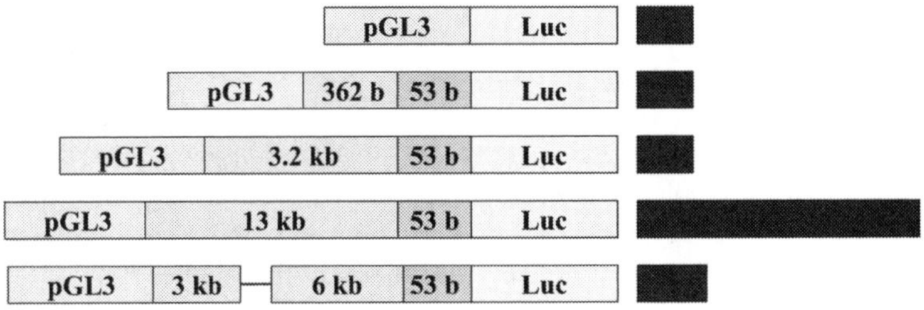

FIGURE 8-3.

An example of the use of a reporter gene assay. Upstream regulatory regions of human CYP3A4, obtained from a genomic clone, were fused to the luciferase gene of a commercial vector (pGL3-Basic). Deletion mutants were constructed and transiently transfected into HepG2 cells. To analyze CYP3A4 inducibility, transfected cells were treated with rifampicin (5 μM) for 48 hours, and luciferase activity compared to that of control (DMSO-treated) cells. The left side of the figure shows the deletion constructs (not to scale) and the right side shows the relative luciferase activity of the corresponding construct. *Note*: A full-color version of this figure appears on the website. (*Adapted from Goodwin, B.; Hodgson, E.; Liddle, C. The orphan human pregnane X receptor mediates the transcriptional activation of CYP3A4 by rifampicin through a distal enhancer module.* Mol. Pharmacol. ***1999,*** *56, 1329–1339.*)

Since a reporter gene assay measures the activity of a protein product, rather than the mRNA per se, it is susceptible to interferences (e.g., by unexpected changes in the stability of the protein). However, the sensitivity and convenience of reporter assays make them ideal for molecular dissection of regulatory sequences. We can cut out a section of the upstream DNA sequences that mediate transcriptional control, and then test whether the induction response is affected. This process of molecular dissection of upstream DNA sequences, using reporter assays, has been used to locate the critical regulatory elements controlling induction of P450 (and other) genes. An example of this application of a reporter assay is shown in figure 8-3.

EUKARYOTIC TRANSCRIPTION REGULATION

The regulation of eukaryotic gene expression is, of course, a topic of vast importance in biology: it underlies the mechanisms of development, differentiation, and response to the environment. Comprehensive discussions of this subject are provided in textbooks of biochemistry or cell biology. Here, we shall only touch on a few fundamental principles.

In prokaryotes, introns do not exist; messages may be mono- or polycistronic (operons); regulatory sequences (promoters, operators) are located immediately upstream of open reading frames; induction of expression may increase transcription rates by factors as high as about 1000, but even uninduced genes are usually expressed at detectable levels. In contrast, in eukaryotes, most genes are composed of several exons split by introns; messages are always monocistronic; regulatory sequences (promoters, enhancers) may be located far upstream (or even downstream) of open reading frames; and induction may increase transcription by factors as high as 10^9, in comparisons between, for example, different cell types in an organism. Connected to this fact is another key difference between pro-karyotes and eukaryotes: eukaryotic RNA polymerase II (which catalyzes transcription of mRNA) can only bind to promoters with the assistance of multiple accessory proteins, termed *transcription factors*. Nevertheless, in both prokaryotes and eukaryotes, proteins act as regulators of tran-scription by the same general mechanism: they sense environmental conditions (e.g., by binding specific chemical ligands), and undergo conformational changes in response; interact with other protein partners; recognize and bind to specific DNA sequences; and modulate the ability of RNA polymerase to initiate transcription. A fundamental feature of such mechanisms, both prokaryotic and eukaryotic, is *cooperativity*. Multiple binding interactions (ligand–protein, protein–DNA, protein–protein) must occur simultaneously for transcription to proceed. Conse-quently, the system switches between "on" and "off" (transcribed or silent) states over a narrow range of external conditions (e.g., ligand concentration, temperature, etc.).

Eukaryotic promoters are located within about 100 bases upstream of transcription start sites. However, regulation of transcription is typically mediated by transcription factors that bind to *enhancer* sequences (*32*, ch. 7). Enhancers are DNA sequence elements that are required for maximal transcription of specific nearby genes, but that may be located hundreds or even thousands of bases from the transcription start sites. Enhancer sequences are recognized by specific transcription factors. Their ability to "act at a distance" is illustrated in figure 8-4. Transcription factors (bound to enhancer sequences) interact with transcription complex proteins (bound to the promoter); the intervening DNA is "looped out,"

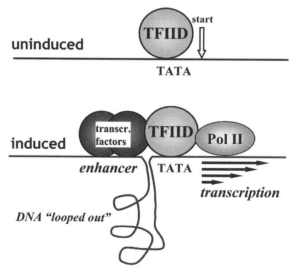

FIGURE 8-4.
Simplified schematic showing the role of transcription factors in enhancing transcription of specific genes. The general transcription factor TFIID binds to eukaryotic promoters. Specific transcription factors bind to enhancer regions, which may be far upstream of genes, and interact with TFIID and RNA polymerase II (Pol II) to stimulate transcription. *Note*: A full-color version of this figure appears on the website.

and the length of the DNA loop is, within wide bounds, immaterial. The relatively large distances between enhancers and the genes they regulate can make the identification of enhancers difficult, and this is a situation where experimental systems such as the reporter assays discussed above prove very valuable. Often, one can play the game in both directions: using the DNA as bait to identify transcription factors or using the binding of the transcription factors to identify critical DNA sequences.

CLONING OF THE ESTROGEN RECEPTOR; DISCOVERY OF "ORPHAN RECEPTORS"

One of the earliest identified and best understood examples of eukaryotic transcriptional regulation is the estrogen receptor system, which mediates the response to the female hormone estrogen. Estrogen acts as a hormonal master switch that induces a large number of genes during mammalian development. Estrogen is a high-affinity ligand for a transcription factor, the estrogen receptor,[5] which is a prototype of a large protein class, the *nuclear receptor superfamily* (*32*, ch. 15). Other members include the glucocorticoid, androgen, progesterone, and retinoic acid receptors. The estrogen (*33, 34*) and retinoic acid (*35*) receptors were cloned in the mid-1980s by Pierre Chambon and colleagues (*36*). Although nuclear receptor proteins are present at very low concentrations (of the order of picomole estrogen receptor per milligram mammary tissue protein), they bind to their cognate hormones (e.g., estrogen) with very high affinities (K_D of the order of 1 nM). Tight binding of physiological ligands facilitated the purification and cloning of nuclear receptor proteins/genes.

As soon as the first members of the nuclear receptor superfamily were cloned and sequenced, it became possible to clone homologous genes/proteins, by hybridization to conserved gene sequences. By such studies, it was soon revealed that mammalian genomes encode many members of this superfamily (approximately 50, in the case of humans). For most of the newly discovered genes/proteins, the corresponding physiological ligands were unknown. These proteins were therefore referred to as "orphan receptors," that is, receptors that had not yet been matched with ligands (*37, 38*). The quest for the identification of the ligands for, and physiological roles of, these receptors became known as "reverse endocrinology," in contrast to "classic" endocrinology (which proceeds from known hormones to their receptor proteins). Reverse endocrinology led, in the 1990s, to the identification of the most important receptors mediating P450 induction.[6] These receptors, including PXR, CAR, and PPAR, described in more detail later in this chapter, had resisted identification by "classic" endocrinology methods. This was mainly because the affinity of binding of most xenobiotics (even potent P450 inducers) to these receptors is much weaker than the interaction of, for example, estrogen with the estrogen receptor.

STRUCTURE OF THE ESTROGEN RECEPTOR

The mechanism of action of the estrogen receptor provides the paradigm for analyzing the biochemistry of other nuclear receptors. All members of the superfamily conform to the same general architecture (figure 8-5);

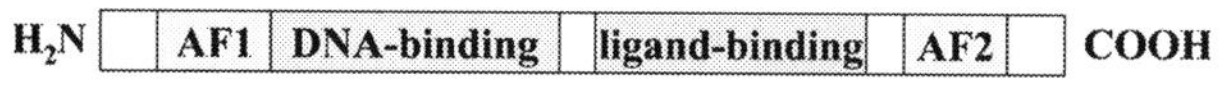

| H₂N | | AF1 | DNA-binding | ligand-binding | AF2 | | COOH |

FIGURE 8-5.

Schematic of the domain structure of nuclear receptor superfamily proteins. AF1 and AF2 are "activation function" domains. *Note*: A full-color version of this figure appears on the website.

see also (*39*, figure 31.22). One domain of the protein recognizes and binds to a specific DNA sequence (typically containing two repeats with the consensus sequence AGGTCA). This domain of the receptor incorporates two "zinc-finger" motifs; within each of these motifs, four conserved cysteine residues bind a Zn^{2+} ion. A second domain (*40*) recognizes and binds a ligand (estradiol, in the case of the estrogen receptor; figure 8-6) and the protein undergoes a conformational change. Consequently, certain protein partners (corepressors) fall off, other protein partners (coactivators) bind, and the receptor dimerizes and assumes a conformation that can bind to its cognate enhancer sequence. (In some cases, activation can also occur without ligand binding, by mechanisms such as receptor phosphorylation.) The dimerization may occur with another molecule of the same receptor, to form a homodimer (as occurs in the case of the estrogen receptor) or with a different nuclear receptor, to form a heterodimer (as in the case of PXR, PPAR, and CAR, each of which forms a heterodimer with RXR; figure 8-7 and table 8-3).

As we have seen, many steroids are potent P450 inducers. So, after the characterization of the receptors for estrogen, glucocorticoids, and other steroid hormones—prototypes of the nuclear receptor superfamily—it was widely anticipated that P450 induction would occur by the same general mechanisms. This proved to be true for most P450 enzymes (but not for the P450 1 family). We first outline the P450 induction processes mediated by members of the nuclear receptor superfamily, leaving the discussion of the AH receptor mechanism to the end (reversing the historical order in which they were discovered).

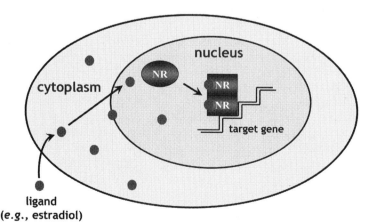

FIGURE 8-6.

Schematic of the mechanism of action of nuclear receptor superfamily transcription factors. Binding of a ligand (e.g., estradiol) induces a conformational change, dimerization, and binding to enhancer sequences. *Note*: A full-color version of this figure appears on the website.

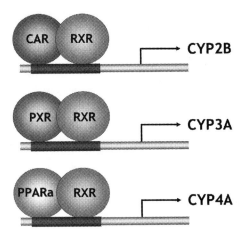

FIGURE 8-7.

P450 induction mediated by nuclear receptor superfamily proteins involves heterodimerization with RXR. *Note*: A full-color version of this figure appears on the website.

RXR AND THE ADOPTION OF THE ORPHAN RECEPTORS

As discussed above, many presumptive nuclear receptor proteins were cloned on the basis of sequence similarity to the estrogen receptor and other steroid hormone receptors. Since their physiological ligands remained unknown, they were called "orphan" receptors (*41*). Recent progress has led to the identification of ligands and physiological roles for many of these orphans, which are therefore considered to be "adopted." The steroid hormone receptors bind endogenous ligands (steroids) with high affinity and bind to DNA as homodimers. In contrast, orphan receptors probably evolved as sensors of dietary lipids and other hydrophobic xenobiotics (*38*). Their ligand-binding affinities are generally weaker (μM rather than nM dissociation constants) and they all bind to enhancers as heterodimers with the partner RXR (figure 8-8). These two groups of nuclear receptors are sometimes distinguished as Class I (steroid receptors; homodimer-forming) and Class II (orphan receptors; heterodimer-forming) (*42*).

The adoption process began with the characterization of RXR, the retinoid X receptor, by Mangelsdorf and co-workers (*43–45*). The term "retinoid X" was applied to this receptor because the identity of its retinoid ligand was not yet clear; 9-*cis*-retinoic acid, a derivative of vitamin A, was shown to be the most potent physiological ligand for RXR, in 1992 (*46*).

Following the characterization of RXR (*47*), the roles of other orphan receptors as mediators of P450 induction were ascertained, using a combination of molecular biological and biochemical strategies. For example, reporter assays were used to identify a phenobarbital-responsive element (PBRE) upstream from the rat P450 2B2 (*48*) and human P450 2B6 genes (*49*) (figure 8-9). (The molecular biological characteristics of these response elements are discussed in detail in a recent review (*50*).) The PBRE DNA sequence was then used to prepare an affinity chromatography medium. Nuclear protein extracts from phenobarbital-treated rat liver were passed through such a column, and western blots showed

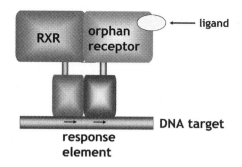

FIGURE 8-8.

Schematic showing the heterodimer of RXR and a nuclear orphan receptor. *Note*: A full-color version of this figure appears on the website.

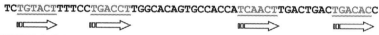

FIGURE 8-9.

The phenobarbital response element upstream (−2235 to −2184) from rat CYP2B2. *Note*: A full-color version of this figure appears on the website. (*Adapted from Trottier, E.; Belzil, A.; Stoltz, C.; Anderson, A. Localization of a phenobarbital-responsive element (PBRE) in the 5′-flanking region of the rat CYP2B2 gene.* Gene **1995**, 158, 263–268.)

that both RXR and the orphan receptor CAR (see table 8-3) were bound by PBRE DNA (*51*).

CAR and PXR proteins bind various drugs and xenobiotics. Moore et al. (*52*) expressed human CAR ligand-binding domain (CAR residues 103–348) in *E. coli* and purified the protein to homogeneity. They designed a scintillation proximity assay (SPA; see sidebar) for measuring ligand binding to CAR. CAR was coupled to SPA beads and [^{3}H]clotrimazole (a broad-spectrum antifungal drug) was bound to the protein. As shown in figure 8-10, unlabelled clotrimazole displaces [^{3}H]clotrimazole from

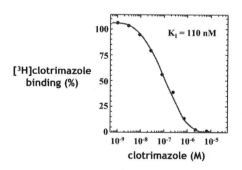

FIGURE 8-10.

Experimental demonstration of binding of a P450 inducer to the nuclear receptor CAR, using a scintillation proximity assay. Purified hCAR ligand-binding domain was immobilized on polyvinyltoluene beads and incubated with 10 nM [^{3}H]clotrimazole, in the presence of increasing concentrations of unlabeled clotrimazole. (*Data from Moore, L. B. et al. Orphan nuclear receptors constitutive androstane receptor and pregnane X receptor share xenobiotic and steroid ligands.* J. Biol. Chem. **2000**, 275, 15122–15127.)

CAR, with the expected kinetics of a ligand-receptor interaction. Similarly, the 3A4 inducer in St. John's wort, hyperforin, binds to PXR with high affinity (53).

PROPERTIES OF THE NUCLEAR RECEPTORS THAT MEDIATE P450 INDUCTION

All of the receptor proteins listed in table 8-3 are evolutionarily related members of the nuclear receptor superfamily. Their individual properties and interactions mediate specific responses to P450 inducers (55). Additional members of the superfamily, such as farnesoid X receptor (FXR) and liver X receptor (LXR), regulate metabolism of cholesterol, bile salts, and other endogenous compounds, but are not strongly associated with P450 induction and not discussed here. All of these proteins are now under intense study, especially with regard to their ligand-binding properties.

CAR

Rodent CAR binds the potent inducer TCPOBOP and activates the P450 2B promoter (56). Surprisingly, phenobarbital itself, the prototypical P450 2B inducer, is not a high-affinity CAR ligand; phenobarbital activates CAR by an indirect mechanism that is still not understood (57). A CAR knockout mouse was reported in 2000 (58). P450 2B expression could not be induced in these animals, following treatment with either TCPOBOP or phenobarbital. Furthermore, the typical liver hypertrophy response to P450 2B inducers is abolished in the CAR knockout animals. CAR knockout mice are also resistant to acetaminophen hepatotoxicity (59) (see chapter 19).

Note that RXR ligands such as 9-*cis*-retinoic acid are not required for activation of CAR (or other nuclear orphan receptors); that is, CAR

▶ **Scintillation Proximity Assay**

The scintillation proximity assay (SPA) has gained popularity for high-throughput screening procedures in drug discovery. In an SPA (54), a protein is linked to polymer microspheres (approximately 5 μm diameter) of polyvinyl-toluene, a solid scintillant. Tritium (^{3}H) beta particles have relatively low energies and can only travel a few micrometers through a solution. Therefore, ^{3}H-labelled molecules that are tightly bound to the SPA beads will produce beta particles that can penetrate into the solid scintillant and generate scintillations; beta particles emitted by molecules in solution will dissipate their energy without producing scintillation photons. ◀

TABLE 8-3.

Nuclear Receptors Involved in P450 Induction

RECEPTOR NAME	SYMBOL	TYPICAL LIGANDS	P450 ENZYMES INDUCED
Retinoid X	RXR	9-*cis*-Retinoic acid	–
Peroxisome proliferator-activated	PPAR	Fatty acids, fibrate drugs	4A
Constitutive androstane	CAR	TCPOBOP	2B
Pregnane X (steroid/xenobiotic)	PXR (SXR)	Steroids	3A

*This list is limited to the most significant forms regulating P450 enzymes involved in xenobiotic metabolism. Many other members of the nuclear receptor protein superfamily exist; about 48 are encoded in the human genome. Multiple forms of RXR (α, β, and γ) and PPAR (α, β (also called δ), and γ) exist. The names of these receptors are often rather obtuse, since they were assigned before their ligand specificities were fully characterized. CAR: the name "constitutive androstane" receptor originated at a time when this receptor was believed to be "constitutive" (active in the absence of ligands), but this terminology is now recognized as a misnomer. The functions of many nuclear receptors (notably, CAR and PXR) overlap ("cross-talk"), so the specificities of P450 induction listed here should not be regarded as absolute. The designation SXR is often used for the human orthologue of rodent PXR, but we will use the term "human PXR" for simplicity. Adapted from Chawla, A.; Repa, J. J.; Evans, R. M.; Mangelsdorf, D. J. Nuclear receptors and lipid physiology: opening the X-files. Science **2001**, 294, 1866–1870.*

dimerizes with RXR even in the absence of retinoids (*60*). Indeed, 9-*cis*-retinoic acid actually *represses* CAR-mediated P450 induction by TCPOBOP in mouse hepatocytes (*61*). This effect may be due to "cross-talk," whereby the retinoid promotes RXR heterodimerization with the retinoic acid receptor, RAR, reducing its availability for binding to CAR.

PXR/SXR

The amino acid sequence of PXR (the human orthologue is sometimes designated SXR) is more similar to that of CAR than to that of any other nuclear receptor, and there is considerable overlap between the actions of PXR and CAR (*62–65*). Mouse PXR knockout animals do not induce P450 3A11 (the major murine hepatic P450 3A enzyme) in response to treatment with dexamethasone or PCN (*66*). The crystal structure of the ligand-binding domain of human PXR (figure 8-11) was reported in 2001 (*67, 68*) both in the presence and absence of a ligand (SR12813, a hypocholesterolemic drug that is a potent P450 3A inducer). The ligand-binding site is larger than observed with typical nuclear receptors. Indeed, the ligand SR12813 occupied multiple binding orientations in the active site. The flexibility of this binding site may explain the broad diversity of P450 3A family inducers. Hyperforin, the active compound of St. John's wort, binds in a single orientation, making multiple polar and hydrophobic contacts to the protein (figure 8-12) (*69*). PXR sequences from different mammals show little variation in the DNA-binding domain but much variation in the ligand-binding domain (figure 8-13). Indeed, these

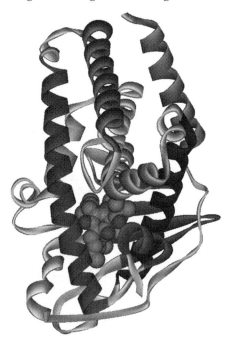

FIGURE 8-11.
Crystal structure of the ligand-binding domain of human PXR protein. Coordinate file: 1M13.pdb. *Note*: A full-color version of this figure appears on the website. (*Watkins, R. E. et al. 2.1 Å crystal structure of human PXR in complex with the St. John's wort compound hyperforin.* Biochemistry **2003**, 42, *1430–1438*.)

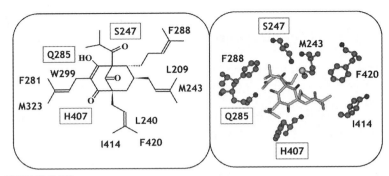

FIGURE 8-12.

Schematic (left) and structural (right) representations of the active site of human PXR ligand-binding domain with bound hyperforin. Amino acid residues interacting with the ligand are indicated; boxed residues form polar (H-bonding) contacts; the remaining residues form van der Waals (hydrophobic) contacts. For clarity, only a subset of the interacting residues are shown in the structural representation; hyperforin is shown as a stick model and protein residues are shown as ball-and-stick models. Coordinate file: 1M13.pdb. *Note:* A full-color version of this figure appears on the website. (*Adapted from Watkins, R. E. et al. 2.1 Å crystal structure of human PXR in complex with the St. John's wort compound hyperforin.* Biochemistry **2003**, *42, 1430–1438.*)

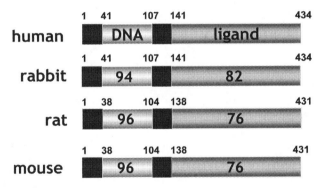

FIGURE 8-13.

Variations in PXR ligand-binding domain sequences are consistent with species differences in response to inducers. The small number above the bar indicates the amino acid residue and the large number on the bar represents % amino acid identity to the human sequence. *Note:* A full-color version of this figure appears on the website. (*Courtesy of Ed LeCluyse, University of North Carolina, Chapel Hill.*)

interspecies differences in PXR structure seem to correlate with P450 induction behavior. For example, rifampicin induces P450 3A4 in humans, but is not an inducer in rats; and rifampicin activates human but not rat PXR (*70*). Bile salts may be among the endogenous ligands of PXR and other nuclear orphan receptors that mediate P450 induction (*71, 72*).

PPAR

Peroxisome-proliferator drugs such as clofibrate induce P450 4 enzymes, as discussed earlier. The nuclear receptor PPARα is required for P450 4A induction in mice, as demonstrated by studies of knockout animals (*73*).

Peroxisome proliferation does not seem to occur in humans, even after treatment with "peroxisome-proliferator" drugs, probably because of inter-species differences in the expression or structure of PPARα. Two additional members of this receptor family exist, PPARγ (74) and PPARδ (75) (also called PPARβ). Recent investigations (76) have revealed roles for PPAR receptors in a host of physiological processes, including regulation of fatty acid catabolism and cholesterol transport, the response to insulin, inflammation, and wound healing (77).

One might have hoped that the ligand binding specificities of purified nuclear receptors would straightforwardly account for the P450 induction activities of xenobiotics. However, making this correlation has not been easy. For example, phenobarbital, as mentioned above, is not a potent ligand for CAR. There may be several reasons for the confusion that presently exists in this regard: (i) the ligand-binding properties of the receptors may be modified by interaction with other protein partners, and these interactions are difficult to replicate with recombinant proteins; (ii) there is considerable cross-talk and overlap among the different receptors; (iii) in some cases, the true receptor ligands may actually be metabolites of the inducers; and (iv) some inducers may affect receptor properties by indirect routes (e.g., altering phosphorylation status), rather than by binding as ligands.

In summary, many nuclear receptors that regulate response to environmental chemicals have been characterized in the past few years, and their pivotal role in P450 induction phenomena has been established. The study of their biochemical properties and physiological functions is still at an early stage and the conclusions presented here are sure to be revised in the near future.

INDUCTION OF THE P450 1 FAMILY ENZYMES

As discussed earlier, PAHs, such as 3-methylcholanthrene (3-MC), were among the first known P450 inducers, and P450 enzymes 1A1 and 1A2 (and, later, 1B1) were identified as the forms inducible by PAH and other planar aromatic compounds. From the outset, it was apparent that P450 family 1 is distinctive, in terms of both P450 protein structure (λ_{max} close to 448 nm; see chapter 7) and mechanism of induction. P450 1 inducers are generally large, planar, hydrophobic molecules, such as PAH and polychlorinated aromatics. We speak of "3-MC-like inducers," and this classification applies to both their structures and effects. This structural consistency contrasts with the wide structural diversity of inducers of other P450 families, notably the PXR ligands that induce P450 3 enzymes, as discussed above. In rats or mice, 3-MC-like inducers cause a great (more than 50-fold) increase in P450 1A1 activity, which is low or undetectable in uninduced animals.

Because of the role of P450 1 enzymes in carcinogen bioactivation, the study of their induction has attracted great interest (78). Several aspects of P450 1 induction expedited its experimental study, leading to the identification of the AH (aromatic hydrocarbon) receptor several years before the other receptors of P450 inducers (discussed above) were dis-covered. First, as mentioned at the beginning of the chapter, TCDD is a highly potent P450 1 inducer, and it is virtually inert (i.e., nonmetabolized).

TCDD and its analogues were used to isolate the cognate receptor protein by direct methods (using the ligand to trap the receptor), in contrast to the "reverse endocrinology" methods used to identify the roles of the nuclear orphan receptors discussed previously. Second, it was recognized that P450 1 induction is genetically polymorphic in mice, and this allowed classic mouse genetics to be applied to the problem. Also, P450 1 induction is readily demonstrated in vitro (e.g., in hepatoma cells).

DISCOVERY OF THE AH RECEPTOR

Some inbred strains of mice (such as strain C57BL/6) are *responsive* to 3-MC. That is, P450 1A1-associated enzyme activities (notably, aryl hydrocarbon hydroxylase) are greatly increased in microsomes prepared from liver of animals exposed to 3-MC or TCDD. Other strains (such as strain DBA/2) are nonresponsive (79): they show no increase in P450 1 activity following exposure to 3-MC. They are also 10- to 100-fold less sensitive to the toxic effects of TCDD. Cross-breeding experiments showed that inducibility (responsiveness) is a simple autosomal dominant Mendelian trait, thereby defining a genetic locus. The receptor presumed to be encoded by this gene was called the AH (for aryl hydrocarbon) receptor (AHR) (80).

The existence of a TCDD-binding protein was first demonstrated biochemically by Alan Poland and colleagues. They showed that when ^{3}H-TCDD is incubated with hepatic cytosol and the proteins are separated by sucrose density-gradient ultracentrifugation, radioactivity associates with a characteristic protein peak (figure 8-14). The affinity of binding can be assessed quantitatively by titrating the cytosol with TCDD. (Conforming to pharmacological practice, we refer to TCDD or other activating AHR ligands as *agonists*.) TCDD binding is characterized by high affinity and saturation kinetics, as expected for a classic ligand–receptor interaction.

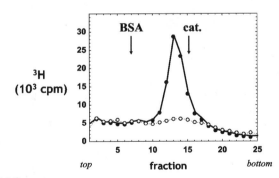

FIGURE 8-14.
Experimental measurement of TCDD binding to the AH receptor. Cytosol from LS180 (human colon carcinoma) cells was incubated with [^{3}H]TCDD (20 nM) either in the presence (open circles) or absence (filled circles) of excess non-labelled competitor (2,3,7,8-tetrachlorodibenzofuran, 2 μM). Linear (10–30%) sucrose gradients were centrifuged at 372,000g for 2 h at 4°C. After centrifugation, fractions (200 μL) were collected and radioactivity measured by scintillation counting. Arrows indicate elution positions of standard marker proteins BSA (bovine serum albumin) and catalase. *Note*: A full-color version of this figure appears on the website. (*Data courtesy of Patricia Harper, Hospital for Sick Children, Toronto.*)

Although the presence of AHR could be demonstrated in this manner, progress toward characterization of protein was long hampered by purification difficulties. The receptor is present in very low concentration, even in the livers of responsive animals. Furthermore, TCDD-binding activity is lost during attempted purification. Poland and colleagues circumvented this obstacle by developing a method for specifically labeling the receptor, based on the use of a *photoaffinity label*. 2-Azido-3-[^{125}I]iodo-7,8-dibromodibenzo-*p*-dioxin, a TCDD analogue (*81*) binds to the receptor much as does TCDD, noncovalently and with high affinity. Irradiation of the agonist–receptor complex with ultraviolet (UV) light activates the azido moiety to a reactive nitrene, which covalently attaches to the adjacent protein (figure 8-15). The resulting radiolabeled receptor could be purified to homogeneity by standard techniques, such as ion-exchange chromatography, reversed-phase HPLC, and SDS-PAGE. A partial N-terminal amino acid sequence was obtained, and, in 1992, the cDNA was cloned (*82, 83*).

The AH receptor is not a member of the nuclear receptor superfamily; it has no homology to proteins such as the estrogen receptor or PXR. AHR is a member of the "PAS family" of proteins, which also includes mammalian Arnt (see below), the drosophila neurogenic protein Sim, and the drosophila circadian rhythm protein Per.[7] PAS proteins are characterized by a region of homology (approximately 250 amino acid residues in

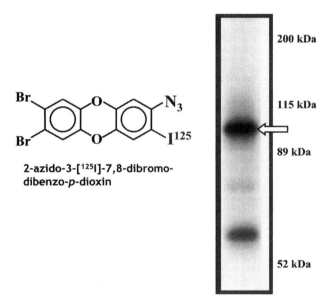

2-azido-3-[^{125}I]-7,8-dibromo-dibenzo-*p*-dioxin

FIGURE 8-15.

Photoaffinity labeling of the AH receptor. The structure of the photoaffinity reagent 2-azido-3-[^{125}I]iodo-7,8-dibromodibenzo-p-dioxin is shown at left. Right: murine AH receptor was expressed in a rabbit reticulocyte in vitro transcription–translation system. Protein extract was separated by SDS-PAGE, labeled, and visualized by autoradiography. *Note*: A full-color version of this figure appears on the website. (*Adapted from Powell-Coffman, J. A.; Bradfield, C. A.; Wood, W. B.* Caenorhabditis elegans *orthologs of the aryl hydrocarbon receptor and its heterodimerization partner the aryl hydrocarbon receptor nuclear translocator.* Proc. Natl. Acad. Sci. USA *1998*, 95, 2844–2849; figure 4.)

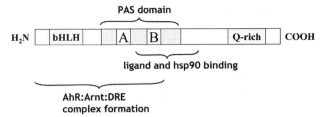

FIGURE 8-16.

Primary structure of the AH receptor protein, illustrating functional domains. *Note*: A full-color version of this figure appears on the website. (*Adapted from Denison, M. S.; Pandini, A.; Nagy, S. R.; Baldwin, E. P.; Bonati, L. Ligand binding and activation of the AH receptor.* Chem. Biol. Interact. ***2002,*** *141, 3–24.*)

length), the *PAS domain* (*84, 85*). In the AHR, the PAS domain plays a role in heterodimer formation and contains the ligand-binding portion of the receptor (figure 8-16). In contrast to nuclear receptor superfamily proteins, which possess a zinc-finger DNA-binding domain motif, PAS proteins have a basic helix-loop-helix (bHLH) motif (*86*). The bHLH motif[8] is a conserved region of about 50 amino acid residues. A short basic region that interacts with the DNA target is followed by two alpha helices connected by a short loop. Pairs of bHLH proteins dimerize via interactions between these helix-loop-helix motifs (*87*, p. 1085).

AHR is found in hepatic cytosol in the ligand-free state. Measurement of the AH receptor's molar mass by ultracentrifugation experiments showed that the cytosolic receptor was much heavier than the expected mass of the AHR protein alone, suggesting that the ligand-binding subunit is complexed to other proteins. In 1988 Gary Perdew (*88*) used the photo-affinity method to label AHR in hepatic cytosol, and then precipitated the AHR by addition of a monoclonal antibody. Electrophoretic and western blotting analysis of the precipitate revealed the presence of the heat shock protein hsp90. Another interacting partner protein was identified in 1997, by application of the yeast two-hybrid screening system; this is a 38 kDa protein called XAP2 (*89*). The present consensus is that the ligand-free receptor is a complex of the AHR itself, two units of the hsp90, and one unit of XAP2 (*90*). These associated proteins stabilize the ligand-free AHR receptor and presumably have additional functions that are not yet understood. After ligand treatment, AHR is found in the nuclear fraction of cells (figure 8-17). Thus, binding of ligand triggers some alteration in receptor function, converting the receptor to a DNA-binding protein. The associated hsp90 and XAP2 proteins dissociate from AHR; it is not yet resolved whether this takes place before or after translocation of the receptor to the nucleus. In the nucleus, AHR heterodimerizes with the partner protein ARNT to form the active DNA-binding transcriptional activator.

ARNT; AHR-MEDIATED INDUCTION OF GENE TRANSCRIPTION

The AH receptor nuclear translocator (ARNT) was cloned and identified as a component of the nuclear form of the AH receptor complex (*91*).

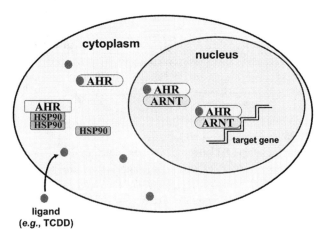

FIGURE 8-17.

Schematic of the mechanism of action of the AH receptor. Hsp90 dissociation may follow, rather than precede, nuclear import of AHR. *Note*: A full-color version of this figure appears on the website. (*Adapted from Gonzalez, F. J.; Fernandez-Salguero, P. The aryl hydrocarbon receptor: studies using the AHR-null mice.* Drug Metab. Dispos. **1998,** 26, 1194–1198.)

(ARNT protein was named for its presumed role in the nuclear translocation of the complex, but this was a misnomer.) ARNT is another member of the PAS family, like AHR. The activated nuclear form of the receptor is a heterodimer of the AHR and ARNT subunits, and possibly additional proteins (*92*).

Like the nuclear receptor superfamily proteins, AHR binds to enhancer sequences upstream of P450 genes: in this case, P450 1 family genes. The DNA sites to which AHR binds were identified by deletion analysis of the regulatory regions upstream from the P450 1A1 gene, in mouse cell lines. A DNA sequence (enhancer element) necessary and sufficient for AHR-mediated induction of P450 1A1 transcription was identified in the 5′-flanking region of this gene. The target contains the core consensus sequence 5′-TNGCGTG-3′. These target regions are known variously as AH-responsive elements (AHREs), dioxin-responsive elements or dioxin-responsive enhancers (DREs), or xenobiotic response elements (XREs) (*93*). At least four XREs are located about −800 to −1200 bp upstream of the murine *P450 1A1* gene (*94*).

In addition to P450 1 family members, transcription of the genes encoding several other enzymes of biotransformation is regulated by AHR, including forms of UDP-glucuronosyltransferase, glutathione transferase, NAD(P)H:quinone oxidoreductase, and aldehyde dehydrogenase. Genes apparently unrelated to xenobiotic metabolism are also controlled by AHR and inducible by TCDD, as revealed by DNA microarray analysis (*95*).

ENDOGENOUS LIGANDS FOR THE AH RECEPTOR

TCDD, the best-known ligand for AHR, is a chlorinated aromatic compound formed by industrial synthesis or combustion; clearly, then, it is not the natural ligand for AHR. Several research groups have hunted for physiological compounds that bind to AHR (*96*). Adachi and colleagues

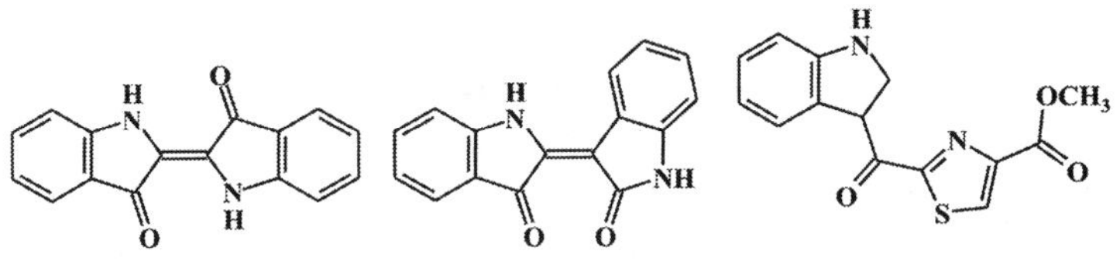

FIGURE 8-18.

Structures of agonists of the AH receptor isolated from human urine (indigo, indirubin) and porcine lung (ITE).

developed a yeast reporter gene assay for AHR ligands and performed bioassay-directed purification of active compounds found in human urine (*97*). Two compounds were isolated and identified: they proved to be *indigo*, the dark blue natural product dye used on fabrics such as blue jeans; and *indirubin*, a by-product of the synthesis of indigo (figure 8-18). Humans are often exposed to these common dye substances, and it is possible that they are also formed endogenously. Indirubin and indigo, like TCDD, induce P450 1A1 expression in rats (*98*).

Song et al. (*99*) used a similar strategy to isolate an AHR ligand from pig lung homogenate. A heroic effort, involving extraction, multiple rounds of HPLC separation, and microscale chemical characterization, including NMR analysis, was required for the purification and identification of 20 μg of the ligand, 2-(indole-3'-carbonyl)-thiazole-4-carboxylic acid methyl ester (ITE; figure 8-18), from 35 kg of lung tissue. ITE proved to be only slightly less potent than TCDD as an AHR ligand. The authors speculate that ITE is formed by condensation of the amino acids tryptophan and cysteine. The origins and biological significance of endogenous TCDD-like ligands are certainly of interest and will be a topic of much study in the future.

THE AH RECEPTOR: STUDIES WITH KNOCKOUT MICE

The use of knockout mice (see sidebar) has yielded further evidence of the physiological roles of the AH receptor (*100, 101*). AHR-deficient mice are viable and are highly resistant to TCDD toxicity, showing that the manifold toxic effects of TCDD are largely or entirely mediated by its binding to the receptor (*102*). This result had been expected but direct proof had been lacking. Benzo[*a*]pyrene (BP) is the prototype PAH carcinogen, metabolically activated to reactive DNA-binding species by P450 1 enzymes. BP is a skin carcinogen in mice. BP, like 3-MC, is an AH receptor agonist and a P450 1 inducer. In AH receptor knockout mice (*103*), BP treatment failed to induce P450 1A1 or 1A2 expression. Subcutaneous injection of BP did not cause any skin tumors in AH receptor knockout mice, even at doses that caused tumors in 100% of AHR-positive mice (both homozygous (+/+) and heterozygous (+/−) genotypes. This finding demonstrates dramatically the importance of the AH receptor in mediating the toxic effects of PAH. However, one should not conclude that the AH receptor is simply a mediator of toxic responses. Homozygous AH receptor knockout mice died at about one year of age, manifesting damage to many organs, including gastric hyperplasia, cardiomyopathy, and T-cell deficiency. These findings show that the receptor plays important roles in the maintenance of many types of cells.

▶ Knockout Mouse Technology

The era of modern molecular biology began with the emergence of techniques for preparing recombinant DNA. Next, specific genes were cloned and sequenced, and methods for expressing recombinant proteins were devised. With the invention of site-directed mutagenesis, it became possible to engineer specific sequence changes into proteins and study their effects on structure and function. Such approaches, while tremendously successful and informative, still leave us quite far removed from the original biological system: when we prepare a recombinant mammalian protein in, say, *E. coli* or yeast cells, we are studying the protein in isolation from its natural context. Classic genetics studied mutations of genes in situ, but mutants could only be obtained by screening or selecting organisms for phenotypes: finding a white-flowered pea plant or a UV-sensitive bacterium. A major advance in molecular biology since the late 1980s has been the emergence of systematic methods for making specific mutations of genes on chromosomes, in their native biological context, rather than working only with genes carried on vectors, such as plasmids or bacteriophage. This is usually done by relying on homologous recombination to replace the normal form of the gene by an engineered mutant form, introduced into the host cell. The most drastic alteration is a null mutation, in which the target gene is either deleted or disrupted by insertion of extraneous DNA: this is a "knockout". Knocking out a specific gene in a cell or organism can provide insight into the gene's normal biological role.

With the complete sequencing of many genomes, biologists are faced with the task of elucidating the functions of many proteins that are presently known only as DNA sequences in a database. Homologous recombination of introduced DNA constructs can be used for efficient generation of gene knockouts in unicellular organisms, including *E. coli* (104) and yeast (105). But how could gene replacement be accomplished in a mammal?

To engineer the genome of an animal, it is necessary to modify the DNA of a cell that can give rise to a gamete. The first successful method (dating to the early 1980s) for generation of transgenic animals was microinjection of DNA directly into the pronucleus of a fertilized mouse ovum (106). Many species of transgenic animals have subsequently been constructed by this route. However, despite its wide applicability, it suffers from major limitations. Integration of the foreign DNA into the chromosome occurs randomly (or at least with no obvious targeting) by nonhomologous (illegitimate) recombination, often at very low frequency. Consequently, this method cannot be used to mutagenize specific genes in the host organism. Also, the expression of the transgene depends on the site of insertion (and the number of inserted copies of the transgene, which often inserts as a concatemer), so phenotypic results are not easily predictable or reproducible.

An alternative route to transgenic animals, using homologous recombination in cultured embryonic stem (ES) cells in vitro, was developed in the late 1980s, notably through the achievements of Mario Capecchi and colleagues (107–110). This technique was made possible by advances in mouse embryology, culminating in the successful culturing of *pluripotent* (i.e., capable of differentiating into any cell type) stem cells derived from preimplantation mouse embryos. These cells can be propagated in vitro, maintaining an undifferentiated state; when they are introduced (by microinjection) into blastocyst stage mouse embryos, they can differentiate and form chimeras with the host embryo (111). In some cases, the ES-derived cell lineage will give rise to gametes, allowing the breeding of a strain whose cells are derived entirely from the ES cells.

The knockout mouse technique (figure 8-19) relies on the genetic manipulation of such ES cells in vitro. A DNA construct is prepared that carries sequences from the endogenous (target) gene, disrupted by the insertion of a gene carrying a selectable marker, usually the *neo* gene; cells carrying *neo* are resistant to the antibiotic G418. Another marker gene, *tk* (*thymidine kinase*) is also present on the construct, but the *tk* gene is *outside* the region of homology. ES cells are transfected with this construct, and, at a certain frequency, homologous recombination events occur, incorporating the construct into the target chromosome. (The mechanism of such homologous recombination is still poorly understood.) The (rare) recombinant cells are selected for, by culturing the cells in medium containing both neomycin and *gancyclovir*. Gancyclovir is a toxic nucleoside analogue; thymidine kinase catalyzes phosphorylation of gancyclovir, so that it is incorporated into newly synthesized DNA, killing the host cell. Consequently, only cells that have incorporated the *neo* gene but *not* the *tk* gene will survive and form colonies. The clones we seek have undergone replacement of the target gene by the knockout construct, effected by homologous recombination. This event will insert the *neo* gene, contained within the region of homology, but not the *tk* gene, which is outside the region of homology. Unwanted clones that have undergone random integration are likely to have integrated both the *neo* and *tk* genes, and will therefore be killed by gancyclovir. Thus, we can positively select in vitro for cells that have undergone the desired knockout event. Such cells, once characterized in vitro, are used to construct the knockout mouse, as follows.

The ES cells are injected into a blastocyst of a mouse strain with a fur color distinct from that of the ES cell animal, giving chimeric blastocysts, which are implanted into a "foster" mouse. The resulting litter is then examined for chimeric mice, which can be distinguished by their "patchy" (mixed) coat color. Chimeric mice are mated and offspring derived from gametes that are in turn derived from the recombinant ES cells are identified (again screening on the basis of coat color). These animals are heterozygous knockouts and inbreeding can be used to produce homozygous knockouts (if such animals are viable).

After more than a decade of application, knockout mouse technology has become routine. Surprisingly, however, the approach has not yet been extended to any other species. This is disappointing, since the rat, in particular, is a model organism of such importance in toxicology. The roadblock has been the failure to isolate pluripotent ES cells with properties equivalent to those of the mouse (112). Differences between rat and mouse embryology may be involved; see Brenin et al. for further discussion (113). The recent successful cloning of rats from adult somatic cells may provide an alternative route to knockout rats (114).

"Conditional" knockout mice are a recent extension of knockout technology, providing a measure of control over the localization of the knockout effect (115). This is done by flanking a target gene with DNA sequences recognized by a specific recombinase enzyme. The transgenic conditional knockout mouse is mated with a second transgenic mouse, which expresses the corresponding recombinase in specific tissues; in the progeny mice, this recombinase acts as a "molecular eraser" and removes the target gene. ◀

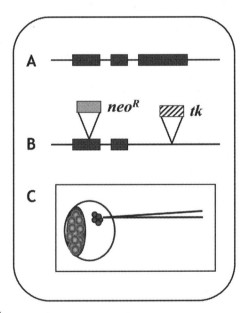

FIGURE 8-19.
Flow chart of the steps required for homologous recombination-mediated gene targeting ("knockouts") in mice. *Note*: A full-color version of this figure appears on the website. (*Adapted from web pages of the Transgenic Mouse Core Facility, University of Virginia.*)

P450 REGULATION BY NONTRANSCRIPTIONAL MECHANISMS

Before leaving the subject of P450 regulation, we should note that transcriptional activation is the major, but not the only, mechanism of regulation of P450 expression. In some cases, mRNA degradation and stabilization may also act as control mechanisms. P450 2E1 is induced by organic solvents, such as ethanol and acetone, and its regulation is effected, at least in part, posttranslationally, by protein stabilization (*116a*).

P450 posttranslational regulation by phosphorylation has also been examined (*116b*).

HUMAN P450 GENETIC VARIATION

In chapter 7, we noted that several human P450 enzymes are genetically polymorphic: allelic variants exist, with markedly altered, or completely absent, enzymatic activity. In several cases, these polymorphisms came to light when occasional individuals responded peculiarly to specific drugs; for example, suffering overdose toxicity because of reduced clearance. In other cases, polymorphisms were uncovered by routine DNA sequencing programs, as part of the human genome project. The list of known human P450 polymorphisms continues to grow, and up-to-date information can be obtained from the P450 Allele Nomenclature Committee internet home page at: http://www.imm.ki.se/CYPalleles/. A sample of the information posted on those pages is shown in table 8-4. Polymorphisms in the gene encoding cytochrome P450 2A6, an enzyme catalyzing nicotine oxidation, influence smoking behaviour (*117a*).

Genes that regulate P450 expression, such as the AH receptor gene, are also polymorphic (*117b*).

There appears to be a greater amount of genetic polymorphism (table 8-5) and a larger number of pseudogenes among P450 families 1–4, chiefly catalyzing xenobiotic metabolism, than among families P450 5–51, chiefly catalyzing metabolism of steroids and other endogenous compounds (*117c*). This difference might yet turn out to be an artifact resulting from increased scientific focus on the former group of enzymes, but it may be real. Perhaps genetic variation among the higher P450 families is more strongly selected against, because of the important physio-logical roles of steroid metabolites.

TABLE 8-4.
Selected Human P450 2A6 Polymorphisms

ALLELE	PROTEIN	NUCLEOTIDE CHANGES	EFFECT	ENZYME ACTIVITY	
				IN VIVO	IN VITRO
*CYP2A6*1A*	CYP2A6.1	None		Normal	Normal
*CYP2A6*1C*	CYP2A6.1	—395G → A; 51A → G; gene conversion in 3′ flanking region			
*CYP2A6*4B*		*CYP2A6* deleted	CYP2A6 deleted	None	
*CYP2A6*4D*		*CYP2A6* deleted	CYP2A6 deleted	None	
*CYP2A6*6*	CYP2A6.6	383G → A	R128Q		Decreased
*CYP2A6*11*	CYP2A6.11	670T → C	S224P	Decreased	Decreased

Data excerpted and adapted from the P450 Allele Nomenclature Committee internet home page. Following human genome conventions, the gene and allele designations are separated by an asterisk and Arabic numerals are used to number the alleles. Upper-case Roman letters are used for subclassification of alleles, as required to identify, for example, combinations of mutations that have already been given allele designations. The wild-type allele is normally designated as *1. Numbering: the A in the initiation codon (ATG) is +1 and the base before that A is −1. Gene conversion (CYP2A6*1C) is an event in which sequence from another gene (in this case, CYP2A7) has replaced the homologous sequence in a gene.

TABLE 8-5.

Some Important Human P450 Polymorphisms

P450 ENZYME	NATURE OF MUTATIONS OR POLYMORPHISMS	FREQUENCY	PHENOTYPIC EFFECTS
1B1	Null alleles	Very rare	Congenital glaucoma
2A6	Several missense alleles	Common, espcially in Oriental populations	Reduced clearance of nicotine
2C9	Several missense alleles; frameshift.	Uncommon	Reduced clearance of tolbutamide
2C19	Several missense alleles; nonsense; splicing defects	Common	Reduced clearance of mephenytoin, diazepam, omeprazole
2D6	Many (>65) missense alleles; also deletions and duplications (*117*)	Common	Reduced clearance of debrisoquine, nicotine, fluoxetine, tricyclic antidepressants, etc.

This is not a complete list; probably, all human P450 genes are polymorphic to some extent. Drugs usually identified with specific polymorphisms are underlined.

Genetic polymorphisms can affect any aspect of the genetic code. Single nucleotide polymorphisms (SNPs) within an open reading frame may result in amino acid substitutions or premature stop codons (nonsense mutations), and they may also affect RNA message stability. SNPs upstream of coding sequences or within introns may alter transcription initiation or regulation, or interfere with splicing. A larger-scale pattern of polymorphism is the deletion or duplication/multiplication of entire genes, and there are several examples of these phenomena affecting human P450 genes, as we discuss next.

Duplication of a gene is likely to result in an approximate doubling of mRNA levels and enzyme activity. This is observed, for example, with P450 2D6. Duplicate (or multiplicate) 2D6 copies are found in some individuals (*118*), who consequently have elevated clearance of drugs such as tricyclic antidepressants. P450 2D6 duplications are particularly common among populations in Saudi Arabia and Ethiopia, and elevated frequencies of this genotype in some European countries, such as Spain, probably reflect the influence of the Muslim expansion into Europe after 700 (*119*).

As with P450 induction and inhibition phenomena, genetic polymorphisms affecting P450 enzymes can have major clinical implications with regard to drug efficacy and safety (*120*). The P450 2D6 (debrisoquine) polymorphism is an important case. Adverse reactions to tricyclic antidepressant drugs are as much as twice as common among individuals with inactive P450 2D6 alleles (*121*). A remarkable and tragic illustration of the impact of the 2D6 polymorphism occurred in Pennsylvania in 1995 (*122, 123*). A nine-year-old boy was under treatment for Tourette's disorder and serious behavioral problems. After prolonged administration of several drugs, including clonidine and fluoxetine, he suffered convulsions and died. Forensic analysis indicated such a high blood level of fluoxetine that the parents were suspected of murder. However, fluoxetine and its metabolite norfluoxetine were present at similar levels, as is expected when metabolism reaches a steady state, after weeks of therapy. And no capsules of drug were present in the stomach, as one would have expected in a case of deliberate overdose. Genetic testing proved that the child was a P450 2D6 poor metabolizer. The parents were exonerated. Probably, several factors contributed to the fatal outcome: simultaneous administration of too many drugs; inadequate clinical management and observation; and insufficient medical awareness of the implications of pharmacokinetic variability.

PHARMACOGENETICS

As we have seen, genetic factors can result in major differences between individuals' metabolism of drugs and xenobiotics. This is not a particularly new observation; it dates back at least to 1960, with the discovery of NAT2 slow acetylators (see chapter 13). However, the development of technologies such as PCR for rapid analysis of DNA sequence variations has expanded our understanding of genetic factors in pharmacology, culminating in the emergence of a new discipline called "pharmacogenetics" accompanied by dedicated conferences and scientific journals. In the popular imagination also, the prospect of genetics-based therapeutics has received much attention. The scenario often presented is of a future medical practice in which individuals would be characterized genetically before the administration of a drug. A physician, consulting the results of this DNA analysis, would then recommend the most appropriate therapy. Certain drugs might be avoided because of an increased risk of side effects, as might occur with poor-metabolizer individuals. In other cases, particular drugs might be recommended because of expected efficacy. The prospect is for reduced incidence of adverse drug reactions and improved therapeutics responses. As one commentator suggested, "to apply ... pharmacogenetic knowledge to clinical practise, specific dosage recommendations based on genotypes will have to be developed to guide the clinician ... Such development will lead to a patient-tailored drug therapy which ... will result in fewer adverse drug reactions" (124).

Genetics-based drug therapy certainly sounds appealing. The deepening scientific understanding of the enzymatic basis of xenobiotic metabolism, which is a principal theme of this textbook, should, one hopes, provide the underpinning for such a pharmacological New Age. However, to date, the impact of pharmacogenetics on clinical practice has been slight (125, 126). At this time, there is only one clinical situation in which genetic testing is mandated before drug therapy: the thiopurine methyltransferase (TPMT) polymorphism (127). TPMT catalyzes an important detoxication step in metabolism of thiopurine anticancer drugs, such as 6-thioguanine. A thiopurine slow-metabolizer phenotype is rather common. These drugs have a relatively narrow therapeutic "window," and an elevated plasma level puts the patient at increased risk of potentially fatal myelosuppression. Preliminary genotyping can identify many of the high-risk patients, and doses can be adjusted accordingly. But the TPMT instance remains exceptional. Even in the case of isoniazid therapy for tuberculosis (see chapter 13), where the genetic basis of increased risk of drug toxicity has been known for decades, drug administration is still performed on a "one dose fits all" basis.

Why has pharmacogenetic testing not been adopted more rapidly into medical practice? First, genetic characterization of individual patients, even with regard to a specific polymorphic enzyme, remains a specialized laboratory analysis. When many different polymorphic alleles of a given gene exist (e.g., *CYP2D6*), a single analysis may not suffice to characterize an individual's status. Complete sequencing of a multi-exon gene is still an ambitious project, at least in terms of routine clinical practice. So the prospect of simply pipetting a drop of blood onto a chip and reading out the results within a few minutes, as conveyed by some media reports, is still a long way off. Genotyping might take several days, and in many clinical situations (e.g., treatment of acute infections), such delay is intolerable.

Furthermore, any specific gene is merely one of a large number of factors affecting individual drug metabolism. Other important factors include diet (especially the use of specific dietary supplements or herbal remedies), age, body mass, simultaneous use of inhibiting or inducing drugs, and so on. The most important hepatic P450 enzyme, 3A4, shows wide interindividual variation in activity, but P450 3A4 genetic polymorphisms account for little or none of this variation (*128*). Research has shown that, in most cases, the genetic, environmental, and physiological determinants of drug response are so complex that it is not useful to adjust drug doses on the basis of any single variable.

There are, as we have noted, certain drugs whose metabolic clearance is determined substantially by a single P450 (or other) enzyme. However, even if we limit our consideration to these drugs, and to genetic determinants of pharmacokinetics, analyzing a single gene is still likely to be insufficient. For example, even the genes that encode regulatory factors, such as PXR (*129*) and the AH receptor (*130*), are themselves polymorphic. And for most drugs, many enzymes contribute to the metabolic fate. Generally, during the drug development process, pharmaceutical companies try to screen out new chemical entities for which a single highly polymorphic enzyme (e.g., P450 2D6) dominates the metabolic fate. The companies are well aware of the potential adverse reactions that might result. As such drugs become less common, the need for pharmacogenetic testing also becomes less.

Why is preliminary genetic testing necessary in the case of 6-thioguanine and TPMT? In this case: (i) treatment can be put off a few days, until genotyping is completed; (ii) there are few, if any, effective alternative drugs; and (iii) the consequences of a TPMT slow metabolizer phenotype can be fatal, because myelosuppression can lead to life-threatening infections (*131*). These considerations do not apply to most drugs. For most pharmaceuticals, the therapeutic index (i.e., the ratio between the toxic dose and the therapeutic dose) is relatively high; side effects are usually controllable; and most drugs have half-lives of only a few hours. So, if a patient encounters toxicity related to unusually elevated plasma levels, the physician can simply reduce the drug dose or lengthen the interval between doses. This sort of empirical approach is sufficient to adjust for most factors that alter drug kinetics; genetic testing is unnecessary.

Since some P450 enzymes catalyze reactions of carcinogen activation or detoxication, P450 polymorphisms might affect individual risk of disease

294 • ENZYMOLOGY OF BIOTRANSFORMATION

due to environmental chemical exposures. Many studies have examined this hypothesis, with regard to, for example, the polymorphism affecting P450 1A1 expression. As yet, there are no unequivocal examples of associations between particular polymorphisms and cancer risk (*132*). The factors that confound the use of pharmacogenetic analyses to predict drug response, as discussed above, also pertain to studies of gene–environment interactions, with the further difficulty that xenobiotic exposures are generally far less well defined than drug exposures.

Notes

1. Agent Orange was named for the colored identification stripe painted on the barrels.

2. A. Poland, personal communication, 2003.

3. These effects appear to be absent in humans.

4. The name is a pun on Southern blots (DNA gels probed with oligonucleotide primers), which were introduced by Edwin Southern.

5. In this context, the term "receptor" refers to the fact that the protein binds a ligand (e.g., estrogen) with high affinity; nuclear receptors should not be confused with membrane-bound (cell surface) receptors, such as the adrenergic receptors.

6. The notable exception to this rule was the identification of the AH receptor, the protein that binds TCDD and mediates induction of P450 1A1 and other P450 1 family enzymes. As we discuss later in this chapter, the AH receptor was discovered by a "forward" search, based on its affinity for TCDD. The AH receptor protein is *not* a member of the nuclear receptor superfamily.

7. Hence the name PAS, for Per-Arnt-Sim.

8. This motif, found in many eukaryotic transcription factors, should not be confused with the similarly named "helix-turn-helix" found in prokaryotic DNA-binding proteins such as the *lac* repressor.

References

1. Spina, E.; Pisani, F.; Perucca, E. Clinically significant pharmacokinetic drug interactions with carbamazepine. An update. *Clin. Pharmacokinet.* **1996**, *31*, 198–214.
2. Durr, D.; Stieger, B.; Kullak-Ublick, G. A.; Rentsch, K. M.; Steinert, H. C.; Meier, P. J.; Fattinger, K. St John's Wort induces intestinal P-glycoprotein/MDR1 and intestinal and hepatic CYP3A4. *Clin. Pharmacol. Ther.* **2000**, *68*, 598–604.
3. Mathijssen, R. H.; Verweij, J.; de Bruijn, P.; Loos, W. J.; Sparreboom, A. Effects of St. John's wort on irinotecan metabolism. *J. Natl. Cancer Inst.* **2002**, *94*, 1247–1249.
4. Ioannides, C. Pharmacokinetic interactions between herbal remedies and medicinal drugs. *Xenobiotica* **2002**, *32*, 451–478.
5. Richardson, H. L.; Stier, A. R.; Borsos-Nachtnebel, E. Liver tumour inhibition and adrenal histologic responses in rats to which 3′-methyl-4-dimethylaminoazobenzene and 20-methyl-cholanthrene were simultaneously administered. *Cancer Res.* **1952**, *12*, 356–361.
6. Conney, A. H. Induction of drug-metabolizing enzymes: a path to the discovery of multiple cytochromes P450. *Annu. Rev. Pharmacol. Toxicol.* **2003**, *43*, 1–30.

7. Birnbaum, L. S.; Tuomisto, J. Non-carcinogenic effects of TCDD in animals. *Food Addit. Contam.* **2000,** *17,* 275–288.

8. Hook, G. E.; Haseman, J. K.; Lucier, G. W. Induction and suppression of hepatic and extrahepatic microsomal foreign-compound-metabolizing enzyme systems by 2,3,7,8-tetrachlorodibenzo-p-dioxin. *Chem. Biol. Interact.* **1975,** *10,* 199–214.

9. Stellman, J. M.; Stellman, S. D.; Christian, R.; Weber, T.; Tomasallo, C. The extent and patterns of usage of Agent Orange and other herbicides in Vietnam. *Nature* **2003,** *422,* 681–687.

10. Signorini, S.; Gerthoux, P. M.; Dassi, C.; Cazzaniga, M.; Brambilla, P.; Vincoli, N.; Mocarelli, P. Environmental exposure to dioxin: the Seveso experience. *Andrologia* **2000,** *32,* 263–270.

11. Alvares, A. P.; Bickers, D. R.; Kappas, A. Polychlorinated biphenyls: a new type of inducer of cytochrome P-448 in the liver. *Proc. Natl. Acad. Sci. USA* **1973,** *70,* 1321–1325.

12. Czygan, P.; Greim, H.; Garro, A. J.; Hutterer, F.; Schaffner, F.; Popper, H.; Rosenthal, O.; Cooper, D. Y. Microsomal metabolism of dimethyl-nitrosamine and the cytochrome P-450 dependency of its activation to a mutagen. *Cancer Res.* **1973,** *33,* 2983–2986.

13. Ames, B. N.; Durston, W. E.; Yamasaki, E.; Lee, F. D. Carcinogens are mutagens: a simple test system combining liver homogenates for activation and bacteria for detection. *Proc. Natl. Acad. Sci. USA* **1973,** *70,* 2281–2285.

14. Elliott, B. M.; Combes, R. D.; Elcombe, C. R.; Gatehouse, D. G.; Gibson, G. G.; Mackay, J. M.; Wolf, R. C. Alternatives to Aroclor 1254-induced S9 in in vitro genotoxicity assays. *Mutagenesis* **1992,** *7,* 175–177.

15. Remmer, H.; Merker, H. J. Drug-induced changes in the liver endoplasmic reticulum: association with drug-metabolizing enzymes. *Science* **1963,** *142,* 1657–1658.

16. Waxman, D. J.; Azaroff, L. Phenobarbital induction of cytochrome P-450 gene expression. *Biochem. J.* **1992,** *281,* 577–592.

17. Orrenius, S.; Ericsson, J. L.; Ernster, L. Phenobarbital-induced synthesis of the microsomal drug-metabolizing enzyme system and its relationship to the proliferation of endoplasmic membranes. A morphological and biochemical study. *J. Cell Biol.* **1965,** *25,* 627–639.

18. Tanaka, T.; Watanabe, J.; Asaka, Y.; Ogawa, R.; Kanamura, S. Quantitative analysis of endoplasmic reticulum and cytochrome P-450 in hepatocytes from rats injected with methylcholanthrene. *Eur. J. Cell Biol.* **1997,** *74,* 20–30.

19. Poland, A.; Mak, I.; Glover, E.; Boatman, R. J.; Ebetino, F. H.; Kende, A. S. 1,4-Bis[2-(3,5-dichloropyridyloxy)]benzene, a potent phenobarbital-like inducer of microsomal monooxygenase activity. *Mol. Pharmacol.* **1980,** *18,* 571–580.

20. Kourounakis, P.; Selye, H.; Tache, Y. Catatoxic steroids. *Adv. Steroid Biochem. Pharmacol.* **1977,** *6,* 35–57.

21. Lieber, C. S.; DeCarli, L. M. Ethanol oxidation by hepatic microsomes: adaptive increase after ethanol feeding. *Science* **1968,** *162,* 917–918.

22. Rubin, E.; Lieber, C. S. Hepatic microsomal enzymes in man and rat: induction and inhibition by ethanol. *Science* **1968,** *162,* 690–691.

23. Hu, Y.; Ingelman-Sundberg, M.; Lindros, K. O. Induction mechanisms of cytochrome P450 2E1 in liver: interplay between ethanol treatment and starvation. *Biochem. Pharmacol.* **1995,** *50,* 155–161.

24. Dzhekova-Stojkova, S.; Bogdanska, J.; Stojkova, Z. Peroxisome prolif- erators: their biological and toxicological effects. *Clin. Chem. Lab. Med.* **2001,** *39,* 468–474.

25. Johnson, E. F.; Palmer, C. N.; Griffin, K. J.; Hsu, M. H. Role of the peroxisome proliferator-activated receptor in cytochrome P450 4A gene regulation. *FASEB J.* **1996,** *10,* 1241–1248.

26. Hoen, P. A.; Bijsterbosch, M. K.; van Berkel, T. J.; Vermeulen, N. P.; Commandeur, J. N. Midazolam is a phenobarbital-like cytochrome P450 inducer in rats. *J. Pharmacol. Exp. Ther.* **2001,** *299,* 921–927.

27. O'Connell, J. The basics of RT-PCR. Some practical considerations. *Methods Mol. Biol.* **2002,** *193,* 19–25.

28. Howbrook, D. N.; van der Valk, A. M.; O'Shaughnessy, M. C.; Sarker, D. K.; Baker, S. C.; Lloyd, A. W. Developments in microarray technologies. *Drug Discov. Today* **2003,** *8,* 642–651.

29. Bartosiewicz, M. J.; Jenkins, D.; Penn, S.; Emery, J.; Buckpitt, A. Unique gene expression patterns in liver and kidney associated with exposure to chemical toxicants. *J. Pharmacol. Exp. Ther.* **2001,** *297,* 895–905.

30. Naylor, L. H. Reporter gene technology: the future looks bright. *Biochem. Pharmacol.* **1999,** *58,* 749–757.

31. Sussman, H. E. Choosing the best reporter assay. *The Scientist* **2001,** *15,* 25.

32. Alberts, B.; Johnson, A.; Lewis, J.; Raff, M.; Roberts, K.; Walter, P. *Molecular Biology of the Cell*; Garland Science: New York, 2002.

33. Green, S.; Walter, P.; Kumar, V.; Krust, A.; Bornert, J. M.; Argos, P.; Chambon, P. Human oestrogen receptor cDNA: sequence, expression and homology to v-erb-A. *Nature* **1986,** *320,* 134–139.

34. Green, S.; Kumar, V.; Krust, A.; Walter, P.; Chambon, P. Structural and functional domains of the estrogen receptor. *Cold Spring Harb. Symp. Quant. Biol.* **1986,** *51,* 751–758.

35. Petkovich, M.; Brand, N. J.; Krust, A.; Chambon, P. A human retinoic acid receptor which belongs to the family of nuclear receptors. *Nature* **1987,** *330,* 444–450.

36. Chambon, P. How I became one of the fathers of a superfamily. *Nat. Med.* **2004,** *10,* 1027–1031.

37. Dumas, B.; Harding, H. P.; Choi, H. S.; Lehmann, K. A.; Chung, M.; Lazar, M. A.; Moore, D. D. A new orphan member of the nuclear hormone receptor superfamily closely related to Rev-Erb. *Mol. Endocrinol.* **1994,** *8,* 996–1005.

38. Chawla, A.; Repa, J. J.; Evans, R. M.; Mangelsdorf, D. J. Nuclear receptors and lipid physiology: opening the X-files. *Science* **2001,** *294,* 1866–1870.

39. Berg, J. M.; Tymoczko, J. L.; Stryer, L. *Biochemistry*; WH Freeman: New York, 2001.

40. Pike, A. C.; Brzozowski, A. M.; Hubbard, R. E. A structural biologist's view of the oestrogen receptor. *J. Steroid Biochem. Mol. Biol.* **2000,** *74,* 261–268.

41. Blumberg, B.; Evans, R. M. Orphan nuclear receptors: new ligands and new possibilities. *Genes Dev.* **1998,** *12,* 3149–3155.

42. Pascussi, J. M.; Gerbal-Chaloin, S.; Drocourt, L.; Maurel, P.; Vilarem, M. J. The expression of CYP2B6, CYP2C9 and CYP3A4 genes: a tangle of networks of nuclear and steroid receptors. *Biochim. Biophys. Acta* **2003,** *1619,* 243–253.

43. Chambon, P. A decade of molecular biology of retinoic acid receptors. *FASEB J.* **1996,** *10,* 940–954.

44. Mangelsdorf, D. J.; Ong, E. S.; Dyck, J. A.; Evans, R. M. Nuclear receptor that identifies a novel retinoic acid response pathway. *Nature* **1990**, *345*, 224–229.

45. Yang, N.; Schule, R.; Mangelsdorf, D. J.; Evans, R. M. Characterization of DNA binding and retinoic acid binding properties of retinoic acid receptor. *Proc. Natl. Acad. Sci. USA* **1991**, *88*, 3559–3563.

46. Heyman, R. A.; Mangelsdorf, D. J.; Dyck, J. A.; Stein, R. B.; Eichele, G.; Evans, R. M.; Thaller, C. 9-*cis*-retinoic acid is a high affinity ligand for the retinoid X receptor. *Cell* **1992**, *68*, 397–406.

47. Bastien, J.; Rochette-Egly, C. Nuclear retinoid receptors and the transcription of retinoid-target genes. *Gene* **2004**, *328*, 1–16.

48. Trottier, E.; Belzil, A.; Stoltz, C.; Anderson, A. Localization of a phenobarbital-responsive element (PBRE) in the 5′-flanking region of the rat CYP2B2 gene. *Gene* **1995**, *158*, 263–268.

49. Sueyoshi, T.; Kawamoto, T.; Zelko, I.; Honkakoski, P.; Negishi, M. The repressed nuclear receptor CAR responds to phenobarbital in activating the human CYP2B6 gene. *J. Biol. Chem.* **1999**, *274*, 6043–6046.

50. Sueyoshi, T.; Negishi, M. Phenobarbital response elements of cytochrome P450 genes and nuclear receptors. *Annu. Rev. Pharmacol. Toxicol.* **2001**, *41*, 123–143.

51. Honkakoski, P.; Zelko, I.; Sueyoshi, T.; Negishi, M. The nuclear orphan receptor CAR-retinoid X receptor heterodimer activates the phenobarbital-responsive enhancer module of the CYP2B gene. *Mol. Cell Biol.* **1998**, *18*, 5652–5658.

52. Moore, L. B.; Parks, D. J.; Jones, S. A.; Bledsoe, R. K.; Consler, T. G.; Stimmel, J. B.; Goodwin, B.; Liddle, C.; Blanchard, S. G.; Willson, T. M.; Collins, J. L.; Kliewer, S. A. Orphan nuclear receptors constitutive androstane receptor and pregnane X receptor share xenobiotic and steroid ligands. *J. Biol. Chem.* **2000**, *275*, 15122–15127.

53. Moore, L. B.; Goodwin, B.; Jones, S. A.; Wisely, G. B.; Serabjit-Singh, C. J.; Willson, T. M.; Collins, J. L.; Kliewer, S. A. St. John's wort induces hepatic drug metabolism through activation of the pregnane X receptor. *Proc. Natl. Acad. Sci. USA* **2000**, *97*, 7500–7502.

54. Cook, N. D. Scintillation proximity assay: a versatile high-throughput screening technology. *Drug Discov. Today* **1996**, *1*, 287–294.

55. Wang, H.; LeCluyse, E. L. Role of orphan nuclear receptors in the regulation of drug-metabolising enzymes. *Clin. Pharmacokinet.* **2003**, *42*, 1331–1357.

56. Swales, K.; Negishi, M. CAR, driving into the future. *Mol. Endocrinol.* **2004**, *18*, 1589–1598.

57. Kakizaki, S.; Yamamoto, Y.; Ueda, A.; Moore, R.; Sueyoshi, T.; Negishi, M. Phenobarbital induction of drug/steroid-metabolizing enzymes and nuclear receptor CAR. *Biochim. Biophys. Acta* **2003**, *1619*, 239–242.

58. Wei, P.; Zhang, J.; Egan-Hafley, M.; Liang, S.; Moore, D. D. The nuclear receptor CAR mediates specific xenobiotic induction of drug metabolism. *Nature* **2000**, *407*, 920–923.

59. Zhang, J.; Huang, W.; Chua, S. S.; Wei, P.; Moore, D. D. Modulation of acetaminophen-induced hepatotoxicity by the xenobiotic receptor CAR. *Science* **2002**, *298*, 422–424.

60. Choi, H. S.; Chung, M.; Tzameli, I.; Simha, D.; Lee, Y. K.; Seol, W.; Moore, D. D. Differential transactivation by two isoforms of the orphan nuclear hormone receptor CAR. *J. Biol. Chem.* **1997**, *272*, 23565–23571.

61. Kakizaki, S.; Karami, S.; Negishi, M. Retinoic acids repress constitutive active receptor-mediated induction by 1,4-*bis*[2-(3,5-dichloropyridyloxy)] benzene of the CYP2B10 gene in mouse primary hepatocytes. *Drug Metab. Dispos.* **2002**, *30*, 208–211.

62. Moore, J. T.; Moore, L. B.; Maglich, J. M.; Kliewer, S. A. Functional and structural comparison of PXR and CAR. *Biochim. Biophys. Acta* **2003**, *1619*, 235–238.

63. Wei, P.; Zhang, J.; Dowhan, D. H.; Han, Y.; Moore, D. D. Specific and overlapping functions of the nuclear hormone receptors CAR and PXR in xenobiotic response. *Pharmacogenomics J.* **2002**, *2*, 117–126.

64. Willson, T. M.; Kliewer, S. A. PXR, CAR and drug metabolism. *Nat. Rev. Drug Discov.* **2002**, *1*, 259–266.

65. Honkakoski, P.; Sueyoshi, T.; Negishi, M. Drug-activated nuclear receptors CAR and PXR. *Ann. Med.* **2003**, *35*, 172–182.

66. Xie, W.; Barwick, J. L.; Downes, M.; Blumberg, B.; Simon, C. M.; Nelson, M. C.; Neuschwander-Tetri, B. A.; Brunt, E. M.; Guzelian, P. S.; Evans, R. M. Humanized xenobiotic response in mice expressing nuclear receptor SXR. *Nature* **2000**, *406*, 435–439.

67. Watkins, R. E.; Wisely, G. B.; Moore, L. B.; Collins, J. L.; Lambert, M. H.; Williams, S. P.; Willson, T. M.; Kliewer, S. A.; Redinbo, M. R. The human nuclear xenobiotic receptor PXR: structural determinants of directed promiscuity. *Science* **2001**, *292*, 2329–2333.

68. Gillam, E. M. The PXR ligand-binding domain: how to be picky and promiscuous at the same time. *Trends Pharmacol. Sci.* **2001**, *22*, 448.

69. Watkins, R. E.; Maglich, J. M.; Moore, L. B.; Wisely, G. B.; Noble, S. M.; Davis-Searles, P. R.; Lambert, M. H.; Kliewer, S. A.; Redinbo, M. R. 2.1 Å crystal structure of human PXR in complex with the St. John's wort compound hyperforin. *Biochemistry* **2003**, *42*, 1430–1438.

70. LeCluyse, E. L. Pregnane X receptor: molecular basis for species differences in CYP3A induction by xenobiotics. *Chem. Biol. Interact.* **2001**, *134*, 283–289.

71. Handschin, C.; Meyer, U. A. Regulatory network of lipid-sensing nuclear receptors: roles for CAR, PXR, LXR, and FXR. *Arch. Biochem. Biophys.* **2005**, *433*, 387–396.

72. Holick, M. F. Stay tuned to PXR: an orphan actor that may not be D-structive only to bone. *J. Clin. Invest.* **2005**, *115*, 32–34.

73. Lee, S. S.; Pineau, T.; Drago, J.; Lee, E. J.; Owens, J. W.; Kroetz, D. L.; Fernandez-Salguero, P. M.; Westphal, H.; Gonzalez, F. J. Targeted disruption of the alpha isoform of the peroxisome proliferator-activated receptor gene in mice results in abolishment of the pleiotropic effects of peroxisome proliferators. *Mol. Cell Biol.* **1995**, *15*, 3012–3022.

74. Tugwood, J. D.; Montague, C. T. Biology and toxicology of PPARγ ligands. *Hum. Exp. Toxicol.* **2002**, *21*, 429–437.

75. Wang, Y. X.; Lee, C. H.; Tiep, S.; Yu, R. T.; Ham, J.; Kang, H.; Evans, R. M. Peroxisome-proliferator-activated receptor delta activates fat metabolism to prevent obesity. *Cell* **2003**, *113*, 159–170.

76. Akiyama, T. E.; Nicol, C. J.; Gonzalez, F. J. On par with PPARs. *Trends Genet.* **2001**, *17*, 310–312.

77. Corton, J. C.; Anderson, S. P.; Stauber, A. Central role of peroxisome proliferator-activated receptors in the actions of peroxisome proliferators. *Annu. Rev. Pharmacol. Toxicol.* **2000**, *40*, 491–518.

78. Nebert, D. W.; Dalton, T. P.; Okey, A. B.; Gonzalez, F. J. Role of aryl hydrocarbon receptor-mediated induction of the CYP1 enzymes in environmental toxicity and cancer. *J. Biol. Chem.* **2004,** *279,* 23847–23850.

79. Chapman, D. E.; Schiller, C. M. Dose-related effects of 2,3,7,8-tetrachlorodibenzo-p-dioxin (TCDD) in C57BL/6J and DBA/2J mice. *Toxicol. Appl. Pharmacol.* **1985,** *78,* 147–157.

80. Poland, A.; Glover, E.; Kende, A. S. Stereospecific, high affinity binding of 2,3,7,8-tetrachlorodibenzo-p-dioxin by hepatic cytosol. Evidence that the binding species is receptor for induction of aryl hydrocarbon hydroxylase. *J. Biol. Chem.* **1976,** *251,* 4936–4946.

81. Poland, A.; Glover, E.; Ebetino, F. H.; Kende, A. S. Photoaffinity labeling of the AH receptor. *J. Biol. Chem.* **1986,** *261,* 6352–6365.

82. Burbach, K. M.; Poland, A.; Bradfield, C. A. Cloning of the AH-receptor cDNA reveals a distinctive ligand-activated transcription factor. *Proc. Natl. Acad. Sci. USA* **1992,** *89,* 8185–8189.

83. Ema, M.; Sogawa, K.; Watanabe, N.; Chujoh, Y.; Matsushita, N.; Gotoh, O.; Funae, Y.; Fujii-Kuriyama, Y. cDNA cloning and structure of mouse putative AH receptor. *Biochem. Biophys. Res. Commun.* **1992,** *184,* 246–253.

84. Pongratz, I.; Antonsson, C.; Whitelaw, M. L.; Poellinger, L. Role of the PAS domain in regulation of dimerization and DNA binding specificity of the dioxin receptor. *Mol. Cell Biol.* **1998,** *18,* 4079–4088.

85. Taylor, B. L.; Zhulin, I. B. PAS domains: internal sensors of oxygen, redox potential, and light. *Microbiol. Mol. Biol. Rev.* **1999,** *63,* 479–506.

86. Atchley, W. R.; Fitch, W. M. A natural classification of the basic helix-loop-helix class of transcription factors. *Proc. Natl. Acad. Sci. USA* **1997,** *94,* 5172–5176.

87. Nelson, D. L.; Cox, M. M. *Lehninger Principles of Biochemistry*; Worth Publishers: New York, 2004.

88. Perdew, G. H. Association of the AH receptor with the 90-kDa heat shock protein. *J. Biol. Chem.* **1988,** *263,* 13802–13805.

89. Ma, Q.; Whitlock, J. P., Jr. A novel cytoplasmic protein that interacts with the AH receptor, contains tetratricopeptide repeat motifs, and augments the transcriptional response to 2,3,7,8-tetrachlorodibenzo-p-dioxin. *J. Biol. Chem.* **1997,** *272,* 8878–8884.

90. Petrulis, J. R.; Perdew, G. H. The role of chaperone proteins in the aryl hydrocarbon receptor core complex. *Chem. Biol. Interact.* **2002,** *141,* 25–40.

91. Hoffman, E. C.; Reyes, H.; Chu, F. F.; Sander, F.; Conley, L. H.; Brooks, B. A.; Hankinson, O. Cloning of a factor required for activity of the AH (dioxin) receptor. *Science* **1991,** *252,* 954–958.

92. Kumar, M. B.; Tarpey, R. W.; Perdew, G. H. Differential recruitment of coactivator RIP140 by AH and estrogen receptors. Absence of a role for LXXLL motifs. *J. Biol. Chem.* **1999,** *274,* 22155–22164.

93. Bacsi, S. G.; Reisz-Porszasz, S.; Hankinson, O. Orientation of the heterodimeric aryl hydrocarbon (dioxin) receptor complex on its asymmetric DNA recognition sequence. *Mol. Pharmacol.* **1995,** *47,* 432–438.

94. Fujisawa-Sehara, A.; Sogawa, K.; Yamane, M.; Fujii-Kuriyama, Y. Characterization of xenobiotic responsive elements upstream from the drug-metabolizing cytochrome P-450c gene: a similarity to glucocorticoid regulatory elements. *Nucleic Acids Res.* **1987,** *15,* 4179–4191.

95. Martinez, J. M.; Afshari, C. A.; Bushel, P. R.; Masuda, A.; Takahashi, T.; Walker, N. J. Differential toxicogenomic responses to 2,3,7,8-tetrachlorodibenzo-p-dioxin in malignant and nonmalignant human airway epithelial cells. *Toxicol. Sci.* **2002,** *69,* 409–423.

96. Denison, M. S.; Nagy, S. R. Activation of the aryl hydrocarbon receptor by structurally diverse exogenous and endogenous chemicals. *Annu. Rev. Pharmacol. Toxicol.* **2003,** *43,* 309–334.

97. Adachi, J.; Mori, Y.; Matsui, S.; Takigami, H.; Fujino, J.; Kitagawa, H.; Miller, C. A., III; Kato, T.; Saeki, K.; Matsuda, T. Indirubin and indigo are potent aryl hydrocarbon receptor ligands present in human urine. *J. Biol. Chem.* **2001,** *276,* 31475–31478.

98. Guengerich, F. P.; Martin, M. V.; McCormick, W. A.; Nguyen, L. P.; Glover, E.; Bradfield, C. A. Aryl hydrocarbon receptor response to indigoids in vitro and in vivo. *Arch. Biochem. Biophys.* **2004,** *423,* 309–316.

99. Song, J.; Clagett-Dame, M.; Peterson, R. E.; Hahn, M. E.; Westler, W. M.; Sicinski, R. R.; DeLuca, H. F. A ligand for the aryl hydrocarbon receptor isolated from lung. *Proc. Natl. Acad. Sci. USA* **2002,** *99,* 14694–14699.

100. Fernandez-Salguero, P. M.; Hilbert, D. M.; Rudikoff, S.; Ward, J. M.; Gonzalez, F. J. Aryl-hydrocarbon receptor-deficient mice are resistant to 2,3,7,8-tetrachlorodibenzo-p-dioxin-induced toxicity. *Toxicol. Appl. Pharmacol.* **1996,** *140,* 173–179.

101. Fernandez-Salguero, P. M.; Ward, J. M.; Sundberg, J. P.; Gonzalez, F. J. Lesions of aryl-hydrocarbon receptor-deficient mice. *Vet. Pathol.* **1997,** *34,* 605–614.

102. Mimura, J.; Fujii-Kuriyama, Y. Functional role of AhR in the expression of toxic effects by TCDD. *Biochim. Biophys. Acta* **2003,** *1619,* 263–268.

103. Shimizu, Y.; Nakatsuru, Y.; Ichinose, M.; Takahashi, Y.; Kume, H.; Mimura, J.; Fujii-Kuriyama, Y.; Ishikawa, T. Benzo[*a*]pyrene carcinogenicity is lost in mice lacking the aryl hydrocarbon receptor. *Proc. Natl. Acad. Sci. USA* **2000,** *97,* 779–782.

104. Datsenko, K. A.; Wanner, B. L. One-step inactivation of chromosomal genes in *Escherichia coli* K-12 using PCR products. *Proc. Natl. Acad. Sci. USA* **2000,** *97,* 6640–6645.

105. Baudin, A.; Ozier-Kalogeropoulos, O.; Denouel, A.; Lacroute, F.; Cullin, C. A simple and efficient method for direct gene deletion in *Saccharomyces cerevisiae. Nucleic Acids Res.* **1993,** *21,* 3329–3330.

106. Gordon, J. W.; Ruddle, F. H. Integration and stable germ line transmission of genes injected into mouse pronuclei. *Science* **1981,** *214,* 1244–1246.

107. Doetschman, T.; Gregg, R. G.; Maeda, N.; Hooper, M. L.; Melton, D. W.; Thompson, S.; Smithies, O. Targetted correction of a mutant HPRT gene in mouse embryonic stem cells. *Nature* **1987,** *330,* 576–578.

108. Capecchi, M. R. Targeted gene replacement. *Sci. Am.* **1994,** *270,* 52–59.

109. Capecchi, M. R. Altering the genome by homologous recombination. *Science* **1989,** *244,* 1288–1292.

110. Mansour, S. L.; Thomas, K. R.; Capecchi, M. R. Disruption of the proto-oncogene int-2 in mouse embryo-derived stem cells: a general strategy for targeting mutations to non-selectable genes. *Nature* **1988,** *336,* 348–352.

111. Kaufman, M. H.; Evans, M. J.; Robertson, E. J.; Bradley, A. Influence of injected pluripotential (EK) cells on haploid and diploid parthenogenetic development. *J. Embryol. Exp. Morphol.* **1984,** *80,* 75–86.

112. Capecchi, M. R. How close are we to implementing gene targeting in animals other than the mouse? *Proc. Natl. Acad. Sci. USA* **2000,** *97,* 956–957.

113. Brenin, D.; Look, J.; Bader, M.; Hubner, N.; Levan, G.; Iannaccone, P. Rat embryonic stem cells: a progress report. *Transplant. Proc.* **1997**, *29*, 1761–1765.

114. Abbott, A. The renaissance rat. *Nature* **2004**, *428*, 464–466.

115. Kuhn, R.; Schwenk, F. Conditional knockout mice. *Methods Mol. Biol.* **2003**, *209*, 159–185.

116. (a) Chien, J. Y.; Thummel, K. E.; Slattery, J. T. Pharmacokinetic consequences of induction of CYP2E1 by ligand stabilization. *Drug Metab. Dispos.* **1997**, *25*, 1165–1175. (b) Oesch-Bartlomowicz, B.; Oesch, F. Phosphorylation of cytochromes P450: first discovery of a posttranslational modification of a drug-metabolizing enzyme. *Biochem. Biophys. Res. Commun.* (in press).

117. (a) Xu, C.; Goodz, S.; Sellers, E. M.; Tyndale, R. F. CYP2A6 genetic variation and potential consequences. *Adv. Drug Deliv. Rev.* **2002**, *54*, 1245–1256. (b) Okey, A. B.; Franc, M. A.; Moffat, I. D.; Tijet, N.; Boutros, P. C.; Korkalainen, M.; Tuomisto, J.; Pohjanvirta, R. Toxicological implications of polymorphisms in receptors for xenobiotic chemicals: the case of the aryl hydrocarbon receptor. *Toxicol. Appl. Pharmacol.* **2005**, *207* (Suppl. 2), 43–51. (c) Ingelman-Sundberg, M.; Rodriguez-Antona, C. Pharmacogenetics of drug-metabolizing enzymes: implications for a safer and more effective drug therapy. *Philos. Trans. R. Soc. Lond. B Biol. Sci.* **2005**, *360*, 1563–1570.

118. Sachse, C.; Brockmöller, J.; Bauer, S.; Roots, I. Cytochrome P450 2D6 variants in a Caucasian population: allele frequencies and phenotypic consequences. *Am. J. Hum. Genet.* **1997**, *60*, 284–295.

119. Ingelman-Sundberg, M.; Oscarson, M.; McLellan, R. A. Polymorphic human cytochrome P450 enzymes: an opportunity for individualized drug treatment. *Trends Pharmacol. Sci.* **1999**, *20*, 342–349.

120. Pillans, P. I. Increasing relevance of pharmacogenetics of drug metabolism in clinical practice. *Intern. Med. J.* **2001**, *31*, 476–478.

121. Chen, S.; Chou, W. H.; Blouin, R. A.; Mao, Z.; Humphries, L. L.; Meek, Q. C.; Neill, J. R.; Martin, W. L.; Hays, L. R.; Wedlund, P. J. The cytochrome P450 2D6 (CYP2D6) enzyme polymorphism: screening costs and influence on clinical outcomes in psychiatry. *Clin. Pharmacol. Ther.* **1996**, *60*, 522–534.

122. Sallee, F. R.; DeVane, C. L.; Ferrell, R. E. Fluoxetine-related death in a child with cytochrome P-450 2D6 genetic deficiency. *J. Child Adolesc. Psychopharmacol.* **2000**, *10*, 27–34.

123. Stipp, D. A DNA tragedy. *Fortune* **2000**, 171–184.

124. Oscarson, M. Pharmacogenetics of drug metabolising enzymes: importance for personalised medicine. *Clin. Chem. Lab Med.* **2003**, *41*, 573–580.

125. Weinshilboum, R.; Wang, L. Pharmacogenomics: bench to bedside. *Nat. Rev. Drug Discov.* **2004**, *3*, 739–748.

126. Lesko, L. J.; Woodcock, J. Opinion: translation of pharmacogenomics and pharmacogenetics: a regulatory perspective. *Nat. Rev. Drug Discov.* **2004**, *3*, 763–769.

127. Weinshilboum, R. Thiopurine pharmacogenetics: clinical and molecular studies of thiopurine methyltransferase. *Drug Metab. Dispos.* **2001**, *29*, 601–605.

128. Lamba, J. K.; Lin, Y. S.; Thummel, K.; Daly, A.; Watkins, P. B.; Ström, S.; Zhang, J.; Schuetz, E. G. Common allelic variants of

cytochrome P4503A4 and their prevalence in different populations. *Pharmacogenetics* **2002,** *12*, 121–132.

129. Zhang, J.; Kuehl, P.; Green, E. D.; Touchman, J. W.; Watkins, P. B.; Daly, A.; Hall, S. D.; Maurel, P.; Relling, M.; Brimer, C.; Yasuda, K.; Wrighton, S. A.; Hancock, M.; Kim, R. B.; Ström, S.; Thummel, K.; Russell, C. G.; Hudson, J. R., Jr.; Schuetz, E. G.; Boguski, M. S. The human pregnane X receptor: genomic structure and identification and functional characterization of natural allelic variants. *Pharmacogenetics* **2001,** *11*, 555–572.

130. Harper, P. A.; Wong, J. Y.; Lam, M. S.; Okey, A. B. Polymorphisms in the human AH receptor. *Chem. Biol. Interact.* **2002,** *141*, 161–187.

131. Lancaster, D. L.; Lennard, L.; Rowland, K.; Vora, A. J.; Lilleyman, J. S. Thioguanine versus mercaptopurine for therapy of childhood lymphoblastic leukaemia: a comparison of haematological toxicity and drug metabolite concentrations. *Br. J. Haematol.* **1998,** *102*, 439–443.

132. Vineis, P. The relationship between polymorphisms of xenobiotic metabolizing enzymes and susceptibility to cancer. *Toxicology* **2002,** *181–182*, 457–462.

INTRODUCTION

Glutathione (GSH, figure 9-1), the tripeptide γ-L-glutamyl-L-cysteinyl-glycine, participates in numerous biochemical processes, especially the maintenance of redox homeostasis and the trapping of electrophiles. In this chapter, we consider many of these reactions, with an emphasis on their chemical mechanisms. Subsequent chapters discuss glutathione transferases (enzymes that catalyze the reactions of GSH with electrophiles) and the toxicological and pharmacological aspects of GSH biochemistry.

OCCURRENCE OF GSH

GSH is the most abundant low-molecular-mass thiol in all mammalian cells (1, 2). The concentrations of GSH in human erythrocytes and in hepatocyte cytosol are approximately 2 mM and 10 mM, respectively. The luminal mucus of the intestine contains up to 0.3 mM GSH, derived from the bile as well as from the food (3). The epithelial lining fluid has a similar GSH content; in the lung alveoli it is less than about 0.5 mM. Extracellular media, such as blood plasma and cerebrospinal fluid, contain lower (micromolar) but still significant concentrations (4).

GSH fulfills many important functions in the cell. In its protective role, GSH defends cellular targets against oxidative and electrophilic chemical species. Another central function is to serve as a reducing cofactor in the biosynthesis of deoxyribonucleotides (5). GSH also contributes to the redox regulation of molecular processes in different cellular compartments (6) and is a carrier of signal molecules such as nitric oxide (7) and certain eicosanoids (8).

ALTERNATIVES TO GSH

Most eukaryotes and many aerobic prokaryotes contain GSH (9). In certain plants, such as the mung bean (*Phaseolus aureus*) and other legumes, the similar compound *homoglutathione*, γ-L-glutamyl-L-cysteinyl-β-alanine (figure 9-1), replaces GSH as the most abundant thiol (10, 11). Functionally, this replacement seems to make little difference, since GSH-dependent enzymes accept homoglutathione as a substitute. Mycobacteria and streptomycetes contain millimolar concentrations of *mycothiol* (figure 9-2) instead of GSH (12). Both GSH S-conjugates and S-conjugates of mycothiol are metabolized to mercapturates, as discussed later in this chapter.

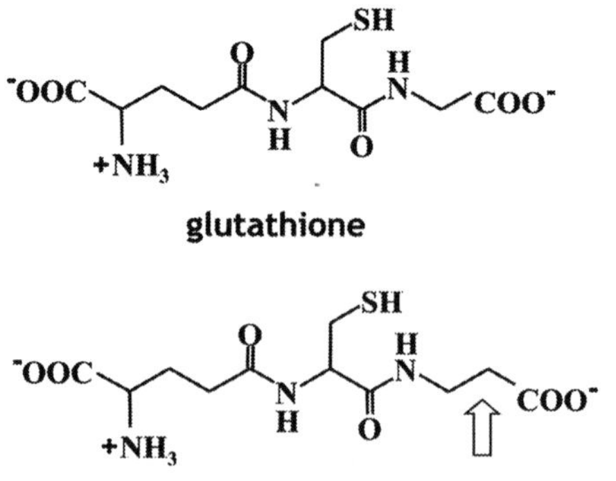

glutathione

homoglutathione

FIGURE 9-1.
Structures of glutathione and homoglutathione.

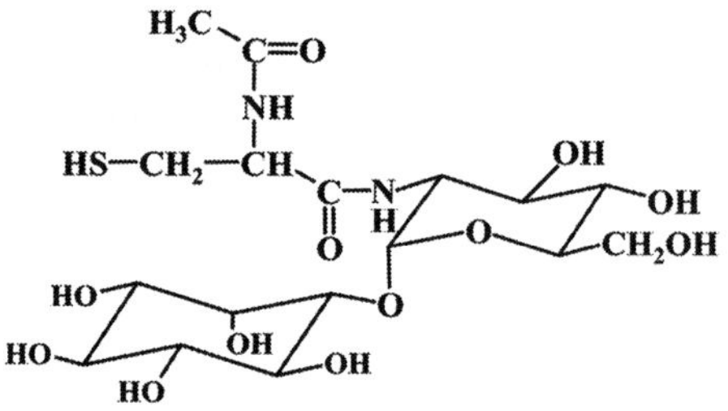

FIGURE 9-2.
The reactive sulfhydryl group of mycothiol can react with electrophiles. The N-acetylcysteinyl residue (upper left) with the conjugated group is cleaved off at the amide bond to the aminosugar and forms a mercapturic acid (*N*-acetyl-*S*-(substituent)-cysteine) and inosityl-glucosamine.

▶ The Repeated Discovery of "Philothion," Alias Glutathione

Elemental sulfur administered to the gastrointestinal tract is converted into sulfate. In the search for a chemical explanation of this transformation, the French researcher J. de Rey-Pailhade discovered "a body of organic origin" capable of producing hydrogen sulfide from sulfur powder (13). In modern terminology, the "body" was a compound, which he named *philothion* owing to its "affinity" (Greek, *philos*) for sulfur (Greek, *thio*). In his most convincing experiments, alcoholic extracts of brewer's yeast were mixed in a flask with sulfur at about 40°C. Hydrogen sulfide, liberated as a gas, rapidly blackened a paper impregnated with lead acetate solution, indicating the formation of lead sulfide. Storage of the philothion extract or treatment with strong acid or base resulted in loss of its reducing power. De Rey-Pailhade also submitted to the French Academy of Sciences his observation that the same philothion, or perhaps a slightly different substance, is present in animal and plant tissues (14). While this is certainly true, his own experimental findings with these crude preparations might have had other explanations.

In the first decade of the 20th century, the presence of sulfhydryl groups in animal tissues was demonstrated by using the reagent sodium nitroprusside, which, in alkaline solution, gives a purple color with thiols. It was originally believed that the amino acid cysteine was responsible for this positive reaction. The British biochemist F. Gowland Hopkins (figure 9-3) rediscovered philothion as a nitroprusside-reactive substance in hot water extracts of liver, kidney, and muscle. He concluded that it accounted for "the whole of the non-protein organically bound sulphur of the cell," and that it was redox active and had "functions in the chemical dynamics of the cell" (15). The substance was purified from yeast, and analysis demonstrated that it contained glutamic acid and cysteine. Hopkins deduced, erroneously, that he had isolated a dipeptide. Recognizing the link to philothion, but also underscoring the presence of glutamic acid linked to a sulfur compound, the peptide was provisionally called *glutathione*. More than a decade of work was needed for Hopkins and other researchers finally to establish the structure of GSH as the *tripeptide* γ-L-glutamyl-L-cysteinylglycine. An historical account of this breakthrough research was published recently (16). Hopkins received the Nobel Prize in Physiology or Medicine in 1929. ◀

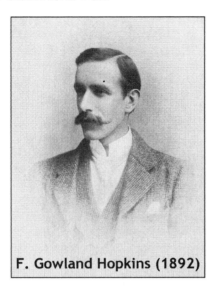

F. Gowland Hopkins (1892)

FIGURE 9-3.
Sir Frederick Gowland Hopkins (1861–1947). *Note*: This figure also appears on the companion website.

CHEMICAL STRUCTURE OF GSH

The structure of GSH demonstrates the unusual feature of a γ-peptide linkage between the N-terminal glutamic acid and the following cysteine residue. The presence of the γ-glutamyl moiety, with its free α-carboxylate group, prevents the hydrolysis of GSH by cellular peptidases that degrade other small peptides. The γ-glutamyl group can be removed by the action of the enzyme γ-glutamyltranspeptidase (EC 2.3.2.4), which is discussed further, later in this chapter.

At physiological pH, GSH carries two negative charges and one positive charge, imparting high solubility in aqueous media. The designation GSH is often used in reaction schemes, with the understanding that "SH" represents the reactive sulfhydryl group whereas "G" embodies the peptide part of the molecule; S-substituted GSH molecules can be denoted GSR, where R is the substituent.

The most prominent chemical feature of the GSH molecule is its functional sulfhydryl (or thiol) group, −SH. The electron cloud surrounding the nucleus of the sulfur atom is highly polarizable. In particular, the ionized thiolate form of GSH is a good *nucleophile* for reactions with electrophilic chemical compounds. The ability of sulfur to donate electrons to other compounds also makes GSH a good *reductant*. The pK_a value of the sulfhydryl group is 9.2. Only a small fraction of GSH is, therefore, in its thiolate anion form at neutral pH. However, some enzymes promote thiolate formation through the binding of GSH, thereby enhancing the reactivity of the molecule; this will be discussed further when we consider glutathione transferase enzymes.

BIOSYNTHESIS OF GSH

The production of GSH in the adult human body has been estimated as about 10 g per day (*17*). GSH biosynthesis (figure 9-4) involves peptide

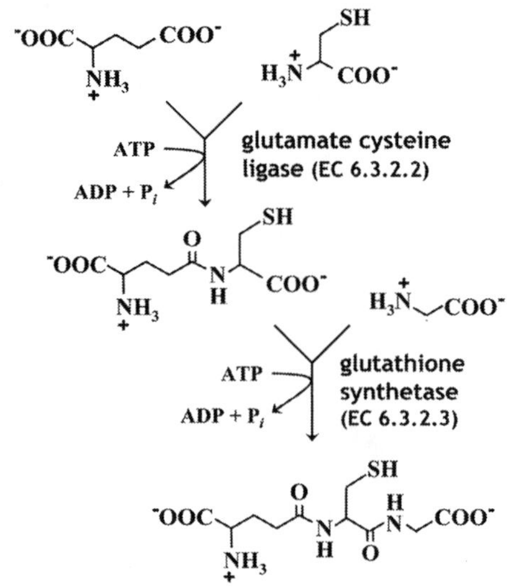

FIGURE 9-4.

The enzymatic steps in the synthesis of glutathione.

bond formation, but does not occur by the ribosomal route of protein synthesis. Instead, the formation of GSH is catalyzed by two specific enzymes (*18*). In the first step, γ-L-glutamyl-L-cysteine is formed from its constituent amino acids, in a reaction catalyzed by *glutamate cysteine ligase* (*γ-glutamylcysteine synthetase*; EC 6.3.2.2). This dipeptide is then linked to glycine by the action of *glutathione synthetase* (EC 6.3.2.3). The enzymes are present in both cytosol and mitochondria. Both of these steps require ATP and Mg^{2+}. Glutamate cysteine ligase activity is rate limiting for GSH biosynthesis and is subject to negative feedback regulation by GSH. By this mechanism, excess production of GSH or accumulation of the intermediate γ-glutamylcysteine is prevented. When GSH is in demand, the enzyme is induced via transcriptional activation of its gene expression. Induction takes place under conditions of oxidative stress or exposure to electrophiles. Induction involves cellular signaling that activates the antioxidant response element (ARE) of the glutamate cysteine ligase gene (*19*). This regulatory mechanism is also used for the control of glutathione transferases and other protective enzymes (see chapter 10). In this way, increased GSH levels contribute to the cellular defense against toxic and mutagenic insults.

If the conversion of γ-glutamylcysteine to GSH is impaired, an alternative pathway takes over, namely its conversion to *5-oxoproline*, catalyzed by *γ-glutamylcyclotransferase* (EC 2.3.2.4; figure 9-5) (*20*). Excessive production of 5-oxoproline occurs in the rare cases of hereditary

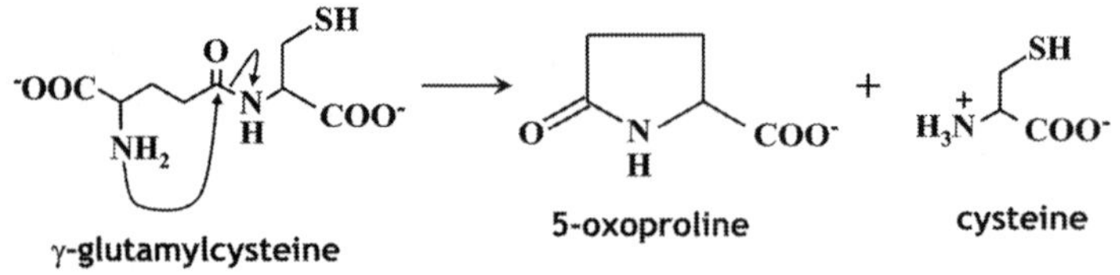

γ-glutamylcysteine   5-oxoproline   cysteine

FIGURE 9-5.

γ-Glutamylcysteine: conversion to 5-oxoproline.

glutathione synthetase deficiency, and is characterized by oxoprolinuria, chronic metabolic acidosis, and neurological disturbances. Patients presenting with glutathione synthetase deficiency have mutations in the protein, leading to loss of catalytic function or decreased stability of the enzyme (21). Complete loss of the glutathione synthetase gene product appears to be lethal.

DEPLETION OF CELLULAR GSH

Both for experimental purposes and in certain therapeutic applications, depletion of cellular GSH may be desirable. Administration of reactive electrophiles may lead to alkylation and other modifications of the thiol group of GSH. The modification is usually accompanied by export of the GSH conjugate from the cell to the surrounding medium, as is discussed further in chapter 11. Diethylmaleate is an activated alkene often used for depletion of GSH in experimental models (figure 9-6). Numerous other electrophilic compounds have the same effect. Foods may also contain reactive chemicals that decrease GSH levels. Their presence in a sample may be quantified as *glutathione-reactive units* (GRU), by measurement of the loss of an added standard amount of GSH; GRU values can range from zero to about 100 nanomole per gram of foodstuff (22).

The synthesis of GSH can be inhibited by *buthionine sulfoximine* (BSO, figure 9-7), an inhibitor with structural similarity to the activated intermediate in the reaction mechanism of glutamate cysteine ligase (18). In experimental systems, suppression of intracellular GSH concentrations by BSO has been observed to make cells more sensitive to ionizing radiation and to certain cytostatic drugs. Such sensitization has been explored for clinical use in cancer therapy. However, this approach is limited by the fact that both normal and tumor cells may be affected: toxicity to normal tissues may override the benefit of making tumor cells more susceptible to killing.

ELEVATION OF CELLULAR GSH

GSH has a pivotal role in the protection of cells against electrophiles and oxidative stress. Can we enhance the GSH levels in an organism, in order to fortify the GSH-dependent defense systems? Enterocytes of the gastrointestinal tract have an active GSH uptake system, suggesting that

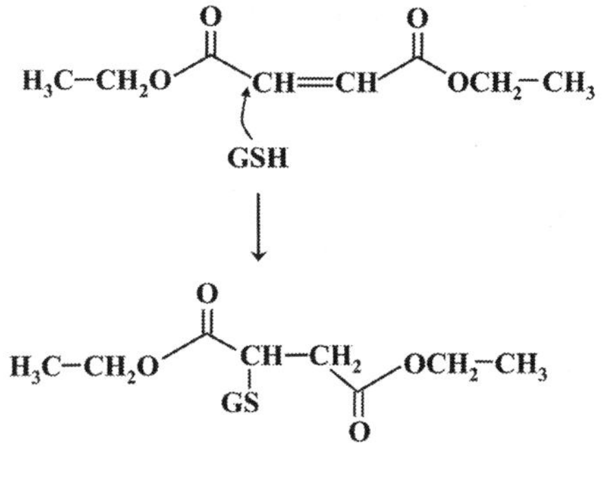

FIGURE 9-6.
Diethylmaleate reaction with glutathione.

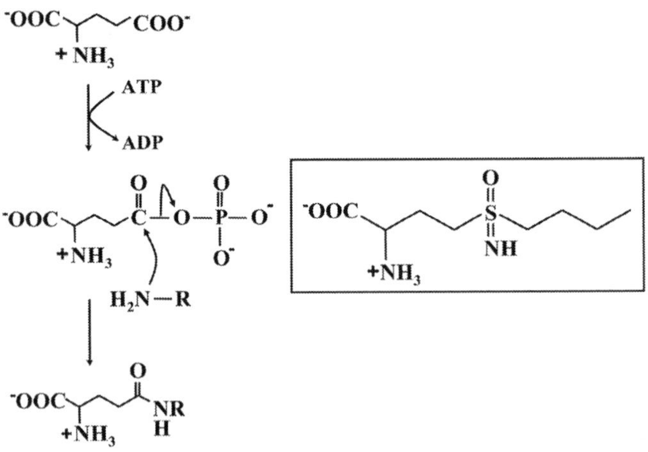

FIGURE 9-7.

The inhibitor buthionine sulfoximine, BSO (inset), mimics the tetrahedral intermediate formed when the activated γ-glutamyl-phosphate in the active site of glutamate cysteine ligase reacts with cysteine.

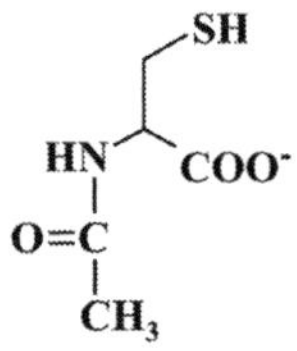

FIGURE 9-8.

N-Acetyl-L-cysteine, a pharmacologically useful GSH precursor.

these cells can make use of ingested GSH, in addition to biliary GSH secreted into the intestine. Nevertheless, most cells are unable to import GSH in intact form, but are dependent on the supply of precursors for GSH biosynthesis.

The sulfur-containing amino acid cysteine is a limiting substrate for GSH biosynthesis and the administration of cysteine precursors is a pharmacological route for GSH replenishment. Cysteine as such is unsuitable, because it is rapidly oxidized to the disulfide cystine, which has low solubility under physiological conditions. Instead, N-acetyl-L-cysteine (figure 9-8) has found clinical use. This compound is intracellularly deacetylated to cysteine and rapidly incorporated into GSH. N-Acetyl-L-cysteine is commonly used to overcome acetaminophen intoxication and its associated hepatic GSH depletion (see chapter 19). L-2-Oxothiazolidine-4-carboxylate, another cysteine precursor, has been found to support GSH biosynthesis in experimental models (figure 9-9).

CHEMICAL REACTIVITY OF GSH

In many respects, GSH has properties typical of other small peptides and low-molecular-mass thiols. An unbuffered aqueous solution of GSH is acidic (similar to a strong carboxylic acid of the same molarity) and the net charge of the tripeptide is −1. The two carboxylate functions have composite macroscopic pK_a values of 2.1 and 3.5 and the ammonium and

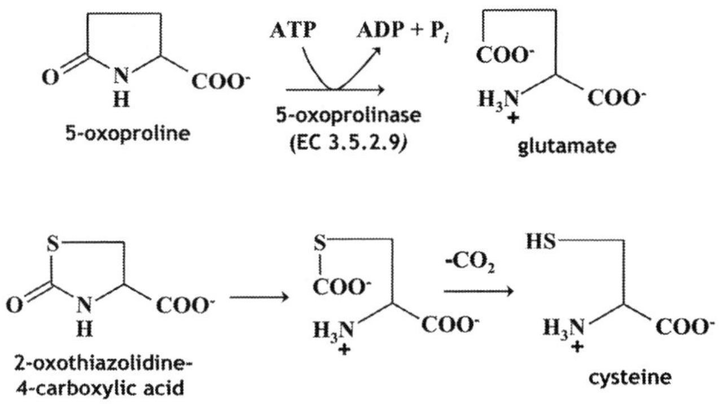

FIGURE 9-9.

L-2-Oxothiazolidine-4-carboxylate is converted to cysteine by the action of 5-oxoprolinase.

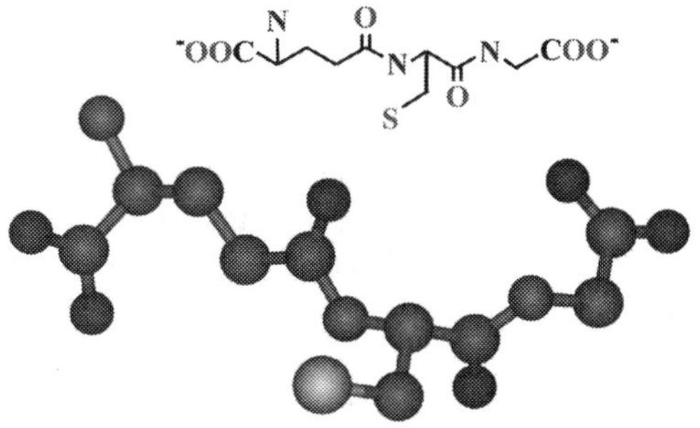

FIGURE 9-10.

Conformation of GSH bound to the active site of crystalline human GST A1-1. Similar conformations have been determined by NMR and theoretical calculations for GSH in free form and bound to other proteins. *Note*: A full-color version of this figure appears on the website. (*Mannervik, B.; Carlberg, I.; Larson, K. Glutathione: general review of mechanism of action. In* Glutathione: Chemical, Biochemical and Medical Aspects; *Dolphin, D., Poulson, R., Avramovic, O., Eds.; John Wiley: New York, 1989; pp. 475–516.*)

thiol groups have pK_a values of 8.7 and 9.6, respectively (*23*). The eight microscopic ionization constants that account for the predominant ionic forms of GSH are influenced by the protonation states of the neighboring residues (up to approximately 0.2 pH units), so unique pK_a values for the individual chemical groups cannot be assigned. Nevertheless, the groups can be ranked in the order of decreasing acidity: α-carboxyl of Glu, carboxyl of Gly, thiol of Cys, and ammonium group of Glu. The macroscopic pK_a of the thiol group, as revealed by its chemical reactivity with electrophiles, is approximately 9.2 (*24*).

The GSH tripeptide has an extended conformation (figure 9-10) that appears to be maintained both in solution and in protein-bound states (*25*). GSH has a zwitterionic N-terminus and a negatively charged C-terminus; the resulting electrical polarity promotes proper orientation of the molecule in protein binding sites, and the charged residues provide potential for ionic interactions with protein side chains.

The sulfhydryl group of GSH undergoes facile oxidation, particularly in its ionized thiolate state. Removal of one electron gives rise to the thiyl radical, GS$^{\bullet}$, which is unstable in free form (26). Further oxidation leads to the sulfenium oxidation state, GS$^+$, which very rapidly combines with a second thiolate to form a disulfide:

$$GS^-(\text{thiolate}) \rightarrow GS^{\bullet}(\text{thiyl radical}) \rightarrow GS^+(\text{sulfenium ion})$$
$$\rightarrow GSSG\,(\text{disulfide})$$

GSH can react with carbon-centered free radicals (R$^{\bullet}$), inactivating these reactive intermediates at the cost of the formation of the thiyl radical species. Christine Winterbourn has suggested that the unpaired electron taken up by GSH can be relayed from the thiyl radical, via a glutathione disulfide radical (GSSG$^{-\bullet}$), to dioxygen (27):

$$R^{\bullet} + GSH \rightarrow RH + GS^{\bullet}$$
$$GS^{\bullet} + GS^- \rightarrow GSSG^{-\bullet}$$
$$GSSG^{-\bullet} + O_2 \rightarrow GSSG + O_2^{-\bullet}$$

The superoxide anion thus formed is finally eliminated by the action of superoxide dismutase (see chapter 1). In this manner, GSH and oxygen jointly act as a "sink" for removing reactive free radicals.

In contrast to this protective function, there is also evidence that the glutathionyl radical, which has a high redox potential (approximately +0.9 V), can abstract hydrogen atoms from bis-allylic sites in polyunsaturated fatty acids (see chapter 1) and thereby act as a prooxidant. In cells exposed to high concentrations of phenol and H_2O_2, which produce large amounts of free radicals via myeloperoxidase activity, the resulting GS$^{\bullet}$ radicals induce phospholipid oxidation and cytotoxicity (28). However, these negative aspects of GSH chemistry are probably only seen under extreme stress conditions: usually, antioxidants (such as ascorbate) inactivate the thiyl radical by reduction before such lipid oxidation events take place.

Glutathione disulfide (GSSG), like GSH, is highly soluble in aqueous media, and does not penetrate biological membranes without the assistance of transport proteins. In the presence of other thiol-containing molecules (RSH), oxidation can lead to mixed disulfides, GSSR. Under conditions of oxidative stress, sulfhydryl groups of some proteins form such mixed disulfides.

(In the literature, glutathione disulfide (GSSG) is often referred as "oxidized glutathione." This is an imprecise designation that should be avoided, because GSH occurs in many oxidized forms. Mixed disulfides of GSH (RSSG), the sulfinic (GSO$_2$H) and sulfonic (GSO$_3$H) acids, as well as S-sulfoglutathione (GSSO$_3$H) are examples of compounds other than GSSG that qualify as "oxidized glutathione.")

GSH is significantly less prone to oxidation than are many other thiols, including the amino acid cysteine. The lability of cysteine is probably related to its capacity to sequester transition metal ions (such as copper and iron), which promote thiol oxidation in aerobic systems. The oxidation product, cystine, may precipitate in tissues and give rise to disease (cystinosis).

The cellular balance between reduced GSH and its disulfide is maintained largely in favor of the reduced form (normally >98%), and the glutathione thiol–disulfide couple, via interchange reactions, serves as a "redox buffer" for other thiols and disulfides. The redox potential of GSH is $-0.24\,V$ at pH 7. The molar ratio between reduced glutathione and its disulfide, 2[GSH]/[GSSG], has been proposed as the best parameter for assessing cellular redox status, and may be a measure of cellular health (29). Among the various conditions of impaired redox homeostasis, HIV infection is associated with a systemic deficiency of GSH, which can be monitored in blood plasma (30).

Biological systems are dynamic, undergoing both temporal and spatial changes of their constituents. This applies also to the cellular distribution of GSH. There is evidence for a gradient of GSH within mammalian cells, with a higher concentration near the nucleus than in other region of the cytoplasmic space (31). This may be the result of perinuclear enrichment of mitochondria, organelles that contain high concentrations of GSH.

GLUTATHIONYLATION AND γ-GLUTAMYL TRANSFER

Oxidative stress is associated with cellular responses that can lead either to proliferation of cells or to their death by apoptosis. GSH and GSH-associated proteins play important roles in these diverging processes (32). The reversible formation of mixed disulfides between GSH and protein sulfhydryl groups has been given particular attention (33). This thioltransferase-catalyzed protein modification may be of general significance in the regulation of cellular functions (34), and has recently been named *glutathionylation*.

In addition to chemistry invoking the sulfhydryl group of GSH, the γ-glutamyl moiety of GSH or GSH conjugates can be transferred to nucleophilic acceptors. The membrane-bound protein γ-*glutamyltranspeptidase*, which was mentioned earlier in the chapter, catalyzes this reaction (figure 9-11). The simplest representative of such a transfer is hydrolysis, in which water is the nucleophile and glutamate is released. Many amino acids and other amino-group-containing substances serve as alternative acceptor substrates in transpeptidation reactions catalyzed by this enzyme (35, 36). γ-Glutamyltranspeptidase is a membrane-bound *ectoenzyme*: it is

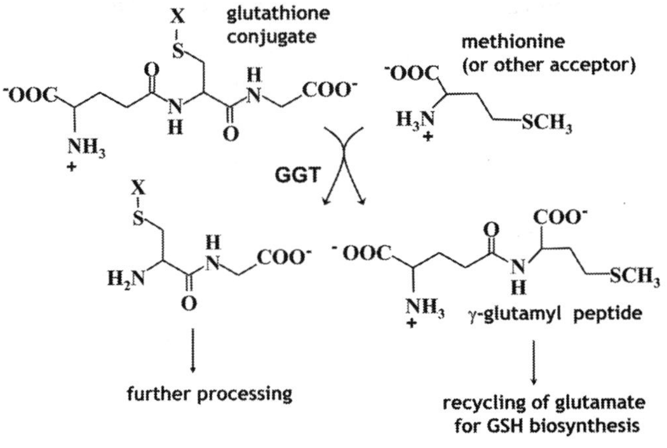

FIGURE 9-11.

γ-Glutamyltranspeptidase is the first enzyme in the pathway from glutathione conjugates to mercapturic acids.

secreted from the cell and acts on its substrates outside the cell membrane (*37*). The transpeptidation reaction is involved in a series of reactions which transport amino acids into cells, a process called the "γ-glutamyl cycle," discussed later in the chapter.

GLUTATHIONE-DISULFIDE REDUCTASE

Numerous metabolic reactions involve GSH as a reductant, and, in most of these, GSH is converted into GSSG. The enzyme responsible for reduction of GSSG is named *glutathione reductase* (*glutathione-disulfide reductase*, EC 1.8.1.7), an intracellular enzyme occurring as ubiquitously as GSH itself. The reaction catalyzed is:

$$GSSG + NADPH + H^+ \rightarrow 2GSH + NADP^+$$

The human enzyme has been investigated in detail and its properties seem to be representative. The enzyme has high specificity towards both the disulfide and the pyridine nucleotide substrate. Among the naturally occurring disulfides, only some mixed disulfides of GSH and related low-molecular-mass thiols can serve as alternative substrates, but the low activities observed are probably not of physiological relevance. Similarly, glutathione reductase has very little activity with NADH rather than NADPH as the reducing substrate.

Glutathione reductase is composed of two identical subunits, and the two equivalent binding sites for GSSG are located at the interfaces between the subunits (figure 9-12) (*38*). Each subunit has a distinct domain with

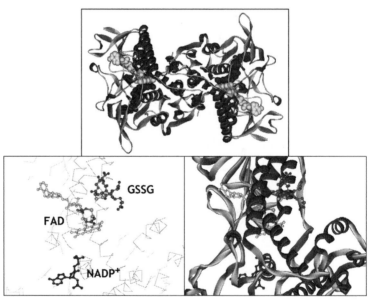

FIGURE 9-12.

Views of human GSSG reductase. Top: the homodimeric enzyme; FAD (yellow) and NADP$^+$ (purple) are shown as space-filling models. Bottom: the active site of the enzyme. FAD (yellow) and NADP$^+$ (purple; partly hidden) are shown as ball-and-stick models, with the protein secondary structure hidden (left) or displayed (right). The nicotinamide moiety of NADP$^+$ is not visible in the crystal structure. *Note*: A full-color version of this figure appears on the website.

a binding site for NADPH. The pyridine nucleotide is bound in an orientation such that the nicotinamide moiety, which carries the reducing equivalents, reaches into the center of the enzyme molecule, towards the GSSG binding site. The reducing equivalents from NADPH are transferred via two adjacent redox-active functional groups of the enzyme: FAD and a disulfide formed by two cysteine residues of the protein. Thus, the electrons originating from NADPH are conducted via FAD to the protein disulfide and finally to GSSG. The reduction of GSSG proceeds in two steps. The first step leads to release of one GSH molecule, with concomitant formation of a mixed disulfide between one of the redox-active cysteine residues of the active site and the other GS–half of the GSSG molecule. The second partial reaction consists of an intramolecular thiol–disulfide interchange reaction, which releases the second GSH molecule from the intermediate mixed disulfide in the active site.

$$\text{Enzyme(SH)}_2 + \text{GSSG} \rightarrow \text{Enzyme} - \text{(SH)} - \text{SSG} + \text{GSH}$$

$$\text{Enzyme} - \text{(SH)} - \text{SSG} \rightarrow \text{Enzyme} - \text{(S)}_2 + \text{GSH}$$

The interaction between the enzyme and GSSG has similarities to the disulfide reductions catalyzed by redox-active proteins such as thioltransferase and thioredoxin (25). The prosthetic group FAD, which serves as a physical barrier between the GSSG- and NADPH-binding sites, provides the electrochemical coupling between the redox chemistry of NADPH and the disulfide reduction.

Two B vitamins, niacin in NADPH and riboflavin in FAD, are required for glutathione reductase catalysis. Nutritional riboflavin deficiency can be monitored by measuring the activity of the enzyme in blood samples (erythrocytes).

Important biochemical reactions usually have backup mechanisms, and this is true of glutathione reductase. Mutant mice found to lack the gene for this enzyme survive, although they are more susceptible to chemical and oxidative insults (39). Clearly, alternative disulfide-reducing pathways must exist.

GSH AS A REDUCTANT

GSH serves as a reductant of many molecules of biological significance, especially those containing scissile sulfur–sulfur or oxygen–oxygen bonds: disulfides and peroxides, respectively. We will consider each of these processes.

Disulfides are formed from low-molecular-mass thiols, polypeptides, and proteins. Intracellular redox conditions normally keep thiols (RSH) predominantly in the reduced form, but oxidative processes generate a continuing flux of disulfides (RSSR). The reduction of disulfides takes place via thiol–disulfide interchange with GSH, with the intermediate formation of a mixed disulfide (GSSR) (40):

$$\text{GSH} + \text{RSSR} \rightarrow \text{GSSR} + \text{RSH}$$

$$\text{GSSR} + \text{GSH} \rightarrow \text{GSSG} + \text{RSH}$$

$$\text{Net: RSSR} + 2\,\text{GSH} \rightarrow 2\,\text{RSH} + \text{GSSG}$$

Thus, a disulfide is converted into the corresponding thiol at the expense of reducing equivalents derived from two GSH molecules. The GSSG formed is reduced via the reaction catalyzed by glutathione reductase, as discussed above. Therefore, the reduction of disulfides is coupled to the reducing equivalents of the pyridine nucleotide pool. NADPH, in turn, is regenerated mainly via the hexose monophosphate shunt (pentose phosphate pathway).

Both of the consecutive thiol–disulfide interchange reactions shown above are catalyzed by *thioltransferase*, a small (approximately 11 kDa) cytosolic protein (*40–42*). The enzyme has broad substrate specificity and is active with naturally occurring symmetrical disulfides (such as cystine and coenzyme A disulfide) and their mixed disulfides with GSH. Even disulfide bonds in proteins may be reduced in the same manner, provided that they are not sterically hindered (*43*). Many enzymes and cellular-signaling proteins require reduced sulfhydryl groups for activity, and are reversibly activated/inactivated by disulfide/thiol interconversion.

In the endoplasmic reticulum (ER) of eukaryotic cells, however, the redox equilibrium is shifted towards oxidation. The more oxidized state of the ER appears to be required for the formation of protein disulfide bonds. The ratio of GSH to GSSG may be only about 1:1 in the ER. This conclusion is based on a study of a synthetic cysteine-containing peptide, which was designed to be glycosylated, and thereby trapped, within the ER (*44*).

S-Sulfo-substituted thiols, such as the naturally occurring S-sulfoglutathione (GSSO$_3^-$), are also reduced via the thioltransferase-catalyzed reaction, to give GSSG and hydrogen sulfite (*45*):

$$GSH + GSSO_3^- \rightarrow GSSG + HSO_3^-$$

Thus, thioltransferase-catalyzed reactions serve to maintain cysteine, coenzyme A, and other important cellular thiols in their reduced state. Sulfhydryl-containing proteins that have been glutathionylated under oxidative conditions can also be reduced (and de-glutathionylated) by the same mechanism.

Originally, only one thioltransferase was recognized (*45*), but it is now known to be related to several other proteins, forming a family of *glutaredoxins* (Grxs), with similarities to thioredoxin (*46*). The differences in their functions have not yet been fully elucidated. Some of the proteins may have more narrow substrate selectivities than the broad-specificity thioltransferase (Grx1).

Hydrogen peroxide (H$_2$O$_2$) is generated as a byproduct of cellular respiration, cytochrome P450-catalyzed reactions, and other oxidative processes linked to oxygen metabolism (see chapter 1). Organic hydroperoxides (ROOH) are formed in tissues and biological fluids by lipid peroxidation and by oxidative damage to nucleic acids. They are also ingested via foodstuffs. Reduction of hydroperoxides is catalyzed by selenium-dependent *glutathione peroxidases* and *peroxiredoxins* (*47*) as well as by glutathione transferases, enzymes that are discussed in the following chapter.

$$ROOH + 2GSH \rightarrow ROH + H_2O + GSSG$$

▶ **Selenium**

Selenium was recognized as an important micronutrient long before it could be linked to any specific biochemical role. Selenium deficiency may lead to muscle disease and increased susceptibility to cancer. In 1973 selenium was found to be an essential component of the enzyme *glutathione peroxidase* (EC 1.11.1.9) isolated from mammalian erythrocytes and other tissues (*49, 50*). Selenium is present in the active-site residue *selenocysteine*, the selenium-containing homologue of cysteine. Glutathione peroxidase is involved in the inactivation of hydrogen peroxide and organic hydroperoxides, which may cause cancer and other degenerative diseases. Consequently, lack of selenium may impair this catalytic function and jeopardize the protection against oxidative stress. However, selenium-deficient mice display severe toxicity at selenium levels above those required to abrogate glutathione peroxidase activity. Additional selenoproteins have subsequently been discovered, contributing to the overall dietary selenium requirement (*51*). A total of 25 mammalian genes have been annotated as encoding selenoproteins.

How is selenocysteine incorporated into glutathione peroxidase? The mechanism incorporation was found to depend on one of the classic "stop" codons (UGA) of the genetic code. In a specific mRNA context (different for prokaryotes and eukaryotes), the UGA codon will be read as selenocysteine. With the aid of a specific tRNA carrying this unusual amino acid, and a cognate translation factor, selenocysteine is incorporated into the polypeptide under construction on the ribosome. Inorganic selenide, in the form of selenophosphate, is introduced by displacement of the oxygen in the side chain of serine bound to a selenocysteine-specific tRNA molecule, thereby forming selenocysteinyl-tRNA in situ. ◀

(Note the formal similarity with disulfide reduction: RSSR + 2GSH → 2RSH + GSSG.)

Nitrogen-containing compounds can also be reduced by GSH; pharmacologically relevant are nitrate esters such as nitroglycerin:

$$RONO_2 + 2GSH \rightarrow ROH + NO_2^- + H^+ + GSSG$$

Similarly, the strong oxidant peroxynitrite (chapter 1) is reduced by GSH (*48*).

SALVAGE OF CELLULAR GSH

Maintenance of the intracellular level of GSH is important to the many essential functions fulfilled by the thiol. Regeneration of GSH from GSSG is afforded by the reaction catalyzed by glutathione reductase (see above). However, both GSH and GSSG can be exported from the cell via members of the MRP family of transporters (*52*) (discussed later in this chapter). Replenishment of the intracellular pool takes place primarily by de novo synthesis of GSH from its constituent amino acids, although this may be limited by the supply of cysteine. Extracellular GSH, GSSG, and glutathione derivatives are degraded by γ-glutamyltranspeptidase on the exterior side of the plasma membrane, as mentioned earlier. Cysteinylglycine released from GSH is hydrolyzed by a cell-surface-associated dipeptidase and the free amino acids are returned to the cytoplasm via amino acid transporters. This biochemical process, the *γ-glutamyl cycle* (*53*), was first described by Alton Meister. GSH is thus recovered in the form of its amino acid building blocks, of which cysteine has particular significance. The importance of γ-glutamyltranspeptidase for maintenance of intracellular GSH is evidenced by inhibition of the enzyme with *acividin*, resulting in GSH depletion; the cysteine precursor 2-oxothiazolidine-4-carboxylate reverses the effect of acividin (*54*).

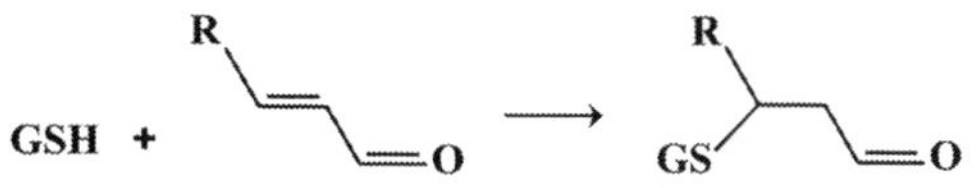

$$\text{GSH} \; + \quad \overset{R}{\diagdown}\!\!\diagup\diagdown\!\!=\!\!\text{O} \quad \longrightarrow \quad \overset{R}{GS\diagup}\!\!\diagdown\!\!\diagup\diagdown\!\!=\!\!\text{O}$$

$$\text{GSH} + \text{CH}_3\text{Cl} \longrightarrow \text{GSCH}_3 + \text{Cl}^- + \text{H}^+$$

FIGURE 9-13.

Addition and substitution reactions of GSH.

GSH CONJUGATIONS

Next, we turn from reductions to the second major class of chemical reactions involving GSH: covalent conjugations with electrophiles. The nucleophilic character of the thiolate group of GSH promotes transfer of negative charge to electrophilic centers. At the extreme, electrons of the sulfur are completely transferred to the recipient molecule, resulting in the reduction of disulfides and other substances, as described above. However, in most cases the shift is not complete, and the donor and acceptor molecules end up as a covalently linked couple sharing an electron pair. There are two main categories of such conjugation reactions: additions and substitutions (figure 9-13). In the first case, the sulfur of GSH adds to a double bond, oxirane ring, or similar structure, resulting in a single product containing all the constituents of the reacting molecules. In the second case, the glutathione thiolate displaces a fragment (e.g., an anion such as a halide) of the electrophilic substrate and is inserted in its place. The net reaction usually involves release of a proton stoichiometric to the one produced in the ionization of GSH to its thiolate.

▶ **Mercapturic Acids are Derived from GSH Conjugates**

In 1879 N-acetyl-S-p-bromophenyl-cysteine (figure 9-14) was isolated from the urine of dogs that had been fed bromobenzene. This metabolite is an example of a *mercapturic acid* (N-acetyl-S-(substituent)-cysteine), so named because, upon treatment with alkali, they decompose to odoriferous mercaptans (thiols). Scientists were puzzled that a simple aromatic compound could be metabolized to a sulfur-containing excretion product. In the late 1950s it was established that mercapturates derive from GSH conjugation. In the case of the unreactive compound bromobenzene, the aromatic hydrocarbon is epoxidized to 1-bromo-3,4-dihydro-3,4-oxybenzene, in a P450-catalyzed process. This reactive epoxide reacts with the thiol group of GSH. The epoxide, as well as the GSH conjugate, is unstable, because the aromatic character of the benzene ring has been eliminated. Aromaticity and stability are regained by the spontaneous elimination of water (figure 9-15). The GSH conjugate is subsequently transformed by the action of γ-glutamyltranspeptidase and dipeptidase, to give the corresponding cysteine conjugate (figures 9-11 and 9-16). The final step in mercapturic acid formation is the acetylation of the amino group of cysteine, a process requiring acetyl-coenzyme A and an N-acetyltransferase. (The mercapturate-forming enzyme is unrelated to the aromatic amine N-acetyltransferase discussed in chapter 13.) ◀

EXAMPLES OF GSH CONJUGATION

Numerous compounds, both of biological and nonbiological origins, can be conjugated with GSH. Sulfur is a "soft" nucleophile (one with easily polarizable electrons (55, p. 505, 56) and preferentially reacts with soft electrophiles. Most electrophilic organic compounds fitting this description

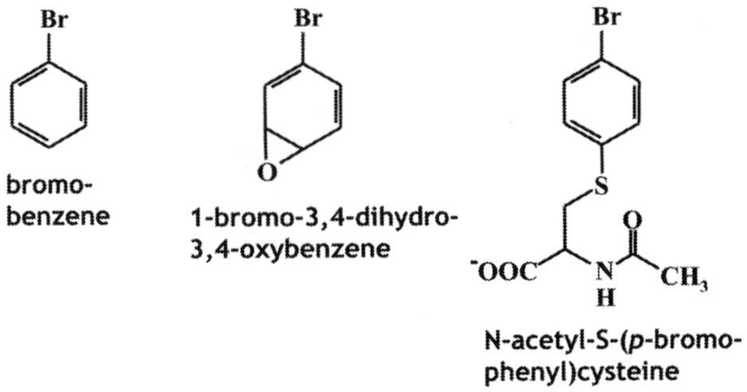

bromo-
benzene

1-bromo-3,4-dihydro-
3,4-oxybenzene

N-acetyl-S-(*p*-bromo-
phenyl)cysteine

FIGURE 9-14.
The mercapturic acid metabolite of bromobenzene (right) is formed by the oxidation of bromobenzene (left) to a reactive epoxide, 1-bromo-3,4-dihydro-3,4-oxybenzene (center), which is trapped by GSH and further metabolized.

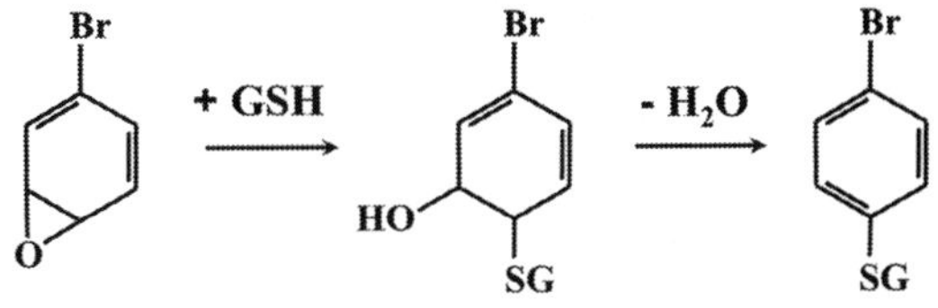

FIGURE 9-15.
Reaction of 1-bromo-3,4-dihydro-3,4-oxybenzene with GSH.

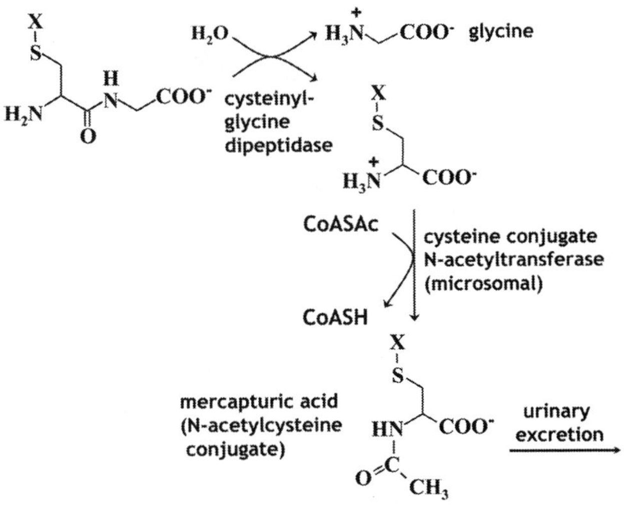

FIGURE 9-16.
The first step of mercapturic acid biosynthesis is shown in figure 9-11. The subsequent steps are illustrated here (see text for further details).

can form GSH conjugates under suitable conditions, unless steric hindrance or other nonelectronic factors are prohibitive. Reaction rates vary greatly, but enzyme catalysis will often accelerate the conjugation. In chapter 10, we discuss glutathione transferases, the enzymes that catalyze these conjugations.

Let us look at some typical examples of GSH conjugates derived from addition reactions. The diuretic drug ethacrynic acid has an activated alkene functionality that reacts with GSH (figure 9-17). Aminochrome is an *ortho*-quinone generated through the oxidation of the neurotransmitter dopamine (figure 9-18). 4-Hydroxy-17β-estradiol, a catechol metabolite of the hormone estradiol, is a suspected mammary carcinogen (*57*); it forms a GSH conjugate via oxidation of the catechol to a reactive *ortho*-quinone (figure 9-19). The carcinogenic fungal toxin aflatoxin is metabolized to a reactive epoxide (see chapters 3 and 7; figure 9-20). Leukotriene C_4 is an eicosanoid, a potent mediator of asthma, inflammation, and other biological responses, which is derived from the oxidation of the polyunsaturated

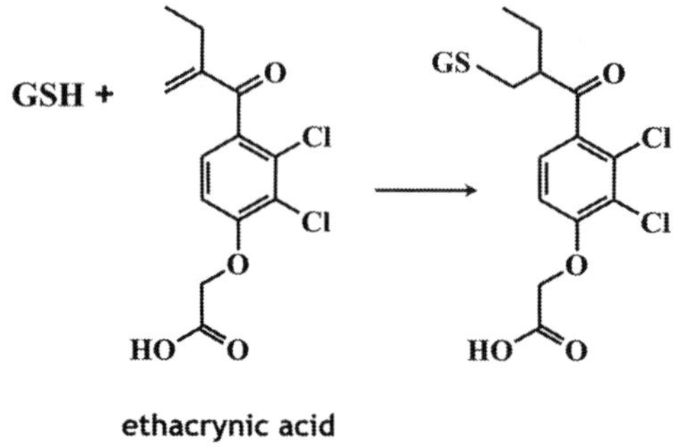

ethacrynic acid

FIGURE 9-17.
Ethacrynic acid.

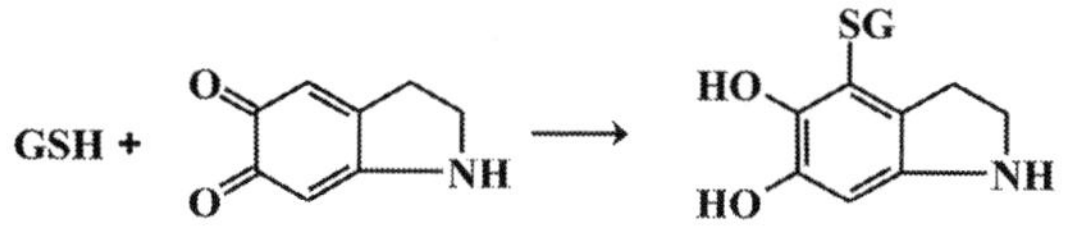

FIGURE 9-18.
Aminochrome, an *ortho*-quinone oxidation product of dopamine, is trapped by GSH.

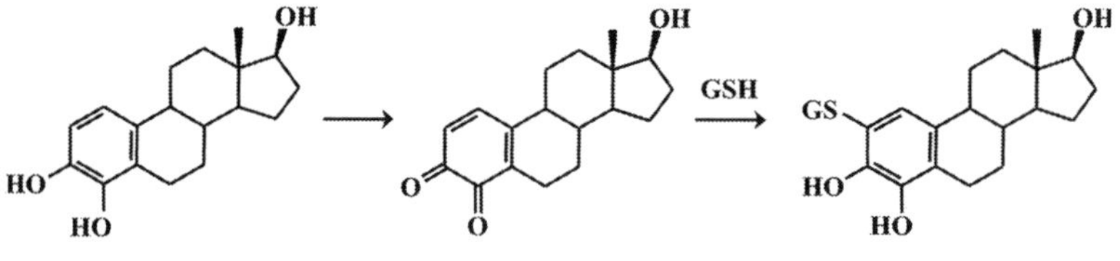

FIGURE 9-19.
Reaction of a catechol estrogen quinone with GSH.

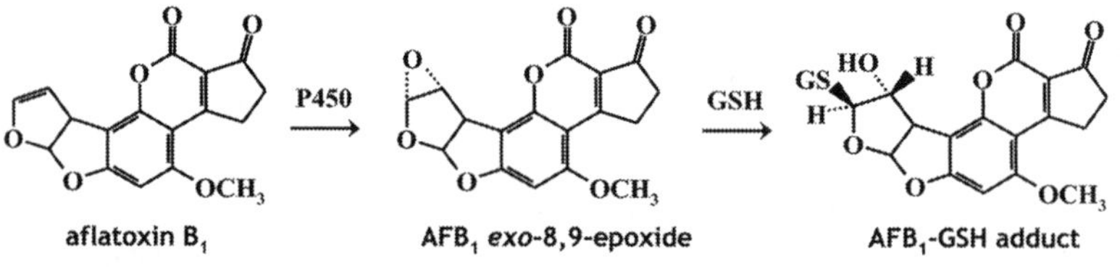

aflatoxin B₁ AFB₁ *exo*-8,9-epoxide AFB₁-GSH adduct

FIGURE 9-20.
Activation of aflatoxin to a reactive epoxide and its reaction with GSH.

fatty acid arachidonic acid; the final step in its biosynthesis is the enzyme-catalyzed reaction of an epoxide with GSH (figure 9-21).

Next, we illustrate some GSH substitution reactions. Hexyl bromide reacts with GSH to give S-hexylglutathione (figure 9-22), which is used as an inhibitor and affinity ligand of glutathione-dependent enzymes (see chapter 10). Menaphthylsulfate is a model compound for carcinogenic benzylic sulfate esters derived from polycyclic aromatic hydrocarbons (see chapter 14; figure 9-23). 2-Cyano-1,3-dimethyl-1-nitrosoguanidine (figure 9-24) mimics the reactivity of the carcinogenic N-nitroso derivative of the antiulcer drug cimetidine; GSH conjugation gives rise to S-nitrosoglutathione (GS–N=O) (58).

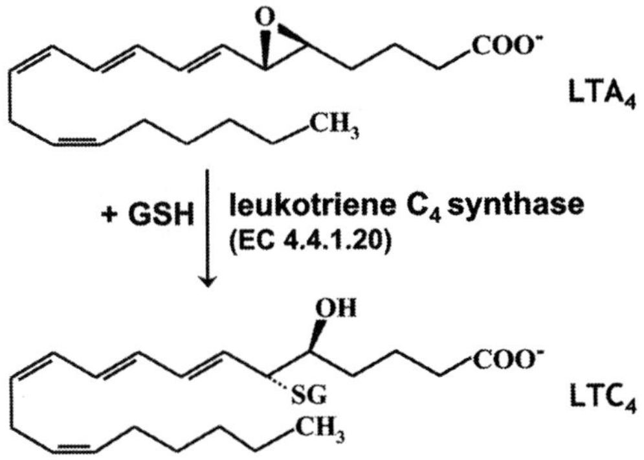

FIGURE 9-21.
Leukotriene A$_4$ (LTA$_4$) is formed from arachidonic acid, in a reaction catalyzed by 5-lipoxygenase, and is then conjugated with GSH to form leukotriene C$_4$ (LTC$_4$).

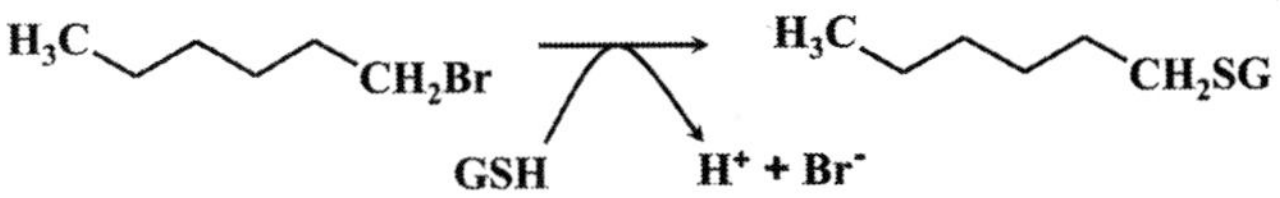

FIGURE 9-22.
Reaction of hexyl bromide with GSH to give S-hexylglutathione.

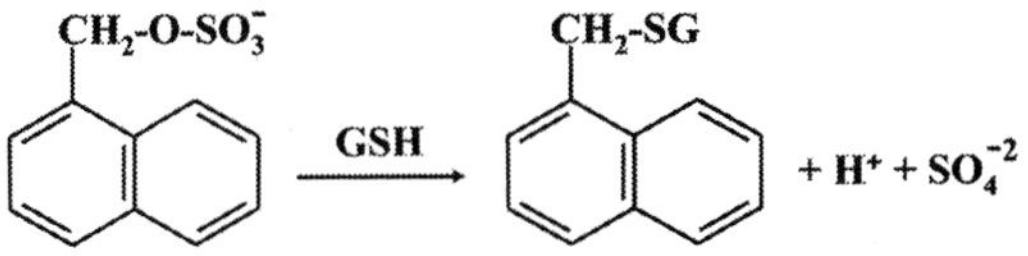

FIGURE 9-23.
Reaction of menaphthylsulfate with GSH.

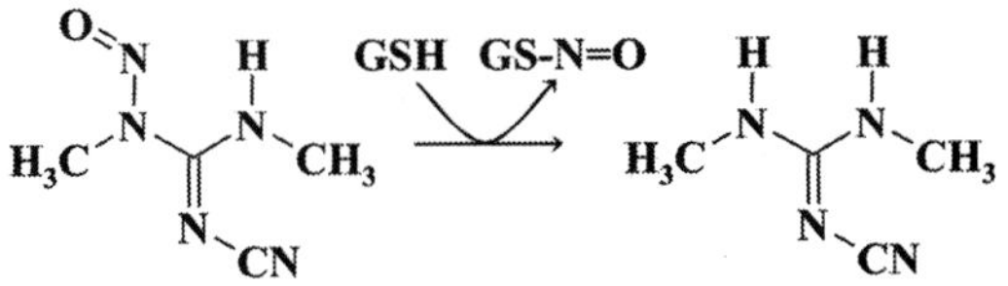

FIGURE 9-24.
Reaction of 2-cyano-1,3-dimethyl-1-nitrosoguanidine with GSH.

MECHANISTIC ASPECTS OF GSH CONJUGATION

In this section, we review the reaction mechanisms by which GSH undergoes substitution and addition reactions. All these conjugation reactions involve the sulfur atom of GSH acting as a nucleophile. The availability of d orbitals in sulfur makes it more potent than oxygen as a nucleophile. Experimental evidence suggests that the thiol group reacts in its ionized thiolate (GS$^-$) form. The undissociated thiol (GSH) is a comparatively poor nucleophile, and reactions of GSH are base-catalyzed when the pH of the reaction medium is lower than the pK_a of the thiol group (9.2). In general, the reactivity of thiols reflects both their basicity and their nucleophilicity. These parameters work in opposite directions, because higher pK_a is associated with greater nucleophilicity, but reduces the proportion of the thiolate anion present at neutral pH. A balance between these contributions is reached when the pK_a is close to the pH at which the reaction is occurring. One of the functions of enzymes catalyzing GSH conjugations is to increase the acidity of the thiol group and thereby promote its ionization.

Bimolecular nucleophilic substitutions (S$_N$2 reactions) are often mechanistically straightforward, proceeding through a transition state in which the negative charge of the sulfur atom is shifted to the leaving group (figure 9-25). When a tetrahedral carbon (e.g., in methyl chloride) is attacked, it is forced into a bipyramidal configuration, with the approaching sulfur in one apical position and the leaving group (chloride) in the other apical position. In the bipyramidal intermediate, negative charge migrates from the thiolate sulfur of GSH to the halide (X) leaving group. The remaining three atoms and the central carbon are coplanar. The progress of the reaction leads to inversion of the stereochemical configuration of the three remaining groups surrounding the central atom. Consequently, if the three groups are different, the S$_N$2 reaction leads to a product with opposite chirality (the so-called "Walden inversion").

The energy barrier to the S$_N$2 transformation is minimized when the attacking sulfur, the electrophilic center (carbon in methyl chloride), and the leaving ligand (chloride in methyl chloride) are arranged in a straight line. In analogy, the thiol–disulfide interchange, which is also an S$_N$2 reaction, involves the reaction of the thiolate with the disulfide bond in a linear fashion, such that the angle S–S–S in the transition state is close to 180°. Most of the negative charge resides with the peripheral sulfur

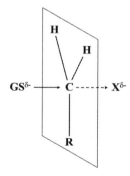

FIGURE 9-25.

Activated complex in the nucleophilic attack of GSH on an alkyl halogenide (R–CH$_2$–X).

atoms as the reaction progresses, and charge is gradually shifted from the attacking nucleophile to the leaving group, with negligible charge at the central sulfur atom (59). In aqueous media, the charges of the peripheral groups can be stabilized by interactions with the solvent, which oppose the chemical transformation by increasing the activation energy of the reaction. Reactions in less polar environments, such as at the active site of an enzyme, are expected to have a decreased energy barrier and an enhanced reaction rate.

Reactions of GSH with hydroperoxides (ROOH) and organic nitrites (RONO) are formally similar to those involving disulfides. They first give rise to unstable intermediates (sulfenic acid and S-nitrosoglutathione, respectively), which can subsequently react with a second GSH molecule to give GSSG:

$$GSH + ROOH \rightarrow GSOH + ROH$$

$$GSOH + GSH \rightarrow GSSG + H_2O$$

$$Net: 2GSH + ROOH \rightarrow GSSG + ROH + H_2O$$

$$GSH + RONO \rightarrow GSNO + ROH$$

$$GSNO + GSH \rightarrow GSSG + HNO$$

$$Net: 2GSH + RONO \rightarrow GSSG + ROH + HNO$$

HNO is nitroxyl (60, 61), the one-electron reduction product of NO.

Substitutions at carbon may also lead to unstable GSH conjugates, which sometimes give rise to products that are more toxic than the parent compound. Reactions with dihalomethanes, such as CH_2Cl_2, will produce S-halomethylglutathione:

$$GSH + CH_2Cl_2 \rightarrow GSCH_2Cl + H^+ + Cl^-$$

which can alkylate DNA or hydrolyze to give the toxic product formaldehyde:

$$GSCH_2Cl + H_2O \rightarrow HCHO + GSH + H^+ + Cl^-$$

Aromatic nucleophilic substitutions (S_NAr) involve attack by the thiolate anion via a reaction trajectory perpendicular to the plane of the aromatic ring of the electrophile. A covalent intermediate (a σ-complex, also known as a "Meisenheimer complex") develops, with concomitant loss of the aromaticity of the ring structure (figure 9-26). The aromatic character

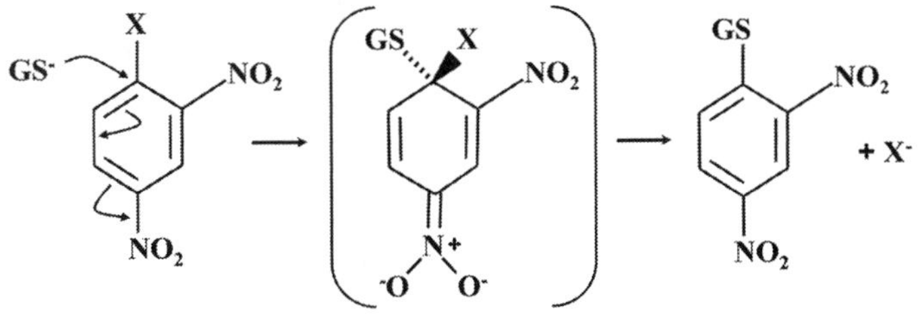

FIGURE 9-26.
Reaction of GSH with a dinitrohalobenzene.

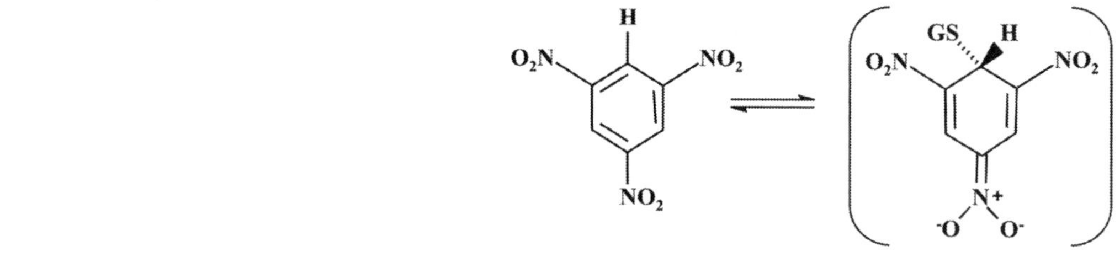

FIGURE 9-27.
Meisenheimer complex formed from GSH and trinitrobenzene.

is regained as the leaving group departs from the σ-complex. The model compound 1,3,5-trinitrobenzene does not possess a proper leaving group and, therefore, is trapped as the intermediate complex (figure 9-27). In this case, the dark red-colored σ-complex is so stable, in the presence of glutathione transferase, that it can be isolated and studied by X-ray crystallography (*62*).

Addition reactions are usually more intricate than substitution reactions. Toxicologically relevant electrophiles undergoing GSH addition (some of which were mentioned previously) include epoxides, activated alkenes, quinones/iminoquinones, and isothiocyanates. Common to the addition reactions is the uptake of a proton by the target substrate (formally, the proton released from the thiol group of GSH). This serves to neutralize the negative charge transferred from the sulfur of GSH in the process of conjugation. In reactions with epoxides, the proton acceptor is oxygen, which acquires a negative charge when the oxirane ring is attacked by the thiolate of glutathione. The reaction with the oxirane structure is sensitive to steric and electronic influences of the substituents on the carbon atoms. Styrene 7,8-oxide is conjugated with GSH at either C7 or C8, but the benzylic C7 position is favored by a factor of about 2, in comparison with the terminal C8 oxirane carbon (*63*). Further, both conjugates occur in *S*- and *R*-enantiomeric forms, which are formed in equal amounts in the nonenzymatic reaction of the racemic epoxide (figure 9-28). In the presence of glutathione transferase, however, the relative amounts of the four diastereomers will be biased in favor of particular isomers, depending on the enzyme used.

The addition of GSH to activated alkenes (typically, α,β-unsaturated carbonyl compounds) is usually referred to as a "Michael addition." (The reaction originally described by A. Michael in 1887 was the formation of a carbon–carbon bond between an acidic methylene carbon and an activated alkene. The designation Michael addition is now generalized to embrace reactions with different nucleophiles, such as GSH, and a variety of compounds with activated double bonds.) An example is the conjugation of acrolein (propen-2-al; figure 9-29). Acrolein (see sidebar on exocyclic DNA adducts in chapter 2) is formed by free radical reactions and oxidative processes in biological systems and is also a product of the activation of the anticancer drug cyclophosphamide. Acrylamide ($CH_2=CH-C(O)-NH_2$) is formed by the Maillard reaction involving asparagine and carbohydrates in the heating of foodstuffs such as potatoes and cereals (*64*). This alkene can also react with bases in DNA and cause mutations. Further biotransformation catalyzed by cytochrome P450 2E1 leads to the more mutagenic epoxide glycidamide (*65, 66*). Both acrylamide and glycidamide

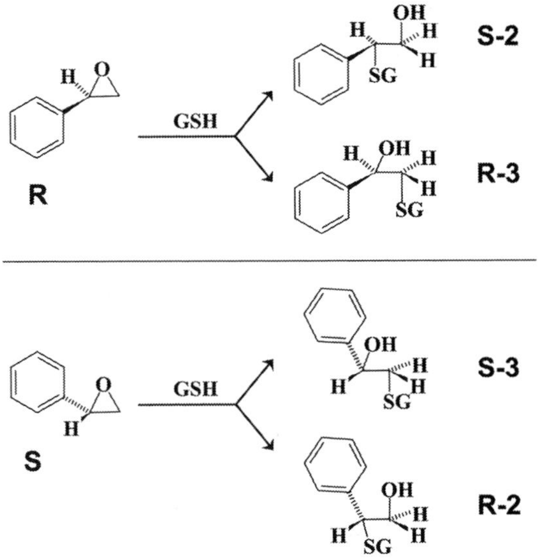

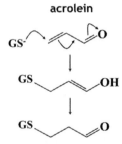

FIGURE 9-28.
Stereo- (R or S) and regio- (proximal C7 or terminal C8) isomeric GSH conjugates formed from R- and S-styrene 7,8-oxide (SO).

FIGURE 9-29.
Reaction of GSH with acrolein.

are conjugated with GSH, but considerably more slowly than acrolein. Measurement of the urinary mercapturic acids of both compounds indicates that, in humans, the major metabolic pathway of acrylamide leads to GSH conjugation without prior epoxidation (67).

The stereochemistry of the addition of a nucleophile to a double bond involves an attack perpendicular to the plane of the sp^2 hybridized electrophilic atom. The approach of the attacking nucleophile may be from "above" or from "below." In the case of acrolein, both approaches yield a product with the same steric configuration around the atom receiving the attack. However, in the higher homologue of acrolein, crotonaldehyde, and other α,β-unsaturated carbonyl compounds, such as the lipid peroxidation product 4-hydroxynonenal (see chapter 1), the β-carbon is a prochiral center: attack from the *si* face will give a chiral product with the opposite steric configuration to that arising from a *re* face attack (figure 9-30). In the absence of steric hindrance from the groups linked to the β-carbon, an uncatalyzed reaction will produce equal proportions of each stereoisomer, but in enzyme-catalyzed reactions, one of the chiral products may be formed exclusively.

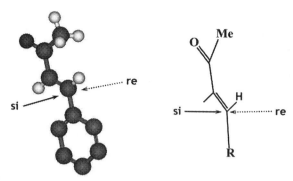

FIGURE 9-30.

Reaction of GSH with α,β-unsaturated carbonyl compounds, such as *trans*-phenylbutenone, can give diasteromeric products. *Note*: A full-color version of this figure appears on the website.

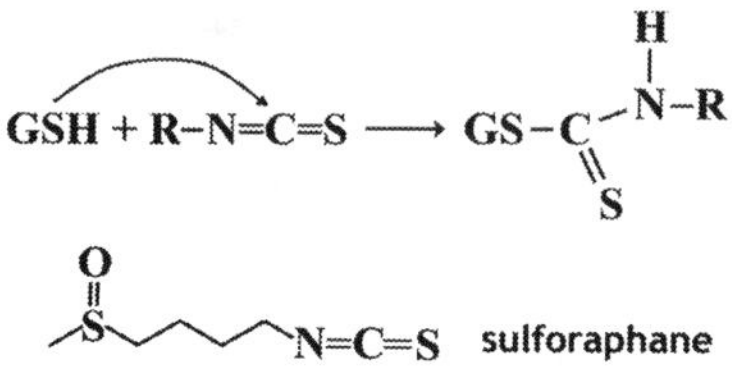

$$GSH + R-N=C=S \longrightarrow GS-C \overset{\overset{\displaystyle H}{|}}{\underset{\overset{\|}{S}}{}} N-R$$

O=S—⌇⌇—N=C=S sulforaphane

FIGURE 9-31.

Organic isothiocyanates are released by hydrolysis of glucosinolates from cruciferous plants and react reversibly with GSH to form dithiocarbamate conjugates. Sulforaphane derives from glucoraphanin and is an inducer of ARE-regulated genes (see chapter 11).

Another addition reaction is the formation of a dithiocarbamate from an isothiocyanate (figure 9-31, upper). Organic isothiocyanates occur abundantly in plants, where they are usually stored as unreactive *glucosinolates*, from which they are released by the action of the enzyme myrosinase (*68*). Even though they generally have been known as toxic substances, many isothiocyanates are now recognized as chemopreventive agents. Sulforaphane (figure 9-31, lower), isolated from broccoli, has been shown to protect against experimental tumors in rats (*69*).

The conjugation of GSH with quinones, and the similar iminoquinones, can be regarded as further examples of Michael addition. In these cases, a glutathionyl hydroquinone derivative is formed, which may be regarded as a reduced quinone (even though the electron pair of the thioether bond, strictly speaking, belongs to the sulfur atom) (figure 9-32). The GSH conjugates of many quinones are prone to oxidation and are more toxic than the parent compounds (*70*). However, in the case of the *ortho*-quinones formed from dopamine and related compounds, GSH conjugation prevents redox cycling and appears to be an important neuroprotective mechanism (*71–73*).

THE MRP FAMILY OF TRANSPORT PROTEINS

Once formed, most glutathione conjugates would be trapped inside the cytoplasm, since their relatively polar character means that they do not readily diffuse across the plasma membrane. This is also true of sulfate and

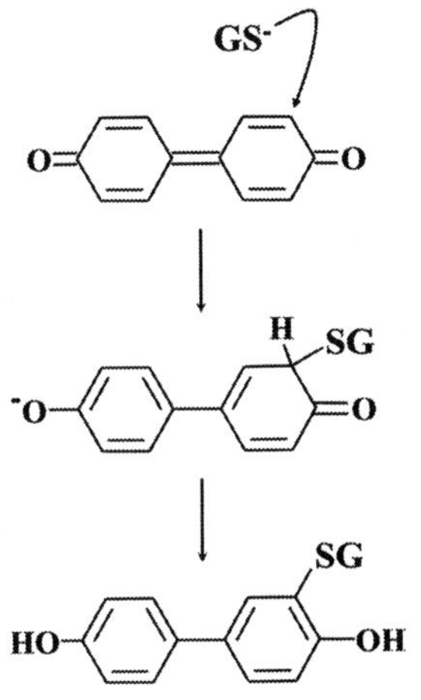

FIGURE 9-32.
The primary product of GSH addition to a quinone isomerizes to give a hydroquinone conjugate.

glucuronic acid conjugates, which are discussed in subsequent chapters. However, a number of integral membrane transporters can bring about an ATP-dependent export of polar conjugates from the cell. The MRP (multidrug resistance-associated protein) family is part of the ABC (ATP-binding cassette) protein superfamily (74), and comprises nine members in humans; several of these are glutathione conjugate efflux pumps (52, 75). The MRP proteins were first identified based on their ability to export anticancer drugs from cells (76). P-glycoprotein (the MDR1 gene product; ABCB1) (77) and MXR protein (mitoxantrone resistance protein; ABCG2) (78), both of which are also ABC superfamily members, were discovered in the same manner.

Another member of this superfamily is the cystic fibrosis transmembrane conductance regulator (CFTR). CFTR is involved in salt and water transport in the respiratory epithelium, and chloride ion conduction through CFTR (79) is essential to fluid secretion by the submucosal glands of the airways. Defects in this protein leads to cystic fibrosis, a lethal autosomal recessive disease (80). Patients present clinically with respiratory malfunction, caused by chronic inflammation and infection of the lung. Interestingly, CFTR also mediates nucleotide-supported GSH efflux from epithelial cells, implicating a role for CFTR in the resistance to oxidative stress in the airways (81). Loss of GSH in the epithelial lining fluid has been suggested as an important contributor to the pathogenesis of cystic fibrosis, and patients have been treated with GSH, in aerosol form, in attempts to suppress the symptoms and the progression of the disease (82).

MRP proteins, like other members of the ABCC subfamily, have two cytoplasmic nucleotide-binding domains (which are highly conserved among ABC proteins) and at least two membrane-spanning domains, each made up of six transmembrane segments. Several MRP family members have an additional membrane-spanning domain of unknown function at the N-terminal end of the protein.

MRP1 (ABCC1) protein is expressed in many normal tissues and carries out the ATP-driven active transport of drugs and xenobiotics conjugated

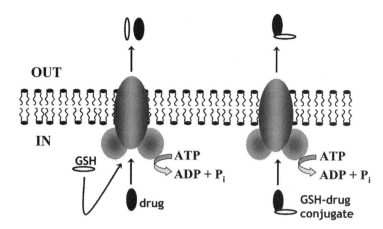

FIGURE 9-33.

Schematic of the actions of MRP as an export pump cotransporting GSH and drugs (left) or transporting GSH conjugates (right).

to glutathione, glucuronic acid, and sulfate, thus preventing their accumulation inside the cell (figure 9-33). MRP1 can also export unconjugated xenobiotics, but cotransport of the drug with glutathione is usually required for it to do so; this finding suggests that the protein has a bipartite ligand-binding site. The MRP2 protein (ABCC2, also known as cMOAT) is expressed at high levels in the apical membrane of canalicular hepatocytes, where its role is to excrete xenobiotics and their conjugates into the bile. Mutations in MRP2 leading to the absence of functional protein in the canalicular membrane in humans result in *Dubin–Johnson syndrome*, a hereditary condition in which conjugates of bilirubin and other compounds are deposited in the liver (*83*).

Detailed information on the nomenclature scheme for human and mouse ABC proteins is provided at: http://www.gene.ucl.ac.uk/nomenclature/genefamily/abc.html.

GSH HOMEOSTASIS

We are now in a position to summarize the metabolic transformations that GSH undergoes in mammalian cells (figure 9-34). Such an overview of GSH turnover was first formulated by Alton Meister. Precursor amino acids are taken up via transporters in the plasma membrane. Meister provided evidence that γ-Glu-amino acids, formed by the action of γ-glutamyltranspeptidase on extracellular GSH and GSH conjugates (including GSSG), are imported as such and subsequently cleaved to release 5-oxoproline and the amino acid (*53*). Glutamic acid is produced by the hydrolytic action of 5-oxoprolinase (EC 3.5.2.9) on 5-oxoproline, which is an amide obtained by cyclization of the γ-glutamyl residue. The GSH synthesized from these imported building blocks is used for reduction of disulfides, hydroperoxides, ribonucleotides, and so on; the GSSG concomitantly formed is reduced back to GSH by the action of glutathione reductase. GSH conjugates are formed from electrophiles by enzymatic or nonenzymatic processes. The GSH derivatives are exported from the cell via integral membrane proteins such as the MRPs. GSSG (which we may

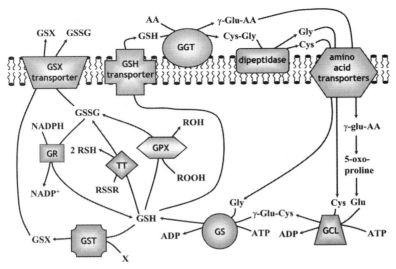

FIGURE 9-34.

Overview of GSH metabolism. The intracellular biochemistry of GSH (lower) is linked via membrane transport processes to extracellular metabolism (upper); GR, glutathione reductase; TT, thioltransferase; GPX, glutathione peroxidase; GST, glutathione transferase; GS, glutathione synthetase; GCL, glutamate cysteine ligase; GGT, γ-glutamyl transpeptidase. The indicated transporters for GSH and GSX may be the same protein, MRP1, in many cell types. (*Modified from Meister, A. Metabolism and function of glutathione. In* Glutathione. Chemical, Biochemical, and Medical Aspects; *Dolphin, D., Poulson, R., Avramovic, O., Eds.; John Wiley: New York, 1989; pp. 367–474; and Dickinson, D. A.; Forman, H. J. Glutathione in defense and signaling: lessons from a small thiol.* Ann. N.Y. Acad. Sci. **2002**, *973, 488–504.*)

regard as a "GSH conjugate" of the glutathione sulfenyl group, GS^+) and GSH itself are also transported out of the cell. This recurring turnover of GSH (Meister's "γ-glutamyl cycle") maintains homeostasis with respect to concentration of the GSH tripeptide as well as to cellular redox balance. The loss of sulfur through the formation of mercapturic acids and other stable end products has to be compensated for, by the input of Cys (or Cys precursors) for GSH replenishment. This metabolic scheme is further complicated by other processes (not shown) that involve GSH (figure 9-34) but do not consume the tripeptide.

An even more complex picture emerges from functional genomics studies of the yeast *Saccharomyces cerevisiae*. Genome-wide screening of yeast deletion mutants identified approximately 270 variants characterized by elevated export of GSH, in comparison with wild-type *S. cerevisiae* cells (*84*). These genes were linked to widely diverse functions, such as nitrogen/carbon source signaling, mitochondrial electron transport, ubiquitin/proteasome processes, transcriptional control, ion transport, and cellular integrity. The strongest effects were associated with late endosome/vacuolar secretory functions. In the mutants tested, GSH excretion was initiated when the intracellular level exceeded the maximal level found in the normal parental yeast cell. Thus, GSH produced intracellularly is cycled, with a low turnover, between the cytoplasm and the extracellular culture medium, and many cellular functions not obviously linked to GSH metabolism can influence GSH homeostasis. Such multifaceted regulatory circuits undoubtedly interconnect numerous cellular components and biochemical processes.

References

1. Reed, D. J. Glutathione: toxicological implications. *Annu. Rev. Pharmacol. Toxicol.* **1990**, *30*, 603–631.

2. Anderson, M. E. Glutathione: an overview of biosynthesis and modulation. *Chem. Biol. Interact.* **1998**, *111–112*, 1–14.

3. Samiec, P. S.; Dahm, L. J.; Jones, D. P. Glutathione S-transferase in mucus of rat small intestine. *Toxicol. Sci.* **2000**, *54*, 52–59.

4. Smith, C. V.; Jones, D. P.; Guenthner, T. M.; Lash, L. H.; Lauterburg, B. H. Compartmentation of glutathione: implications for the study of toxicity and disease. *Toxicol. Appl. Pharmacol.* **1996**, *140*, 1–12.

5. Holmgren, A. Hydrogen donor system for *Escherichia coli* ribonucleoside-diphosphate reductase dependent upon glutathione. *Proc. Natl. Acad. Sci. USA* **1976**, *73*, 2275–2279.

6. Forman, H. J.; Fukuto, J. M.; Torres, M. Redox signaling: thiol chemistry defines which reactive oxygen and nitrogen species can act as second messengers. *Am. J. Physiol. Cell Physiol.* **2004**, *287*, C246-C256.

7. Napoli, C.; Ignarro, L. J. Nitric oxide-releasing drugs. *Annu. Rev. Pharmacol. Toxicol.* **2003**, *43*, 97–123.

8. Murphy, R. C.; Zarini, S. Glutathione adducts of oxyeicosanoids. *Prostaglandins Other Lipid Mediat.* **2002**, *68–69*, 471–482.

9. Fahey, R. C. Novel thiols of prokaryotes. *Annu. Rev. Microbiol.* **2001**, *55*, 333–356.

10. Carnegie, P. R. Structure and properties of a homologue of glutathione. *Biochem. J.* **1963**, *89*, 471–478.

11. Iturbe-Ormaetxe, I.; Heras, B.; Matamoros, M. A.; Ramos, J.; Moran, J. F.; Becana, M. Cloning and functional characterization of a homoglutathione synthetase from pea nodules. *Physiol. Plant* **2002**, *115*, 69–73.

12. Newton, G. L.; Fahey, R. C. Mycothiol biochemistry. *Arch. Microbiol.* **2002**, *178*, 388–394.

13. de Rey-Pailhade, J. Sur un corps d'origine organiques hydrogénant le soufre à froid. *Compt. Rend.* **1888**, *106*, 1683–1684.

14. de Rey-Pailhade, J. Nouvelles recherches physiologiques sur la substance organique hydrogénant le soufre à froid. *Compt. Rend.* **1888**, *107*, 43–44.

15. Hopkins, F. G. An autoxidisable constituent of the cell. *Biochem. J.* **1921**, *15*, 286–305.

16. Simoni, R. D.; Hill, R. L.; Vaughan, M. On glutathione: II. A thermostable oxidation–reduction system (Hopkins, F. G.; Dixon, M. *J. Biol. Chem.* **1922**, *54*, 527–563). *J. Biol. Chem.* **2002**, *277*, e13.

17. Meister, A. Glutathione metabolism. *Methods Enzymol.* **1995**, *251*, 3–7.

18. Meister, A. Metabolism and function of glutathione. In *Glutathione. Chemical, Biochemical, and Medical Aspects*; Dolphin, D., Poulson, R., Avramovic, O., Eds.; John Wiley:, New York, 1989; pp. 367–474.

19. Nguyen, T.; Sherratt, P. J.; Pickett, C. B. Regulatory mechanisms controlling gene expression mediated by the antioxidant response element. *Annu. Rev. Pharmacol. Toxicol.* **2003**, *43*, 233–260.

20. Bridges, R. J.; Meister, A. γ-Glutamyl amino acids. Transport and conversion to 5-oxoproline in the kidney. *J Biol. Chem.* **1985**, *260*, 7304–7308.

21. Njålsson, R.; Carlsson, K.; Olin, B.; Carlsson, B.; Whitbread, L.; Polekhina, G.; Parker, M. W.; Norgren, S.; Mannervik, B.; Board, P. G.; Larsson, A. Kinetic properties of missense mutations in patients with glutathione synthetase deficiency. *Biochem. J.* **2000,** *349,* 275–279.

22. He, M.; Openo, K.; McCullough, M.; Jones, D. P. Total equivalent of reactive chemicals in 142 human food items is highly variable within and between major food groups. *J. Nutr.* **2004,** *134,* 1114–1119.

23. Fuhr, B. J.; Rabenstein, D. L. Nuclear magnetic resonance studies of the solution chemistry of metal complexes: IX. The binding of cadmium, zinc, lead, and mercury by glutathione. *J. Am. Chem. Soc.* **1973,** *95,* 6944–6950.

24. Pettersson, P. L.; Mannervik, B. The role of glutathione in the isomerization of Δ5-androstene-3,17-dione catalyzed by human glutathione transferase A1-1. *J. Biol. Chem.* **2001,** *276,* 11698–11704.

25. Mannervik, B.; Carlberg, I.; Larson, K. Glutathione: general review of mechanism of action. In *Glutathione: Chemical, Biochemical and Medical Aspects*; Dolphin, D., Poulson, R., Avramovic, O., Eds.; John Wiley:, New York, 1989; pp. 475–516.

26. Josephy, P. D.; Rehorek, D.; Janzen, E. G. Electron spin resonance spin trapping of thiyl radicals from the decomposition of thionitrites. *Tetrahedron Lett.* **1984,** *25,* 1685–1688.

27. Winterbourn, C. C. Superoxide as an intracellular radical sink. *Free Radic. Biol. Med.* **1993,** *14,* 85–90.

28. Borisenko, G. G.; Martin, I.; Zhao, Q.; Amoscato, A. A.; Tyurina, Y. Y.; Kagan, V. E. Glutathione propagates oxidative stress triggered by myeloperoxidase in HL-60 cells. Evidence for glutathionyl radical-induced peroxidation of phospholipids and cytotoxicity. *J. Biol. Chem.* **2004,** *279,* 23453–23462.

29. Schafer, F. Q.; Buettner, G. R. Redox environment of the cell as viewed through the redox state of the glutathione disulfide/glutathione couple. *Free Radic. Biol. Med.* **2001,** *30,* 1191–1212.

30. Herzenberg, L. A.; De Rosa, S. C.; Dubs, J. G.; Roederer, M.; Anderson, M. T.; Ela, S. W.; Deresinski, S. C. Glutathione deficiency is associated with impaired survival in HIV disease. *Proc. Natl. Acad. Sci. USA* **1997,** *94,* 1967–1972.

31. Söderdahl, T.; Enoksson, M.; Lundberg, M.; Holmgren, A.; Ottersen, O. P.; Orrenius, S.; Bolcsfoldi, G.; Cotgreave, I. A. Visualization of the compartmentalization of glutathione and protein-glutathione mixed disulfides in cultured cells. *FASEB J.* **2003,** *17,* 124–126.

32. Cotgreave, I. A.; Gerdes, R. G. Recent trends in glutathione biochemistry: glutathione–protein interactions: a molecular link between oxidative stress and cell proliferation? *Biochem. Biophys. Res. Commun.* **1998,** *242,* 1–9.

33. Thomas, J. A.; Poland, B.; Honzatko, R. Protein sulfhydryls and their role in the antioxidant function of protein S-thiolation. *Arch. Biochem. Biophys.* **1995,** *319,* 1–9.

34. Mannervik, B.; Axelsson, K. Role of cytoplasmic thioltransferase in cellular regulation by thiol–disulphide interchange. *Biochem. J.* **1980,** *190,* 125–130.

35. Hanigan, M. H. γ-Glutamyl transpeptidase, a glutathionase: its expression and function in carcinogenesis. *Chem. Biol. Interact.* **1998,** *111–112,* 333–342.

36. Castonguay, R.; Lherbet, C.; Keillor, J. W. Kinetic studies of rat kidney γ-glutamyltranspeptidase deacylation reveal a general base-catalyzed mechanism. *Biochemistry* **2003,** *42,* 11504–11513.

37. Ingbar, D. H.; Hepler, K.; Dowin, R.; Jacobsen, E.; Dunitz, J. M.; Nici, L.; Jamieson, J. D. γ-Glutamyl transpeptidase is a polarized alveolar epithelial membrane protein. *Am. J Physiol.* **1995**, *269*, L261–L271.

38. Schirmer, R.H.; Krauth-Siegel, R. L.; Schulz, G. E. Glutathione reductase. In *Glutathione. Chemical, Biochemical, and Clinical Aspects*; Dolphin, D., Poulson, R., Avramovic, O., Eds.; John Wiley:, New York, 1989; pp. 553–596.

39. Rogers, L. K.; Tamura, T.; Rogers, B. J.; Welty, S. E.; Hansen, T. N.; Smith, C. V. Analyses of glutathione reductase hypomorphic mice indicate a genetic knockout. *Toxicol. Sci.* **2004**, *82*, 367–373.

40. Askelöf, P.; Axelsson, K.; Eriksson, S.; Mannervik, B. Mechanism of action of enzymes catalyzing thiol-disulfide interchange. Thioltransferases rather than transhydrogenases. *FEBS Lett.* **1974**, *38*, 263–267.

41. Qiao, F.; Xing, K.; Liu, A.; Ehlers, N.; Raghavachari, N.; Lou, M. F. Human lens thioltransferase: cloning, purification, and function. *Invest Ophthalmol. Vis. Sci.* **2001**, *42*, 743–751.

42. Xing, K.; Lou, M. F. The possible physiological function of thioltransferase in cells. *FASEB J.* **2003**, *17*, 2088–2090.

43. Mannervik, B.; Axelsson, K.; Sundewall, A. C.; Holmgren, A. Relative contributions of thioltransferase- and thioredoxin-dependent systems in reduction of low-molecular-mass and protein disulphides. *Biochem. J.* **1983**, *213*, 519–523.

44. Hwang, C.; Sinskey, A. J.; Lodish, H. F. Oxidized redox state of glutathione in the endoplasmic reticulum. *Science* **1992**, *257*, 1496–1502.

45. Axelsson, K.; Eriksson, S.; Mannervik, B. Purification and characterization of cytoplasmic thioltransferase (glutathione:disulfide oxidoreductase) from rat liver. *Biochemistry* **1978**, *17*, 2978–2984.

46. Fernandes, A. P.; Holmgren, A. Glutaredoxins: glutathione-dependent redox enzymes with functions far beyond a simple thioredoxin backup system. *Antioxid. Redox Signal.* **2004**, *6*, 63–74.

47. Rhee, S. G.; Kang, S. W.; Chang, T. S.; Jeong, W.; Kim, K. Peroxiredoxin, a novel family of peroxidases. *IUBMB Life* **2001**, *52*, 35–41.

48. Balazy, M.; Kaminski, P. M.; Mao, K.; Tan, J.; Wolin, M. S. S-Nitroglutathione, a product of the reaction between peroxynitrite and glutathione that generates nitric oxide. *J. Biol. Chem.* **1998**, *273*, 32009–32015.

49. Rotruck, J. T.; Pope, A. L.; Ganther, H. E.; Swanson, A. B.; Hafeman, D. G.; Hoekstra, W. G. Selenium: biochemical role as a component of glutathione peroxidase. *Science* **1973**, *179*, 588–90.

50. Flohé, L.; Gunzler, W. A.; Schock, H. H. Glutathione peroxidase: a selenoenzyme. *FEBS Lett.* **1973**, *32*, 132–134.

51. Diwadkar-Navsariwala, V.; Diamond, A. M. The link between selenium and chemoprevention: a case for selenoproteins. *J. Nutr.* **2004**, *134*, 2899–2902.

52. Kruh, G. D.; Belinsky, M. G. The MRP family of drug efflux pumps. *Oncogene* **2003**, *22*, 7537–7552.

53. Griffith, O. W.; Bridges, R. J.; Meister, A. Evidence that the γ-glutamyl cycle functions in vivo using intracellular glutathione: effects of amino acids and selective inhibition of enzymes. *Proc. Natl. Acad. Sci. USA* **1978**, *75*, 5405–5408.

54. Liu, R. M.; Hu, H.; Robison, T. W.; Forman, H. J. Differential enhancement of γ-glutamyl transpeptidase and γ-glutamylcysteine synthetase by

tert-butylhydroquinone in rat lung epithelial L2 cells. *Am. J. Respir. Cell Mol. Biol.* **1996**, *14*, 186–191.

55. Carroll, F. A. *Perspectives on Structure and Mechanism in Organic Chemistry*; Brooks/Cole: Pacific Grove, 1998.

56. Hartman, P. E.; Shankel, D. M. Antimutagens and anticarcinogens: a survey of putative interceptor molecules. *Environ. Mol. Mutagen.* **1990**, *15*, 145–182.

57. Rogan, E. G.; Cavalieri, E. L. Estrogen metabolites, conjugates, and DNA adducts: possible biomarkers for risk of breast, prostate, and other human cancers. *Adv. Clin. Chem.* **2004**, *38*, 135–149.

58. Jensen, D. E.; Belka, G. K. Enzymic denitrosation of 1,3-dimethyl-2-cyano-1-nitrosoguanidine in rat liver cytosol and the fate of the immediate product S-nitrosoglutathione. *Biochem. Pharmacol.* **1997**, *53*, 1279–1295.

59. Fernandes, P. A.; Ramos, M. J. Theoretical insights into the mechanism for thiol/disulfide exchange. *Chem. Eur. J.* **2004**, *10*, 257–266.

60. Fukuto, J. M.; Dutton, A. S.; Houk, K. N. The chemistry and biology of nitroxyl (HNO): a chemically unique species with novel and important biological activity. *Chembiochem.* **2005**, *6*, 612–619.

61. Fukuto, J. M.; Switzer, C.; Miranda, K. M.; Wink, D. A. Nitroxyl (HNO): chemistry, biochemistry, and pharmacology. *Ann. Rev. Pharmacol. Toxicol.* **2005**, *45*, 335–355.

62. Ji, X.; Armstrong, R. N.; Gilliland, G. L. Snapshots along the reaction coordinate of an S_NAr reaction catalyzed by glutathione transferase. *Biochemistry* **1993**, *32*, 12949–12954.

63. Dostal, L. A.; Guthenberg, C.; Mannervik, B.; Bend, J. R. Stereoselectivity and regioselectivity of purified human glutathione transferases pi, alpha-epsilon, and mu with alkene and polycyclic arene oxide substrates. *Drug Metab. Dispos.* **1988**, *16*, 420–424.

64. Tareke, E.; Rydberg, P.; Karlsson, P.; Eriksson, S.; Törnqvist, M. Analysis of acrylamide, a carcinogen formed in heated foodstuffs. *J. Agric. Food Chem.* **2002**, *50*, 4998–5006.

65. Besaratinia, A.; Pfeifer, G. P. Genotoxicity of acrylamide and glycidamide. *J. Natl. Cancer Inst.* **2004**, *96*, 1023–1029.

66. Besaratinia, A.; Pfeifer, G. P. DNA adduction and mutagenic properties of acrylamide. *Mutat. Res.* **2005**, *580*, 31–40.

67. Boettcher, M. I.; Schettgen, T.; Kutting, B.; Pischetsrieder, M.; Angerer, J. Mercapturic acids of acrylamide and glycidamide as biomarkers of the internal exposure to acrylamide in the general population. *Mutat. Res.* **2005**, *580*, 167–176.

68. Shapiro, T. A.; Fahey, J. W.; Wade, K. L.; Stephenson, K. K.; Talalay, P. Chemoprotective glucosinolates and isothiocyanates of broccoli sprouts: metabolism and excretion in humans. *Cancer Epidemiol. Biomarkers Prev.* **2001**, *10*, 501–508.

69. Zhang, Y.; Kensler, T. W.; Cho, C. G.; Posner, G. H.; Talalay, P. Anticarcinogenic activities of sulforaphane and structurally related synthetic norbornyl isothiocyanates. *Proc. Natl. Acad. Sci. USA* **1994**, *91*, 3147–3150.

70. Bolton, J. L.; Trush, M. A.; Penning, T. M.; Dryhurst, G.; Monks, T. J. Role of quinones in toxicology. *Chem. Res. Toxicol.* **2000**. *13*, 135–160.

71. Baez, S.; Segura-Aguilar, J.; Widersten, M.; Johansson, A. S.; Mannervik, B. Glutathione transferases catalyse the detoxication of oxidized metabolites (*o*-quinones) of catecholamines and may serve as an

antioxidant system preventing degenerative cellular processes. *Biochem. J.* **1997**, *324*, 25–28.

72. Dagnino-Subiabre, A.; Cassels, B. K.; Baez, S.; Johansson, A. S.; Mannervik, B.; Segura-Aguilar, J. Glutathione transferase M2-2 catalyzes conjugation of dopamine and dopa *o*-quinones. *Biochem. Biophys. Res. Commun.* **2000**, *274*, 32–36.

73. Segura-Aguilar, J.; Baez, S.; Widersten, M.; Welch, C. J.; Mannervik, B. Human class Mu glutathione transferases, in particular isoenzyme M2-2, catalyze detoxication of the dopamine metabolite aminochrome. *J. Biol. Chem.* **1997**, *272*, 5727–5731.

74. Jones, P. M.; George, A. M. The ABC transporter structure and mechanism: perspectives on recent research. *Cell. Mol. Life Sci.* **2004**, *61*, 682–699.

75. Haimeur, A.; Conseil, G.; Deeley, R. G.; Cole, S. P. The MRP-related and BCRP/ABCG2 multidrug resistance proteins: biology, substrate specificity and regulation. *Curr. Drug Metab.* **2004**, *5*, 21–53.

76. Litman, T.; Druley, T. E.; Stein, W. D.; Bates, S. E. From MDR to MXR: new understanding of multidrug resistance systems, their properties and clinical significance. *Cell. Mol. Life Sci.* **2001**, *58*, 931–959.

77. Szakacs, G.; Chen, G. K.; Gottesman, M. M. The molecular mysteries underlying P-glycoprotein-mediated multidrug resistance. *Cancer Biol. Ther.* **2004**, *3*, 382–384.

78. Schinkel, A. H.; Jonker, J. W. Mammalian drug efflux transporters of the ATP binding cassette (ABC) family: an overview. *Adv. Drug Deliv. Rev.* **2003**, *55*, 3–29.

79. Riordan, J. R. Assembly of functional CFTR chloride channels. *Annu. Rev. Physiol.* **2005**, *67*, 701–718.

80. McAuley, D. F.; Elborn, J. S. Cystic fibrosis: basic science. *Paediatr. Respir. Rev.* **2000**, *1*, 93–100.

81. Kogan, I.; Ramjeesingh, M.; Li, C.; Kidd, J. F.; Wang, Y.; Leslie, E. M.; Cole, S. P.; Bear, C. E. CFTR directly mediates nucleotide-regulated glutathione flux. *EMBO J.* **2003**, *22*, 1981–1989.

82. Day, B. J. Glutathione: a radical treatment for cystic fibrosis lung disease? *Chest* **2005**, *127*, 12–14.

83. König, J.; Nies, A. T.; Cui, Y. H.; Leier, I.; Keppler, D. Conjugate export pumps of the multidrug resistance protein (MRP) family: localization, substrate specificity, and MRP2-mediated drug resistance. *Biochim. Biophys. Acta* **1999**, *1461*, 377–394.

84. Perrone, G. G.; Grant, C. M.; Dawes, I. W. Genetic and environmental factors influencing glutathione homeostasis in *Saccharomyces cerevisiae*. *Mol. Biol. Cell* **2005**, *16*, 218–230.

DISCOVERY OF GLUTATHIONE TRANSFERASES

In chapter 9 we studied the chemistry of the conjugation of glutathione (GSH) with electrophiles. Now, we examine the family of enzymes that catalyze these conjugations: the glutathione transferases (*1*). Two research groups reported independently, in 1961, that GSH conjugation of xenobiotics (bromosulfophthalein (*2, 3*), figure 10-1; or halobenzenes (*4*)) was catalyzed by an enzyme found in the cytosolic fraction of rat liver. The laboratory of Eric Boyland in London, U.K., pursued the investigations, using numerous electrophilic compounds as substrates, and obtained evidence for the existence of several forms of glutathione transferase (GST). These activities were named GSH S-aryltransferase, GSH alkyltransferase, GSH S-epoxidetransferase, and so on, according to their assumed substrate specificities. Boyland's group thus established that an exceedingly broad range of electrophiles can serve as substrates for enzymatic GSH conjugation (*5*). Electrophiles are often cytotoxic, mutagenic, and carcinogenic compounds, and we now know that their conjugation to GSH is the cell's major defense against them. Particularly noteworthy was Boyland's discovery that GSH conjugation was involved in the biotransformation and inactivation of arene oxides, formed by the cytochrome P450-catalyzed oxidation of polycyclic aromatic hydrocarbons such as benzo[*a*]pyrene (*6*) (see chapter 18). At that time, however, high-resolution methods of protein purification were not commonly used and characterization of the various enzymes catalyzing GSH conjugations remained nebulous.

Improved enzyme preparations and the monitoring of enzyme activity with alternative substrates were key to clarifying the multiplicity of GSH transferases and their substrate selectivity profiles. Gradient elution of ion-exchange columns, isoelectric focusing, and chromatofocusing techniques were used to resolve GST isoenzymes from rat liver and many other tissues (*7, 8*). An important tool was the "universal" GST substrate 1-chloro-2, 4-dinitrobenzene (CDNB; figure 10-2) (*9*), introduced by J. N. Smith and coworkers:

$$1\text{-Chloro-2,4-dinitrobenzene} + GSH \rightarrow$$
$$S\text{-2,4-dinitrophenylglutathione} + H^+ + Cl^-$$

The finding that CDNB, an "aryl electrophile," was a substrate for most GSTs studied[1] made the name "GSH S-aryltransferase" unsuitable, since this label applied to numerous enzymes. Indeed, GSTs generally displayed overlapping substrate specificities. GSTs were found not only in the cytoplasm but also in hepatic mitochondrial and microsomal fractions. A distinct rat liver "microsomal" GST was finally isolated by Ralf

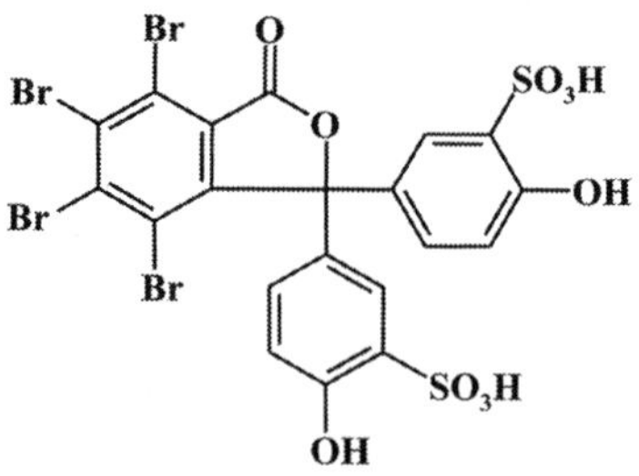

FIGURE 10-1.
Bromosulfophthalein, the first GST substrate used.

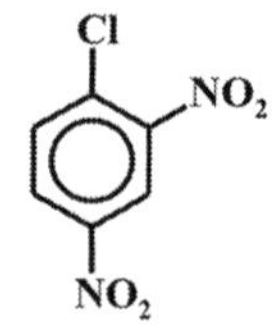

FIGURE 10-2.
1-Chloro-2,4-dinitrobenzene an easily monitored GST substrate.

Morgenstern and found to be structurally unrelated to the soluble GSTs (*10*).

GST: CLASSIFICATION AND NOMENCLATURE

Advances in genomics have facilitated the identification and classification of the multiple forms of soluble GST, as has been true for other families of drug-metabolizing enzymes. The *GST* genes encode proteins belonging to a superfamily of enzymes that are, first and foremost, regarded as detoxication enzymes (*11, 12*). Some of the enzymes have also adopted alternative functions, serving, for example, as eye lens crystallins (*13*), steroid double-bond isomerase (*14*), or components of cellular signaling pathways (*15*), as we discuss later. When necessary, the GST nomenclature can be supplemented with other names that reflect more accurately the primary biological function of a particular member of the superfamily. We first consider the soluble mammalian GSTs, which are expressed mainly in the cytoplasm but also in other cellular compartments, such as the nucleoplasm.

GSTs do not possess a diagnostic spectral signature comparable to the P450 chromophore, and the variety of chemical reactions catalyzed by GSTs makes it rather difficult to decide on an appropriate systematic name for the enzymes. The Enzyme Commission has assigned the name "RX: glutathione R-transferase" (EC 2.5.1.18) and recommends the trivial name "glutathione transferase" (without the prefix "S"). The commonly used term "glutathione S-transferase" is a misnomer, since the sulfur atom per se is not transferred; rather, it is the glutathionyl group, GS^- (or, equivalently, the R-substituent of RX), which is transferred. (In fact, most reactions with substrates of biological origin are additions rather than substitutions ("transfers"). Enzymes catalyzing additions (or, considered in the reverse direction, eliminations) should correctly be classified as lyases rather than as transferases, according to the Enzyme Commission guidelines.) The abbreviation GST is commonly used and will also be used here.

The concept of *isoenzyme* should, strictly speaking, be applied to enzymes that occur in multiple forms and catalyze the same reaction, for example, the different lactate dehydrogenases of heart and skeletal muscle (*16, 17*). This common catalytic function does not apply to the GSTs, which have distinct, if largely overlapping, substrate specificities. The term isoenzyme could perhaps be appropriate for variant GSTs derived from the same gene, by subunit swapping or alternative splicing. However, it is generally best to avoid the designation "isoenzyme"; if GSTs are related, we can describe them as members of a given GST class. Similar issues arise in the nomenclature of P450 enzymes (see chapter 7).

HUMAN GLUTATHIONE TRANSFERASES

A nomenclature system for human GSTs has been adopted, with new members of the superfamily added as they have been discovered (*18*). The soluble GSTs are subdivided into classes based on sequence similarities (table 10-1). The classes are designated by the *names* of the Greek letters: Alpha, Mu, Pi, and so on, abbreviated in Roman capitals: A, M, P, and so on. (The Greek characters should not be used, since they are not compatible with computational bioinformatics tools.) A given class may contain one or several protein sequences (protein subunits); within the class, proteins are numbered using Arabic numerals. Members of a given class may be more than 90% sequence identical. A tentative lower limit of 50% sequence identity is used to define members of a given class of mammalian GSTs. By this criterion, all of the functional human *GST* genes are clustered on separate chromosomes in a class-wise manner, and this genomic distribution lends strong support to the classification system. Furthermore, the exon/intron structures of genes belonging to the various classes show distinctive differences, including variations in the numbers of exons and introns.

As an example of the nomenclature, the gene for the Mu class subunit 1 is written *GSTM1* (italicized). GSTs are dimeric proteins. The homodimeric protein composed of two copies of subunit 1 of the Mu class is called GST M1-1 (the protein name is not italicized). Heterodimeric structures within the same class can also occur; the enzyme composed of subunits 1 and 2 in the Alpha class is called GST A1-2.

The microsomal GST and its related membrane-bound proteins (*19a*) are structurally distinct from the soluble GSTs. They form a separate superfamily called "MAPEG" (membrane-associated proteins in eicosanoid and glutathione metabolism; table 10-2). The membrane-bound GSTs are designated MGST followed by an Arabic numeral. In cases where a physiological substrate is well defined, the enzyme is named accordingly. An example is leukotriene C_4 synthase.

GLUTATHIONE TRANSFERASES FROM OTHER SPECIES

GSTs from other mammals have been named in a manner similar to that used for the human enzymes (*19b*). For example, the gene *gsta1* in the mouse

TABLE 10-1.

Human Soluble Glutathione Transferases, Classes, and Chromosomal Locations of Their Genes

ENZYME DESIGNATION	CLASS	GENE LOCUS	CHROMOSOME BAND
GST A1-1	Alpha[a]	GSTA1	6p12
GST A2-2		GSTA2	
GST A3-3		GSTA3	
GST A4-4		GSTA4	
GST M1-1	Mu	GSTM1	1p13
GST M2-2		GSTM2	
GST M3-3		GSTM3	
GST M4-4		GSTM4	
GST M5-5		GSTM5	
GST P1-1	Pi	GSTP1	11q13
GST T1-1	Theta	GSTT1	22q11.2
GST T2-2		GSTT2	
GST K1-1	Kappa[b]	GSTK1	7q35
GST Z1-1	Zeta	GSTZ1	14q24.3
GST O1-1	Omega	GSTO1	10q24.3
GST O2-2		GSTO2	
PGD2/GST S1-1$_c$	Sigma[c]	PGD2	4q22.3

[a]*A fifth, possibly functional, Alpha-class gene GSTA5 on human chromosome 6 has been recognized (NP_714543), but a corresponding expressed protein has yet to be demonstrated.*

[b]*The Kappa GST is structurally distinct from the other GSTs in the table. Like the other GST proteins, it forms a dimer, but the secondary structural elements of its subunit have been permutated. Instead of the canonical N-terminal α/β-domain followed by an all α-helical domain, GST K1-1 has the α-helical domain inserted in the α/β-domain (78). This topology has previously been noted in glutaredoxin-2.*

[c]*The Sigma-class enzyme is known as the glutathione-dependent prostaglandin D2 synthase.*

TABLE 10-2.

Membrane-Associated Proteins in Eicosanoid and Glutathione Metabolism (MAPEG)

PROTEIN	GENE DESIGNATION
Microsomal glutathione transferase 1	MGST1
Microsomal glutathione transferase 2	MGST2
Microsomal glutathione transferase 3	MGST3
Leukotriene C$_4$ synthase	LTC4S
Prostaglandin E synthase (microsomal glutathione transferase 1-like)	MGST-L1
5-Lipoxygenase activating protein	FLAP

encodes subunit 1 of the Alpha class. (By convention, *mouse* genes are designated by *lower case*, whereas *human* genes are written in *CAPITAL LETTERS*.) A review listing the current and previous designations for rat and mouse GSTs is available (*11*); a web site for the mouse GSTs is found at the following URL: http://www.people.virginia.edu/~wrp/gst_mouse.html.

When there is a need to distinguish GSTs from different species, a prefix is added; mGST A1-1 and rGST A1-1 are enzymes from the mouse and the rat, respectively. This distinction may be important, since there is no strict one-to-one correspondence between the subunits from different species. Intriguingly, GSTs with the same name from different species do not always have similar functional properties. Also, a given class can have different numbers of genes, even in related species: for example, humans and rats have a single Pi-class gene, *GSTP1*, whereas mice have two, *gstp1* and *gstp2*.

GSTs have been found in aerobic organisms ranging from prokaryotes to multicellular eukaryotes. Some of them are highly divergent from the mammalian GSTs and are assigned to classes other than those already mentioned. Classes Phi and Tau are prevalent in plants and are apparently plant specific (*20, 21*). In many genomes that have been analyzed in their entirety, 20–60 genes have been annotated as *GSTs*. An example of a large superfamily is found in rice (*Oryza sativa*), in which 59 putative GST genes and 2 pseudogenes have been recognized (*20*). Many GST genes occur in clusters, suggesting their origin by successive gene duplications.

Finally, a metalloenzyme catalyzing the conjugation of glutathione with the antibiotic fosfomycin has been isolated from bacteria in clinical samples. This glutathione transferase, FosA, is a dimeric metal-dependent protein, structurally unrelated to either the soluble or membrane-bound mammalian GSTs (*22*). FosA is not encoded in the human genome, but it has a protein fold similar to the human glutathione-linked metalloenzyme, glyoxalase I (*23*).

GST: STRUCTURE

Soluble GSTs

As mentioned above, GST molecules are composed of equal-sized subunits; the soluble enzymes are dimers of approximately 25 kDa subunits. Isolated monomers would presumably be catalytically inactive; an engineered GST P1 monomer has no detectable enzyme activity (*24*). Generally, the functional properties (catalytic efficiency with different substrates; inhibition characteristics) of a given subunit in a cytosolic GST dimer are largely independent of the neighboring subunit (whether identical or nonidentical) (*25, 26*). However, under some conditions, functional cooperativity between the subunits emerges (*27–29*).

The three-dimensional structures of numerous GSTs have been determined by X-ray crystallography. Despite low similarity in amino acid sequences, the tertiary and quaternary structures of GSTs are remarkably similar. Figure 10-3 shows the "canonical fold" of representative GST subunits of the major mammalian classes, Alpha, Mu, Pi, and Theta and illustrates the consistent location of the bound GSH tripeptide. The fold of the polypeptide chain of a subunit is very similar for all four structures, but significant changes occur in the active site region.

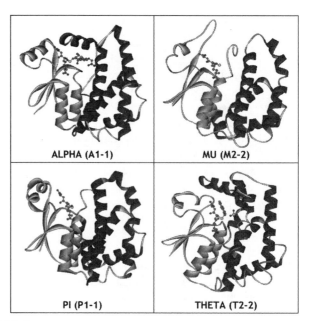

FIGURE 10-3.

Subunit structures of representative human GST enzymes. The thioredoxin-like N-terminal domains, which provide most of the interactions with GSH, are rendered blue. The ligands bound are GSH (in Mu and Pi) and GSH conjugates of ethacrynic acid (Alpha) or menaphthylsulphate (Theta). The second, all-helical, domain provides most of the contacts with the electrophilic substrate and is rendered red. The long red helices contribute to the subunit-subunit interface of the dimeric protein. Structure files are: GST A1-1, 1GSE; GST M2-2, 1HNC; GST P1-1; 6GSS; GST T2-2, 3LJR. *Note*: A full-color version of this figure appears on the website.

An individual GST subunit is built of two domains. The N-terminal domain comprises the first approximately 80 residues and is essentially an α/β structure (*30*, pp. 30–39). This domain harbors the GSH-binding site ("G-site"). The second domain is an α-structure, composed of five or six α-helices. This domain contributes most of the interactions responsible for binding of the electrophilic substrate. With the exception of the Kappa class (discussed later), the subunits of soluble GSTs, ranging from bacteria to insects and plants, are folded and assembled into dimers in the same manner. Structure-based alignment and comparison of GST subunits from numerous classes demonstrate the overall similarities as well as the structural variations of the active-site region that determine their catalytic differences (*31, 32*). GST active sites are discussed in a later section of this chapter.

The two subunits of the GST dimer are related to one another by a two-fold symmetry axis and each subunit contains an active site (figure 10-4). The two active sites are 15 to 20 Å apart. A ligand bound in one active site is, therefore, not close to a ligand bound to the other site (i.e., in the neighboring subunit). In some GSTs, the γ-glutamyl or the glycine portion of GSH bound to the active site of one subunit interacts, via an ionic bond, with a residue in the neighboring subunit; the function of this interaction is not clear.

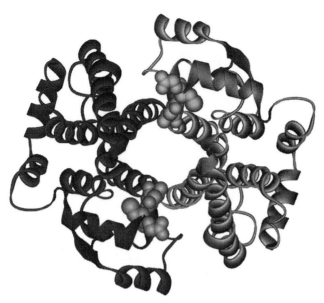

FIGURE 10-4.
GSTs are homodimers; human GST A1-1 is shown from "above" with the (identical) subunits colored red or blue and the bound GSH in space-filling representation.; Structure file 1GSE. *Note*: A full-color version of this figure appears on the website.

Among the few amino acids that are strongly conserved in the GST superfamily are structural core residues that form the *N-cap folding motif*, Ser-X-X-Asp or Thr-X-X-Asp, flanked by hydrophobic residues, called the *hydrophobic staple motif*. In addition, a Gly residue located three residues away in the direction of the N-terminus is maintained in this structural module. These features are important for proper folding of the polypeptide chain and have consequently been safeguarded in evolution (*33, 34*).

Membrane-Bound GSTs

The members of the MAPEG family are membrane bound and their structures are not known in great detail. The "microsomal" enzyme MGST1, which is abundant in both the endoplasmic reticulum and outer membrane of mitochondria, has been studied by electron crystallography. So far, the two-dimensional crystals of the enzyme in complex with phosphatidylcholine have been analyzed to 3 Å resolution in projection (*35*) and a preliminary three-dimensional structure has been determined at 6 Å resolution (*36, 37*). The protein is a trimer of identical 17 kDa subunits; each subunit contains a four-helix bundle penetrating the membrane. The binding site for GSH is located on the cytosolic side of the membrane. Only one GSH molecule per homotrimer is bound at a time, even though all three subunits span the phospholipid bilayer. A cysteine residue (Cys-49 in the rat enzyme) on the same cytosolic side reacts with alkylating and oxidizing agents and may serve a sensor of chemical stress. Modification of this residue by certain agents enhances the enzyme's catalytic activity by an order of magnitude.

Other members of the MAPEG family have similar-sized polypeptide chains (approximately 140–160 residues). Multiple sequence alignment and hydropathy analysis suggest that they have protein folds similar to that of MGST1, including the four membrane-spanning helices (*38*). A structural study of LTC$_4$ synthase (*39*) supports this notion.

The structure of the manganese-dependent GST, FosA, has been determined for both a plasmid-encoded (*40*) and a genomically encoded protein (*41*). The fold has no similarity to any of the canonical GSTs or the MAPEG structure, but resembles glyoxalase I and the estradiol dioxygenase, as well as other members of the vicinal oxygen chelate (VOC) superfamily (*42*).

GST: ASSAYS

GSTs have evolved, under selective pressure, to catalyze the inactivation of noxious electrophilic substances, many of which occur naturally in biological systems. These substrates include epoxides, activated alkenes, and organic hydroperoxides, which are unavoidably generated when organic molecules are exposed to molecular oxygen. Since GSH reacts with many classes of electrophiles (see chapter 9) and GSTs recognize many different substrates, the enzymes can be assayed in many ways. Note that many GST-catalyzed reactions proceed at detectable rates even in the absence of enzyme, a factor that limits the sensitivity of some GST assays.

A convenient, although nonphysiological, substrate is CDNB, mentioned earlier in this chapter. The formation of the GSH conjugate of CDNB can be measured spectrophotometrically at 340 nm, the wavelength at which the thioether product, *S*-2,4-dinitrophenylglutathione, has maximal absorbance. This is the most common method for determining GST activity. However, some GSTs have low or undetectable activity with CDNB.

Many other GST substrates have chromophores that allow spectrophotometric assay of enzyme activity (*43*, *44*), for example epoxy-*para*-nitrophenoxypropane (EPNP; figure 10-5). In some cases, GSTs also catalyze reactions in which GSH serves as reductant and is oxidized to GSSG. An important example is the reduction of hydroperoxides:

$$ROOH + 2GSH \rightarrow ROH + H_2O + GSSG$$

(the "nonselenium glutathione peroxidase" reaction). Such reactions can be coupled to the glutathione reductase-catalyzed reduction of GSSG and monitored by following the oxidation of NADPH at 340 nm. The same coupled assay can be used for monitoring the reduction of disulfides and nitrate esters. Fluorometry is an alternative to absorbance spectroscopy, if the substrate is fluorescent or fluorogenic. Monochlorobimane gives strong fluorescence when conjugated with GSH (*45*).

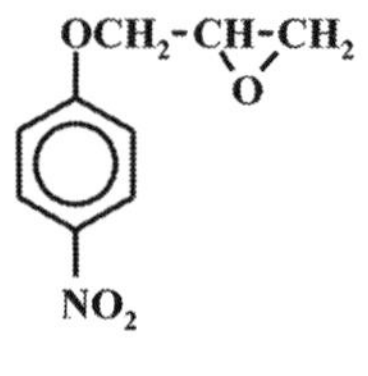

FIGURE 10-5.

Epoxy-*para*-nitrophenoxypropane, a chromogenic epoxide substrate.

Certain biologically relevant substrates, such as activated alkenes, organic isothiocyanates, and *ortho*-quinones, have absorption spectra that change upon conjugation with GSH, but these substances are useful only for certain enzymes and are not "universal" GST substrates. Substitution reactions of GSH are accompanied by proton release, which, in media with low buffer capacity, can be measured directly (electrochemically) or monitored via a pH indicator.

For a large number of reactions catalyzed by GSTs, simple spectro-photometric assays are not available, and one must rely on separation of the substrates and products by chromatography, electrophoresis, or solvent partitioning. High-performance liquid chromatography (HPLC) is often used. Radioactively labeled GSH or xenobiotic substrate can be employed. As with any reaction, one has the choice of measuring product formation or reactant consumption.

The most general assay method is to follow the consumption of GSH; consumption of GSH is common to all conjugation and redox reactions catalyzed by GSTs. However, experience shows that this is practical only for reactions with a low nonenzymatic contribution and high enzyme activity.

GST: PURIFICATION, RECOMBINANT GSTs, AND GST FUSION PROTEINS

In mammalian tissues, some GSTs are very abundant and can be purified to homogeneity by ion-exchange chromatography, gel filtration, and other traditional purification methods. Several percent of the cytosolic protein fraction of liver is composed of soluble GSTs and MGST1 makes up a similar proportion of the membrane proteins in the microsomes. Many GSTs bind tightly to immobilized GSH derivatives and can therefore be purified by affinity chromatography, exploiting the specific recognition of the γ-glutamylcysteinylglycine peptide by the GSTs. Suitable affinity matrices include S-hexylglutathione-Sepharose (*46*) and glutathione-Sepharose (*47*) (figure 10-6). Under favorable conditions, a single step of affinity purification may isolate the bound GSTs from essentially all other proteins in the sample. However, these affinity matrices have somewhat different selectivities and not all GSTs bind to them. Also, some non-GST proteins, for example glyoxalase I, display affinity for the matrices; a particularly tightly binding protein is *macrophage migration inhibitory factor*, which occurs in significant concentrations in some tumor cells (*48*).

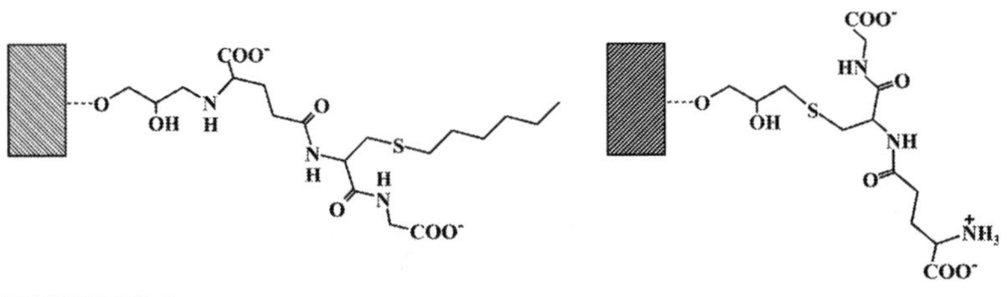

FIGURE 10-6.

Affinity matrices for GST purification. S-Hexyl-glutathione (left) and GSH (right) have been coupled to epoxy-activated Sepharose (boxes).

The different GST enzymes can be separated by means of a high-resolution technique, such as chromatofocusing or preparative isoelectric focusing (*49*). For analytical purposes, HPLC has proved useful for separation and quantification of the different GST subunits obtained by affinity chromatography (*50*). Two-dimensional electrophoresis combined with microsequencing of peptides and immunoanalysis (*48*) was a forerunner to current proteomics approaches. Liquid chromatography in combination with mass spectrometry represents a further development in the analysis of GST expression in tissue samples (*51–53*).

The introduction, in the late 1980s, of recombinant DNA methods for the heterologous expression of GSTs in *E. coli* (*54*) has given a major impetus to protein functional and structural studies. Numerous GSTs have been expressed in good yield, facilitating crystallographic and spectroscopic investigations. With human GST M2-2, for example, expression levels may reach 12% of the soluble protein in the bacterial host (*55*). In cases when insufficient yields are encountered, silent mutations in the DNA may boost expression. Recombinant GSTs can also be furnished with a histidine tag (usually six His residues in the N- or C-terminus), in order to allow purification by Ni(II)-IMAC (immobilized-metal affinity chromatography) (*56*).

The facile expression and high solubility of GSTs make GST fusions very useful for the purification of recalcitrant proteins and for other applications in molecular cell biology (*57*). Complete systems for expression and purification of recombinant GST fusion proteins are available commercially. The system most commonly used is based on an expression plasmid encoding a GST from the parasite *Schistosoma japonicum* (*58*); the target protein-coding sequence is fused to the GST cDNA. The fusion protein is usually soluble and can be purified by GSH affinity chromatography. An analytical application of GST fusion technology is the *GST pull-down assay*: biomolecules interacting with the target protein fused to GST are isolated via immunoadsorption to anti-GST antibodies or through other methods recognizing the GST moiety. (As a consequence of the popularity of these technologies, many of the papers selected by computerized literature searches with the keywords "glutathione transferase" are not studies of GSTs per se, but papers in which GST-fusion technology has been applied to other proteins.)

ACTIVE SITE OF GST

Many mammalian GST enzymes have been studied in great detail and found to have exquisite specificity for the tripeptide GSH. No alternative thiol occurring in the cell can serve as a substitute. The high specificity of GSTs for GSH is associated with the N-terminal domain, composed of β-strands sandwiched between two α-helices on the core side and one α-helix on the surface side of the protein. This region also contains a characteristic proline residue in *cis* conformation that is highly conserved among GSTs and related proteins, such as thioredoxin and thioredoxin-like proteins. In GSTs, the conserved *cis*-proline makes possible a sharp turn of the polypeptide backbone that facilitates the formation of two hydrogen bonds between the main chain of the protein and the cysteinyl moiety of GSH (figure 10-7).

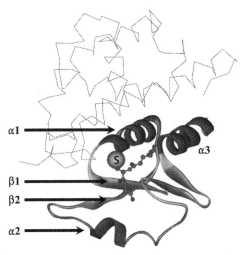

FIGURE 10-7.
Active site of GST M2-2 showing the G-site in the thioredoxin-like domain with the sulfur (yellow) of bound GSH (ball and stick) near the N-terminus of the α1-helix; the second domain of the subunit is rendered as a Cα trace. Structure file: 1HNC. *Note*: A full-color version of this figure appears on the website.

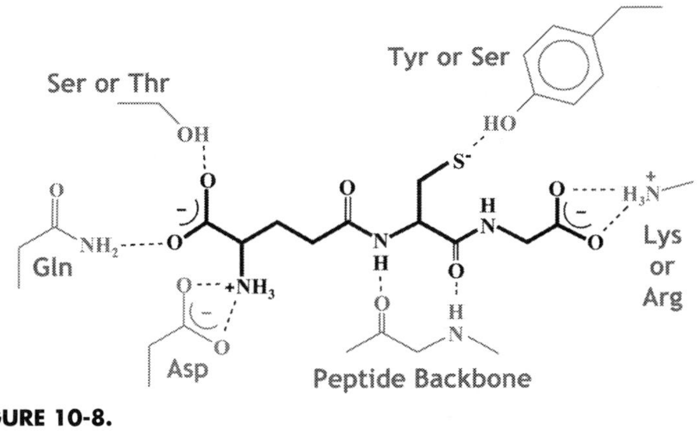

FIGURE 10-8.
The GSH-binding sites of GSTs from the Alpha, Mu, Pi, and Theta classes. *Note*: A full-color version of this figure appears on the website.

G-site

The binding pocket for GSH has been called the "G-site." There are many variations on a common theme, but the first structures analyzed, which represent mammalian classes Alpha, Mu, Pi, and Theta, share the features shown in figure 10-8. Multiple polar bonds contribute to the binding of the charged tripeptide. A tyrosine residue located with its hydroxyl group within hydrogen bonding distance from the GSH sulfur atom is important for catalysis (figure 10-9). In many other GST classes, such as Theta, Zeta, Phi, and Tau, the hydrogen bonding hydroxyl group is provided by the side chain of a serine residue rather than a tyrosine. A third variation is found in the bacterial Beta- and mammalian Omega-class enzymes: a cysteine residue forms a mixed disulfide with GSH in the active site (*31*). None of these G-site residues appears to be responsible for the ionization of the

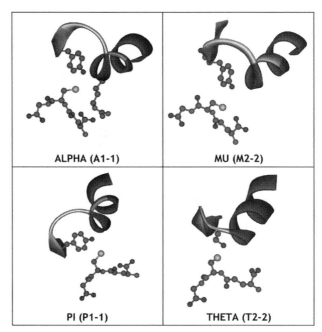

FIGURE 10-9.
GSH bound at the active site of GSTs from four classes, showing the hydroxyl-carrying residue donating a hydrogen bond to the sulfur of GSH in front of the α1 helix. Structure files are: GST A1-1, 1PKW; GST M2-2, 1HNC; GST P1-1, 6GSS; GST T2-2; 3LJR. *Note:* A full-color version of this figure appears on the website.

thiol group of GSH; instead, ionization may be promoted by the proximity of the positive end of the dipole formed by the α1-helix (figure 10-7).

H-site

A hydrophobic binding site called the H-site governs the binding of the diverse electrophilic substrates upon which GSTs act (figure 10-3). In contrast to the G-site, the H-site varies significantly from enzyme to enzyme. The H-site is built primarily from three or four separate segments of the primary structure: the loop between the β1-strand and the α1-helix, a portion of a central helix, α4, and a section of the C-terminal region (see figure 10-9) are the main contributors. They are brought together in the folded protein and form a pocket adjacent to the G-site. The site has some structural flexibility; especially the mobile residues of the C-terminus may allow an induced fit of the substrate to the enzyme.

Several examples show that the peptide segments forming the H-site are the primary determinants of substrate specificity. The catalytic activity of GST A1-1 with alkenals is modest, but exchange of H-site amino acids by site-directed mutagenesis enhanced this activity to the high level that characterizes GST A4-4 (*59*). Similarly, GST A2-2 has been transmuted into an efficient steroid isomerase mimicking GST A3-3 (*60*). Remodeling of the H-site is, therefore, thought to be a major evolutionary mechanism for responding to the challenges presented by novel toxic substances. Even though the H-site residues provide the primary binding contacts with the substrate, additional residues remote from the active site often govern

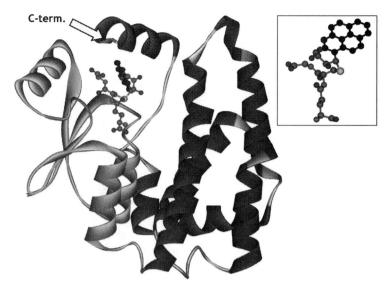

FIGURE 10-10.
Benzo[*a*]pyrene dihydrodiol epoxide (BPDE)–GSH adduct bound in the H-site of an Alpha class mouse GST enzyme; structure file: 1F3B. The inset shows a close-up view of the GSH–BPDE adduct, roughly perpendicular to the view shown in the main figure. *Note*: A full-color version of this figure appears on the website.

TABLE 10-3.
Human GSTs Displaying High Catalytic Activity With Particular Functional Groups

SUBSTRATE CLASS	ENZYME
Epoxides	GST M1-1
Activated alkenes	GST A4-4
ortho-Quinones	GST M2-2
Organic hydroperoxides	GST A1-1

catalytic efficiency. This observation may be explained by the idea that the rate-limiting step in enzyme catalysis may involve conformational changes of the protein or may be controlled by product release, not solely by catalytic chemistry (*61*).

Attempts have been made to correlate the sequence-based classification of GSTs with their activity against the reactive groups of their favored substrates. However, the dramatic alterations of substrate selectivity that may be caused even by single point mutations in GSTs make such generalizations futile. As is also observed with the cytochrome P450 proteins, some of the more abundant enzymes are broad-specificity general catalysts, whereas other forms have evolved to catalyze more specific reactions. Nevertheless, some of the human GSTs are recognized as highly active with particular functional groups of endogenous substrates (table 10-3).

INHIBITION OF GST

GSTs have affinity for a broad range of chemical structures, particularly those enzymes that have a role in the general detoxication of electrophiles. Many compounds can act as inhibitors by competing with GST substrates. GST inhibitors can rationally be divided into molecules that bind to the active site, *endo-inhibitors*, and those that bind outside the active site, *exo-inhibitors*. The endo-inhibitors can be further subdivided based on their binding to the G-site, the H-site, or both sites. G-site inhibition is restricted mainly to compounds with structural similarity to the GSH molecule. This is not a trivial statement, since the γ-glutamyl portion of the peptide moiety is a key determinant for binding, and peptide analogues lacking this part generally do not bind tightly (*62*). The criteria for high affinity to the H-site cannot be readily generalized, since the binding characteristics vary from enzyme to enzyme and the binding pocket has structural flexibility. Hydrophobicity promotes binding and increased potency is usually afforded by an increased chain length of hydrophobic S-alkyl substituents (*8*). The temperature dependence of the inhibition constants demonstrates that the increased affinity is entropy- rather than enthalpy-driven, as is characteristic of hydrophobic interactions (*63*).

S-Substituted GSH derivatives combine affinities for the neighboring G- and H-sites. The peptide moiety anchors the inhibitor specifically in the G-site and the S-substituent provides additional binding affinity via the H-site. This combined effect may be regarded as loss of entropy caused by covalent linking of the hydrocarbon to the peptide, since the two parts, separated, do not strongly inhibit GSTs. However, there is more than entropy loss contributing to high affinity binding. Such synergistic effects do not necessarily require a covalent link between the ligands occupying the G- and the H-sites. A rat Mu-class GST was found to be more strongly inhibited by the antiinflammatory drug indomethacin at high concentrations of the substrate CDNB than at low concentrations (*64*). Conformational changes in the enzyme induced by substrates and inhibitors are probable explanations.

Organotin compounds exemplify the rule that GSTs can be inhibited differentially, by potencies that vary by more than four orders of magnitude (table 10-4). These compounds are valuable experimental tools demonstrating the possibility of discriminating among different GSTs. The usefulness of organotin GST inhibitors in cellular systems is unclear, however, since they are also potent inducers of apoptosis via cytochrome c release and the caspase cascade (*65*).

Inhibitors of GSTs have possible applications as antiparasitic drugs, in counteracting insect resistance to pesticides, and as cytostatic drugs in cancer cells.

▶ GSTs as Targets for Antimalarial Agents

Malaria is the most ubiquitous parasitic disease in the human population, affecting up to 500 million individuals worldwide (*66*) and causing approximately 2 million deaths per year (see also chapter 16). The human parasite, *Plasmodium falciparum*, is transmitted by an insect vector such as the mosquito *Anopheles gambiae*. The parasite propagates in the erythrocytes of its hosts, where it is nourished by the abundant hemoglobin protein, leaving hemin as a toxic byproduct. Hemin has prooxidant activity, presenting an oxidative stress challenge to the parasite.

Two approaches to combat malaria appear possible: targeting the parasite in infected individuals (67) and tackling the mosquito vector. Studies of the genome of *P. falciparum* have identified a single GST; its crystal structure shows an open active-site topology that may be favorable for rational design of parasite-selective drugs (68). Is inhibition of the GST detrimental to the parasite? This remains to be seen, but it is believed that the protein provides protection against the oxidative challenges in the cellular environment of the parasite. The GST is highly abundant in the parasite and may act as a detoxication protein both by sequestering free hemin and by catalyzing the inactivation of toxic products of oxidative stress.

The genome of *Anopheles gambiae* has 31 genes annotated as GST genes (69). Only 9 of the 31 putative GST genes are singletons, and the majority of them occur in clusters of 5 to 11 genes, suggesting multiple gene duplications in their evolution. The control of the malaria insect vector by DDT initiated in the middle of the 1900s raised hopes for the eradication of the disease. However, the rapid development of insecticide resistance was a severe setback. Eight anopheles GST genes colocalize to one of the major genetic loci for DDT resistance, and it is thought that the insecticide has imposed recent selective pressure for gene multiplication. At least one of the encoded GSTs is catalyzing the detoxication of DDT (70). Others may have roles in cellular defense against the oxidative stress often mounted in association with the development of drug resistance. Although DDT has now been largely abandoned, in favor of pyrethroids, detailed understanding of the genetic basis of insecticide resistance may help in monitoring its evolution in the insect population and afford new biochemical tools for controlling the malaria vector. ◀

TABLE 10-4.

Inhibition of Human GSTs by Organotin Compounds

GST	TRIETHYLTIN BROMIDE	TRIPHENYLTIN CHLORIDE
P1-1	3.5	7
M1-1	4.1	0.3
M2-2	3.7	0.7
M5-5	0.14	0.04
A1-1	6	–
O1-1	No inhibition	–
Z1-1	3000	51
T1-1	1400	470
A3-3	8.6	0.6

The values represent inhibition constants K_i (μM).

A. Musungu and B. Mannervik, unpublished.

Note the differential effects of the two inhibitors on the various enzymes.

GST: CATALYTIC MECHANISM

Sulfhydryl groups are weak acids and a central feature of the catalytic activity of GSTs is the activation of GSH. The pK_a of the GSH sulfhydryl is lowered from 9.2 (aqueous solution) to a value below 7 in the active site. Exactly what aspects of the enzyme–GSH interaction accomplish this shift are not known, but proximity to the positive end of the α1-helix dipole is probably a contributing factor. The first step in the catalytic cycle is, therefore, the release of a proton to form the thiolate anion of glutathione (GS⁻). Perhaps surprisingly, the nucleophilic active-site residue (Tyr or Ser) juxtaposed to the sulfur of glutathione is not directly involved in this ionization; mutation of Tyr 9 to Phe in Alpha class GSTs has no major effect of the pK_a value of the sulfhydryl group (71). Instead, these nucleophilic residues promote catalysis by orienting the bonding orbitals of the sulfur for facile attack on the second substrate. For most GSTs, this occurs via hydrogen bonding from a hydroxyl group of Tyr or Ser. In some GSTs (e.g., the Omega and the bacterial Beta class GSTs), as mentioned earlier in this chapter, a covalent disulfide bond is formed between glutathione and the active-site Cys. The precise orientation of the reactants forming the activated complex in enzyme catalysis has been described by Daniel E. Koshland as "orbital steering" (72). Another way of expressing the steric positioning of reactants effected by the enzyme is selection of the subpopulation of substrate molecules with the "near attack conformation" preceding the transition state (73). Guiding the sulfur-orbitals to accomplish a favorable reaction trajectory appears to be a key feature of the G-site of GSTs.

In the steroid double-bond isomerization reaction catalyzed by some Alpha class GSTs (14, 71), the role of the thiolate of glutathione is to serve as a base, abstracting a proton from the steroid substrate. In this case, the proton is the electrophilic center under attack, rather than carbon or a heteroatom, as in most GST substrates.

In aqueous media, hydration of the sulfur atom may attenuate the reactivity of glutathione. Binding of the thiolate to the G-site removes the inhibitory effect of the water molecules and lowers the activation energy for the reaction with the second substrate. The interaction with the nucleo-philic active-site residue may facilitate the desolvation of the sulfur (74).

The chemistry of a GST-catalyzed reaction can be regarded as an attack by an electrophilic center on the reactive sulfur atom of glutathione. It is generally assumed that an important contributor to enzyme catalysis is transition-state stabilization, based on recognition and high-affinity binding of an activated complex. The diverse substrate selectivities displayed by different GSTs presumably rely on the varied abilities of different active sites to accommodate particular transition-state structures. Dis-crimination among alternative substrates is not based on simple com-plementarity between a preformed active site and the selected substrate, since the H-site has structural flexibility and may enclose the substrate in a binding process involving structural adjustments that increase the affinity. Such ligand-induced fit is common to many enzymes interacting with their substrates, as well as to receptors binding their cognate agonists. Indeed, in broad-specificity GSTs, it appears that electrophilic substrates can bind in the H-site in more than one orientation. This is consistent with the notion that one and the same GST may be active with substrates differing widely in size and molecular properties. Nevertheless, the H-site is more elaborate than a flexible hydrophobic cavity, since GSTs, like P450 enzymes, display different substrate selectivity profiles, including regio- and stereospecificity. Topological and conformational constraints in the H-site, and their spatial relationship to the sulfur of GSH in the G-site, govern the productive binding of the second substrate that is necessary for catalysis to occur.

Transition-state stabilization and product formation are crucial to the catalytic process, but many GSTs acting on their most active substrates are not rate-limited by the chemical transformations. Instead conformational transitions and product release limit the catalytic turnover. Numerous GST substrates are large hydrophobic molecules and their GSH conjugates can bind with high affinity to both the H-site and the G-site. Tight-binding GSH conjugates may not only impede catalysis by slow product release, but also cause progressive inhibition of the enzyme, since product concentration increases with time. Product inhibition has consequences for the overall capacity of GSTs to serve in cellular detoxication and this may (at least partly) explain why such high GST protein concentrations are present in liver and many other tissues.

GSTs: EVOLUTION

The molecules of biological systems can be considered as being assembled from a limited number of building blocks. This principle applies at every structural level. All intermediary metabolites can be derived from the combination and transformation of a few dozen simple molecules. All proteins are built from 21 amino acids (and their chemically modified forms) linked into polypeptides. Fusions and recombinations of DNA fragments have gradually caused the expansion of genes, enabling them to encode larger and larger protein structures. Duplication of genes is an important mechanism of evolutionary diversification. Following duplication, one of the gene copies can continue to carry information for the original biological function, while the other copy can be "tried out" for novel purposes. Short sequences that fold into stable secondary and tertiary structures are key elements in protein structure. Larger proteins can be assembled from such "folding modules," each composed of a few α-helices, β-strands, or both.

Among the GSH-dependent enzymes, the structure of the human glyoxalase I subunit bears evidence of duplications of an α/β-motif (23). Glyoxalase I catalyzes the reaction of glutathione with methylglyoxal (H_3C–C(O)–CH=O). In the structure of yeast (*Saccharomyces cerevisiae*) glyoxalase I, this duplication is reduplicated in the same polypeptide chain, thus presenting a "molecular fossil" of sequential duplications and fusions (75). As mentioned earlier, glyoxalase I belong to the VOC superfamily, of which the metallo-GST FosA is also a member. This relationship provides a clue to the evolutionary ancestry of this GST.

Soluble GSTs share the structural α/β-fold originally discovered in structural studies of thioredoxin. Even before any GST structures had been determined, it was suggested that the evolutionary origin of GSTs lay in the fusion between a GSH-binding module and components that conferred the characteristic enzymatic properties of the different enzymes (76). The proposed "primordial GSH binding module" remains unknown, but the suggestion received independent support from the finding that the selenium-dependent glutathione peroxidase (GPX1) contains a thioredoxin-like region similar to that of glutaredoxin (77). Indeed, this GSH-binding α/β-fold has now been recognized in all soluble GSTs, with the exception of the unrelated protein FosA.

Most soluble GSTs seem to have arisen through the addition of an essentially all-α-helical C-terminal portion onto the thioredoxin-like domain. An important exception is the mitochondrial Kappa GST, in which the α-helical domain is inserted after α2 in the first α/β-motif (78). This divergence has a structural counterpart in the bacterial proteins glutaredoxin 2 (79) and the disulfide isomerase DsbA. In retrospect, this should not be surprising, considering the origin of mitochondria as prokaryotic symbionts. In all of these structural variants based on the

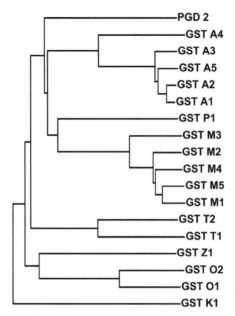

FIGURE 10-11.
Phylogenetic tree of soluble human GST subunits. The Kappa enzyme GST K1-1 is an outlier in which the secondary structure elements of the canonical GST structure have been rearranged in the sequence. PGD2 is prostaglandin D2 synthase.

thioredoxin-like fold, the sulfur of GSH (or the redox active disulfide or selenium in redoxins and GPXs, respectively) is maintained in a position that can be activated by the dipole of an α-helix. This conservation of a topologically equivalent α-helix possessing the ability to activate the thiol may represent biochemical mechanism-driven evolution (80, 81).

The nature of the "ancestral GST" is unknown, but many suggestions have been made about the phylogeny of the GST superfamily. Pemble and Taylor proposed that the Theta class preceded the evolution of the Alpha, Mu, and Pi classes, which are not present in plants (82). Clearly, a separate evolutionary branch led to the Tau and Phi classes, which have abundant members in many plants, but do not exist in animals (20). The Theta and Zeta classes are represented in both animals and plants, and thus have a monophyletic origin closer to the ancestral GST. On the basis of known sequences of human soluble GSTs, a phylogenetic tree can be constructed (figure 10-11). Comparative genomics based on further advances in genome sequencing will help to clarify GST phylogeny and increase our understanding of the various biological functions of the proteins.

Protein engineering studies have shown that point mutations, interchange of chain segments, and other structural rearrangements can give rise to altered substrate selectivities in the GSTs. Stochastic mutations generate ensembles of variants from which GSTs with novel properties can be selected. In addition to exon shuffling as a possible evolutionary mechanism, certain organisms utilize alternative splicing to generate, from a single gene, variant GSTs with different substrate selectivities (83, 84). This is the case for the malaria vector Anopheles as well as for a human parasite, the filarial nematode *Onchocerca volvulus* (85).

▶ **Alternative Splicing**

Many of the genes encoding proteins that participate in the biotransformation of xenobiotics occur in multigene families, and, by virtue of complementary functional properties, they form ensembles of enzymes or transporters capable of handling a vast number of alternative substrates. This functional multiplicity is clearly advantageous for detoxication and elimination of noxious agents of different chemical structures and origins. However, the cell has the capacity to further enhance its functions by rearrangement of its genetic information. Most eukaryotic genes are composed of protein-encoding exons separated by introns, and the latter are spliced out from the pre-mRNA in the course of its nuclear maturation for export to the ribosomes and subsequent translation. The exons of a given gene are not necessarily combined in a single arrangement, but may be assembled such that one, or several, of them is omitted in the processing of the pre-mRNA, a phenomenon called "alternative splicing."

By this mechanism, a single gene can give rise to more that one protein species, thereby broadening its functional expression. Recent estimates suggest that at least 70% of human pre-mRNAs from multiexon genes undergo alternative splicing (86, 87). Alternative splicing is observed in the UDPGT 1 enzyme family (see chapter 12) and the xenobiotic receptors CAR (88) and PXR (89) (see chapter 8). ◀

ALTERNATIVE ROLES OF GSTs

GSTs have acquired biochemical functions in addition to their well-established role in the cellular defense against toxic electrophiles. The evolution of GSTs illustrates what is true for many protein superfamilies: once a stable structural scaffold with adequate functional plasticity has been obtained, it is modified and used over and over again for novel tasks. In the words of Francois Jacob, "Nature is a tinkerer" (90).

Indeed, recent research has revealed that many proteins serve functions other than those with which they were originally identified. In some cases protein evolution, alternative splicing or proteolysis provide modified structures with novel functions. However, in other instances the very same structure seems to play alternative biological roles. A person who holds two different jobs, one during the day and another at night, is said to be "moonlighting," and these dual-function proteins have been termed "moonlighting proteins" (91).

In 1977 Paul Talalay and co-workers (92) found that a hepatic Alpha class GST catalyzes the double-bond isomerization of Δ^5-androstene-3,17-dione to Δ^4-androstene-3,17-dione (figure 10-12). This is a step in the biosynthesis of steroid sex hormones. Johansson and Mannervik later found that a different enzyme, GST A3-3, expressed in human steroidogenic tissues such as placenta, adrenal gland, testis, and ovary, is significantly more efficient with both Δ^5-androstene-3,17-dione and Δ^5-pregnene-3,20-dione (14). The high steroid isomerase activity of GST A3-3 and its tissue distribution suggest an important role in hormone biosynthesis.

The Sigma class GST S1-1 catalyzes the conversion of prostaglandin H2 into prostaglandin D2 and is, therefore, also known as prostaglandin D synthase, EC 5.3.99.2 (93, 94). GST P1-1 has isomerase activity with 13-*cis*-retinoic acid (95), which is transformed into all-*trans*-retinoic acid. Another *cis–trans* isomerase activity is associated with the Zeta-class enzyme GST Z1-1. This enzyme catalyzes the isomerization of maleyl-acetoacetate into fumarylacetoacetate, the penultimate step (of a total of six) in the catabolism of the aromatic amino acids phenylalanine and tyrosine (figures 10-13 and 10-14) (96). Disruption of the *GSTZ1* gene in the mouse is not necessarily lethal, but young animals fed phenylalanine die, with pathological changes to the liver and spleen (97).

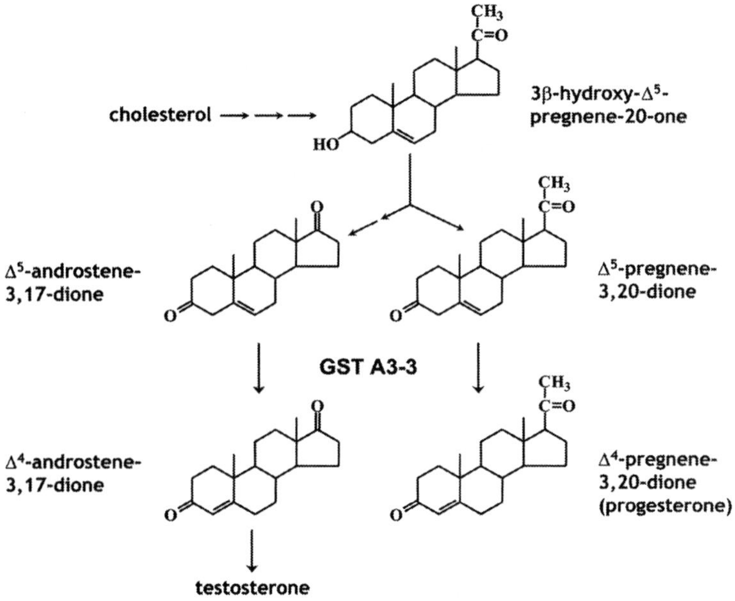

FIGURE 10-12.
Double-bond isomerizations in steroid biosynthesis efficiently catalyzed by GST A3-3; see text for details.

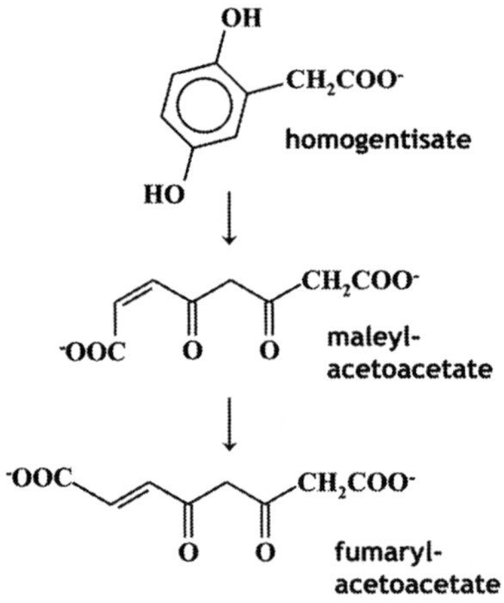

FIGURE 10-13.
Isomerization of maleylacetoacetate to fumarylacetoacetate in tyrosine catabolism.

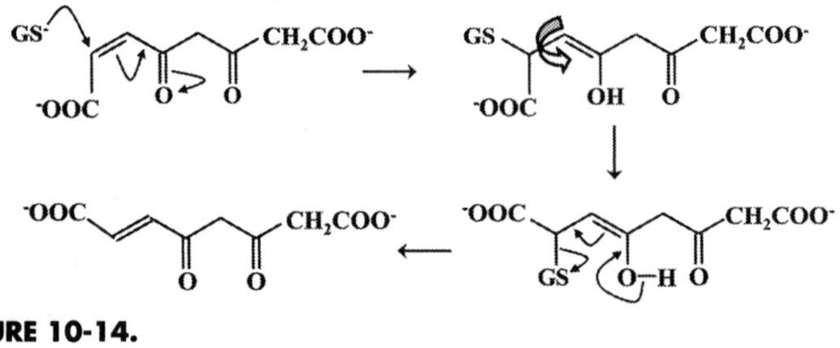

FIGURE 10-14.
Catalytic role of GSH in the isomerization of maleylacetoacetate to fumarylacetoacetate.

GST AS A BINDING PROTEIN

GSTs have repeatedly been rediscovered in new contexts. The research groups of Ketterer, Litwack, and Arias independently found an abundant protein in liver with the ability to bind hydrophobic substances such as azodyes, steroids, and bilirubin. They concluded that they were working on the same protein and named it "ligandin," recognizing its capacity to bind numerous organic ligands in a manner reminiscent of albumin's action in blood plasma (98). Experiments with isolated cells demonstrated that ligandin was capable of facilitated transport of some organic molecules across the plasma membrane. The protein was subsequently identified with an Alpha-class GST (99), now called GST A1-3 in rats and GST A1-1 in humans. The biological importance of this intracellular binding function is still somewhat uncertain, but it may be associated with the active transport of molecules effected by MRPs (see chapter 9) and other ATP-driven membrane pumps.

NONCATALYTIC FUNCTIONS OF GSTs IN THE EYE

Two carotenoid compounds, lutein and zeaxanthin, are present in the macula of the human eye, where they fulfill protective functions. Their concentrations at the fovea are in the millimolar range. A specific macular zeaxanthin-binding protein was purified and identified as GST P1-1 (100). Immunohistochemical analysis of the human retina demonstrated high levels of GST P1-1 in the parafoeval plexiform layers in good correlation with the known distribution of the macular carotenoid pigments. Thus, in addition to the Alpha-class proteins just mentioned, a Pi-class GST also may serve as a physiologically important binding protein.

In the lenses of cephalopod (squid, octopus) eyes—but not in mammalian eyes, which evolved independently—GSTs have been adopted as structural proteins, crystallins (13). The catalytic GST function has been lost by an insertion of a peptide segment between the conserved α-4 and α-5 helices in the structure, which otherwise resembles the canonical GST fold. This results in a very closed conformation around the putative active site, despite overall topological similarities with the Sigma-class structure (101). The digestive gland of the cephalopod (which has liver-like functions) contains homologous GSTs with high enzymatic activity. The high solubility and optical transparency of GSTs apparently make them suitable as crystallins.

GSH AND GSTs IN CELLULAR SIGNALING

Inactivation of Signal Substances

GSH and GSTs appear to have at least two functions in the cellular signaling of chemical stress. One role is the chemical transformation of molecules that serve as messengers of oxidative stress and other insults. Another is the regulation of signal transduction via protein–protein interactions.

Several products of lipid peroxidation are not only toxic agents per se, but also elicit cellular responses, such as chemotaxis, apoptosis, and transcriptional activation. We are reminded of well-recognized signaling molecules such as prostaglandins, leukotrienes, and thromboxanes that arise from arachidonic acid and related polyunsaturated fatty acids (*102, 103*), but which are not usually regarded as toxins. 13-Oxooctadecadienoic acid, a reactive 2,4-dienenone derived from linoleic acid, impinges on cell proliferation and differentiation. The disposition of this bioactive compound involves GSH conjugation and export of the conjugate, thus terminating its action (*104*).

4-Hydroxynonenal (HNE), a major end product of lipid peroxidation (see chapter 1), occurs in submicromolar concentration in human plasma and increases during oxidative stress caused by inflammation, exposure to pollutants, and other prooxidative conditions. This toxic compound results from oxidative degradation of arachidonic acid in biological membranes and has multiple cellular effects. Several lines of evidence suggest that HNE is a key signaling molecule that links oxidative stress and redox regulation of cellular processes (*105*). Many apoptosis-causing agents induce lipid peroxidation and HNE formation, and there is evidence that HNE serves as an intermediary that translates the oxidative stress into an apoptotic response. Like other 4-hydroxyalkenals, HNE is efficiently conjugated and inactivated by GST A4-4 (*106–109*). Scavenging of HNE by GSH conjugation and export from the cell counteract apoptosis. In fact, an increase of the intracellular concentration of GST A4-4 can cause transformation and immortalization of cells in tissue culture (*110*).

Thus, GSTs can take part in signaling by modulating the concentration of effector molecules and eliminating their activity through metabolism, in a manner similar to the action of acetylcholine esterase, which degrades the neurotransmitter substance acetylcholine. In fact, many, if not most, GST substrates can activate the transcription factor Nrf2, thereby eliciting upregulation of GST genes via the antioxidant response elements (ARE). An electrophile that is not inactivated sufficiently rapidly will induce the transcription and biosynthesis of GSTs. This feedback control appears to be a device suited to adjust the biochemical defense to the cell's requirements.

Binding to Stress-Activated Protein Kinases

Eukaryotic organisms ranging from nematodes to humans can respond to chemical and physical stress via signals sent from the cell surface to intracellular compartments. GSTs may participate in cell signaling pathways (*111*) (figures 10-15 and 10-16). Key players in intracellular signal transduction are *stress-activated protein kinases* belonging to the family of mitogen-activated protein (MAP) kinases. Three mammalian genes encode alternative forms of c-Jun N-terminal kinase (JNK), and these proteins, depending on cellular context and available protein substrates, regulate pathways leading either to apoptosis or to cellular proliferation and differentiation (*112*). The JNK homologues extracellular signal-regulated kinase (Erk) and p38 (38 kDa protein kinase) are downstream catalysts in these signaling cascades (*113*). Phosphorylation of transcription factors, for example, c-Jun and c-Fos, which dimerize to form activator protein-1 (AP-1), enhances transcription via binding to cognate nucleotide sequences in promoters of targeted genes. Translocation of JNK into mitochondria will cause phosphorylation of the Bcl-2 family members, which govern the balance between proapoptotic and antiapoptotic processes.

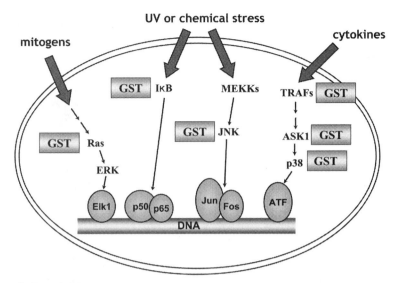

FIGURE 10-15.

Binding studies suggest that GSTs may selectively combine with stress-activated protein kinases and other intracellular proteins, thereby affecting downstream transcriptional regulation of gene expression. Some of the components of the cellular signaling pathways that may be affected by interactions with GSTs are indicated. *Note*: A full-color version of this figure appears on the website.

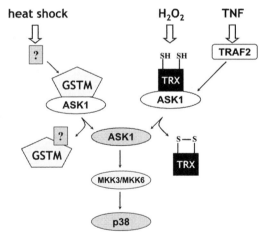

FIGURE 10-16.

Participation of GST M1-1 in the cellular response to heat shock, via dissociation from an inhibitory complex with apoptosis signal-regulating kinase 1 (ASK1). Activated ASK1 protein phosphorylates the downstream mitogen-activated protein (MAP) kinase kinases 3 and 6, which in turn activate p38. The heat-responsive pathway is distinct from the sensing of oxidative stress (H_2O_2) via release of ASK from the inhibitory complex with thioredoxin, which also enables signaling by tumor necrosis factor (TNF) via TNF receptor-associated factor 2 (TRAF2). (*Adapted from Dorion, S.; Lambert, H.; Landry, J. Activation of the p38 signaling pathway by heat shock involves the dissociation of glutathione S-transferase Mu from Ask1.* J. Biol. Chem. **2002**, 277, 30792–30797.) *Note*: A full-color version of this figure appears on the website.

GSTs bind to components of cellular signaling pathways (protein–protein interactions). GST P1-1 forms a complex with JNK1 (*114*) and thereby inhibits its kinase activity (*15*). The regulatory role of GST P1-1 may be linked to oxidative stress, which leads to dissociation of the complex and consequent activation of JNK. Similarly, mouse GST M1-1 can bind to apoptosis signal-regulating kinase 1 (ASK1), thereby suppressing its basal kinase activity (*115*). The complex between GST M1-1 and ASK1 dissociates (by an unknown mechanism) when cells are exposed to heat shock (44°C), but not when subjected to H_2O_2 (oxidative stress). In contrast, ASK1 complexed with thioredoxin is activated by the oxidation and release of thioredoxin, thereby enabling TRAF2 binding (figure 10-16). Thus, two different pathways responding to disparate forms of cellular stress (heat shock and oxidative stress) converge at the same kinase, which in turn activates p38 (via MAP kinase kinases 3 and 6). In this scheme GST M1-1 is a component of a cellular device sensing heat shock (*115*).

A general search for amino acid sequences binding to human GSTs identified a peptide with affinity for GST A1-1. The peptide sequence was similar to a portion of the primary structure of tumor necrosis factor (TNF) receptor-associated factor (TRAF4) (*111*). This finding suggests that ASK1 can be activated by TNFα via members of the TRAF family (*116*).

The interactions between GSTs and signaling kinases indicate essential roles of GSTs in the regulation of cell proliferation and apoptosis. Other proteins with which GSTs might interact include the members of the protein families related to IκB, Ras, and p38 (figure 10-15). GST–protein interactions are not limited to mammalian tissues, but have counterparts in insects and other organisms. Four alternatively spliced variants of an *Anopheles dirus* GST had differential effects on JNK (*114*). A proteomics approach based on immobilized nematode GST similarly identified JNK as a binding partner (*117*). In addition, many other types of proteins were found to have affinity for the GST. Some of these appear to reflect the genes influencing GSH homeostasis in yeast, as was mentioned in chapter 9 (*118*).

How do GSTs sense the stress signals that affect their interactions with kinases? This is not yet known, but many GSTs have conserved Cys residues that can react with oxidants or electrophiles and thereby sense chemical stress. Modification of a sulfhydryl group can cause conformational changes that might affect the GST's affinity for its partner protein. Recognition of the roles of GSTs in cellular signaling extends the scope of GST biochemistry to critical events in the transcriptional regulation of gene expression in response to toxic insults.

Note

1. Since the 1970s many GSTs have been discovered that have no significant activity with CDNB. Therefore, the description of CDNB as a "universal" GST substrate was mistaken.

References

1. Hayes, J. D.; Flanagan, J. U.; Jowsey, I. R. Glutathione transferases. *Ann. Rev. Pharmacol. Toxicol.* **2005**, *45*, 51–88.

2. Combes, B.; Stakelum, G. S. A liver enzyme that conjugates sulfo-bromophthalein sodium with glutathione. *J. Clin. Invest.* **1961**, *40*, 981–988.

3. Sano, K.; Totsuka, Y.; Ikegami, Y.; Uesugi, T. Metabolism of sulphobromophthalein I: positional isomers of sulphobromophthalein monoglutathione conjugate. *J. Pharm. Pharmacol.* **2001**, *53*, 1015–1020.

4. Boyland, E.; Booth, J.; Sims, P. An enzyme from rat liver catalyzing conjugations with glutathione. *Biochem. J.* **1961**, *79*, 516–524.

5. Chasseaud, L. F. The role of glutathione and glutathione S-transferases in the metabolism of chemical carcinogens and other electrophilic agents. *Adv. Cancer Res.* **1979**, *29*, 175–274.

6. Boyland, E.; Chasseaud, L. F. The role of glutathione and glutathione S-transferases in mercapturic acid biosynthesis. *Adv. Enzymol. Relat Areas Mol. Biol.* **1969**, *32*, 173–219.

7. Habig, W. H.; Pabst, M. J.; Jakoby, W. B. Glutathione S-transferases. The first enzymatic step in mercapturic acid formation. *J. Biol. Chem.* **1974**, *249*, 7130–7139.

8. Askelöf, P.; Guthenberg, C.; Jakobson, I.; Mannervik, B. Purification and characterization of two glutathione S-aryltransferase activities from rat liver. *Biochem. J.* **1975**, *147*, 513–522.

9. Clark, A. G.; Smith, J. N.; Speir, T. W. Cross-specificity in some vertebrate and insect glutathione-transferases with methyl parathion (dimethyl *p*-nitrophenyl phosphorothionate), 1-chloro-2,4-dinitro-benzene and *S*-crotonyl-*N*-acetylcysteamine as substrates. *Biochem. J.* **1973**, *135*, 385–392.

10. Morgenstern, R.; Guthenberg, C.; DePierre, J. W. Microsomal glutathione S-transferase. Purification, initial characterization and demonstration that it is not identical to the cytosolic glutathione S-transferases A, B and C. *Eur. J. Biochem.* **1982**, *128*, 243–8.

11. Hayes, J. D.; Pulford, D. J. The glutathione S-transferase supergene family: regulation of GST and the contribution of the isoenzymes to cancer chemoprotection and drug resistance. *Crit. Rev. Biochem. Mol. Biol.* **1995**, *30*, 445–600.

12. Armstrong, R. N. Structure, catalytic mechanism, and evolution of the glutathione transferases. *Chem. Res. Toxicol.* **1997**, *10*, 2–18.

13. Tomarev, S. I.; Chung, S.; Piatigorsky, J. Glutathione S-transferase and S-crystallins of cephalopods: evolution from active enzyme to lens-refractive proteins. *J. Mol. Evol.* **1995**, *41*, 1048–1056.

14. Johansson, A.-S.; Mannervik, B. Human glutathione transferase A3-3, a highly efficient catalyst of double-bond isomerization in the biosynthetic pathway of steroid hormones. *J. Biol. Chem.* **2001**, *276*, 33061–33065.

15. Adler, V.; Yin, Z.; Fuchs, S. Y.; Benezra, M.; Rosario, L.; Tew, K. D.; Pincus, M. R.; Sardana, M.; Henderson, C. J.; Wolf, C. R.; Davis, R. J.; Ronai, Z. Regulation of JNK signaling by GSTp. *EMBO J.* **1999**, *18*, 1321–1334.

16. Markert, C. L.; Møller, F. Multiple forms of enzymes: tissue, ontogenetic, and species specific patterns. *Proc. Natl. Acad. Sci. USA* **1959**, *45*, 753–763.

17. Cahn, R. D.; Kaplan, N. O.; Levine, L.; Zwilling, E. Nature and development of lactic dehydrogenases. *Science* **1962**, *136*, 962–969.

18. Mannervik, B.; Awasthi, Y. C.; Board, P. G.; Hayes, J. D.; Di Ilio, C.; Ketterer, B.; Listowsky, I.; Morgenstern, R.; Muramatsu, M.; Pearson, W. R.; Pickett, C. B.; Sato, K.; Widersten, M.; Wolf, C. R. Nomenclature for human glutathione transferases. *Biochem. J.* **1992**, *282*, 305–306.

19. (a) Jakobsson, P. J.; Thorén, S.; Morgenstern, R.; Samuelsson, B. Identification of human prostaglandin E synthase: a microsomal, glutathione-dependent, inducible enzyme, constituting a potential novel drug target. *Proc. Natl. Acad. Sci. USA* **1999**, *96*, 7220–7225. (b) Mannervik, B.; Board, P. G.; Hayes, J. D.; Listowsky, I.; Pearson, W. R. Nomenclature for mammalian soluble glutathione transferases. *Methods Enzymol.* **2005**, *401*, 1–8.

20. Soranzo, N.; Sari Gorla, M.; Mizzi, L.; De Toma, G.; Frova, C. Organisation and structural evolution of the rice glutathione S-transferase gene family. *Mol. Genet. Genomics* **2004**, *271*, 511–521.

21. Dixon, D. P.; Davis, B. G.; Edwards, R. Functional divergence in the glutathione transferase superfamily in plants. Identification of two classes with putative functions in redox homeostasis in *Arabidopsis thaliana*. *J. Biol. Chem.* **2002**, *277*, 30859–30869.

22. Bernat, B. A.; Laughlin, L. T.; Armstrong, R. N. Fosfomycin resistance protein (FosA) is a manganese metalloglutathione transferase related to glyoxalase I and the extradiol dioxygenases. *Biochemistry* **1997**, *36*, 3050–3055.

23. Cameron, A. D.; Olin, B.; Ridderström, M.; Mannervik, B.; Jones, T. A. Crystal structure of human glyoxalase I: evidence for gene duplication and 3D domain swapping. *EMBO J.* **1997**, *16*, 3386–3395.

24. Abdalla, A. M.; Bruns, C. M.; Tainer, J. A.; Mannervik, B.; Stenberg, G. Design of a monomeric human glutathione transferase GSTP1, a structurally stable but catalytically inactive protein. *Protein Eng.* **2002**, *15*, 827–834.

25. Danielson, U. H.; Mannervik, B. Kinetic independence of the subunits of cytosolic glutathione transferase from the rat. *Biochem. J.* **1985**, *231*, 263–267.

26. Tahir, M. K.; Mannervik, B. Simple inhibition studies for distinction between homodimeric and heterodimeric isoenzymes of glutathione transferase. *J. Biol. Chem.* **1986**, *261*, 1048–1051.

27. Caccuri, A. M.; Antonini, G.; Ascenzi, P.; Nicotra, M.; Nuccetelli, M.; Mazzetti, A. P.; Federici, G.; Lo Bello, M.; Ricci, G. Temperature adaptation of glutathione S-transferase P1-1. A case for homotropic regulation of substrate binding. *J. Biol. Chem.* **1999**, *274*, 19276–19280.

28. Xiao, B.; Singh, S. P.; Nanduri, B.; Awasthi, Y. C.; Zimniak, P.; Ji, X. Crystal structure of a murine glutathione S-transferase in complex with a glutathione conjugate of 4-hydroxynon-2-enal in one subunit and glutathione in the other: evidence of signaling across the dimer interface. *Biochemistry* **1999**, *38*, 11887–11894.

29. Lien, S.; Gustafsson, A.; Andersson, A.-K.; Mannervik, B. Human glutathione transferase A1-1 demonstrates both half-of-the-sites and all-of-the-sites reactivity. *J. Biol. Chem.* **2001**, *276*, 35599–35605.

30. Petsko, G. A.; Ringe, D. *Protein Structure and Function*; New Series Press: London, 2004.

31. Board, P. G.; Coggan, M.; Chelvanayagam, G.; Easteal, S.; Jermiin, L. S.; Schulte, G. K.; Danley, D. E.; Hoth, L. R.; Griffor, M. C.; Kamath, A. V.; Rosner, M. H.; Chrunyk, B. A.; Perregaux, D. E.; Gabel, C. A.; Geoghegan, K. F.; Pandit, J. Identification, characterization, and crystal structure of the Omega class glutathione transferases. *J. Biol. Chem.* **2000**, *275*, 24798–24806.

32. Thom, R.; Cummins, I.; Dixon, D. P.; Edwards, R.; Cole, D. J.; Lapthorn, A. J. Structure of a Tau class glutathione S-transferase from wheat active in herbicide detoxification. *Biochemistry* **2002,** *41*, 7008–7020.

33. Cocco, R.; Stenberg, G.; Dragani, B.; Rossi Principe, D.; Paludi, D.; Mannervik, B.; Aceto, A. The folding and stability of human Alpha class glutathione transferase A1-1 depend on distinct roles of a conserved N-capping box and hydrophobic staple motif. *J. Biol. Chem.* **2001,** *276*, 32177–32183.

34. Kong, G. K.; Polekhina, G.; McKinstry, W. J.; Parker, M. W.; Dragani, B.; Aceto, A.; Paludi, D.; Principe, D. R.; Mannervik, B.; Stenberg, G. Contribution of glycine 146 to a conserved folding module affecting stability and refolding of human glutathione transferase P1-1. *J. Biol. Chem.* **2003,** *278*, 1291–1302.

35. Schmidt-Krey, I.; Murata, K.; Hirai, T.; Mitsuoka, K.; Cheng, Y.; Morgenstern, R.; Fujiyoshi, Y.; Hebert, H. The projection structure of the membrane protein microsomal glutathione transferase at 3 Å resolution as determined from two-dimensional hexagonal crystals. *J Mol. Biol.* **1999,** *288*, 243–253.

36. Schmidt-Krey, I.; Mitsuoka, K.; Hirai, T.; Murata, K.; Cheng, Y.; Fujiyoshi, Y.; Morgenstern, R.; Hebert, H. The three-dimensional map of microsomal glutathione transferase 1 at 6 Å resolution. *EMBO J* **2000,** *19*, 6311–6316.

37. Holm, P. J.; Morgenstern, R.; Hebert, H. The 3-D structure of microsomal glutathione transferase 1 at 6 Å resolution as determined by electron crystallography of p22(1)2(1) crystals. *Biochim. Biophys. Acta* **2002,** *1594*, 276–285.

38. Jakobsson, P. J.; Morgenstern, R.; Mancini, J.; Ford-Hutchinson, A.; Persson, B. Common structural features of MAPEG: a widespread superfamily of membrane associated proteins with highly divergent functions in eicosanoid and glutathione metabolism. *Protein Sci.* **1999,** *8*, 689–692.

39. Schmidt-Krey, I.; Kanaoka, Y.; Mills, D. J.; Irikura, D.; Haase, W.; Lam, B. K.; Austen, K. F.; Kuhlbrandt, W. Human leukotriene C4 synthase at 4.5 Å resolution in projection. *Structure (Camb.)* **2004,** *12*, 2009–2014.

40. Pakhomova, S.; Rife, C. L.; Armstrong, R. N.; Newcomer, M. E. Structure of fosfomycin resistance protein FosA from transposon Tn2921. *Protein Sci.* **2004,** *13*, 1260–1265.

41. Rife, C. L.; Pharris, R. E.; Newcomer, M. E.; Armstrong, R. N. Crystal structure of a genomically encoded fosfomycin resistance protein (FosA) at 1.19 Å resolution by MAD phasing off the L-III edge of Tl(+). *J. Am. Chem. Soc.* **2002,** *124*, 11001–11003.

42. Armstrong, R. N. Mechanistic diversity in a metalloenzyme superfamily. *Biochemistry* **2000,** *39*, 13625–13632.

43. Habig, W. H.; Jakoby, W. B. Assays for differentiation of glutathione S-transferases. *Methods Enzymol.* **1981,** *77*, 398–405.

44. Mannervik, B.; Jemth, P. Measurements of glutathione transferases. In *Current Protocols in Toxicology*; Maines, M. D., Costa, L. G., Reed, D. J., Sassa, S., Sipes, I. G., Eds.; John Wiley: New York, 1999; pp. 6.4.1–6.4.10.

45. Eklund, B. I.; Edalat, M.; Stenberg, G.; Mannervik, B. Screening for recombinant glutathione transferases active with monochlorobimane. *Anal. Biochem.* **2002,** *309*, 102–108.

46. Aronsson, A.-C.; Mannervik, B. Characterization of glyoxalase I purified from pig erythrocytes by affinity chromatography. *Biochem. J.* **1977,** *165,* 503–509.

47. Simons, P. C.; Vander Jagt, D. L. Purification of glutathione S-transferases by glutathione-affinity chromatography. *Methods Enzymol.* **1981,** *77,* 235–237.

48. Hao, X.-Y.; Widersten, M.; Ridderström, M.; Hellman, U.; Mannervik, B. Co-variation of glutathione transferase expression and cytostatic drug resistance in HeLa cells: establishment of class Mu glutathione transferase M3-3 as the dominating isoenzyme. *Biochem. J.* **1994,** *297,* 59–67.

49. Jensson, H.; Ålin, P.; Mannervik, B. Glutathione transferase isoenzymes from rat liver cytosol. *Methods Enzymol.* **1985,** *113,* 504–507.

50. Ostlund Farrants, A. K.; Meyer, D. J.; Coles, B.; Southan, C.; Aitken, A.; Johnson, P. J.; Ketterer, B. The separation of glutathione transferase subunits by using reverse-phase high-pressure liquid chromatography. *Biochem. J.* **1987,** *245,* 423–428.

51. Rowe, J. D.; Nieves, E.; Listowsky, I. Subunit diversity and tissue distribution of human glutathione S-transferases: interpretations based on electrospray ionization-MS and peptide sequence-specific antisera. *Biochem. J.* **1997,** *325,* 481–486.

52. Zhang, F.; Bartels, M. J.; Stott, W. T. Quantitation of human glutathione S-transferases in complex matrices by liquid chromatography/tandem mass spectrometry with signature peptides. *Rapid Commun. Mass Spectrom.* **2004,** *18,* 491–498.

53. Burns, S. A.; Hong, Y. J.; Mitchell, A. E. Direct liquid chromatography-mass spectrometry method for the detection of glutathione S-transferase isozymes and investigation of their expression in response to dietary flavone. *J. Chromatogr. B* **2004,** *809,* 331–337.

54. Board, P. G.; Pierce, K. Expression of human glutathione S-transferase 2 in *Escherichia coli.* Immunological comparison with the basic glutathione S-transferases isoenzymes from human liver. *Biochem. J.* **1987,** *248,* 937–941.

55. Johansson, A. S.; Bolton-Grob, R.; Mannervik, B. Use of silent mutations in cDNA encoding human glutathione transferase M2-2 for optimized expression in *Escherichia coli. Protein Expr. Purif.* **1999,** *17,* 105–112.

56. Chaga, G.; Widersten, M.; Andersson, L.; Porath, J.; Danielson, U. H.; Mannervik, B. Engineering of a metal coordinating site into human glutathione transferase M1-1 based on immobilized metal ion affinity chromatography of homologous rat enzymes. *Protein Eng.* **1994,** *7,* 1115–1119.

57. Hengen, P. N. Methods and reagents. Purification of GST fusion proteins. *Trends Biochem. Sci.* **1996,** *21,* 400–401.

58. Smith, D. B.; Johnson, K. S. Single-step purification of polypeptides expressed in *Escherichia coli* as fusions with glutathione S-transferase. *Gene* **1988,** *67,* 31–40.

59. Nilsson, L. O.; Gustafsson, A.; Mannervik, B. Redesign of substrate-selectivity determining modules of glutathione transferase A1-1 installs high catalytic efficiency with toxic alkenal products of lipid peroxidation. *Proc. Natl. Acad. Sci. USA* **2000,** *97,* 9408–9412.

60. Pettersson, P. L.; Johansson, A.-S.; Mannervik, B. Transmutation of human glutathione transferase A2-2 with peroxidase activity into an efficient steroid isomerase. *J. Biol. Chem.* **2002,** *277,* 30019–30022.

61. Codreanu, S. G.; Ladner, J. E.; Xiao, G.; Stourman, N. V.; Hachey, D. L.; Gilliland, G. L.; Armstrong, R. N. Local protein dynamics and catalysis: detection of segmental motion associated with rate-limiting product release by a glutathione transferase. *Biochemistry* **2002**, *41*, 15161–15172.

62. Burg, D.; Mulder, G. J. Glutathione conjugates and their synthetic derivatives as inhibitors of glutathione-dependent enzymes involved in cancer and drug resistance. *Drug Metab. Rev.* **2002**, *34*, 821–863.

63. Satoh, K. Weak electrophile selective characteristics of the rat preneoplastic marker enzyme glutathione S-transferase P-form, GST-P (7-7): a theory of linear free energy relationships for evaluation of the active site hydrophobicity of isoenzymes. *Carcinogenesis* **1998**, *19*, 1665–1671.

64. Danielson, U. H.; Mannervik, B. Paradoxical inhibition of rat glutathione transferase 4-4 by indomethacin explained by substrate-inhibitor-enzyme complexes in a random-order sequential mechanism. *Biochem. J.* **1988**, *250*, 705–711.

65. Stridh, H.; Orrenius, S.; Hampton, M. B. Caspase involvement in the induction of apoptosis by the environmental toxicants tributyltin and triphenyltin. *Toxicol. Appl. Pharmacol.* **1999**, *156*, 141–146.

66. Snow, R. W.; Guerra, C. A.; Noor, A. M.; Myint, H. Y.; Hay, S. I. The global distribution of clinical episodes of *Plasmodium falciparum* malaria. *Nature* **2005**, *434*, 214–217.

67. Krauth-Siegel, R. L.; Bauer, H.; Schirmer, R. H. Dithiol proteins as guardians of the intracellular redox milieu in parasites: old and new drug targets in trypanosomes and malaria-causing plasmodia. *Angew. Chem. Int. Ed Engl.* **2005**, *44*, 690–715.

68. Fritz-Wolf, K.; Becker, A.; Rahlfs, S.; Harwaldt, P.; Schirmer, R. H.; Kabsch, W.; Becker, K. X-Ray structure of glutathione S-transferase from the malarial parasite *Plasmodium falciparum*. *Proc. Natl. Acad. Sci. USA* **2003**, *100*, 13821–13826.

69. Ranson, H.; Claudianos, C.; Ortelli, F.; Abgrall, C.; Hemingway, J.; Sharakhova, M. V.; Unger, M. F.; Collins, F. H.; Feyereisen, R. Evolution of supergene families associated with insecticide resistance. *Science* **2002**, *298*, 179–181.

70. Ranson, H.; Rossiter, L.; Ortelli, F.; Jensen, B.; Wang, X.; Roth, C. W.; Collins, F. H.; Hemingway, J. Identification of a novel class of insect glutathione S-transferases involved in resistance to DDT in the malaria vector *Anopheles gambiae*. *Biochem. J.* **2001**, *359*, 295–304.

71. Pettersson, P. L.; Mannervik, B. The role of glutathione in the isomerization of Δ5-androstene-3,17-dione catalyzed by human glutathione transferase A1-1. *J. Biol. Chem.* **2001**, *276*, 11698–11704.

72. Mesecar, A. D.; Stoddard, B. L.; Koshland, D. E., Jr. Orbital steering in the catalytic power of enzymes: small structural changes with large catalytic consequences. *Science* **1997**, *277*, 202–206.

73. Bruice, T. C.; Lightstone, F. C. Ground state and transition state contributions to the rates of intramolecular and enzymatic reactions. *Acc. Chem. Res.* **1999**, *32*, 127–136.

74. Gustafsson, A.; Etahadieh, M.; Jemth, P.; Mannervik, B. The C-terminal region of human glutathione transferase A1-1 affects the rate of glutathione binding and the ionization of the active-site Tyr9. *Biochemistry* **1999**, *38*, 16268–16275.

75. Ridderström, M.; Mannervik, B. The primary structure of monomeric yeast glyoxalase I indicates a gene duplication resulting in two similar

segments homologous to the subunit of dimeric human glyoxalase I. *Biochem. J.* **1996**, *316*, 1005–1006.

76. Mannervik, B. The isoenzymes of glutathione transferase. *Adv. Enzymol. Relat Areas Mol. Biol.* **1985,** *57*, 357–417.

77. Mannervik, B.; Carlberg, I.; Larson, K. Glutathione: general review of mechanism of action. In *Glutathione: Chemical, Biochemical and Medical Aspects*; Dolphin, D., Poulson, R., Avramovic, O., Eds.; John Wiley: New York, 1989; pp. 475–516.

78. Ladner, J. E.; Parsons, J. F.; Rife, C. L.; Gilliland, G. L.; Armstrong, R. N. Parallel evolutionary pathways for glutathione transferases: structure and mechanism of the mitochondrial class Kappa enzyme rGSTK1-1. *Biochemistry* **2004,** *43*, 352–361.

79. Fernandes, A. P.; Holmgren, A. Glutaredoxins: glutathione-dependent redox enzymes with functions far beyond a simple thioredoxin backup system. *Antioxid. Redox Signal.* **2004,** *6*, 63–74.

80. Babbitt, P. C.; Gerlt, J. A. Understanding enzyme superfamilies. Chemistry as the fundamental determinant in the evolution of new catalytic activities. *J. Biol. Chem.* **1997,** *272*, 30591–30594.

81. Gerlt, J. A.; Babbitt, P. C. Divergent evolution of enzymatic function: mechanistically diverse superfamilies and functionally distinct supra-families. *Annu. Rev. Biochem.* **2001,** *70*, 209–246.

82. Pemble, S. E.; Taylor, J. B. An evolutionary perspective on glutathione transferases inferred from class-theta glutathione transferase cDNA sequences. *Biochem. J.* **1992,** *287*, 957–963.

83. Ranson, H.; Collins, F.; Hemingway, J. The role of alternative mRNA splicing in generating heterogeneity within the *Anopheles gambiae* class I glutathione S-transferase family. *Proc. Natl. Acad. Sci. USA* **1998,** *95*, 14284–14289.

84. Jirajaroenrat, K.; Pongjaroenkit, S.; Krittanai, C.; Prapanthadara, L.; Ketterman, A. J. Heterologous expression and characterization of alternatively spliced glutathione S-transferases from a single *Anopheles* gene. *Insect Biochem. Mol. Biol.* **2001,** *31*, 867–875.

85. Kampkotter, A.; Volkmann, T. E.; de Castro, S. H.; Leiers, B.; Klotz, L. O.; Johnson, T. E.; Link, C. D.; Henkle-Duhrsen, K. Functional analysis of the glutathione S-transferase 3 from *Onchocerca volvulus* (Ov-GST-3): a parasite GST confers increased resistance to oxidative stress in *Caenorhabditis elegans. J. Mol. Biol.* **2003,** *325*, 25–37.

86. Johnson, J. M.; Castle, J.; Garrett-Engele, P.; Kan, Z.; Loerch, P. M.; Armour, C. D.; Santos, R.; Schadt, E. E.; Stoughton, R.; Shoemaker, D. D. Genome-wide survey of human alternative pre-mRNA splicing with exon junction microarrays. *Science* **2003,** *302*, 2141–2144.

87. Lareau, L. F.; Green, R. E.; Bhatnagar, R. S.; Brenner, S. E. The evolving roles of alternative splicing. *Curr. Opin. Struct. Biol.* **2004,** *14*, 273–282.

88. Auerbach, S. S.; Ramsden, R.; Stoner, M. A.; Verlinde, C.; Hassett, C.; Omiecinski, C. J. Alternatively spliced isoforms of the human constitutive androstane receptor. *Nucleic Acids Res.* **2003,** *31*, 3194–3207.

89. Lamba, V.; Yasuda, K.; Lamba, J. K.; Assem, M.; Davila, J.; Ström, S.; Schuetz, E. G. PXR (NR1I2): splice variants in human tissues, including brain, and identification of neurosteroids and nicotine as PXR activators. *Toxicol. Appl. Pharmacol.* **2004,** *199*, 251–265.

90. Jacob, F. Evolution and tinkering. *Science* **1977,** *196*, 1161–1166.

91. Copley, S. D. Enzymes with extra talents: moonlighting functions and catalytic promiscuity. *Curr. Opin. Chem. Biol.* **2003,** *7*, 265–272.

92. Benson, A. M.; Talalay, P.; Keen, J. H.; Jakoby, W. B. Relationship between the soluble glutathione-dependent Δ^5-3-ketosteroid isomerase and the glutathione S-transferases of the liver. *Proc. Natl. Acad. Sci. USA* **1977**, *74*, 158–162.

93. Meyer, D. J.; Thomas, M. Characterization of rat spleen prostaglandin H D-isomerase as a sigma-class GSH transferase. *Biochem. J.* **1995**, *311*, 739–742.

94. Kanaoka, Y.; Ago, H.; Inagaki, E.; Nanayama, T.; Miyano, M.; Kikuno, R.; Fujii, Y.; Eguchi, N.; Toh, H.; Urade, Y.; Hayaishi, O. Cloning and crystal structure of hematopoietic prostaglandin D synthase. *Cell* **1997**, *90*, 1085–1095.

95. Chen, H.; Juchau, M. R. Recombinant human glutathione S-transferases catalyse enzymic isomerization of 13-*cis*-retinoic acid to all-*trans*-retinoic acid in vitro. *Biochem. J.* **1998**, *336*, 223–226.

96. Blackburn, A. C.; Woollatt, E.; Sutherland, G. R.; Board, P. G. Characterization and chromosome location of the gene GSTZ1 encoding the human Zeta class glutathione transferase and maleylacetoacetate isomerase. *Cytogenet. Cell Genet.* **1998**, *83*, 109–114.

97. Lim, C. E.; Matthaei, K. I.; Blackburn, A. C.; Davis, R. P.; Dahlstrom, J. E.; Koina, M. E.; Anders, M. W.; Board, P. G. Mice deficient in glutathione transferase zeta/maleylacetoacetate isomerase exhibit a range of pathological changes and elevated expression of alpha, mu, and pi class glutathione transferases. *Am. J. Pathol.* **2004**, *165*, 679–693.

98. Litwack, G.; Ketterer, B.; Arias, I. M. Ligandin: a hepatic protein which binds steroids, bilirubin, carcinogens and a number of exogenous organic anions. *Nature* **1971**, *234*, 466–467.

99. Habig, W. H.; Pabst, M. J.; Fleischner, G.; Gatmaitan, Z.; Arias, I. M.; Jakoby, W. B. The identity of glutathione S-transferase B with ligandin, a major binding protein of liver. *Proc. Natl. Acad. Sci. USA* **1974**, *71*, 3879–3882.

100. Bhosale, P.; Larson, A. J.; Frederick, J. M.; Southwick, K.; Thulin, C. D.; Bernstein, P. S. Identification and characterization of a Pi isoform of glutathione S-transferase (GSTP1) as a zeaxanthin-binding protein in the macula of the human eye. *J. Biol. Chem.* **2004**, *279*, 49447–49454.

101. Chuang, C. C.; Wu, S. H.; Chiou, S. H.; Chang, G. G. Homology modeling of cephalopod lens S-crystallin: a natural mutant of sigma-class glutathione transferase with diminished endogenous activity. *Biophys. J.* **1999**, *76*, 679–690.

102. Samuelsson, B.; Dahlén, S. E.; Lindgren, J. A.; Rouzer, C. A.; Serhan, C. N. Leukotrienes and lipoxins: structures, biosynthesis, and biological effects. *Science* **1987**, *237*, 1171–1176.

103. Simmons, D. L.; Botting, R. M.; Hla, T. Cyclooxygenase isozymes: the biology of prostaglandin synthesis and inhibition. *Pharmacol. Rev.* **2004**, *56*, 387–437.

104. Bull, A. W.; Seeley, S. K.; Geno, J.; Mannervik, B. Conjugation of the linoleic acid oxidation product, 13-oxooctadeca-9,11-dienoic acid, a bioactive endogenous substrate for mammalian glutathione transferase. *Biochim. Biophys. Acta* **2002**, *1571*, 77–82.

105. Awasthi, Y. C.; Yang, Y.; Tiwari, N. K.; Patrick, B.; Sharma, A.; Li, J.; Awasthi, S. Regulation of 4-hydroxynonenal-mediated signaling by glutathione S-transferases. *Free Radic. Biol. Med.* **2004**, *37*, 607–619.

106. Ålin, P.; Danielson, U. H.; Mannervik, B. 4-Hydroxyalk-2-enals are substrates for glutathione transferase. *FEBS Lett.* **1985**, *179*, 267–270.

107. Stenberg, G.; Ridderström, M.; Engström, A.; Pemble, S. E.; Mannervik, B. Cloning and heterologous expression of cDNA encoding class alpha rat glutathione transferase 8-8, an enzyme with high catalytic activity towards genotoxic alpha,beta-unsaturated carbonyl compounds. *Biochem. J.* **1992,** *284,* 313–319.

108. Hubatsch, I.; Ridderström, M.; Mannervik, B. Human glutathione transferase A4-4: an alpha class enzyme with high catalytic efficiency in the conjugation of 4-hydroxynonenal and other genotoxic products of lipid peroxidation. *Biochem. J.* **1998,** *330,* 175–179.

109. Singhal, S. S.; Zimniak, P.; Sharma, R.; Srivastava, S. K.; Awasthi, S.; Awasthi, Y. C. A novel glutathione S-transferase isozyme similar to GST 8-8 of rat and mGSTA4-4 (GST 5.7) of mouse is selectively expressed in human tissues. *Biochim. Biophys. Acta* **1994,** *1204,* 279–286.

110. Sharma, R.; Brown, D.; Awasthi, S.; Yang, Y.; Sharma, A.; Patrick, B.; Saini, M. K.; Singh, S. P.; Zimniak, P.; Singh, S. V.; Awasthi, Y. C. Transfection with 4-hydroxynonenal-metabolizing glutathione S-transferase isozymes leads to phenotypic transformation and immortalization of adherent cells. *Eur. J. Biochem.* **2004,** *271,* 1690–1701.

111. Edalat, M.; Persson, M. A.; Mannervik, B. Selective recognition of peptide sequences by glutathione transferases: a possible mechanism for modulation of cellular stress-induced signaling pathways. *Biol. Chem.* **2003,** *384,* 645–651.

112. Lin, A. Activation of the JNK signaling pathway: breaking the brake on apoptosis. *Bioessays* **2003,** *25,* 17–24.

113. Roux, P. P.; Blenis, J. ERK and p38 MAPK-activated protein kinases: a family of protein kinases with diverse biological functions. *Microbiol. Mol. Biol. Rev.* **2004,** *68,* 320–344.

114. Udomsinprasert, R.; Bogoyevitch, M. A.; Ketterman, A. J. Reciprocal regulation of glutathione S-transferase spliceforms and the *Drosophila* c-Jun N-terminal kinase pathway components. *Biochem. J.* **2004,** *383,* 483–490.

115. Cho, S. G.; Lee, Y. H.; Park, H. S.; Ryoo, K.; Kang, K. W.; Park, J.; Eom, S. J.; Kim, M. J.; Chang, T. S.; Choi, S. Y.; Shim, J.; Kim, Y.; Dong, M. S.; Lee, M. J.; Kim, S. G.; Ichijo, H.; Choi, E. J. Glutathione S-transferase mu modulates the stress-activated signals by suppressing apoptosis signal-regulating kinase 1. *J. Biol. Chem.* **2001,** *276,* 12749–12755.

116. Hoeflich, K. P.; Yeh, W. C.; Yao, Z.; Mak, T. W.; Woodgett, J. R. Mediation of TNF receptor-associated factor effector functions by apoptosis signal-regulating kinase-1 (ASK1). *Oncogene* **1999,** *18,* 5814–5820.

117. Greetham, D.; Morgan, C.; Campbell, A. M.; van Rossum, A. J.; Barrett, J.; Brophy, P. M. Evidence of glutathione transferase complexing and signaling in the model nematode *Caenorhabditis elegans* using a pull-down proteomic assay. *Proteomics* **2004,** *4,* 1989–1995.

118. Perrone, G. G.; Grant, C. M.; Dawes, I. W. Genetic and environmental factors influencing glutathione homeostasis in *Saccharomyces cerevisiae*. *Mol. Biol. Cell* **2005,** *16,* 218–230.

11

▷

Glutathione

and

Glutathione

Transferases:

Toxicological

and

Pharmacological

Aspects

MOLECULAR TOXICOLOGY OF GSH CONJUGATION

The previous two chapters have presented the biochemistry of glutathione (GSH) and some of the enzymes of glutathione-dependent metabolism, especially the glutathione transferases (GSTs). In this chapter we delve into aspects of molecular toxicology and physiology in which glutathione conjugation plays an important role. A major theme is exploration of the factors (developmental, nutritional, genetic, etc.) that influence the expression of GST enzymes. We also examine the roles of GSH and GSTs in cancer prevention and treatment.

GSTs AND OXIDATIVE STRESS

Detoxication mechanisms must be very general in order for cells to cope with the myriad of toxic molecules that arise from endogenous and exogenous compounds. The formation of endogenous substrates for GSTs is linked to oxygen metabolism. That is, many of the important electrophilic functionalities of substrate molecules—including epoxides, activated alkenes, and hydroperoxides—can arise in the cell by oxidative processes. As with cytochrome P450, this may be a reason why multiple forms of GST, with overlapping and complementary substrate specificities, have evolved. Figure 11-1 shows some of the toxic products that arise from oxidative stress to membrane lipids, DNA, and catecholamines. Many of these products have been discussed in earlier chapters (see chapters 1, 3, 9, etc.). Inactivation of these reactive compounds is essential to protect the organism against degenerative processes. In human medicine, oxidative stress is implicated in many pathological conditions, for example, vascular disorders, inflammation, cataract, Alzheimer's disease, and Parkinson's disease (see chapter 1).

The various forms of GSTs have different catalytic efficiencies with these endogenous toxicants, as noted in chapter 10. Lipid peroxidation of polyunsaturated fatty acids, such as arachidonic acid, gives rise to 4-hydroxynonenal and other α,β-unsaturated carbonyl compounds. GST A4-4, encoded in human, rat, and mouse genes, is distinguished by particularly high activity with 4-hydroxynonenal. Clear evidence for the protective effect of this GST has been obtained by experiments with mice in which the *GSTA4* gene has been disrupted. Animals deficient in GST A4-4 have a reduced life span and are more sensitive to prooxidants such as paraquat (*1*). 4-Hydroxynonenal is also one of the reactive substances formed in oxidative processes associated with the etiology of neurodegenerative diseases such as Parkinson's disease (*2*) and Alzheimer's

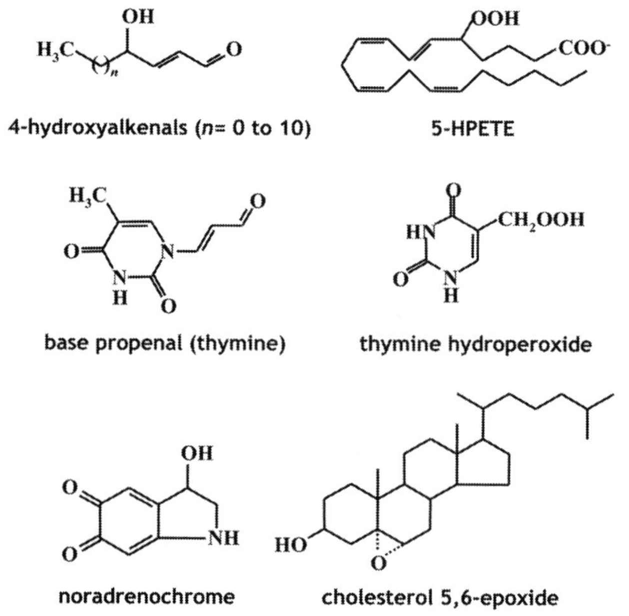

FIGURE 11-1.

Some toxic products arising from oxidative stress to cellular components, such as membranes, DNA, and catecholamines.

disease (*3*). GST P1-1 is the most active human GST with respect to propen-2-al (acrolein) and base-substituted propenals (*4*), oxidative degradation products of nucleic acids (see chapter 2).

Human GST M2-2 has high activity in the conjugation of *ortho*-quinones derived from catecholamines, such as dopamine, dopa, epinephrine, and norepinephrine (figures 11-2 and 11-3). Some quinones are readily reduced by flavoproteins, and their reduced products (hydroquinones) can be reoxidized by dioxygen; this redox cycling process generates reactive oxygen species (see chapter 1). However, the GSH conjugates formed from *ortho*-quinones of dopamine and related compounds are more resistant to such redox cycling. GST M2-2 is present in the substantia nigra and other parts of the brain that are relevant to Parkinson's disease. GSH conjugation can therefore protect the brain, and other tissues, against *ortho*-quinones formed from catecholamines under conditions of oxidative stress (*5–7*). Dopamine-induced oxidative toxicity may contribute to neurodegenerative diseases (*8*) and schizophrenia (*9*).

Organic hydroperoxides are important products of oxidative processes in biological tissues. Polyunsaturated fatty acids are particularly vulnerable to reactive oxygen species and give rise to hydroperoxide derivatives in the form of phospholipids, free fatty acids, and their degradation products. Phospholipid and fatty acid hydroperoxides are highly active as substrates for human GST A1-1 and GST A2-2 (*10*). In addition, hydroperoxides of cholesterol or DNA bases may be reduced by GSTs (*11, 12*). By this "non-selenium GSH peroxidase" activity, GSTs complement the function of the selenium-dependent GSH peroxidases (see chapter 9).

Next, we examine the conjugation of some xenobiotics with GSH.

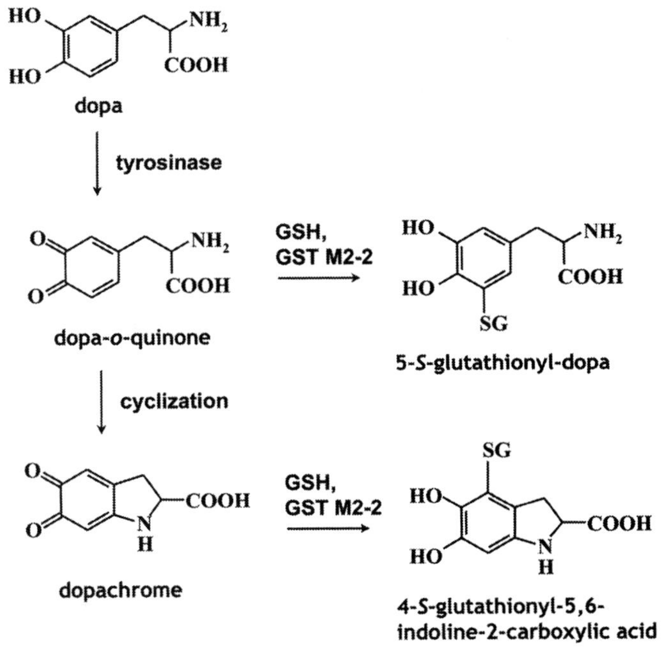

FIGURE 11-2.

GSH, GST, and the formation of neurotoxic *ortho*-quinones. Tyrosinase, which catalyzes the formation of dihydroxyphenylalanine (dopa) from tyrosine, also produces the corresponding dopa-*ortho*-quinone. The amino group of dopa-*ortho*-quinone can undergo Michael addition to the ring structure and, upon further oxidation, a second *ortho*-quinone, dopachrome, is formed. Both *ortho*-quinones can be reduced to their semiquinone forms by flavoproteins, such as NADPH-cytochrome P450 reductase (*continued in figure 11-3*).

GSH, GSTs, AND THE BIOTRANSFORMATION OF CARCINOGENIC EPOXIDES

As discussed earlier in this text (e.g., chapter 2), most chemical carcinogens are genotoxic electrophiles that react with the bases or the sugar–phosphate backbone of DNA. The carcinogens may be intrinsically reactive, but, in most cases, they are activated by metabolism. Ionizing radiation and ultraviolet (UV) light also give rise to reactive free radicals and other electrophilic chemical species. Often, the attack of such reactive species on DNA can be intercepted by reactions with intracellular GSH. Some of these inactivation reactions may be spontaneous and nonenzymatic, but, in most cases, GSH-linked enzymes are involved.

The metabolism and bioactivation of the carcinogenic benzo[*a*]pyrene is discussed in detail in chapter 18. The ultimate carcinogen is believed to be the 7,8-dihydrodiol-9,10-epoxide (BPDE), which binds to guanine residues in DNA. Of the four diastereomeric forms of BPDE, (+) *anti*-BPDE has the highest carcinogenicity. This stereoisomer is a substrate for GSTs (*13*) and experiments with isolated hepatocytes from the rat show that a dose of this dihydrodiol epoxide is almost completely converted into the GSH conjugate (*14*). The biological damage is done by the small

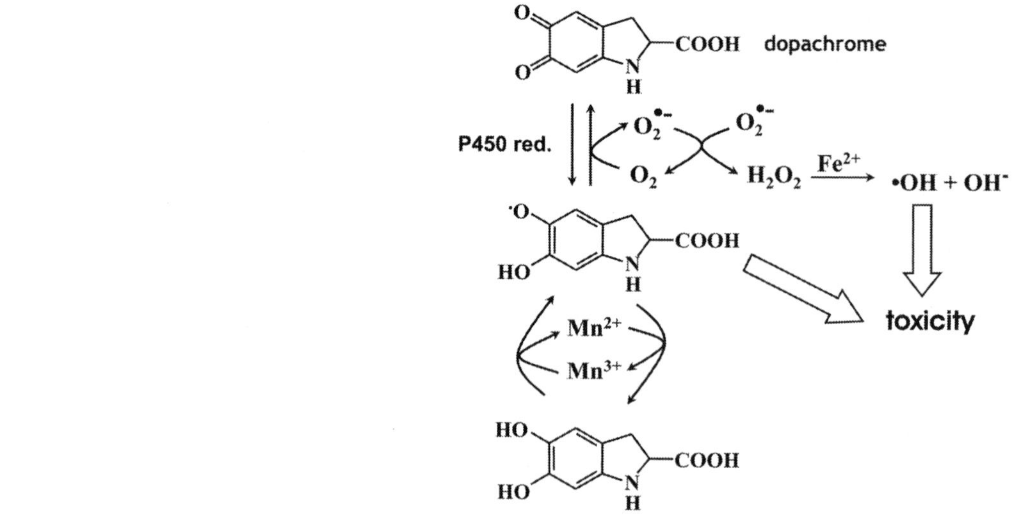

FIGURE 11-3.

GSH, GST, and the formation of neurotoxic *ortho*-quinones (*continued from figure 11-2*). Semiquinones react with dioxygen to form superoxide anion and other reactive oxygen species. GST M2-2 prevents the formation of reactive oxygen species by catalyzing the conjugation of dopa-*ortho*-quinone to give the product 5-glutathionyl dopa and of dopachrome to give 4-*S*-glutathionyl-5,6-indoline-2-carboxylate. The conjugation reactions compete with the one-electron quinone reductions and prevent the formation of reactive oxygen species.

portion of the dose that escapes conjugation with GSH or hydrolysis by water, and survives to react with DNA. The conjugation of BPDE serves as a prototype for the inactivation of many carcinogenic epoxides arising from polycyclic aromatic hydrocarbons. The GSH conjugation is catalyzed by several GSTs, including members of the Alpha, Mu, and Pi classes (*15, 16*). Their catalytic efficiencies differ, as do their regio- and stereoselectivities with respect to the oxirane (epoxide) functional group. In the mouse, a particularly active Alpha-class enzyme, GST A1-1, has been identified, and the structure of its complex with the product (i.e., the conjugate of GSH and BPDE) has been determined (*17*) (see figure 10-10). The mobile $\alpha 9$ helix of the C-terminus of the GST shifts to enclose the substrate tightly in the H-site, and an Arg side chain in the helix folds over the aromatic substrate molecule and contributes to the opening of the oxirane ring.

Aflatoxin B_1, one of the most potent liver carcinogens known, is a mycotoxin produced by the mold *Aspergillus flavus*, which grows on peanuts and grains stored under warm, humid conditions (*18*). Dietary exposure to aflatoxin B_1, in combination with chronic hepatitis caused by virus infections, is a major cause of liver cancer in parts of China and Africa (see chapter 5). Like benzo[*a*]pyrene, aflatoxin B_1 is activated to the ultimate carcinogen, the *exo*-8,9-epoxide (see figure 9-20), through cytochrome-P450-mediated oxygenation. This reactive epoxide is highly unstable and will rapidly be hydrolyzed, unless it has reacted with a nucleophilic group

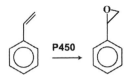

FIGURE 11-4.
Oxidation of styrene catalyzed by cytochrome P450.

of DNA or another cellular component. GST-catalyzed GSH conjugation plays an important role in the biotransformation of aflatoxin. An Alpha-class GST found in the mouse efficiently catalyzes the inactivation of the carcinogen, but rats do not constitutively express an enzyme with a corresponding high activity (19). This probably accounts for the much greater sensitivity to aflatoxin hepatocarcinogenesis of rats, compared to mice. The mercapturate metabolite of aflatoxin can be used as a biomarker to monitor human exposure to the toxin (20).

Styrene is an aromatic liquid used in very large quantities (millions of tons per year) as a raw material for plastics manufacturing. Accidental environmental releases of styrene have occurred repeatedly. In November 2000 a tanker ship carrying 4000 tonnes of styrene sank in the English Channel, leaking much of its cargo into the sea. Another large marine discharge took place in Zhanjiang, China, in March 1995. Styrene is epoxidized by the cytochrome P450 system, producing the mutagenic and carcinogenic metabolite styrene 7,8-oxide (figure 11-4). The benzylic carbon of styrene oxide is a chiral atom and the epoxide occurs as the *R*- and *S*-stereoisomers. Four distinct GSH conjugates (two pairs of enantiomers) can be formed by the attack of GSH at either carbon (7 or 8) of the oxirane rings of the two epoxide stereoisomers (21) (see figure 9-28). This addition reaction exemplifies the possibility of forming alternative regio- and stereoisomers, as is the case for most epoxides. Another well-known example is the formation of four isomeric GSH conjugates of the polycyclic aromatic hydrocarbon metabolite 7,8-benzo[*a*]pyrene dihydrodiol 9,10-epoxide (BPDE; see chapter 18).

GSTs differ in their stereoselectivities for epoxide substrates, so the yields of the isomeric conjugates will not be equal. Human GST M1-1, which has the highest catalytic efficiency with styrene 7,8-oxide, favors the *S*- rather than the *R*-enantiomer of the substrate, and catalyzes the addition of GSH to both C7 and C8. In contrast, human GST P1-1 catalyzes the addition of GSH almost exclusively to the terminal C8 position.

GSTs AFFORD RESISTANCE TO HERBICIDES AND PESTICIDES

Some agricultural herbicides may be inactivated by GST-catalyzed GSH conjugation. A typical example is *atrazine* (2-chloro-4-(ethylamino)-6-(isopropylamino)-*s*-triazine) (22), a triazine used for postemergence control of weeds in corn and other crops (figure 11-5). Seeds of the crop to be cultivated can be pretreated with a "safener," or antidote, to increase resistance to subsequent contact with the herbicide. In the case of corn (maize, *Zea mays*), the safener *N,N*-diallyl-2,2-dichloroacetamide

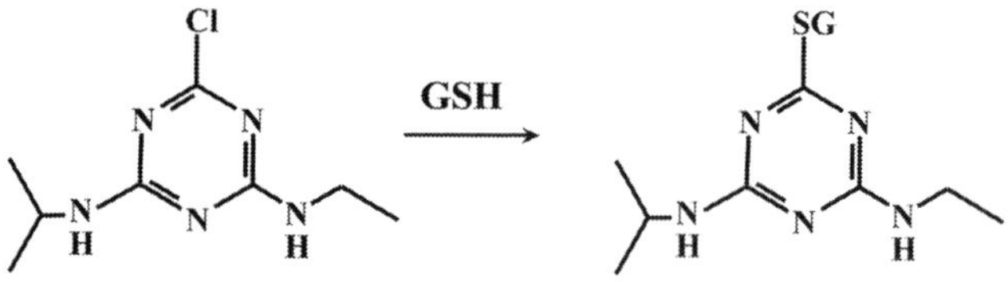

FIGURE 11-5.

The herbicide atrazine undergoes a GST-catalyzed substitution of Cl to form a GSH conjugate.

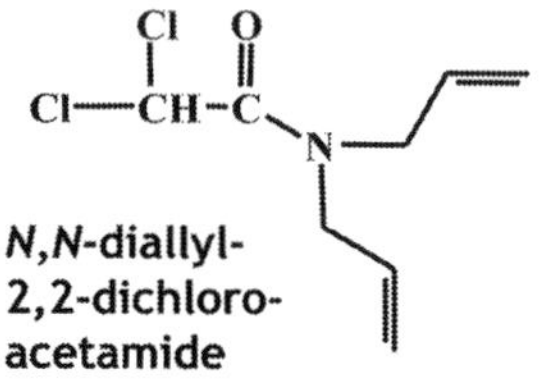

N,N-diallyl-
2,2-dichloro-
acetamide

FIGURE 11-6.

N,N-Diallyl-2,2-dichloro-acetamide.

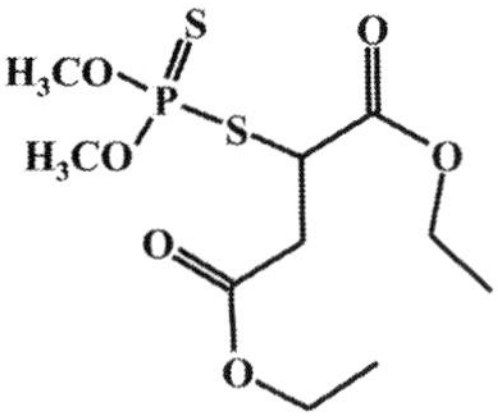

FIGURE 11-7.

Malathion.

(figure 11-6) induces the expression of a novel form of GST, which is undetectable in the untreated seedlings. This is a typical example of the acquisition of resistance to xenobiotics through increasing the intracellular concentrations of a particular form of GST.

Insects treated with insecticides can also develop resistance against the toxic agent, by production of increased concentrations of GST. We have previously mentioned that DDT is inactivated by a GST-catalyzed reaction (see sidebar on malaria in chapter 10). Among the insecticides used in large scale to control pests are organophosphorus compounds, which target acetylcholine esterase in the insect nervous system; examples are malathion (figure 11-7) and methyl parathion (figure 11-8) (*23*). These compounds are bioactivated by oxidative desulfuration, catalyzed by cytochrome P450 to generate the phosphoryl (oxon) derivative that blocks the active-site serine of acetylcholine esterase. In mammals, paraoxonase in blood plasma and tissues hydrolyze and inactivate the reactive intermediate. An alternative detoxication reaction is the O-dealkylation of the organophosphate catalyzed by GSTs. In humans GST T1-1 has particularly prominent

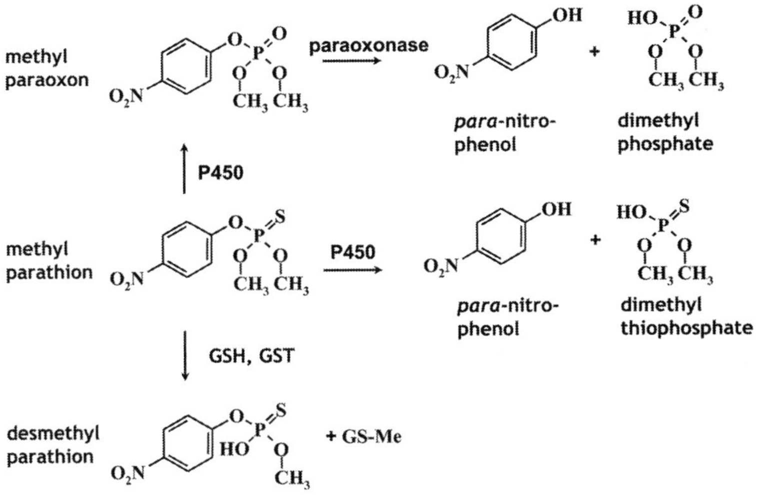

FIGURE 11-8.
Metabolism of methyl parathion; see text for details.

activity with methyl parathion (*24*). Studies on animals or animal cells in tissue culture have similarly demonstrated that cellular resistance to toxic agents can arise by a wide range of chemical substances that induce GST expression.

BIOACTIVATION AND GSH CONJUGATION OF PHARMACEUTICAL DRUGS

Inhibitors of nucleotide biosynthesis (*25*, pp. 876–878) are important cancer chemotherapeutic drugs. 6-Mercaptopurine (figure 11-9) and 6-thioguanine are purine antimetabolites used in the treatment of leukemias. Gertrude Elion and George Hitchings were awarded the Nobel Prize in Medicine or Physiology, 1988, for the development of these drugs (*26, 27*) in the early 1950s. *Azathioprine* is a derivative of 6-mercaptopurine (*28, 29*). Its bone marrow toxicity, an undesirable side effect, has been turned to advantage for suppression of the immune system

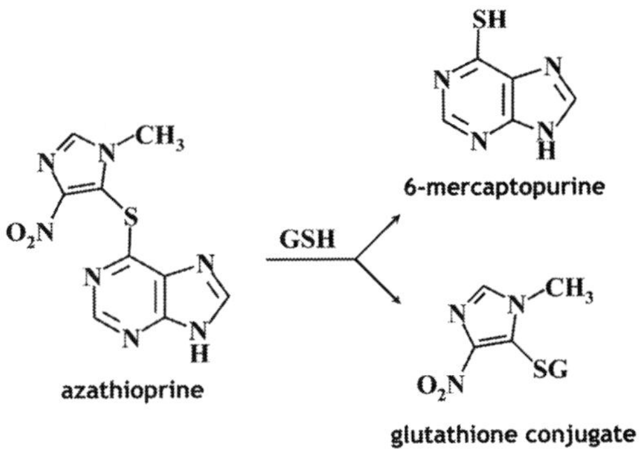

FIGURE 11-9.
GSH-dependent metabolism of azathioprine, releasing the pharmacologically active 6-mercaptopurine.

TABLE 11-1.

Examples of Drugs That Form GSH-Reactive Metabolites

COMPOUND	STRUCTURAL CLASS	REACTIVE METABOLITE
Acetaminophen	Anilide	Quinoneimine
Amodiaquine	Aniline derivative	Quinoneimine
Carbamazepine	Benzene rings	Arene oxide
Clozapine	Fused azaheterocycle	Nitrenium ion
Diclofenac	Aniline derivative	Quinoneimine
Felbamate	Michael acceptor	Atropaldehyde
Imipramine	Benzene rings	Arene oxide
Indomethacin	Indole	Iminoquinone
Pioglitazone	Glitazone	α-Keto-isocyanate
Rosiglitazone	Glitazone	α-Keto-isocyanate
Sulfamethoxazole	Aniline	Nitrosoamine
Valproic acid	Fatty acids	α,β-Unsaturated carbonyl

Adapted from Soglia, J. R.; Harriman, S. P.; Zhao, S.; Barberia, J.; Cole, M. J.; Boyd, J. G.; Contillo, L. G. The development of a higher throughput reactive intermediate screening assay incorporating micro-bore liquid chromatography-micro-electrospray ionization-tandem mass spectrometry and glutathione ethyl ester as an in vitro conjugating agent. J. Pharm. Biomed. Anal. **2004,** 36, 105–116.

in organ transplantation (*30*). Chemical blocking of the SH group of the purine drug reduces its systemic toxicity, and the intracellular reaction of GSH with carbon 5 in the imidazole ring liberates the pharmacologically active agent. Based on the same principle, 2-acetylvinyl derivatives of thiopurines have been developed for possible use as GSH-activated prodrugs (*31*).

Many other pharmaceutical drugs form reactive metabolites that can be conjugated with GSH; if they escape conjugation, toxicity may result. (Nevertheless, we should resist the temptation to ascribe all drug toxicities to the formation of reactive metabolites: see following sidebar.) Some examples of drugs that form GSH-reactive metabolites are given in table 11-1 (*32*).

Acetaminophen (Tylenol^{TM}) is a very widely used analgesic drug (see chapter 19). The mechanism of acetaminophen hepatotoxicity has been studied extensively. Acetaminophen is metabolized to *N*-acetyl-*p*-benzoquinoneimine by cytochrome P450 2E1-catalyzed oxidation (chapter 7). *N*-Acetyl-*p*-benzoquinoneimine, like other quinonoid structures (figure 11-10), can be conjugated with GSH (*33*). At high doses, liver cells become totally depleted of GSH, and *N*-acetyl-*p*-benzoquinoneimine binds covalently to proteins. The major target in proteins is the thiol group of cysteine residues (*34*). In experimental animals, the time course of liver damage following drug administration indicates that injury follows GSH depletion, in particular from the mitochondrial pool (*35*). Administration of *N-acetyl-L-cysteine* (see chapter 9), which replenishes GSH stores, protects against acetaminophen toxicity (*36*). Diclofenac and indomethacin are further examples of drugs that are metabolically transformed to GSH-reactive quinoneimine products.

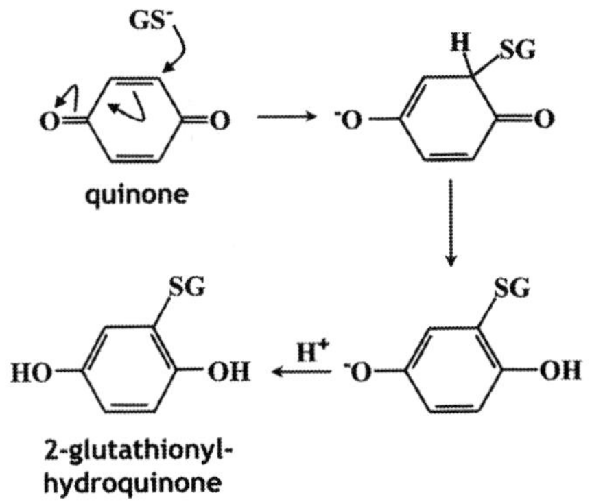

FIGURE 11-10.

Reaction of GSH with quinones.

▶ **Are Most Toxicities Caused by Reactive Metabolites?**

Many of the chemical toxicities discussed in this book are attributed to reactive metabolites. But is a metabolite always the culprit? Given the broad implications, it is important to evaluate the validity of this generalization. Without question, reactive metabolites do play a central role in many toxicities, including some of the best characterized instances. Some of the toxicities occur acutely and can be reproduced in animal species. The facility of the animal model is conducive to a thorough evaluation of the mechanism. Furthermore, in many (but certainly not all) cases, the hallmarks of reactive metabolite-mediated toxicity are distinctive. For example, hepatotoxicity induced by acetaminophen (see chapter 19), bromobenzene (37, 38), the fungal product aflatoxin (39), or the insecticidal plant natural product precocene (40) is characterized by zonal coagulative necrosis with inflammation, often preceded by depletion of cellular nucleophiles such as GSH. This outcome of the toxicological evaluation of a new chemical entity (NCE) will inevitably trigger mechanistic research evaluating the possible involvement of reactive metabolites. Experimental evidence linking a metabolite to such toxicity is usually considered "publishable" in the scientific literature. The notion that "most toxicities are caused by metabolites" may be partly due to such publication bias, as well as to insufficient evaluation of alternative mechanisms. The marketplace failure of a registered drug due to a previously unrecognized idiosyncratic drug reaction (41) often draws wide publicity. In retrospective analyses, reactive metabolites may be attributed as causative factors of such drug reactions.

Bearing these considerations in mind, does the extensive literature on reactive-metabolite-mediated toxicity reflect its true overall incidence? This author's perspective suggests that it does not. An enormous effort is expended toward discovery of NCEs in the pharmaceutical industry and almost half of drug attrition is related to adverse effects. However, a retrospective examination of one pharmaceutical company's causes of toxicological failures indicated that fewer than 20% of toxicities could be attributed either to reactive metabolites or to metabolites with undesired pharmacology. This analysis is consistent with my own experience. During my own experience in the drug development business, hepatotoxicity was the most commonly observed preclinical adverse effect. Nevertheless, these toxicities rarely resembled that found with classic reactive metabolite-mediated hepatotoxicants. Despite the high level of toxicologically related failures, a recent literature search of 1465 citations in the leading toxicology journals revealed no reports of hepatotoxicity attributable to reactive metabolites, and only three citations describing reactive metabolites of pharmaceutical NCEs.

If most toxicities are not, in fact, due to metabolites (whether reactive or stable), then what are the causes of toxicity, and why would metabolites be so frequently impugned? In developing a new drug, one usually relies on screening information, suggesting specificity for the desired target (e.g., enzyme). But the number of molecular targets actually screened during drug development is only a tiny fraction of the number of potential unintended interactions (which is at least as large as the number of human proteins, perhaps 50,000). Even considering only the classes of proteins that are conventionally used as drug targets (G-protein-coupled receptors, protein kinases, nuclear hormone receptors, ion channels, etc.), one would anticipate that there are at least 5000 "pharmacological targets" in the human genome. And this analysis does not consider other potential binding sites that might give rise to pharmacological responses. Thus, tens of thousands of possible unanticipated interactions will not have been tested prior to preclinical evaluation of even the most "specific" pharmacological agent.

continues next page

continued from previous page

Interspecies differences can also cloud the interpretation of a drug's specificity. While a particular NCE may appear to be specific when tested against a panel of expressed human proteins, interspecies differences in binding site structure may lead to unexpected interactions in preclinical animal models. Thus, for example, a NCE may appear not to interact with human chemokine receptors, but might have relatively high affinity in the mouse, leading to an unanticipated inflammatory response during preclinical testing.

Beyond this, even the interaction of a molecule with its intended molecular target may give rise to unanticipated effects. The full range of effects that a pharmacological target may impinge upon is often not fully recognized. Species differences in a response mediated through the same pathway are often noted. For example, inhibition of the rate-limiting step in cholesterol synthesis (catalyzed by the enzyme hydroxymethylglutaryl-CoA reductase) leads to cholesterol lowering in humans and is the mechanism of action of the blockbuster "statin" drugs. However, inhibition of the same enzyme in rodents produces a profound upregulation of the enzyme (42) along with hepatic hypertrophy. "Target-based" toxicity is probably a more common occurrence than is generally appreciated. Wider use of transgenic and knockout animals may offer more insight into such mechanisms in the future.

One common basis for assigning the cause of an adverse effect to a metabolite is an observed time difference between the onset of effects and the parent molecule's systemic exposure. That is, the onset of biological effects may lag behind drug exposure and extend beyond the drug's presence in the circulation. Undoubtedly, these observations are cause for further investigation of a long-lasting metabolite. A "hysteresis" in the plasma concentration versus biological effect time course is also commonly observed with responses requiring depletion of cellular intermediates (in the case of enzyme inhibition) or intracellular signaling pathways (in the case of receptor-driven effects). Thus, a careful consideration of toxic mechanism as well as metabolite time-course is essential for proper interpretation of etiology.

Vast numbers of NCEs fail in development because of adverse effects. Unfortunately, these causes are often poorly studied and inadequately understood. Much of the information that is obtained is not published, so that myriad causes of failure never reach the scientific literature. While it is likely that reactive metabolites play a causal role in many idiosyncratic toxicities of registered drugs, these events are probably notorious more from the spectacle of their failure than from their frequency.[1]

GSH AND NITRIC OXIDE

The discovery of the physiological significance of the diatomic molecule nitric oxide (NO) has opened up new vistas in biochemistry and medicine (see chapter 1). NO is an important biological signal molecule, which acts locally on cells near its site of release. (This mode of signaling is called *paracrine*, in distinction to the classic *endocrine* signaling exerted by hormones, which are carried by the circulatory system to their targets.) NO is generated from the amino acid arginine by the action of the enzyme nitric oxide synthase (NOS) (43). The enzyme occurs in inducible (iNOS) and constitutively expressed forms (eNOS and nNOS, found in epithelial cells and the nervous system, respectively). NO regulates the action of guanylate cyclase, and thereby stimulates pharmacological responses, such as the relaxation of vascular smooth muscle. As this muscle relaxes, the blood vessel, which it surrounds, dilates, and blood pressure drops. This action of NO explains the long-known pharmacological activity of glyceryltrinitrate (nitroglycerin), a coronary vasodilator, which releases NO in vivo (44). NO-releasing derivatives of nonsteroidal antiinflammatory drugs (NSAIDs, e.g., aspirin) and other compounds are currently being developed, because the NO released counters the toxic side effects of the parental drug (45). NO also has biological functions related to cytotoxicity and apoptosis. The simple NO molecule has complex redox chemistry associated with many normal and pathophysiological processes. Free NO is short-lived, and

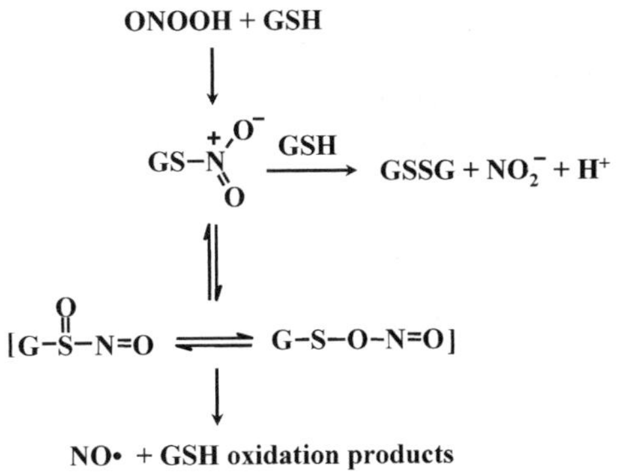

$$ONOOH + GSH$$

$$\downarrow$$

$$GS-\overset{+}{\underset{O}{N}}\overset{O^-}{\underset{\parallel}{}} \xrightarrow{\text{GSH}} GSSG + NO_2^- + H^+$$

$$\updownarrow$$

$$[G-\overset{O}{\underset{\parallel}{S}}-N=O \rightleftharpoons G-S-O-N=O]$$

$$\downarrow$$

$$NO\bullet + GSH \text{ oxidation products}$$

FIGURE 11-11.

Reaction of GSH with peroxynitrite.

thiols, in particular GSH, are important endogenous carriers of NO, in the form of S-nitroso derivatives (*46*).

Organic nitrites (RONO) react with GSH to form *S-nitrosoglutathione* (GSNO). *S*-Nitrosothiols (also called thionitrites: R–S–N=O, the esters of thionitrous acid, H–S–N=O) are more stable than NO and can function as molecular reservoirs and carriers of the NO group. By facile transnitrosation NO can be relayed between the sulfur atoms of different thiols, including proteins. *S*-Nitrosothiols are ubiquitous in biological systems, and, like NO, have vasodilator and other biological activities. For example, the spontaneous apoptosis of blood monocytes, which is necessary for the normal turnover of the cells, is suppressed by *S*-nitrosothiols. This inhibitory effect is linked to S-nitrosylation of thiol groups in caspase-3 and caspase-9 in the intrinsic apoptotic pathways (*47*). Given the abundance of GSH in tissues, GSNO has particular prominence in the physiological reactions of NO, but little is known about the biosynthesis and turnover of this important GSH derivative (*48*). The S-nitro derivative of GSH, $GSNO_2$, may also have metabolic importance; $GSNO_2$ is formed as a product of peroxynitrite detoxication (figure 11-11) and can undergo redox chemistry to form GSNO and free NO (*49*).

TOXICATION OF XENOBIOTICS BY GSH CONJUGATION

The majority of GSH-linked reactions serve the function of detoxication, but, in a limited number of cases, toxicity is *increased* by formation of a GSH conjugate (*50–52*). GST M1-1 and GST T1-1 enzymes are absent in many individuals in the human population, as discussed later in this chapter. Perhaps these genetic polymorphisms are maintained by selective pressures due to exposure to dietary components that produce toxic products in reactions catalyzed by these enzymes. Ethylene dibromide (EDB), a compound used as a fumigant and insecticide, is converted by GSH conjugation into a reactive conjugate which cyclizes to form an episulfonium ion alkylating agent, as discussed in chapter 15.

Dichloromethane (methylene chloride, a common industrial and laboratory solvent) is far less toxic than carbon tetrachloride or chloroform, but its reaction with GSH yields formaldehyde (*53*), via the intermediate

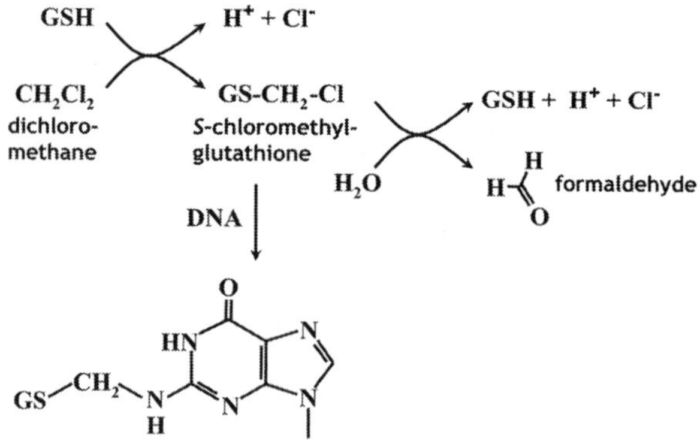

FIGURE 11-12.
GSH and dichloromethane metabolism; see text for details.

S-(chloromethyl) glutathione (figure 11-12). Both the GSH conjugate (54, 55) and formaldehyde are reactive and potentially tumorigenic. Therefore, GSH conjugation of dichloromethane leads to toxication. In contrast, the conjugation of (mono)chloromethane is a detoxication reaction. Among the human enzymes, GST T1-1 is particularly active with the small haloalkane molecules.

▶ **Cysteine Conjugates and Smelly Thiols**

Sulfur-containing compounds are notoriously odorous, contributing to the characteristic scents of onions (56) and skunks (57). Many sulfur-containing secondary metabolites arise from S-alkylated cysteine derivatives by the action of the cysteine conjugate β-lyase. In some noteworthy cases, microbial lyases act on odorless compounds to release smelly thiols. Felinine (S-(3-hydroxy-1,1-dimethylpropyl)-L-cysteine), the major amino acid in cat urine (58), gives rise to the key odoriferous compound 3-methyl-3- mercaptobutan-1-ol by the lyase reaction. Fresh human sweat is almost odorless, but microbial activities release odoriferous steroids and short, branched-chain fatty acids. Individuals with a dense population of corynebacteria on the skin of the armpit (axilla) develop strong axillary odor due to the bacterial expression of β-lyases that catalyze the formation of at least four foul-smelling mercaptoalkanols (sulfanylalkanols) from the corresponding cysteine conjugates (59). The substrates in axillary secretions were traced to Michael adducts to the cysteinyl sulfur of α,β-unsaturated compound such as alken-2-als. One of the most potent odorants was 3-mercaptopentan-1-ol (figure 11-13), which has an odor described as "onion-like," and which can be detected by humans at a concentration of only 2 pg per liter air (typical aroma chemicals have threshold values in the range of nanograms per liter).

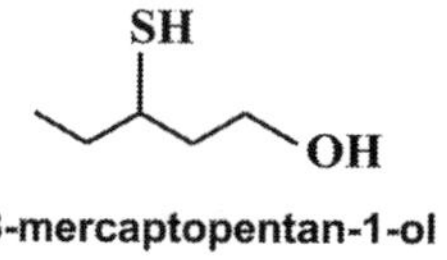

3-mercaptopentan-1-ol

FIGURE 11-13.
3-Mercaptopentan-1-ol. ◀

TISSUE DISTRIBUTION OF GSTs

The distribution of GSTs differs from tissue to tissue and expression of GSTs in a given tissue varies both temporally and topographically. Knowledge of this distribution is important, since the enzymes have different substrate specificities, and the occurrence of a given GST will influence the cellular inactivation capacity toward diverse electrophilic toxic chemicals. The absence of particular enzymes may predispose tissues to organ-selective toxicity. For example, absence of GST M1-1, which generally has high activity with epoxides, may render an organ susceptible to the genotoxic effects of this class of compounds.

In humans, GSTs A1-1 and A2-2 are remarkably abundant in liver and kidney, where they account for more than 2% of the soluble protein. GST P1-1 is present in most tissues, including placenta (from which it derives its name) and erythrocytes (60), but not in normal adult hepatocytes. GSTs M3-3 and M5-5 are especially prominent in testis and brain (61), whereas GST A3-3 is primarily found in steroidogenic organs such as placenta, ovary, testis, and adrenal gland (62). Fetal and adult tissues differ markedly in GST expression. For example, GST P1-1 is abundant in fetal liver (63) but is downregulated in the time period preceding birth (64).

At the histological level, the GST expression differs among cell types in the same tissue. Thus, even though hepatocytes are lacking GST P1-1 (in rats and humans, but not in mice), this enzyme is present in significant amounts in the bile duct epithelium of adult liver. In the kidney, adjacent epithelial cells have been observed to differ in their expression of some (but not all) GSTs (65). Such "mosaicity" indicates temporal changes reflecting cellular activities related to proliferation, apoptosis, or other processes. In the colon, inflammation, as well as the intestinal bacterial flora, upregulate some GSTs and downregulate others.

In the subcellular compartments, there are also spatial and temporal differences in the distribution of GSTs. Most "soluble" GSTs are present in the cytoplasm, as distinct from MGST1 and other MAPEG members, which occur in cellular membranes. GST K1-1 has been found in the matrix of mitochondria and peroxisomes, but other soluble GSTs are also present there. Phosphorylation has been reported as a posttranslational mechanism for import of GST A4-4 to the mitochondrion (66). Immunohistochemistry and electron microscopy have shown that the nucleoplasm, but not the nucleolus, may contain soluble GSTs that were originally identified in the cytoplasm. Again, the nuclear localization appears to have temporal variations.

Compilations of reported tissue distributions have been made (67–69), but the records are still incomplete. The tools of proteomics will be helpful in preparing more comprehensive inventories.

GST INDUCTION

Inducibility appears to be a common feature among GSTs and has been observed in many species, including mammals, insects, and plants. Only certain forms of GST are induced by a given compound. As with P450 enzymes, substrates (or their metabolic precursors) often induce enzymes that catalyze their biotransformation. In many instances, GSTs that are not expressed constitutively will be produced following administration of the inducer. Induction is reversible: the level of an enzyme returns to its original level after removal of the inducer.

GST gene expression can be induced by a variety of chemical agents, including many inducers of cytochrome P450s (see chapter 8) and other drug-metabolizing enzymes. Well-studied GST inducers in mammals include phenobarbital, 3-methylcholanthrene, and TCDD. Regulation of

GST gene expression occurs at the transcriptional level and can involve the aryl hydrocarbon receptor (AhR), AhR nuclear translocator protein (ARNT), and a regulatory DNA sequence in the promoter region of the gene (70) (see chapter 8). Perhaps more important for GSTs is an alternative induction mechanism involving the so-called antioxidant response element, ARE. Like the genes of many other enzymes responding to cellular oxidative stress and electrophiles, GST genes carry an ARE nucleotide sequence, with the consensus sequence 5′-TGACNNNGC-3′ (N = any nucleotide) in the promoter region (71). The term ARE is somewhat misleading, since many inducers acting on the ARE are electrophiles rather than antioxidants. The alternative designation "electro-phile response element," ErRE, is therefore sometimes used (72). In addition to GSTs, quinone reductase, glutamate cysteine ligase, glutathione reductase, and many other enzymes are induced via transcriptional activation mediated by AREs in the 5′ flanking regions of their genes (73). As a consequence, a variety of proteins that are needed in the cellular protection against oxidative stress and electrophiles are coordinately expressed.

Electrophilic substrates of GSTs are particularly prominent inducers of the GST genes. This observation is probably fundamental to the understanding of the cellular defense mechanisms. Most of these inducers act primarily via transcriptional activation of ARE. Paul Talalay and co-workers developed an in vitro assay based on measuring quinone reductase induction in microtiter-plate cultures of mouse cells. They observed that most electrophiles exert their effect via the ARE (74). Induction is dependent on reactions of the inducer with sulfhydryl groups of the cytosolic zinc protein Keap1, which occurs in a complex with the transcription factor Nrf2 in the cytoplasm (75). Modification of Keap1 results in liberation of Nrf2, which is transferred to the nucleus and effects activation of ARE-regulated genes (76). Nfr2 is a basic region-leucine zipper (bZIP) protein, and as such expected to bind as a dimer to ARE. However, it is not clear whether Nfr2 forms a homodimer, or dimerizes with another bZIP family member. The formation of alternative heterodimers would be a possible mechanism for differential control among ARE-regulated genes. In any case, Keap1 acts as a cytoplasmic sensor of electrophiles and oxidants and translates the toxic insults into nuclear transcriptional activation of target genes.

Many inducers, including isothiocyanates, are electrophiles that reversibly combine with the sulfhydryl group of GSH via GST-catalyzed reactions (77). Their actions, therefore, can be modulated by the intra-cellular GSH concentration and GST composition and it is possible that GSTs can deliver the effector groups from their GSH conjugates to Keap1. Some food substances are strong GST inducers, including organic isothiocyanates (e.g., sulforaphane in broccoli; figure 11-14) (78) and activated alkenes (e.g., curcumin in turmeric (79)), and GST induction

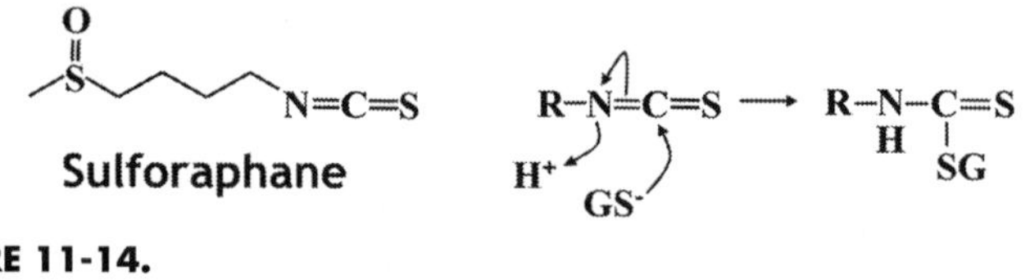

Sulforaphane

FIGURE 11-14.
Reaction of GSH with sulforaphane, forming a dithiocarbamate.

may account for some anticancer effects of diet (*80*), as discussed in the sidebar on fruits and vegetables.

▶ Fruits and Vegetables, Phytochemicals, and Human Cancer Risk

The clinical manifestation of tumors is usually preceded by years or even decades of "silent" disease, involving a series of genetic events, which promote cellular transformation and the selection of increasingly malignant subpopulations (cancer progression) (*81*). The long time period between initiation of cancer and its clinical consequences suggests that there may be opportunities to delay or prevent the process.

Many epidemiological studies have shown an association between a diet rich in fruits and vegetables and decreased risk of cancer. As dietary vegetable intake increases from 100 to 400 g per day, the incidences of cancers of the mouth, esophagus, stomach, colon, and lung are reduced by roughly 50%. However, the mechanism of this protective effect remains uncertain; multiple factors are likely to be involved. The antioxidant properties of nutrients and phytochemicals (natural products present in plant foods) probably contribute to cancer protection. Dietary phytochemicals can also alter xenobiotic metabolism and interact with dietary and environmental carcinogens in the body, for example, gastrointestinal tract and lung carcinogens, such as polycyclic aromatic hydrocarbons (PAH; see chapter 18), heterocyclic amines (see chapter 17), and nitrosamines (see chapter 7). These carcinogens can be formed during the preservation and cooking of foods, especially muscle meats. A diet high in fruits and vegetables usually means a diet lower in meat consumption, thereby reducing exposure to meat-associated carcinogens. However, animal experiments also indicate a protective effect of dietary fruits or vegetables against treatment with various carcinogens: plant-based foods may contain active chemoprotective components.

Phytochemicals can alter xenobiotic metabolism in several ways. Many phytochemicals induce P450 enzymes (*82*) by activation of the receptors discussed in chapter 8 (e.g., AHR, CAR, PXR). For example, feeding rats 1% dietary turmeric (a spice present in curry) induces lung and stomach CYP 1A enzymes about two-fold, indicating a weak activation of the AHR. Of course, such induction might increase carcinogen bioactivation rather than (or in addition to) detoxication. PAH carcinogens themselves are very effective P450 inducers, as discussed earlier in this chapter. Vegetables and cooked meats are often consumed together. In that circumstance, phytochemicals can compete with PAH binding to AHR and thereby *decrease* the level of P450 1A induction in the stomach and lung by these carcinogens (*83*). Phytochemicals can also modulate xenobiotic metabolism by competitive inhibition of P450 enzyme activities. For example, broccoli isothiocyanates and turmeric curcumins have IC_{50} values for P450 2E1 and 1A enzymes in the low micromolar range (*83*).

Phytochemicals can also induce the expression of GSTs and UDP-glucuronosyltransferases (UDPGTs). Consumption of cruciferous vegetables, such as brussels sprouts, induces UDPGT and thereby protects against heterocyclic amine-induced carcinogenesis in rats (*84*). Organosulfur compounds from garlic induce the expression of GSTs and mitigate PAH carcinogenicity in rats (*85*).

Aflatoxin exposure, in association with prevalent hepatitis, is the probable cause of high levels of liver cancer in many tropical regions, as already discussed. Dietary garlic can have multiple effects on aflatoxin metabolism. In rats, garlic induces P450 3A2, which bioactivates aflatoxin, but also induces P450 3A1, 1A, and 2B enzymes, which can detoxify aflatoxin. Garlic components also induce the expression of GST, which increases the detoxication of electrophilic aflatoxin metabolites. Garlic phytochemicals can also competitively inhibit P450 enzymes. The net result of these interactions is that dietary garlic significantly decreases aflatoxin-induced hepatocarcinogenesis in rodents (*85*) and it may also have protective effects in humans.

PAH (see chapter 18) are formed during combustion of tobacco leaves and tobacco-specific nitrosamines are formed in reactions between nitrite (enhanced by crop fertilization) and nicotine, while the tobacco leaves cure. These two classes of carcinogens are thought to account for most of the lung carcinogenic activity of tobacco smoke. High dietary vegetable intake is associated with decreased lung cancer incidence in cigarette smokers. Antioxidant activity of β-carotene was postulated to be a protective mechanism, and two large randomized, double-blinded, placebo-controlled intervention trials (one in Finland and the other in the United States) were initiated (*86*). Startlingly, both studies observed a significant *increase* in lung cancer incidence in the β-carotene intervention groups. Very high intakes of β-carotene induce P450 enzymes (*87*), which might provide a mechanism for the observed increase in lung cancer. Nevertheless, high vegetable intake was still protective within the β-carotene-supplemented group, which suggests that some protective dietary components were still active, even in the presence of "toxic" levels of β-carotene. Further work with rodent and in vitro models showed that phytochemicals from vegetables and spices are able to inhibit the P450 enzymes that bioactivate PAH and tobacco-specific nitrosamines.

continues next page

continued from previous page

Phytochemicals are natural, rather than human-made, compounds, but they can still be regarded as xenobiotics, which undergo oxidative and conjugative metabolism in much the same manner as do drugs and carcinogens. Many of the beneficial effects of phytochemicals probably result from competitive interactions with carcinogens in the diet, potent agents which are present at trace concentrations. These interactions may be merely fortuitous; perhaps they also reflect the coevolution of humans and their cultivated crops. In either case, it is important to remember the nature of our relationship with phytochemicals when one purifies these products into a concentrated form, where supraphysiological exposure is likely. The toxic potential of nutraceutical products and herbal remedies must not be ignored (88).

Chemoprevention by nonnutritional substances is another approach to reducing cancer-related mortality. The drug oltipraz (figure 11-15) has been used in prospective chemopreventive trials in a region of China where dietary aflatoxin B_1 is a major risk factor for liver cancer (89–91).[2]

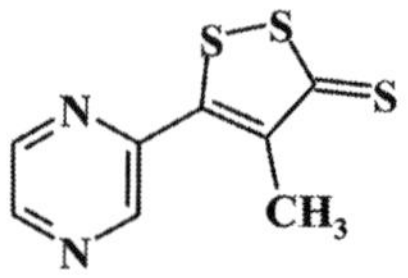

FIGURE 11-15.
Oltipraz. ◀

HORMONAL CONTROL OF GST EXPRESSION

The transcription of GST genes is affected by hormones and other physiological signal substances. Surgical removal of endocrine glands causes alterations in the relative amounts of different forms of GST in various organs. A particularly striking example is the regulation of the Pi-class GST in mouse liver. Although hepatocytes of rat or human origin do not contain significant amounts of GST P1-1, adult male mice express this enzyme as one of the major hepatic forms. Females and young males have approximately ten-fold lower cytosolic concentrations of this enzyme (92). When the young males reach puberty, GST P1-1 increases to the high levels of adult males. Castration of adult males reduces the enzyme concentration to that of the juvenile and administration of testosterone brings the concentration up to that of the adult. Hypophysectomy of rats causes dramatic changes of GST expression in both adrenal glands and liver (93, 94). Significantly, the effects on the six GSTs examined were different, such that the levels of some GSTs were upregulated while others were downregulated or unchanged. Further, a sexual dimorphism in hepatic GST expression has been demonstrated, with higher expression levels of at least one Alpha- and two Mu-class members in males than in female rats.

Continuous infusion of growth hormone (via minipumps) caused a feminization of the GST expression pattern in male rats (93). A high basal level of growth hormone also resulted in a feminine pattern of expression of cytochrome P450 (95, 96). In hypophysectomized males, coadministration of thyroxine and cortisone acetate with growth hormone is necessary for the complete feminization, indicating that the levels of several hormones regulating cellular GST expression are influenced by the pituitary gland. Studies of animals or cells in tissue culture have demonstrated that a variety of other mediators of cellular signaling, such as interferon and retinoic acid, also affect the cellular concentrations of GSTs.

GST POLYMORPHISMS

So far, we have addressed many factors affecting GST expression, including development, tissue distribution, cellular and subcellular characteristics, and regulation by inducers and hormones. Now we turn to a discussion of genetic polymorphisms of the GSTs.

Two genes, *GSTM1* and *GSTT1*, are frequently missing in human individuals. In persons of European descent, approximately 50% have a *GSTM1*-null genotype (*97*). In some Oceanic regions, almost all individuals lack the *GSTM1* gene. The *GSTT1*-null genotype is found in 10–20% of Europeans and about 50% of Asians. Figure 11-16 shows the structure of the human GST Mu locus on chromosome 1. As shown in figure 11-17, some individuals lack the *GSTM1* gene entirely, whereas a few carry two copies. These alterations in copy number are possibly a consequence of misaligned crossing over between chromosomes, a process made facile by the high degree of sequence identity among the multiple Mu-class genes. Why *GSTM1*, in particular, should be subject to frequent loss/duplication is not known.

Neither the *GSTM1*-null nor the *GSTT1*-null genotype has unmistakable phenotypic consequences. Nevertheless, many experimental studies indicate that the absence of GST M1-1 makes cells more vulnerable to DNA damage and chromosomal aberrations following exposure to genotoxic epoxides. Individuals defective in both genes often stand out in epidemiological studies as being at higher risk for certain cancers and other diseases (see sidebar on molecular epidemiology, chapter 13).

Besides the total absence of certain GST genes, variations in the coding regions and promoter regions are also known, and may account for much of the interindividual variation in GST expression in the humans population (*98*). Why do strong ethnic differences exist in GST polymorphism

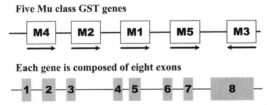

FIGURE 11-16.
Structure of the human Mu-class GST gene locus on chromosome 1.

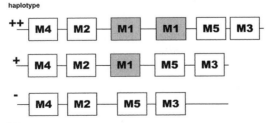

FIGURE 11-17.
Haplotypes of the human Mu-class GST gene locus, showing variation in the number of copies of the *GSTM1* gene. *Note*: A full-color version of this figure appears on the website.

frequencies? One possible explanation is distinct dietary factors. GST-catalyzed activation of an as-yet-unidentified human dietary toxicant may be a cause of the high frequency of the *GSTM1*- or *GSTT1*-null alleles. In contrast, some Saudi Arabian individuals have three or more copies of the *GSTM1* gene; in the same population, some individuals have up to 13 copies of one of the cytochrome P450 2D6 genes (see chapter 8). Perhaps the beneficial effect of detoxication of some substances needs to be balanced against the adverse effect of activation of other compounds to which humans are exposed.

MALIGNANT TRANSFORMATION AND GSTs IN CANCER CELLS

The transformation of normal cells into a malignant state is accompanied by alterations in their profiles of gene expression. In comparison to normal tissues, tumor cells often have elevated concentrations of GSH and glyoxalase I as well as altered levels of various GSTs (*99*). Many (although far from all) tumors have significantly increased expression of GST P1-1 in comparison with the surrounding normal tissue (*100, 101*). Other GSTs may be downregulated in comparison with the normal phenotype. In human breast tissue, the GST P1-1 expression by epithelial cells progressively decreases as normal epithelium dedifferentiates into preneoplastic and neoplastic lesions. Such GST P1-1 downregulation is particularly prominent in prostate cancer (see sidebar on epigenetic regulation of GST P1-1 in cancer cells).

Tumor cells are largely dependent on glycolysis for their supply of ATP, whereas normal cells mainly rely on mitochondrial oxidative phosphorylation. Glycolysis generates toxic methylglyoxal as an obligatory byproduct of the triose phosphate isomerase reaction, which suggests the need of increased amounts of glyoxalase I for detoxication of methylglyoxal. Increased concentrations of GSH and GSTs may be a reflection of the general "resistance phenotype" characterizing many tumor cells. Considering the additional roles of GSTs in cellular signaling and other processes, altered GST levels may have implications other than those directly linked to inactivation of noxious chemical agents.

▶ **Epigenetic Regulation of GST P1-1 in Cancer Cells**

A common covalent modification of DNA in eukaryotes is the enzyme-catalyzed methylation of the C5 position of cytosine, as discussed in chapter 3. This modification is a form of epigenetic change, that is, an alteration that affects phenotype but does not alter the sequence of a gene. Somatic methylation of cytosine residues at CpG dinucleotides can be an important step in tumorigenesis, for example, by silencing the expression of tumor suppressor genes (*102*).

Among the genes that undergo hypermethylation in CpG islands is the *GSTP1* gene in prostate cancer cells (*103*). This promoter hypermethylation is the most common epigenetic event known in human prostate carcinogenesis and has, therefore, been proposed as a clinically useful biomarker. The phenomenon appears to indicate the transition from proliferative inflammatory atrophy and neoplastic transformation to cancer (*104*). The effect of the hypermethylation is to recruit methylated-DNA binding proteins, repressing transcription and leading to a complete loss of GST P1-1 expression in the tumor. The general significance of this process in carcinogenesis is unclear, since many tumor cells overexpress GST P1-1. However, for human prostate cancer, it has been suggested that loss of GST P1-1 represents a significant growth advantage, because inhibition of JNK activity will be relaxed. The resulting JNK activation leads to genetic instability and enhanced redundancy in survival pathways that maintain the proliferation of the cancer cells (*104*). This may be the case also for other human neoplasias, such as breast cancer and malignant melanoma.

In rat liver, genotoxic agents induce the formation of foci of transformed cells and preneoplastic nodules (105). These pathological changes are accompanied by a dramatic increase of GST P1-1 expression, rising from undetectable levels to become one of the most abundant proteins in the transformed cells (106, 107). This response in GST P1-1 expression has not been observed in corresponding lesions in human liver, but the rat model has still been found useful in the screening of chemical compounds for genotoxic effects (108). Foci formed in the liver of animals treated with a genotoxic agent are clearly visualized by immunohistochemistry based on antibodies directed against GST P1-1. ◀

GSTs AND TUMOR RESISTANCE TO CYTOSTATIC DRUGS

Many anticancer drugs cause covalent damage to biological macromolecules, including DNA. The basis of their chemotherapeutic action is a rather nonselective activity against rapidly dividing cells based on indirect or direct inhibition of mitosis. Bifunctional agents, such as the nitrogen mustards and platinum compounds (e.g., cisplatin (*cis*-diamminedichloroplatinum(II); figure 11-18) (*109*) can cause covalent cross-linking of the polynucleotide strands of DNA. Not surprisingly, all of these electrophilic agents react with GSH, and GSH conjugation may play an important role in their pharmacology. GSH interferes with DNA modification by reacting with the electrophilic functional groups of the drugs. Administration of BSO, which inhibits GSH biosynthesis and, therefore, lowers the intracellular concentration of GSH, makes tumor cells more sensitive to treatment with these agents.

The cytotoxic effects of anthraquinone drugs, such as adriamycin (figure 11-19) and doxorubicin, probably result from the generation of free radicals and reactive oxygen species by redox cycling mechanisms (*110*) (see chapter 1). GSH may counteract toxicity by scavenging free radicals and by reducing hydroperoxides. Accumulation of GST P1-1 in the nucleus of cancer cells that are resistant to doxorubicin has been noted, and a role of the nuclear GST in scavenging products of lipid peroxidation products that form exocyclic deoxyguanosine adducts (see chapter 2) has been suggested as an explanation for the resistance (*111*).

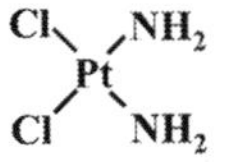

FIGURE 11-18.
Cisplatin.

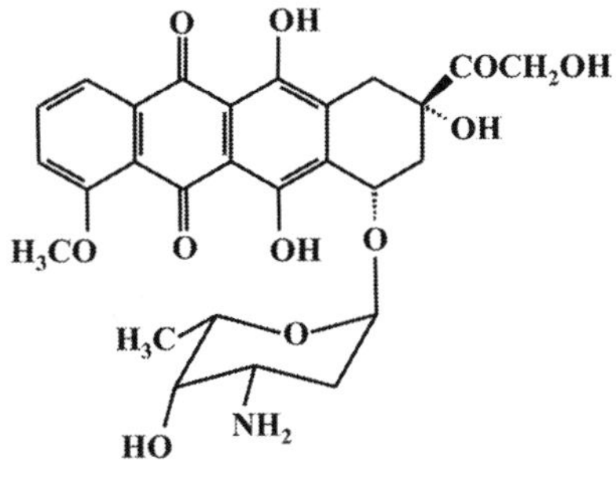

FIGURE 11-19.
Adriamycin.

Although the role of GSH in the inactivation of cytostatic drugs is well established, the contribution of GSTs has been more difficult to assess. Tumor cells with intrinsic (e.g., malignant melanoma (99)) or acquired drug resistance (cf. (112)) often overexpress GSTs, in particular GST P1-1. The increased GST level in tumors may confer a selective growth advantage, that is, a greater capacity to inactivate cytostatic drugs.

Propenal (acrolein) has already been mentioned on several occasions in this text as a product of lipid peroxidation and other oxidative processes. Propenal is also formed in the metabolic activation of the cancer chemotherapeutic agent cyclophosphamide. Cyclophosphamide is hydroxylated by cytochrome P450 (113); propenal is released (114) when the ultimate cytostatic metabolite, the alkylating agent phosphorodiamidate mustard, is formed (figure 11-20). Bleomycin (figure 11-21) is another important anticancer agent; it is one component of the drug "cocktail" used to treat testicular cancer, with highly successful results (115). Base propenals are formed from the action of bleomycin on DNA (116). Propenal and base propenals (figure 11-1) are cytotoxic compounds that react with DNA and proteins; they are efficiently inactivated by human GST P1-1.

In vitro experiments with purified GSTs have demonstrated some enzymatic activities with respect to alkylating cytostatic drugs (117) (see chapter 15). Human Alpha-class GST A1-1 is active with chlorambucil and melphalan. The Mu-class GSTs M2-2 and M3-3, and most significantly the Theta-class GST T1-1, have activity with BCNU (118). However, the comparatively low catalytic activities of GSTs with most cytostatic drugs have led investigators to question the importance of these enzyme-catalyzed detoxication reactions.

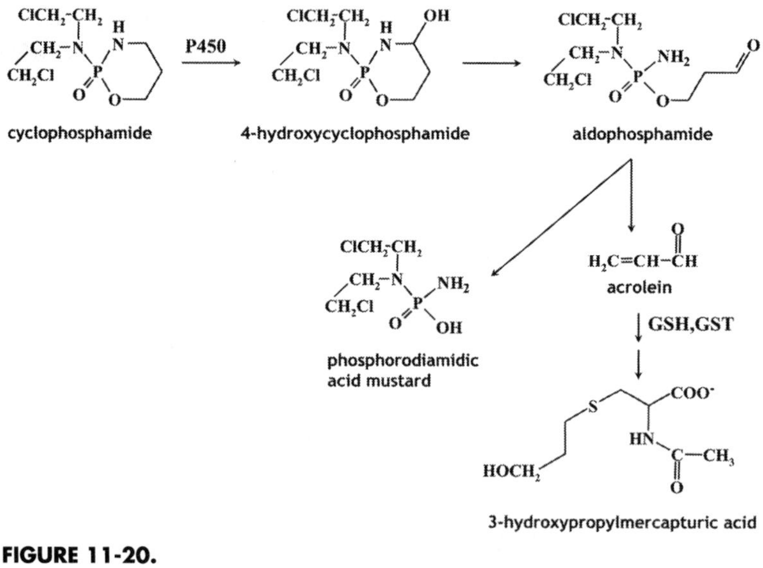

FIGURE 11-20.

Cyclophosphamide is bioactivated through hydroxylation, catalyzed by cytochrome P450, to give a product that decomposes into the bifunctional alkylating agent phosphorodiamide and the toxic acrolein. Acrolein is conjugated with GSH and finally excreted via the mercapturic acid pathway.

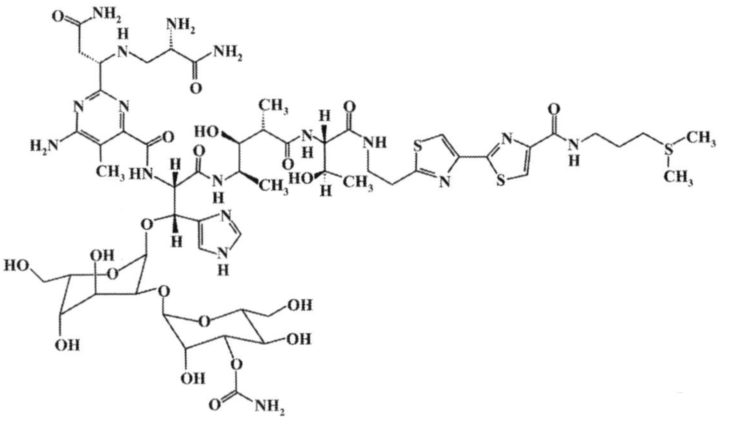

FIGURE 11-21.
Bleomycin.

Indirect evidence for a significant role of GSTs in drug resistance includes the observation that tumor cells often express high intracellular concentrations of both GSH and GSTs, which may compensate for the intrinsically low catalytic activities. Downregulation of GST mRNA by antisense complementary DNA sensitizes cells to anticancer drugs (*119*). Furthermore, transfection of cDNA encoding particular GSTs into tumor cells in vitro provides increased intracellular concentrations of the corresponding enzymes and collateral increase in drug resistance.

Experiments with cells overexpressing both GST A1-1 and the transport protein MRP1 (see chapter 9) demonstrate that they act synergistically to provide resistance against chlorambucil, although not to some other alkylating agents (*120*). Similar protective effects of other GSTs, in combination with MRPs, have been demonstrated (*121, 122*). The finding that both enzyme and transporter need to be present for optimal protective effect indicates that it is necessary not only to express a GST with the required catalytic efficiency, but also to have a mechanism for disposing of the product, which would otherwise inhibit the enzyme (*123*).

With respect to the clinical treatment of tumors, it is unlikely that GSTs or other possible resistance factors would be the only components that govern resistance to chemotherapy. Cancer cells, like normal cells, can protect themselves by a variety of mechanisms, and drug resistance has to be overcome by simultaneous targeting of several of these biochemical defenses.

▶ **Gene Therapy for Cancer**

In the treatment of cancer patients, we hope to target the malignant cells while sparing normal tissues. Ideally, the distinctive phenotype of cancer cells should provide a basis for treatment selectivity. One recent approach to this problem is to employ gene transfer into selected cells, in order to enhance the phenotypic differences. Expression of cytotoxic cytokines or functional tumor suppressor proteins in cancer cells can be considered. Another approach would be to alter the phenotype of drug resistance either in the tumor or in normal cells. Several alternative routes for the administration of therapeutic proteins and/or DNA are available. Viral vectors of genes, as well as liposomes and aerosols for proteins and DNA are currently being tested (*124*).

Some anticancer agents are prodrugs bioactivated in the tissues of a patient. This is the case for cyclophosphamide, which is hydroxylated by cytochrome P450s, as noted above, and also for certain quinones that are reduced by quinone reductase (*125*). An increase of these activating enzymes in the tumor or in its

continues next page

continued from previous page

vicinity would increase the concentration of the activated drug at its intended site of action, without a corresponding increase in toxicity to vulnerable nontumor cells, such as stem cells of the bone marrow or epithelial cells of the intestinal tract (*126*). For maximal efficacy, it will be necessary to optimize the properties of both the prodrug (*127*) and the enzyme (*128*).

Another strategy would be to furnish sensitive normal cells with a protective enzyme, in order to reduce toxicity to vulnerable tissues. For example, a GST enzyme capable of inactivating an alkylating agent might provide protection of the bone marrow. ◀

PHARMACOLOGICAL INHIBITION OF GST

A potentially useful approach to improve the efficacy of cancer chemotherapy would be to thwart resistance mechanisms in the tumor cells. As noted earlier, cellular resistance to certain drugs can be diminished by lowering the intracellular concentration of GSH, by administration of inhibitors of GSH biosynthesis or compounds that deplete the GSH pool. For attempts at overcoming drug resistance caused by GSTs, compounds which are already used as drugs (for other applications) have been tried. Among such compounds, ethacrynic acid (chapter 9), a diuretic drug, has been tested in a clinical trial (*129*). Ethacrynic acid is a good inhibitor of all GSTs so far investigated, and may also serve as an alternative substrate, in particular for GST P1-1 (*130, 131*). In fact, ethacrynic acid has three coincident effects: inhibition of GSTs, depletion of GSH by serving as GST substrate, and forming an ethacrynic acid conjugate that is even more inhibitory than the parent compound. Unfortunately, the diuretic properties of ethacrynic acid limit its usefulness.

Rational design of GST inhibitors, based on structural similarities to the GSH molecule, has been attempted. Such inhibitors would, of course, be targeted to the G-site and would compete with GSH, thereby inhibiting the enzymatic reaction. S-Substituents on GSH that bind to the adjacent hydrophobic H-site of the enzyme increase the affinity of the inhibitor for the enzyme (*132*). In the search for inhibitors, a very wide range of chemical compounds has been investigated. For structure-based rational design of inhibitors, one must appreciate that the GST structure is not rigid, but undergoes conformational transitions that contribute to the overall thermodynamics of ligand binding. This is the case for human GST P1-1, in which the α2-helix has a flexible structure that becomes less flexible upon GSH derivative binding (*133, 134*).

A serious limitation for the application of inhibitors based on the GSH structure is that the charged peptide structure does not freely permeate cell membranes, and only a very limited number of cell types have a transport system for uptake of GSH. In order to circumvent this problem, one or both of the carboxyl groups of GSH have been esterified with alcohols such

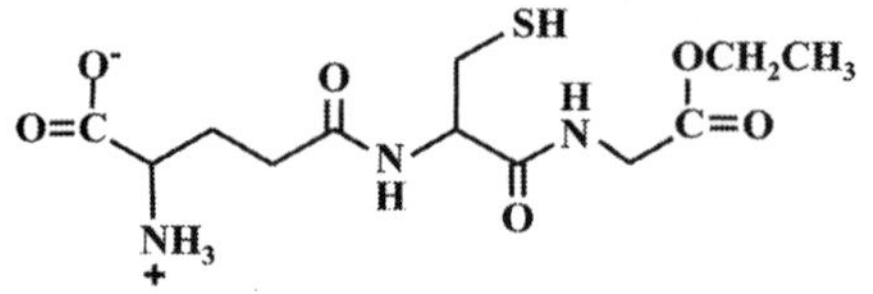

FIGURE 11-22.
Glutathione monoethyl ester.

as ethanol (figure 11-22) (*135*). By blocking the negatively charged carboxylate groups, the molecule is made more lipid-soluble than GSH. The compound is more easily taken up by cells, and the ester bonds of the carboxyl groups are then hydrolyzed by intracellular esterases. Another obstacle is the susceptibility of the γ-glutamyl group to cleavage by γ-glutamyltranspeptidase, which may cause inactivation of the inhibitor. This problem has been approached by the design of peptidomimetic GSH analogues, in which the scissile peptide bonds have been replaced by peptidase-stable linkages (*136*).

Intracellular levels of resistance factors might also be lowered by administration of antisense oligonucleotide derivatives. The antisense molecule is expected to hybridize with its cognate mRNA, thereby inhibiting translation as well as increasing the rate of degradation of the mRNA (*137*). A powerful alternative to the original antisense methodology is *RNA interference* (RNAi), a natural mechanism of gene regulation (discovered in 1998 (*138*)) that has been adopted for the silencing of gene expression (*139, 140*). Short double-stranded RNA fragments (about 23 base pairs; called "small interfering RNA," siRNA) are used to build up an intracellular complex with specific proteins called RISC (RNA-induced silencing complex). RISC, activated by ATP, can repress expression of gene sequences complementary to the siRNA in three ways: digestion of the mRNA, inhibition of its ribosomal translation, or blocking the transcription of the corresponding gene in the chromatin. When long double-stranded RNA appears in the cell, it is cut by an RNAse called Dicer (*141*) into siRNA duplexes, which are built into RISC. Synthetic siRNA molecules, designed for downregulation of targeted genes, can be transfected into cells, either directly or transcribed from transfected vectors.

GST-ACTIVATED PRODRUGS

One further approach to exploit tumor-specific expression of GSTs is the use of prodrugs that can be activated by a GST expressed at high levels in the tumor. Such "mechanism-based" or "suicide" inhibition exploits the catalytic potential of the enzyme to generate toxic compounds in situ. GSH-based prodrugs that release alkylating agents through the action of GSTs have been designed (*142*). Attachment of the GSH backbone to a phosphoramide mustard, similar to the anticancer drug cyclophosphamide mentioned earlier, is expected to target the release of the alkylating agent preferentially to cells with high GST activity. Phenylglycine in the C-terminus of the tripeptide gives selectivity for GST P1-1 (figure 11-23).

Many human tumor cells express high levels of GST P1-1 (*143*), as noted above, and this observation was the basis for the development of Telcyta^{TM}, a GST P1-1-activated phosphoramide prodrug (*144*). By means of this tumor-supported activation, the cytotoxic phosphoramide mustard can be delivered at the site of its intended action. However, essentially all prostate cancers, >80% of liver cancers, and >30% of breast cancers do not express GST P1-1, because of somatic hypermethylation of CpG islands in the *GSTP1* gene, as mentioned earlier (*145*).

Anticancer drugs based on the 2-crotonyloxymethyl-2-cycloalkenone structure are also activated by GSH conjugation, forming a toxic exocyclic enone that appears to be causing the tumoricidal effect (figure 11-24).

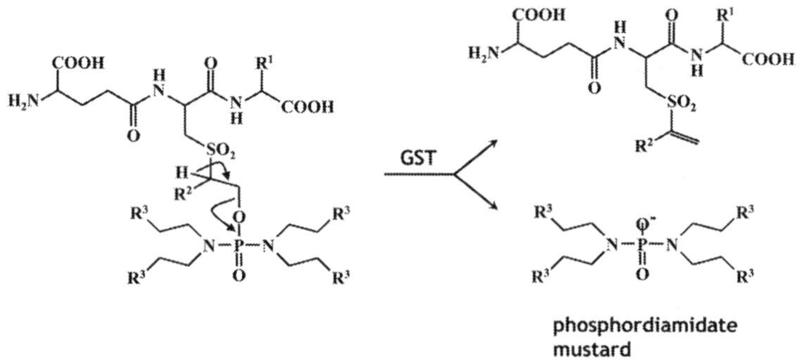

FIGURE 11-23.
GSH-derived cytostatic prodrugs that bind to GSTs in target cells and release the alkylating phosphorodiamide (compare cyclophosphamide). The variant with $R^1 = $ phenyl, $R^2 = H$, $R^3 = $ 2-chloroethyl (Telcyta^{TM}) is in clinical testing.

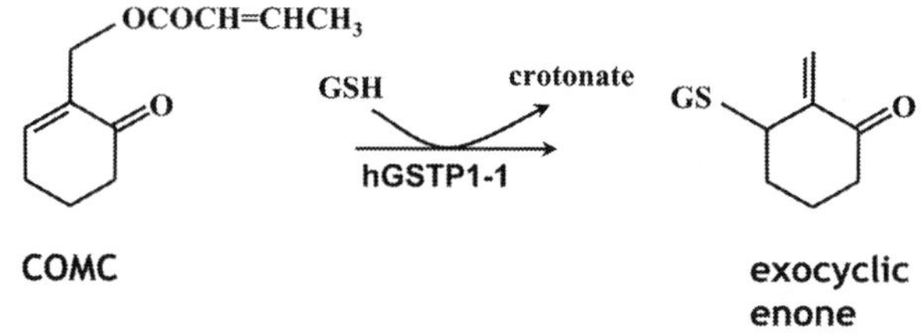

FIGURE 11-24.
GSH-dependent metabolism of 2-crotonyloxymethyl-2-cycloalkenones; see text for details.

In this case, the potentiation of the drug is catalyzed by several GSTs in addition to GST P1-1, with GST A4-4 showing the highest catalytic efficiency (*146*).

Adverse side effects are often a limiting factor in cancer chemotherapy with cytostatic drugs. Toxicity to rapidly dividing cells in the bone marrow, intestinal epithelium, and so on is dose-limiting and may also be directly life-threatening to the patient. Administration of an enzyme that could protect normal sensitive cells, in connection with chemotherapy, could allow treatment with higher doses, and, consequently, more effective eradication of tumor cells. Furthermore, the enzyme could reduce some of the undesired side effects and make the therapy more tolerable.

ENGINEERING OF GSTs FOR NOVEL FUNCTIONS

The naturally evolved GST protein framework has adequate stability and solubility for the further evolution of new functions. The creation of mutations in an evolved scaffold is a robust approach that minimizes the risks of unfavorable folding and low stability of the resulting structure. Repeated use of existing structural modules appears to be the paradigm for natural evolution of proteins and a powerful rationale for directed evolution in vitro.

Various approaches have been employed to adapt GSTs for novel functions (*147*). Structure-based rational redesign of GSTs supports the notion that specific substrate recognition depends on interactions with residues in the H-site (*148, 149*). One can also tailor new chemical functionalities into the active site, to achieve desired catalytic properties. A His residue in the H-site of GST A1-1 enables thiolesterase activity (*150*), and replacement of the active-site Ser in GST T2-2 by selenocysteine affords glutathione peroxidase activity (*151*). Site-specific replacements of Tyr by fluorinated Tyr derivatives in the active site of GST A1-1 have also been accomplished (*152*). The rational approach to structural and functional variability is consequently applicable to chemical functionalities beyond the strict limitations of the genetic code.

Even though it is sometimes possible, by rational redesign, to engineer desired catalytic properties into a protein structure, there is still a lack of fundamental understanding and of accurate methods for the prediction of function. Amino acid residues far away from the active site may be of major significance for enzymatic activity, and this effect is very difficult to model. For these reasons, stochastic methods are generally more effective than rational redesign in producing the targeted function. In this approach, libraries of randomly generated mutants are created, from which individuals with the desired characteristics are isolated. DNA shuffling (*153*) is a powerful method for producing recombined peptide segments, especially "family shuffling" of fragments from structurally related sequences (*154*). (The name recalls the shuffling of a deck of playing cards.) Recombination of stochastically generated fragments of the parental DNA gives rise to a library of variant DNA sequences, which encode variant protein structures expressed in *E. coli* or other host cells. From the recombinant sequences in the library, those that express improved protein functions are chosen for further rounds of DNA shuffling among the isolated variants. This procedure is reiterated until a satisfactory result has been obtained. DNA shuffling has similarities to genetic recombination processes that drive the natural evolution of proteins.

Under favorable circumstances, proteins with desired properties can be selected from the library by providing an essential property for survival of the host cell. This could be an enzyme inactivating a noxious agent that would otherwise kill the cell. Alternatively, the targeted protein may have selectable properties that could be identified by chemical or physical methods. However, the most general procedure is to screen the library by testing every member, or a sample of library members, for the desired function (high-throughput screening).

In the screening of GST mutant libraries, one may measure activities of the mutants with several substrates, owing to the broad specificity of GSTs. Compounds undergoing different chemical reactions, such as additions and substitutions, can be assayed in parallel. For a given mutant, the activity values obtained with the different substrates can be considered as a point in a multidimensional "substrate–activity space." For example, measurements with three alternative substrates (dichloromethane (DCM), 4-nitrophenethyl bromide (NPB), and 1,2-epoxy-3-(4-nitrophenoxy)propane (EPNP)) can be represented in three dimensions. The graph (*155*) (figure 11-25) shows that, in the projection of the points onto the two-dimensional plane of the two alkyl halide substrates, mutants that have activity with DCM also have highly correlated activity with NPB. In the third dimension represented by the epoxide substrate EPNP, the points

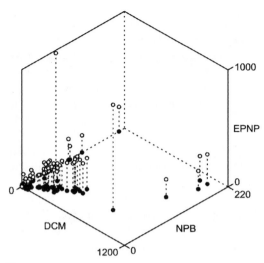

FIGURE 11-25.

Three-dimensional representation (circles) of substrate–activity space for recombinant Theta-class GSTs sampled from a library of mutants. Each GST variant was assayed with three alternative substrates, DCM, NPB, and EPNP and the values plotted; projections onto the two-dimensional subspace (DCM/NPB) are shown as dots. (*Reproduced from Larsson, A. K.; Emrén, L. O.; Bardsley, W. G.; Mannervik, B. Directed enzyme evolution guided by multidimensional analysis of substrate-activity space. Protein Eng. Des. Sel.* **2004**, *17, 49–55. Copyright Oxford University Press.*)

are more divergent. Using multivariate analysis, the mutants can be assigned to clusters, based on defined properties, and subgroups of mutants can be isolated for further evolution in an alternative direction. For example, one cluster could be suited for enhanced alkyltransferase activity while another could be further evolved for addition of GSH to epoxides.

Clusters of mutants can be chosen in each generation to serve as progenitors for the following generation of mutants. This recursive process of mutagenesis and identification of mutants with enhanced properties can be repeated for further optimization. Similar to the breeding of plants and animals, it may be advantageous to choose not only the "best" individual to parent the next generation, but also to broaden the genetic background by inclusion of additional mutants. In this manner, deleterious inbreeding is offset. The naturally occurring GSTs bear evidence of catalytic versatility, indicating that the GST structure can be tailored for novel functions by protein evolution.

Notes

1. Scott J. Grossman, Vice President, Pharmaceutical Candidate Optimization, BMS Pharmaceutical Research Institute.

2. James Kirkland, Dept. of Human Biology and Nutritional Sciences, University of Guelph.

References

1. Engle, M. R.; Singh, S. P.; Czernik, P. J.; Gaddy, D.; Montague, D. C.; Ceci, J. D.; Yang, Y.; Awasthi, S.; Awasthi, Y. C.; Zimniak, P.

Physiological role of mGSTA4-4, a glutathione S-transferase metabolizing 4-hydroxynonenal: generation and analysis of mGsta4 null mouse. *Toxicol. Appl. Pharmacol.* **2004,** *194,* 296–308.

2. Zarkovic, K. 4-Hydroxynonenal and neurodegenerative diseases. *Mol. Aspects Med.* **2003,** *24,* 293–303.

3. Picklo, M. J.; Montine, T. J.; Amarnath, V.; Neely, M. D. Carbonyl toxicology and Alzheimer's disease. *Toxicol. Appl. Pharmacol.* **2002,** *184,* 187–197.

4. Berhane, K.; Widersten, M.; Engström, A.; Kozarich, J. W.; Mannervik, B. Detoxication of base propenals and other alpha, beta-unsaturated aldehyde products of radical reactions and lipid peroxidation by human glutathione transferases. *Proc. Natl. Acad. Sci. USA* **1994,** *91,* 1480–1484.

5. Baez, S.; Segura-Aguilar, J.; Widersten, M.; Johansson, A.-S.; Mannervik, B. Glutathione transferases catalyse the detoxication of oxidized metabolites (*o*-quinones) of catecholamines and may serve as an antioxidant system preventing degenerative cellular processes. *Biochem. J.* **1997,** *324,* 25–28.

6. Segura-Aguilar, J.; Baez, S.; Widersten, M.; Welch, C. J.; Mannervik, B. Human class Mu glutathione transferases, in particular isoenzyme M2-2, catalyze detoxication of the dopamine metabolite aminochrome. *J. Biol. Chem.* **1997,** *272,* 5727–5731.

7. Dagnino-Subiabre, A.; Cassels, B. K.; Baez, S.; Johansson, A.-S.; Mannervik, B.; Segura-Aguilar, J. Glutathione transferase M2-2 catalyzes conjugation of dopamine and dopa *o*-quinones. *Biochem. Biophys. Res. Commun.* **2000,** *274,* 32–36.

8. Asanuma, M.; Miyazaki, I.; Ogawa, N. Dopamine- or L-DOPA-induced neurotoxicity: the role of dopamine quinone formation and tyrosinase in a model of Parkinson's disease. *Neurotox. Res.* **2003,** *5,* 165–176.

9. Grima, G.; Benz, B.; Parpura, V.; Cuenod, M.; Do, K. Q. Dopamine-induced oxidative stress in neurons with glutathione deficit: implication for schizophrenia. *Schizophr. Res.* **2003,** *62,* 213–224.

10. Zhao, T.; Singhal, S. S.; Piper, J. T.; Cheng, J.; Pandya, U.; Clark-Wronski, J.; Awasthi, S.; Awasthi, Y. C. The role of human glutathione S-transferases hGSTA1-1 and hGSTA2-2 in protection against oxidative stress. *Arch. Biochem. Biophys.* **1999,** *367,* 216–224.

11. Ketterer, B.; Meyer, D. J. Glutathione transferases: a possible role in the detoxication and repair of DNA and lipid hydroperoxides. *Mutat. Res.* **1989,** *214,* 33–40.

12. Bao, Y.; Jemth, P.; Mannervik, B.; Williamson, G. Reduction of thymine hydroperoxide by phospholipid hydroperoxide glutathione peroxidase and glutathione transferases. *FEBS Lett.* **1997,** *410,* 210–212.

13. Robertson, I. G.; Guthenberg, C.; Mannervik, B.; Jernström, B. Differences in stereoselectivity and catalytic efficiency of three human glutathione transferases in the conjugation of glutathione with 7β, 8α-dihydroxy-9α,10α-oxy-7,8,9,10-tetrahydrobenzo(a)pyrene. *Cancer Res.* **1986,** *46,* 2220–2224. 2220–2224.

14. Jernström, B.; Martinez, M.; Svensson, S. A.; Dock, L. Metabolism of benzo[a]pyrene-7,8-dihydrodiol and benzo[a]pyrene-7,8-dihydrodiol-9,10-epoxide to protein-binding products and glutathione conjugates in isolated rat hepatocytes. *Carcinogenesis* **1984,** *5,* 1079–1085.

15. Sundberg, K.; Widersten, M.; Seidel, A.; Mannervik, B.; Jernström, B. Glutathione conjugation of bay- and fjord-region diol epoxides of

polycyclic aromatic hydrocarbons by glutathione transferases M1-1 and P1-1. *Chem. Res. Toxicol.* **1997,** *10*, 1221–1227.

16. Sundberg, K.; Johansson, A.-S.; Stenberg, G.; Widersten, M.; Seidel, A.; Mannervik, B.; Jernström, B. Differences in the catalytic efficiencies of allelic variants of glutathione transferase P1-1 towards carcinogenic diol epoxides of polycyclic aromatic hydrocarbons. *Carcinogenesis* **1998,** *19*, 433–436.

17. Gu, Y.; Singh, S. V.; Ji, X. Residue R216 and catalytic efficiency of a murine class alpha glutathione S-transferase toward benzo[*a*]pyrene 7(R),8(S)-diol 9(S), 10(R)-epoxide. *Biochemistry* **2000,** *39*, 12552–12557.

18. Busby, W. F., Jr.; Woosley, R. L. Aflatoxins. In *Chemical Carcinogens*; Searle, C. E., Ed.; American Chemical Society: Washington, DC, 1984; pp. 945–1136.

19. Hayes, J. D.; Judah, D. J.; McLellan, L. I.; Neal, G. E. Contribution of the glutathione S-transferases to the mechanisms of resistance to aflatoxin B_1. *Pharmacol. Ther.* **1991,** *50*, 443–472.

20. Walton, M.; Egner, P.; Scholl, P. F.; Walker, J.; Kensler, T. W.; Groopman, J. D. Liquid chromatography electrospray-mass spectrometry of urinary aflatoxin biomarkers: characterization and application to dosimetry and chemoprevention in rats. *Chem. Res. Toxicol.* **2001,** *14*, 919–926.

21. Dostal, L. A.; Guthenberg, C.; Mannervik, B.; Bend, J. R. Stereo-selectivity and regioselectivity of purified human glutathione transferases pi, alpha-epsilon, and mu with alkene and polycyclic arene oxide substrates. *Drug Metab. Dispos.* **1988,** *16*, 420–424.

22. Ware G. W. *Pesticides: Theory and Application*; WH Freeman: San Francisco, 1983.

23. Leng, G.; Lewalter, J. Role of individual susceptibility in risk assessment of pesticides. *Occup. Environ. Med.* **1999,** *56*, 449–453.

24. Abel, E. L.; Bammler, T. K.; Eaton, D. L. Biotransformation of methyl parathion by glutathione S-transferases. *Toxicol. Sci.* **2004,** *79*, 224–32.

25. Nelson, D. L.; Cox, M. M. *Lehninger Principles of Biochemistry*; Worth Publishers: New York, 2004.

26. Elion, G. B. The purine path to chemotherapy. *Science* **1989,** *244*, 41–47.

27. Colvin, M. Gertrude Belle Elion (1918–1999). *Science* **1999,** *284*, 1480.

28. Elgemeie, G. H. Thioguanine, mercaptopurine: their analogs and nucleosides as antimetabolites. *Curr. Pharm. Des.* **2003,** *9*, 2627–2642.

29. Cara, C. J.; Pena, A. S.; Sans, M.; Rodrigo, L.; Guerrero-Esteo, M.; Hinojosa, J.; Garcia-Paredes, J.; Guijarro, L. G. Reviewing the mechanism of action of thiopurine drugs: towards a new paradigm in clinical practice. *Med. Sci. Monit.* **2004,** *10*, RA247–RA254.

30. Chan, G. L.; Canafax, D. M.; Johnson, C. A. The therapeutic use of azathioprine in renal transplantation. *Pharmacotherapy* **1987,** *7*, 165–177.

31. Gunnarsdottir, S.; Rucki, M.; Elfarra, A. A. Novel glutathione-dependent thiopurine prodrugs: evidence for enhanced cytotoxicity in tumor cells and for decreased bone marrow toxicity in mice. *J Pharmacol. Exp. Ther.* **2002,** *301*, 77–86.

32. Soglia, J. R.; Harriman, S. P.; Zhao, S.; Barberia, J.; Cole, M. J.; Boyd, J. G.; Contillo, L. G. The development of a higher throughput reactive intermediate screening assay incorporating micro-bore liquid chromatography-micro-electrospray ionization-tandem mass spectrometry and glutathione ethyl ester as an in vitro conjugating agent. *J. Pharm. Biomed. Anal.* **2004,** *36*, 105–116.

33. McGirr, L. G.; Subrahmanyam, V. V.; Moore, G. A.; O'Brien, P. J. Peroxidase-catalyzed-3-(glutathion-S-yl)-p,p'-biphenol formation. *Chem. Biol. Interact.* **1986**, *60*, 85–99.

34. Hoffmann, K. J.; Streeter, A. J.; Axworthy, D. B.; Baillie, T. A. Identification of the major covalent adduct formed in vitro and in vivo between acetaminophen and mouse liver proteins. *Mol. Pharmacol.* **1985**, *27*, 566–573.

35. Savides, M. C.; Oehme, F. W.; Nash, S. L.; Leipold, H. W. The toxicity and biotransformation of single doses of acetaminophen in dogs and cats. *Toxicol. Appl. Pharmacol.* **1984**, *74*, 26–34.

36. Hazelton, G. A.; Hjelle, J. J.; Klaassen, C. D. Effects of cysteine pro-drugs on acetaminophen-induced hepatotoxicity. *J. Pharmacol. Exp. Ther.* **1986**, *237*, 341–349.

37. Koen, Y. M.; Williams, T. D.; Hanzlik, R. P. Identification of three protein targets for reactive metabolites of bromobenzene in rat liver cytosol. *Chem. Res. Toxicol.* **2000**, *13*, 1326–1335.

38. Koen, Y. M.; Hanzlik, R. P. Identification of seven proteins in the endoplasmic reticulum as targets for reactive metabolites of bromobenzene. *Chem. Res. Toxicol.* **2002**, *15*, 699–706.

39. Luyendyk, J. P.; Copple, B. L.; Barton, C. C.; Ganey, P. E.; Roth, R. A. Augmentation of aflatoxin B1 hepatotoxicity by endotoxin: involvement of endothelium and the coagulation system. *Toxicol. Sci.* **2003**, *72*, 171–181.

40. Ravindranath, V.; Boyd, M. R.; Jerina, D. M. Hepatotoxicity of precocene I in rats. Role of metabolic activation in vivo. *Biochem. Pharmacol.* **1987**, *36*, 441–446.

41. Uetrecht, J. P. Is it possible to more accurately predict which drug candidates will cause idiosyncratic drug reactions? *Curr. Drug Metab.* **2000**, *1*, 133–141.

42. Ness, G. C.; Eales, S.; Lopez, D.; Zhao, Z. Regulation of 3-hydroxy-3-methylglutaryl coenzyme A reductase gene expression by sterols and nonsterols in rat liver. *Arch. Biochem. Biophys.* **1994**, *308*, 420–425.

43. Marletta, M. A. Nitric oxide synthase structure and mechanism. *J. Biol. Chem.* **1993**, *268*, 12231–12234.

44. Smith, R. P.; Wilcox, D. E. Toxicology of selected nitric oxide-donating xenobiotics, with particular reference to azide. *Crit. Rev. Toxicol.* **1994**, *24*, 355–377.

45. Napoli, C.; Ignarro, L. J. Nitric oxide-releasing drugs. *Annu. Rev. Pharmacol. Toxicol.* **2003**, *43*, 97–123.

46. Foster, M. W.; McMahon, T. J.; Stamler, J. S. S-Nitrosylation in health and disease. *Trends Mol. Med.* **2003**, *9*, 160–168.

47. Zeigler, M. M.; Doseff, A. I.; Galloway, M. F.; Opalek, J. M.; Nowicki, P. T.; Zweier, J. L.; Sen, C. K.; Marsh, C. B. Presentation of nitric oxide regulates monocyte survival through effects on caspase-9 and caspase-3 activation. *J. Biol. Chem.* **2003**, *278*, 12894–12902.

48. Liu, Z.; Rudd, M. A.; Freedman, J. E.; Loscalzo, J. S-Transnitrosation reactions are involved in the metabolic fate and biological actions of nitric oxide. *J. Pharm. Exp. Ther.* **1998**, *284*, 526–534.

49. Balazy, M.; Kaminski, P. M.; Mao, K.; Tan, J.; Wolin, M. S. S-Nitroglutathione, a product of the reaction between peroxynitrite and glutathione that generates nitric oxide. *J. Biol. Chem.* **1998**, *273*, 32009–32015.

50. Dekant, W.; Vamvakas, S. Glutathione-dependent bioactivation of xenobiotics. *Xenobiotica* **1993**, *23*, 873–887.

51. Monks, T. J.; Anders, M. W.; Dekant, W.; Stevens, J. L.; Lau, S. S.; van Bladeren, P. J. Glutathione conjugate mediated toxicities. *Toxicol. Appl. Pharmacol.* **1990,** *106*, 1–19.

52. Dekant, W., Ed. *Conjugation-Dependent Carcinogenicity and Toxicity of Foreign Compounds*; Academic Press: New York, 2003.

53. Casanova, M.; Bell, D. A.; Heck, H. D. Dichloromethane metabolism to formaldehyde and reaction of formaldehyde with nucleic acids in hepatocytes of rodents and humans with and without glutathione S-transferase T1 and M1 genes. *Fundam. Appl. Toxicol.* **1997,** *37*, 168–180.

54. Marsch, G. A.; Mundkowski, R. G.; Morris, B. J.; Manier, M. L.; Hartman, M. K.; Guengerich, F. P. Characterization of nucleoside and DNA adducts formed by S-(1-acetoxymethyl)glutathione and implications for dihalomethane-glutathione conjugates. *Chem. Res. Toxicol.* **2001,** *14*, 600–608.

55. Guengerich, F. P. Activation of dihaloalkanes by thiol-dependent mechanisms. *J. Biochem. Mol. Biol.* **2003,** *36*, 20–27.

56. Griffiths, G.; Trueman, L.; Crowther, T.; Thomas, B.; Smith, B. Onions: a global benefit to health. *Phytother. Res.* **2002,** *16*, 603–615.

57. Wood, W. F.; Sollers, B. G.; Dragoo, G. A. Volatile components in defensive spray of the hooded skunk, *Mephitis macroura. J. Chem. Ecol.* **2002,** *28*, 1865–1870.

58. Hendriks, W. H.; Moughan, P. J.; Tarttelin, M. F.; Woolhouse, A. D. Felinine: a urinary amino acid of *Felidae. Comp Biochem. Physiol. B Biochem. Mol. Biol.* **1995,** *112*, 581–588.

59. Natsch, A.; Gfeller, H.; Gygax, P.; Schmid, J.; Acuna, G. A specific bacterial aminoacylase cleaves odorant precursors secreted in the human axilla. *J. Biol. Chem.* **2003,** *278*, 5718–5727.

60. Guthenberg, C.; Mannervik, B. Glutathione S-transferase (transferase pi) from human placenta is identical or closely related to glutathione S-transferase (transferase rho) from erythrocytes. *Biochim. Biophys. Acta* **1981,** *661*, 255–260.

61. Rowe, J. D.; Nieves, E.; Listowsky, I. Subunit diversity and tissue distribution of human glutathione S-transferases: interpretations based on electrospray ionization-MS and peptide sequence-specific antisera. *Biochem. J.* **1997,** *325*, 481–486.

62. Johansson, A.-S.; Mannervik, B. Human glutathione transferase A3-3, a highly efficient catalyst of double-bond isomerization in the biosynthetic pathway of steroid hormones. *J. Biol. Chem.* **2001,** *276*, 33061–33065.

63. Guthenberg, C.; Warholm, M.; Rane, A.; Mannervik, B. Two distinct forms of glutathione transferase from human foetal liver. Purification and comparison with isoenzymes isolated from adult liver and placenta. *Biochem. J.* **1986,** *235*, 741–745.

64. Strange, R. C.; Davis, B. A.; Faulder, C. G.; Cotton, W.; Bain, A. D.; Hopkinson, D. A.; Hume, R. The human glutathione S-transferases: developmental aspects of the GST1, GST2, and GST3 loci. *Biochem. Genet.* **1985,** *23*, 1011–1028.

65. Rozell, B.; Hansson, H. A.; Guthenberg, C.; Tahir, M. K.; Mannervik, B. Glutathione transferases of classes alpha, mu and pi show selective expression in different regions of rat kidney. *Xenobiotica* **1993,** *23*, 835–849.

66. Robin, M. A.; Prabu, S. K.; Raza, H.; Anandatheerthavarada, H. K.; Avadhani, N. G. Phosphorylation enhances mitochondrial targeting

of GSTA4-4 through increased affinity for binding to cytoplasmic Hsp70. *J. Biol. Chem.* **2003,** *278*, 18960–18970.

67. Mannervik, B.; Widersten, M. Human glutathione transferases: classification, tissue distribution, structure, and functional properties. In *Advances in Drug Metabolism in Man*; Pacifici, G. M., Fracchia, G. N., Eds.; European Commission: Luxembourg, 1995; pp. 407–459.

68. Raijmakers, M. T.; Steegers, E. A.; Peters, W. H. Glutathione S-transferases and thiol concentrations in embryonic and early fetal tissues. *Hum. Reprod.* **2001,** *16*, 2445–2450.

69. Hayes, J. D.; Pulford, D. J. The glutathione S-transferase supergene family: regulation of GST and the contribution of the isoenzymes to cancer chemoprotection and drug resistance. *Crit. Rev. Biochem. Mol. Biol.* **1995,** *30*, 445–600.

70. Rushmore, T. H.; King, R. G.; Paulson, K. E.; Pickett, C. B. Regulation of glutathione S-transferase Ya subunit gene expression: identification of a unique xenobiotic-responsive element controlling inducible expression by planar aromatic compounds. *Proc. Natl. Acad. Sci. USA* **1990,** *87*, 3826–3830.

71. Rushmore, T. H.; Morton, M. R.; Pickett, C. B. The antioxidant responsive element. Activation by oxidative stress and identification of the DNA consensus sequence required for functional activity. *J. Biol. Chem.* **1991,** *266*, 11632–11639.

72. Friling, R. S.; Bensimon, A.; Tichauer, Y.; Daniel, V. Xenobiotic-inducible expression of murine glutathione S-transferase Ya subunit gene is controlled by an electrophile-responsive element. *Proc. Natl. Acad. Sci. USA* **1990,** *87*, 6258–6262.

73. Nguyen, T.; Sherratt, P. J.; Pickett, C. B. Regulatory mechanisms controlling gene expression mediated by the antioxidant response element. *Annu. Rev. Pharmacol. Toxicol.* **2003,** *43*, 233–260.

74. Dinkova-Kostova, A. T.; Fahey, J. W.; Talalay, P. Chemical structures of inducers of nicotinamide quinone oxidoreductase 1 (NQO1). *Methods Enzymol.* **2004,** *382*, 423–448.

75. Motohashi, H.; Yamamoto, M. Nrf2-Keap1 defines a physiologically important stress response mechanism. *Trends Mol. Med.* **2004,** *10*, 549–557.

76. Wakabayashi, N.; Dinkova-Kostova, A. T.; Holtzclaw, W. D.; Kang, M. I.; Kobayashi, A.; Yamamoto, M.; Kensler, T. W.; Talalay, P. Protection against electrophile and oxidant stress by induction of the phase 2 response: fate of cysteines of the Keap1 sensor modified by inducers. *Proc. Natl. Acad. Sci. USA* **2004,** *101*, 2040–2045.

77. Kolm, R. H.; Danielson, U. H.; Zhang, Y.; Talalay, P.; Mannervik, B. Isothiocyanates as substrates for human glutathione transferases: structure–activity studies. *Biochem. J.* **1995,** *311*, 453–459.

78. Talalay, P.; Dinkova-Kostova, A. T.; Holtzclaw, W. D. Importance of phase 2 gene regulation in protection against electrophile and reactive oxygen toxicity and carcinogenesis. *Adv. Enzyme Regul.* **2003,** *43*, 121–134.

79. Awasthi, S.; Pandya, U.; Singhal, S. S.; Lin, J. T.; Thiviyanathan, V.; Seifert, W. E., Jr.; Awasthi, Y. C.; Ansari, G. A. Curcumin–glutathione interactions and the role of human glutathione S-transferase P1-1. *Chem. Biol. Interact.* **2000,** *128*, 19–38.

80. Duvoix, A.; Morceau, F.; Delhalle, S.; Schmitz, M.; Schnekenburger, M.; Galteau, M. M.; Dicato, M.; Diederich, M. Induction of apoptosis by

curcumin: mediation by glutathione S-transferase P1-1 inhibition. *Biochem. Pharmacol.* **2003,** *66,* 1475–1483.

81. Zhang, Y.; Gordon, G. B. A strategy for cancer prevention: stimulation of the Nrf2-ARE signaling pathway. *Mol. Cancer Ther.* **2004,** *3,* 885–893.

82. Steinkellner, H.; Rabot, S.; Freywald, C.; Nobis, E.; Scharf, G.; Chabicovsky, M.; Knasmuller, S.; Kassie, F. Effects of cruciferous vegetables and their constituents on drug metabolizing enzymes involved in the bioactivation of DNA-reactive dietary carcinogens. *Mutat. Res.* **2001,** *480–481,* 285–297.

83. Thapliyal, R.; Maru, G. B. Inhibition of cytochrome P450 isozymes by curcumins in vitro and in vivo. *Food Chem. Toxicol.* **2001,** *39,* 541–547.

84. Kassie, F.; Uhl, M.; Rabot, S.; Grasl-Kraupp, B.; Verkerk, R.; Kundi, M.; Chabicovsky, M.; Schulte-Hermann, R.; Knasmuller, S. Chemoprevention of 2-amino-3-methylimidazo[4,5-*f*]quinoline (IQ)-induced colonic and hepatic preneoplastic lesions in the F344 rat by cruciferous vegetables administered simultaneously with the carcinogen. *Carcinogenesis* **2003,** *24,* 255–261.

85. Guyonnet, D.; Belloir, C.; Suschetet, M.; Siess, M. H.; Le Bon, A. M. Mechanisms of protection against aflatoxin B1 genotoxicity in rats treated by organosulfur compounds from garlic. *Carcinogenesis* **2002,** *23,* 1335–1341.

86. Omenn, G. S.; Goodman, G. E.; Thornquist, M. D.; Balmes, J.; Cullen, M. R.; Glass, A.; Keogh, J. P.; Meyskens, F. L., Jr.; Valanis, B.; Williams, J. H., Jr.; Barnhart, S.; Cherniack, M. G.; Brodkin, C. A.; Hammar, S. Risk factors for lung cancer and for intervention effects in CARET, the Beta-Carotene and Retinol Efficacy Trial. *J. Natl. Cancer Inst.* **1996,** *88,* 1550–1559.

87. Paolini, M.; Antelli, A.; Pozzetti, L.; Spetlova, D.; Perocco, P.; Valgimigli, L.; Pedulli, G. F.; Cantelli-Forti, G. Induction of cytochrome P450 enzymes and over-generation of oxygen radicals in β-carotene supplemented rats. *Carcinogenesis* **2001,** *22,* 1483–1495.

88. Talalay, P.; Talalay, P. The importance of using scientific principles in the development of medicinal agents from plants. *Acad. Med.* **2001,** *76,* 238–247.

89. Jacobson, L. P.; Zhang, B. C.; Zhu, Y. R.; Wang, J. B.; Wu, Y.; Zhang, Q. N.; Yu, L. Y.; Qian, G. S.; Kuang, S. Y.; Li, Y. F.; Fang, X.; Zarba, A.; Chen, B.; Enger, C.; Davidson, N. E.; Gorman, M. B.; Gordon, G. B.; Prochaska, H. J.; Egner, P. A.; Groopman, J. D.; Munoz, A.; Helzlsouer, K. J.; Kensler, T. W. Oltipraz chemoprevention trial in Qidong, People's Republic of China: study design and clinical outcomes. *Cancer Epidemiol. Biomarkers Prev.* **1997,** *6,* 257–265.

90. Kensler, T. W.; He, X.; Otieno, M.; Egner, P. A.; Jacobson, L. P.; Chen, B.; Wang, J. S.; Zhu, Y. R.; Zhang, B. C.; Wang, J. B.; Wu, Y.; Zhang, Q. N.; Qian, G. S.; Kuang, S. Y.; Fang, X.; Li, Y. F.; Yu, L. Y.; Prochaska, H. J.; Davidson, N. E.; Gordon, G. B.; Gorman, M. B.; Zarba, A.; Enger, C.; Munoz, A.; Helzlsouer, K. J. Oltipraz chemoprevention trial in Qidong, People's Republic of China: modulation of serum aflatoxin albumin adduct biomarkers. *Cancer Epidemiol. Biomarkers Prev.* **1998,** *7,* 127–134.

91. Kensler, T. W.; Egner, P. A.; Wang, J. B.; Zhu, Y. R.; Zhang, B. C.; Lu, P. X.; Chen, J. G.; Qian, G. S.; Kuang, S. Y.; Jackson, P. E.; Gange, S. J.; Jacobson, L. P.; Munoz, A.; Groopman, J. D. Chemoprevention of hepatocellular carcinoma in aflatoxin endemic areas. *Gastroenterology* **2004,** *127,* S310–S318.

92. Hatayama, I.; Satoh, K.; Sato, K. Developmental and hormonal regulation of the major form of hepatic glutathione S-transferase in male mice. *Biochem. Biophys. Res. Commun.* **1986**, *140*, 581–588.

93. Staffas, L.; Mankowitz, L.; Söderström, M.; Blanck, A.; Porsch-Hallström, I.; Sundberg, C.; Mannervik, B.; Olin, B.; Rydström, J.; DePierre, J. W. Further characterization of hormonal regulation of glutathione transferase in rat liver and adrenal glands. Sex differences and demonstration that growth hormone regulates the hepatic levels. *Biochem. J.* **1992**, *286*, 65–72.

94. Mankowitz, L.; Castro, V. M.; Mannervik, B.; Rydström, J.; DePierre, J. W. Increase in the amount of glutathione transferase 4-4 in the rat adrenal gland after hypophysectomy and down-regulation by subsequent treatment with adrenocorticotrophic hormone. *Biochem. J.* **1990**, *265*, 147–154.

95. Mode, A.; Norstedt, G.; Simic, B.; Eneroth, P.; Gustafsson, J. Å. Continuous infusion of growth hormone feminizes hepatic steroid metabolism in the rat. *Endocrinology* **1981**, *108*, 2103–2108.

96. Mode, A.; Wiersma-Larsson, E.; Ström, A.; Zaphiropoulos, P. G.; Gustafsson, J. Å. A dual role of growth hormone as a feminizing and masculinizing factor in the control of sex-specific cytochrome P-450 isozymes in rat liver. *J. Endocrinol.* **1989**, *120*, 311–317.

97. Johansson, A.-S.; Mannervik, B. Interindividual variability of glutathione transferase expression. In *Interindividual Variability in Drug Metabolism*; Pacifici, G. M., Fracchia, G. N., Eds.; Taylor & Francis: London, 2001, pp. 460–519.

98. Coles, B. F.; Kadlubar, F. F. Detoxification of electrophilic compounds by glutathione S-transferase catalysis: determinants of individual response to chemical carcinogens and chemotherapeutic drugs? *Biofactors* **2003**, *17*, 115–130.

99. Mannervik, B.; Castro, V. M.; Danielson, U. H.; Tahir, M. K.; Hansson, J.; Ringborg, U. Expression of class Pi glutathione transferase in human malignant melanoma cells. *Carcinogenesis* **1987**, *8*, 1929–1932.

100. Lewis, A. D.; Forrester, L. M.; Hayes, J. D.; Wareing, C. J.; Carmichael, J.; Harris, A. L.; Mooghen, M.; Wolf, C. R. Glutathione S-transferase isoenzymes in human tumours and tumour derived cell lines. *Br. J. Cancer* **1989**, *60*, 327–331.

101. Kelley, M. K.; Engqvist-Goldstein, A.; Montali, J. A.; Wheatley, J. B.; Schmidt, D. E.; Jr.; Kauvar, L. M. Variability of glutathione S-transferase isoenzyme patterns in matched normal and cancer human breast tissue. *Biochem. J.* **1994**, *304*, 843–848.

102. Jones, P. A.; Baylin, S. B. The fundamental role of epigenetic events in cancer. *Nat. Rev. Genet.* **2002**, *3*, 415–428.

103. Nakayama, M.; Gonzalgo, M. L.; Yegnasubramanian, S.; Lin, X.; De Marzo, A. M.; Nelson, W. G. GSTP1 CpG island hypermethylation as a molecular biomarker for prostate cancer. *J. Cell Biochem.* **2004**, *91*, 540–552.

104. Nelson, W. G.; De Marzo, A. M.; Isaacs, W. B. Prostate cancer. *N. Engl. J. Med.* **2003**, *349*, 366–381.

105. Solt, D. B.; Medline, A.; Farber, E. Rapid emergence of carcinogen-induced hyperplastic lesions in a new model for the sequential analysis of liver carcinogenesis. *Am. J. Pathol.* **1977**, *88*, 595–618.

106. Eriksson, L. C.; Sharma, R. N.; Roomi, M. W.; Ho, R. K.; Farber, E.; Murray, R. K. A characteristic electrophoretic pattern of cytosolic

polypeptides from hepatocyte nodules generated during liver carcinogenesis in several models. *Biochem. Biophys. Res. Commun.* **1983,** *117,* 740–745.

107. Kitahara, A.; Satoh, K.; Nishimura, K.; Ishikawa, T.; Ruike, K.; Sato, K.; Tsuda, H.; Ito, N. Changes in molecular forms of rat hepatic glutathione S-transferase during chemical hepatocarcinogenesis. *Cancer Res.* **1984,** *44,* 2698–2703.

108. Satoh, K.; Kitahara, A.; Soma, Y.; Inaba, Y.; Hatayama, I.; Sato, K. Purification, induction, and distribution of placental glutathione transferase: a new marker enzyme for preneoplastic cells in the rat chemical hepatocarcinogenesis. *Proc. Natl. Acad. Sci. USA* **1985,** *82,* 3964–3968.

109. Abrams M.J. The chemistry of platinum antitumour agents. In *The Chemistry of Antitumour Agents*; Wilman, D. E. V., Ed.: Chapman and Hall: New York, 1990; pp. 331–341.

110. Myers, C.; Gianni, L.; Zweier, J.; Muindi, J.; Sinha, B. K.; Eliot, H. Role of iron in adriamycin biochemistry. *Fed. Proc.* **1986,** *45,* 2792–2797.

111. Kamada, K.; Goto, S.; Okunaga, T.; Ihara, Y.; Tsuji, K.; Kawai, Y.; Uchida, K.; Osawa, T.; Matsuo, T.; Nagata, I.; Kondo, T. Nuclear glutathione S-transferase pi prevents apoptosis by reducing the oxidative stress-induced formation of exocyclic DNA products. *Free Radic. Biol. Med.* **2004,** *37,* 1875–1884.

112. Tsuchida, S.; Sato, K. Glutathione transferases and cancer. *Crit. Rev. Biochem. Mol. Biol.* **1992,** *27,* 337–384.

113. Rooney, P. H.; Telfer, C.; McFadyen, M. C.; Melvin, W. T.; Murray, G. I. The role of cytochrome P450 in cytotoxic bioactivation: future therapeutic directions. *Curr. Cancer Drug Targets.* **2004,** *4,* 257–265.

114. Takamoto, S.; Sakura, N.; Namera, A.; Yashiki, M. Monitoring of urinary acrolein concentration in patients receiving cyclophosphamide and ifosphamide. *J. Chromatogr. B Analyt. Technol. Biomed. Life Sci.* **2004,** *806,* 59–63.

115. Einhorn, L. H. Curing metastatic testicular cancer. *Proc. Natl. Acad. Sci. USA* **2002,** *99,* 4592–4595.

116. Rashid, R.; Langfinger, D.; Wagner, R.; Schuchmann, H. P.; von Sonntag, C. Bleomycin versus OH-radical-induced malonaldehydic-product formation in DNA. *Int. J. Radiat. Biol.* **1999,** *75,* 101–109.

117. Ciaccio, P. J.; Tew, K. D.; LaCreta, F. P. Enzymatic conjugation of chlorambucil with glutathione by human glutathione S-transferases and inhibition by ethacrynic acid. *Biochem. Pharmacol.* **1991,** *42,* 1504–1507.

118. Lien, S.; Larsson, A.-K.; Mannervik, B. The polymorphic human glutathione transferase T1-1, the most efficient glutathione transferase in the denitrosation and inactivation of the anticancer drug 1,3-bis (2-chloroethyl)-1-nitrosourea. *Biochem. Pharmacol.* **2002,** *63,* 191–197.

119. Ban, N.; Takahashi, Y.; Takayama, T.; Kura, T.; Katahira, T.; Sakamaki, S.; Niitsu, Y. Transfection of glutathione S-transferase (GST)-pi antisense complementary DNA increases the sensitivity of a colon cancer cell line to adriamycin, cisplatin, melphalan, and etoposide. *Cancer Res.* **1996,** *56,* 3577–3582.

120. Morrow, C. S.; Smitherman, P. K.; Diah, S. K.; Schneider, E.; Townsend, A. J. Coordinated action of glutathione S-transferases (GSTs) and multidrug resistance protein 1 (MRP1) in antineoplastic drug detoxification. Mechanism of GST A1-1- and MRP1-associated resistance to

chlorambucil in MCF7 breast carcinoma cells. *J. Biol. Chem.* **1998,** *273,* 20114–20120.

121. O'Brien, M.; Kruh, G. D.; Tew, K. D. The influence of coordinate overexpression of glutathione phase II detoxification gene products on drug resistance. *J. Pharmacol. Exp. Ther.* **2000,** *294,* 480–487.

122. Depeille, P.; Cuq, P.; Mary, S.; Passagne, I.; Evrard, A.; Cupissol, D.; Vian, L. Glutathione S-transferase M1 and multidrug resistance protein 1 act in synergy to protect melanoma cells from vincristine effects. *Mol. Pharmacol.* **2004,** *65,* 897–905.

123. Smitherman, P. K.; Townsend, A. J.; Kute, T. E.; Morrow, C. S. Role of multidrug resistance protein 2 (MRP2, ABCC2) in alkylating agent detoxification: MRP2 potentiates glutathione S-transferase A1-1-mediated resistance to chlorambucil cytotoxicity. *J. Pharmacol. Exp. Ther.* **2004,** *308,* 260–267.

124. Gautam, A.; Waldrep, J. C.; Densmore, C. L. Aerosol gene therapy. *Mol. Biotechnol.* **2003,** *23,* 51–60.

125. Rooseboom, M.; Commandeur, J. N.; Vermeulen, N. P. Enzyme-catalyzed activation of anticancer prodrugs. *Pharmacol. Rev.* **2004,** *56,* 53–102.

126. Kirn, D.; Niculescu-Duvaz, I.; Hallden, G.; Springer, C. J. The emerging fields of suicide gene therapy and virotherapy. *Trends Mol. Med.* **2002,** *8,* 68–73.

127. Denny, W. A. Prodrugs for gene-directed enzyme-prodrug therapy (suicide gene therapy). *J. Biomed. Biotechnol.* **2003,** *2003,* 48–70.

128. Chen, C. S.; Lin, J. T.; Goss, K. A.; He, Y. A.; Halpert, J. R.; Waxman, D. J. Activation of the anticancer prodrugs cyclophosphamide and ifosfamide: identification of cytochrome P450 2B enzymes and site-specific mutants with improved enzyme kinetics. *Mol. Pharmacol.* **2004,** *65,* 1278–1285.

129. Tew, K. D.; Dutta, S.; Schultz, M. Inhibitors of glutathione S-transferases as therapeutic agents. *Adv. Drug Deliv. Rev.* **1997,** *26,* 91–104.

130. Ranganathan, S.; Ciaccio, P. J.; Tew, K. D. Principles of drug modulation applied to glutathione S-transferases. In *Structure and Function of Glutathione Transferases*; Tew, K. D., Pickett, C. B., Mantle, T. J., Mannervik, B., Hayes, J. D., Eds.; CRC Press: Boca Raton, FL, 1993; pp. 249–256.

131. Hansson, J.; Berhane, K.; Castro, V. M.; Jungnelius, U.; Mannervik, B.; Ringborg, U. Sensitization of human melanoma cells to the cytotoxic effect of melphalan by the glutathione transferase inhibitor ethacrynic acid. *Cancer Res.* **1991,** *51,* 94–98.

132. Burg, D.; Mulder, G. J. Glutathione conjugates and their synthetic derivatives as inhibitors of glutathione-dependent enzymes involved in cancer and drug resistance. *Drug Metab. Rev.* **2002,** *34,* 821–863.

133. Oakley, A. J.; Lo Bello, M.; Ricci, G.; Federici, G.; Parker, M. W. Evidence for an induced-fit mechanism operating in pi class glutathione transferases. *Biochemistry* **1998,** *37,* 9912–9917.

134. Hitchens, T. K.; Mannervik, B.; Rule, G. S. Disorder-to-order transition of the active site of human class Pi glutathione transferase, GST P1-1. *Biochemistry* **2001,** *40,* 11660–11669.

135. Puri, R. N.; Meister, A. Transport of glutathione, as γ-glutamylcysteinyl-glycyl ester, into liver and kidney. *Proc. Natl. Acad. Sci. USA* **1983,** *80,* 5258–5260.

136. Burg, D.; Filippov, D. V.; Hermanns, R.; van der Marel, G. A.; van Boom, J. H.; Mulder, G. J. Peptidomimetic glutathione analogues as novel γ-GT-stable GST inhibitors. *Bioorg. Med. Chem.* **2002**, *10*, 195–205.

137. Kalota, A.; Shetzline, S. E.; Gewirtz, A. M. Progress in the development of nucleic acid therapeutics for cancer. *Cancer Biol. Ther.* **2004**, *3*, 4–12.

138. Fire, A.; Xu, S.; Montgomery, M. K.; Kostas, S. A.; Driver, S. E.; Mello, C. C. Potent and specific genetic interference by double-stranded RNA in *Caenorhabditis elegans*. *Nature* **1998**, *391*, 806–811.

139. Hannon, G. J. RNA interference. *Nature* **2002**, *418*, 244–251.

140. Hannon, G. J.; Rossi, J. J. Unlocking the potential of the human genome with RNA interference. *Nature* **2004**, *431*, 371–378.

141. Kolb, F. A.; Zhang, H.; Jaronczyk, K.; Tahbaz, N.; Hobman, T. C.; Filipowicz, W. Human dicer: purification, properties, and interaction with PAZ PIWI domain proteins. *Methods Enzymol.* **2005**, *392*, 316–336.

142. Satyam, A.; Hocker, M. D.; Kane-Maguire, K. A.; Morgan, A. S.; Villar, H. O.; Lyttle, M. H. Design, synthesis, and evaluation of latent alkylating agents activated by glutathione S-transferase. *J. Med. Chem.* **1996**, *39*, 1736–1747.

143. Castro, V. M.; Söderström, M.; Carlberg, I.; Widersten, M.; Platz, A.; Mannervik, B. Differences among human tumor cell lines in the expression of glutathione transferases and other glutathione-linked enzymes. *Carcinogenesis* **1990**, *11*, 1569–1576.

144. Morgan, A. S.; Sanderson, P. E.; Borch, R. F.; Tew, K. D.; Niitsu, Y.; Takayama, T.; Von Hoff, D. D.; Izbicka, E.; Mangold, G.; Paul, C.; Broberg, U.; Mannervik, B.; Henner, W. D.; Kauvar, L. M. Tumor efficacy and bone marrow-sparing properties of TER286, a cytotoxin activated by glutathione S-transferase. *Cancer Res.* **1998**, *58*, 2568–2575.

145. Lin, X.; Nelson, W. G. Methyl-CpG-binding domain protein-2 mediates transcriptional repression associated with hypermethylated GSTP1 CpG islands in MCF-7 breast cancer cells. *Cancer Res.* **2003**, *63*, 498–504.

146. Hamilton, D. S.; Zhang, X.; Ding, Z.; Hubatsch, I.; Mannervik, B.; Houk, K. N.; Ganem, B.; Creighton, D. J. Mechanism of the glutathione transferase-catalyzed conversion of antitumor 2-crotonyloxymethyl-2-cycloalkenones to GSH adducts. *J. Am. Chem. Soc.* **2003**, *125*, 15049–15058.

147. Ivarsson, Y.; Mackey, A. J.; Edalat, M.; Pearson, W. R.; Mannervik, B. Identification of residues in glutathione transferase capable of driving functional diversification in evolution. A novel approach to protein redesign. *J. Biol. Chem.* **2003**, *278*, 8733–8738.

148. Nilsson, L. O.; Gustafsson, A.; Mannervik, B. Redesign of substrate-selectivity determining modules of glutathione transferase A1-1 installs high catalytic efficiency with toxic alkenal products of lipid peroxidation. *Proc. Natl. Acad. Sci. USA* **2000**, *97*, 9408–9412.

149. Pettersson, P. L.; Johansson, A.-S.; Mannervik, B. Transmutation of human glutathione transferase A2-2 with peroxidase activity into an efficient steroid isomerase. *J. Biol. Chem.* **2002**, *277*, 30019–30022.

150. Hederos, S.; Broo, K. S.; Jakobsson, E.; Kleywegt, G. J.; Mannervik, B.; Baltzer, L. Incorporation of a single His residue by rational design enables thiol-ester hydrolysis by human glutathione transferase A1-1. *Proc. Natl. Acad. Sci. USA* **2004**, *101*, 13163–13167.

151. Ren, X.; Jemth, P.; Board, P. G.; Luo, G.; Mannervik, B.; Liu, J.; Zhang, K.; Shen, J. A semisynthetic glutathione peroxidase with high catalytic efficiency. Selenoglutathione transferase. *Chem. Biol.* **2002,** *9*, 789–794.

152. Thorson, J. S.; Shin, I.; Chapman, E.; Stenberg, G.; Mannervik, B.; Schulz, P. G. Analysis of the role of the active site tyrosine in human glutathione transferase A1-1 by unnatural amino acid mutagenesis. *J. Am. Chem. Soc.* **1998,** *120*, 451–452.

153. Stemmer, W. P. C. Rapid evolution of a protein in vitro by DNA shuffling. *Nature* **1994,** *370*, 389–391.

154. Crameri, A.; Raillard, S. A.; Bermudez, E.; Stemmer, W. P. C. DNA shuffling of a family of genes from diverse species accelerates directed evolution. *Nature* **1998,** *391*, 288–291.

155. Larsson, A.-K.; Emrén, L. O.; Bardsley, W. G.; Mannervik, B. Directed enzyme evolution guided by multidimensional analysis of substrate–activity space. *Protein Eng. Des. Sel.* **2004,** *17*, 49–55.

UDP-GLUCURONIC ACID

In this chapter we discuss conjugation with sugars (*glycosylation* or *glyco-sidation*), an important pathway of xenobiotic metabolism. Conjugation of lipophilic compounds to a sugar derivative usually results in a great increase in water solubility. For example, nucleosides are the water-soluble ribose glycosides of the hydrophobic nucleic acid bases. Glucuronic acid is the sugar commonly used for the glycosidation of xenobiotics by humans and UDP-glucuronic acid (UDPGA) is the activated donor of this sugar moiety.

UDPGA is biosynthesized from glucose and UTP (figure 12-1). Glucose-1-phosphate (the product of glycogen phosphorolysis) is coupled to UTP to give UDP-glucose. UDP-glucose can be used for the synthesis of glycogen or other activated sugars; two NAD^+-dependent oxidations convert UDP-glucose to the sugar acid, UDPGA.

GLUCURONIDE FORMATION

Glucuronic acid conjugation is one of the most important pathways for biotransformation of many foreign substances, including natural products (e.g., morphine), pollutants (e.g., aromatic amines, hydroxylated metabolites of polycyclic aromatic hydrocarbons), and drugs (e.g., acetaminophen, irinotecan). This pathway accounts for more than one-third of all conjugation reactions involved in drug metabolism (*1*). In addition, several endogenous lipophilic compounds (bilirubin, bile salts, steroid hormones, etc.) are metabolized by conjugation to glucuronic acid.

Glucuronide formation is a specific example of glycosylation. We refer to the nonsugar substrate as an *aglycone* (Greek, "without sugar"); the product glycoside is a β-D-glucopyranosiduronic acid (glucuronide). The enzymes that catalyze these conjugations are called UDP-glucuronosyl-transferases (UGTs; EC 2.4.1.17). Glucuronides are recognized by the biliary and renal organic anion transport systems, which enable their secretion into the bile or urine. Addition of glucuronic acid to a xenobiotic radically changes the structure of the molecule and alters its biological activity. Usually, the activity of the aglycone is reduced or abolished, due to reduction in affinity for the biological target (and facilitation of excretion). Therefore, glucuronide formation is mainly (but not exclusively) a detoxication process leading to inactive metabolites.

Since the systematic name for the enzymes catalyzing glucuronide formation is "glucuronosyltransferase," we prefer to denote the process "glucuronosylation." However, the synonymous term "glucuronidation" is also very widely used.

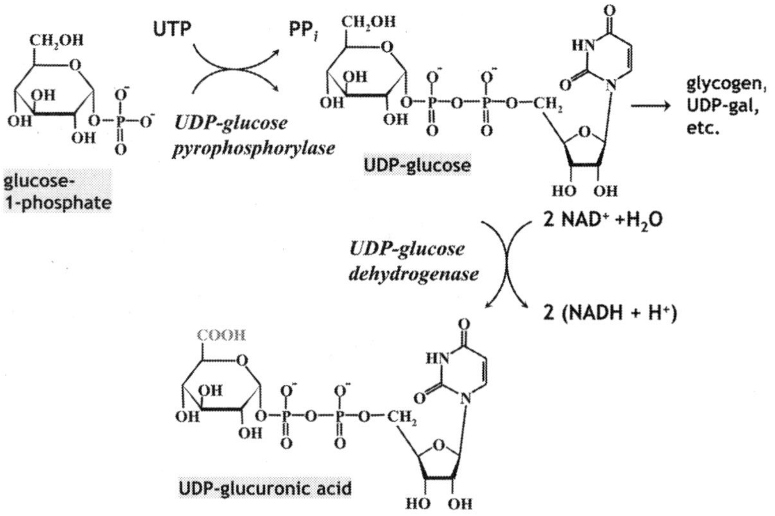

FIGURE 12-1.
Biosynthesis of UDP-glucuronic acid.

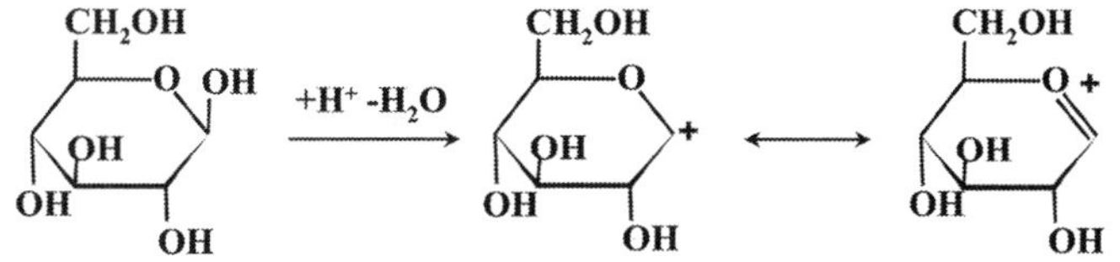

FIGURE 12-2.
The anomeric carbon of a sugar is the principal site of attack by nucleophiles.

Glucuronosylation proceeds by the enzyme-catalyzed attack of a nucleophile (typically, a hydroxyl or amino function) on the anomeric carbon atom (C-1) of UDPGA (figures 12-2 and 12-3). The anomeric carbon is electrophilic because of resonance stabilization of cationic intermediates at this position. Therefore, reactions at the anomeric carbon atom are central to sugar chemistry. The glucuronosylation reaction is an S_N2-type displacement reaction, with UDP as the leaving group. The reaction proceeds with inversion of optical configuration at the anomeric carbon atom (figure 12-4; see also chapter 9). Thus, UDPGA has an α-configuration but the product glycoside is of β-configuration. The resulting glucuronides contain the D-glucopyranuronosyl radical linked to −OR, −SR, −NRR', or −CR.

CLASSES OF GLUCURONIDES

The most common glucuronides are formed at the nucleophilic oxygens of hydroxyl or carboxylic acid groups, yielding ether (figure 12-5) or ester (figure 12-6) glucuronides, respectively. O-Glucuronide conjugates can also be formed from hydroxylamines; an example is the metabolite of a piperazine oral hypoglycemic agent shown in figure 12-7.

Glucuronosylation of primary or secondary amines yields N-glucuronides (cf. nucleosides). With tertiary amines, a positively charged

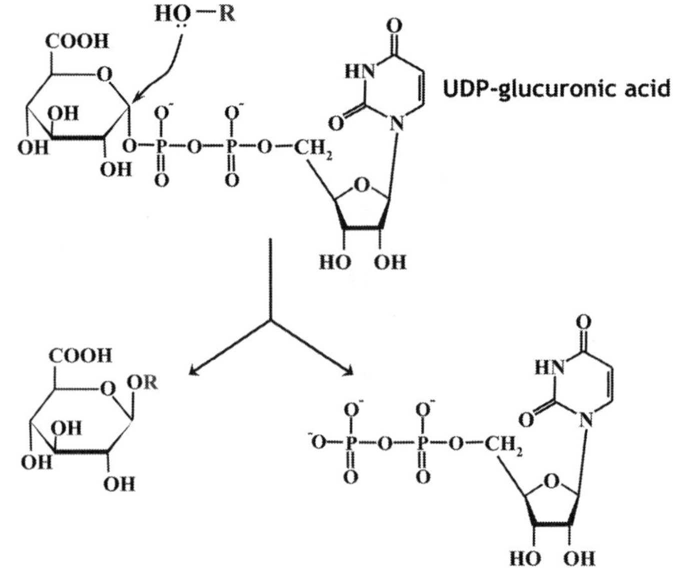

FIGURE 12-3.
The general reaction catalyzed by UDP-glucuronosyltransferases.

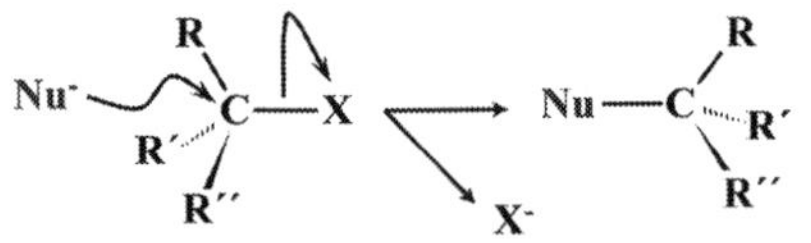

FIGURE 12-4.
Inversion of configuration during an S_N2 reaction.

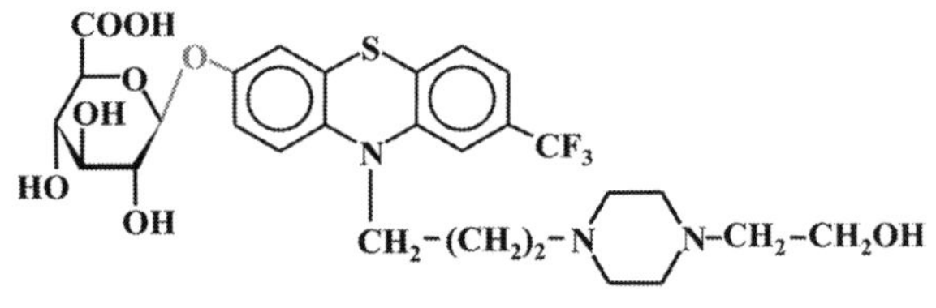

FIGURE 12-5.
An ether glucuronide, 7-hydroxyfluphenazine glucuronide. (*Jackson, C. J.; Hubbard, J. W.; Midha, K. K. Biosynthesis and characterization of glucuronide metabolites of fluphenazine: 7-hydroxyfluphenazine glucuronide and fluphenazine glucuronide.* Xenobiotica **1991**, 21, 383–393.)

N^+-glucuronide is formed (figure 12-8) (*2*). *C*-Glucuronides are very rare (*3–5*). One example is the *C*-glucuronide metabolite of the antiinflammatory drug phenylbutazone (figure 12-9). In this case, the central carbon atom of the β-diketone unit of the heterocyclic ring is nucleophilic, since the carbanion is stabilized by resonance.

Glucuronosylation is the first example of a conjugation reaction that we will examine in this book. In the following chapters we look at sulfonation and acetylation (see table 12-1). These processes are among those that R. T. Williams called "Phase 2" biotransformations. However, we wish to

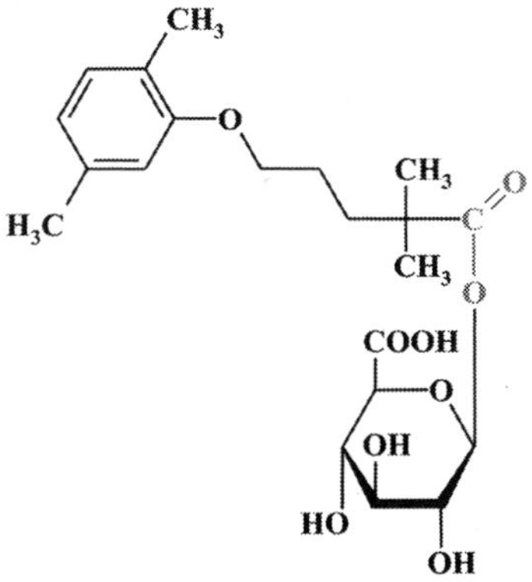

FIGURE 12-6.
An ester (acyl) glucuronide; a metabolite of the hypolipidemic agent gemfibrozil. (*Thomas, B. F.; Burgess, J. P.; Coleman, D. P.; Scheffler, N. M.; Jeffcoat, A. R.; Dix, K. J. Isolation and identification of novel metabolites of gemfibrozil in rat urine.* Drug Metab. Dispos. **1999**, 27, *147–157.*)

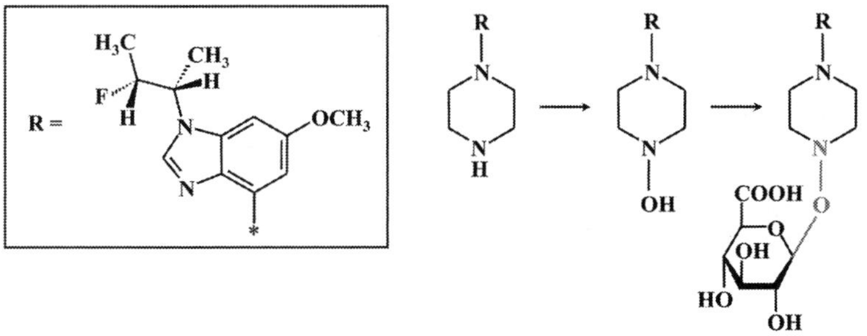

FIGURE 12-7.
Formation of an *N,O*-glucuronide metabolite of a proposed hypoglycemic drug, 9-[(1*S*,2*R*)-2-fluoro-1-methylpropyl]-2-methoxy-6-(1-piperazinyl) purine hydrochloride. (*Miller, R. R.; Doss, G. A.; Stearns, R. A. Identification of a hydroxylamine glucuronide metabolite of an oral hypoglycemic agent.* Drug Metab. Dispos. **2004**, 32, *178–185.*)

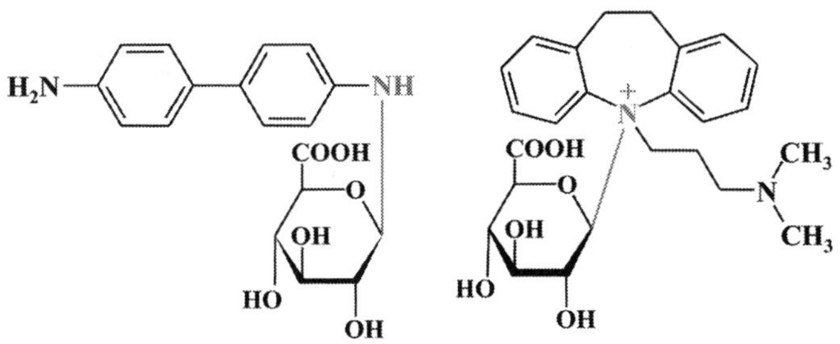

FIGURE 12-8.
N-Glucuronides. Left: metabolite of the aromatic amine carcinogen benzidine; right: *N*⁺-glucuronide metabolite of the antidepressant drug imipramine. (*Left: Babu, S. R.; Lakshmi, V. M.; Hsu, F. F.; Zenser, T. V.; Davis, B. B. Role of N-glucuronidation in benzidine-induced bladder cancer in dog.* Carcinogenesis **1992**, 13, *1235–1240; right: Green, M. D.; Bishop, W. P.; Tephly, T. R. Expressed human UGT1.4 protein catalyzes the formation of quaternary ammonium-linked glucuronides.* Drug Metab. Dispos. **1995**, 23, *299–302.*)

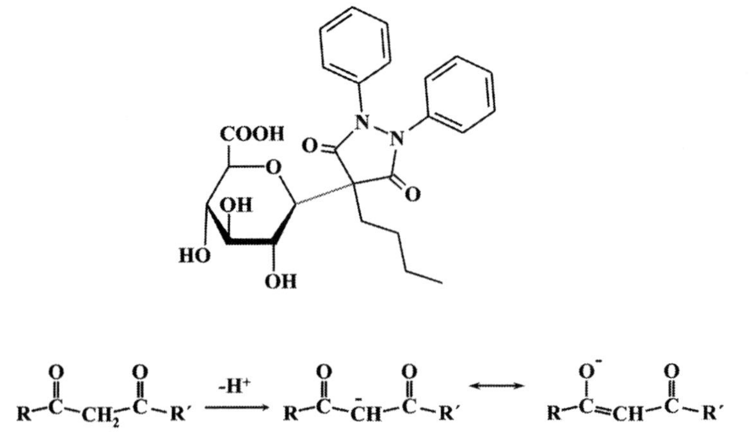

FIGURE 12-9.

A *C*-glucuronide formed from the antiinflammatory drug phenylbutazone. Lower: the nucleophilicity of the β-diketone carbon is enhanced by resonance stabilization.

TABLE 12-1.

Selected Enzymes of Xenobiotic Conjugation

REACTION	ENZYME	ACTIVATED DONOR
Glucuronide formation	Glucuronosyltransferase	UDP-glucuronic acid
Sulfation	Sulfotransferase	3′-Phosphoadenosine-5′-phosphosulfate
Methylation	Methyltransferase	*S*-Adenosylmethionine
Acetylation	Acetyltransferase	Acetylcoenzyme A

distinguish between these synthetic conjugations[1] (and a few others, such as methylation and amino acid conjugation) and the reactions of xenobiotics with water or glutathione (also classified as "Phase 2" reactions). In each of the synthetic conjugations, the conjugating group is introduced via an electrophilic activated donor that reacts with nucleophilic centers in xenobiotic substrates. The reactions catalyzed by glutathione transferases and epoxide hydrolase, in contrast, involve the reaction of a xenobiotic electrophile (such as an epoxide or alkylating agent) with an endogenous nucleophile (glutathione or water).

CHEMICAL ANALYSIS OF GLUCURONIDES

How are glucuronide metabolites analyzed and identified? Extraction of glucuronides from biological fluids and gas chromatography/mass spectrometry (GC/MS) separation are difficult, due to the high polarity and low volatility of the conjugates. However, enzymatic hydrolysis of the glucuronides, liberating the aglycones, can often be achieved. The aglycones are then analyzed. β-Glucuronidase from *E. coli* is commonly used for this purpose. (Similar difficulties arise in the analysis of sulfates.

In that case, the enzyme arylsulfatase (from the snail *Helix pomatia*) is often capable of releasing the parent compound.) However, some glucuronides fail to be cleaved. Most researchers are turning to mass spectrometry methods that allow the analysis of glucuronide conjugates without prior hydrolysis. Soft ionization modes (*6*, pp. 297–299), such as chemical ionization, fast atom bombardment (*7*), electrospray (*8*), and laser desorption ionization techniques have been applied successfully.

GLUCURONIDATION OF ENDOGENOUS COMPOUNDS: HEME CATABOLISM

The degradation of heme is an important example of the role of glucuronosylation in the metabolism of endogenous metabolites. In adult humans, red blood cells are turned over at a rate of more than one million cells per second. The catabolism of the hemoglobin of the red cells removed from circulation generates several hundred milligrams of heme per day. Free heme is toxic (perhaps because it is a catalyst of oxygen radical production (*9*)) and must be catabolized. Heme oxygenase (EC 1.14.99.3) is a microsomal enzyme found in the macrophage, hepatocyte, and spleen cell. All these cells are involved in the breakdown of aged or damaged red cells. Heme oxygenase (*10*) catalyzes the remarkable process illustrated in figure 12-10. Reducing equivalents are supplied by NADPH-cytochrome P450 reductase and molecular oxygen is incorporated into the substrate (cf. cytochrome P450). Two isozymes of human heme oxygenase exist (*11*). One form (HO-2) is constitutive and the other (HO-1) is induced by environmental stresses, including heat shock and heavy metal

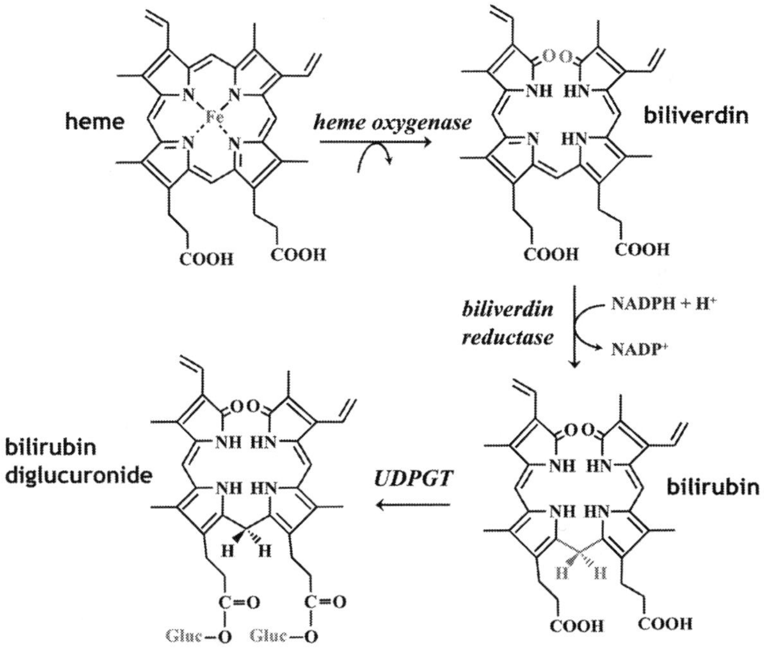

FIGURE 12-10.

Heme catabolism. (The complete stoichiometry of the heme oxygenase-catalyzed reaction is not shown.) *Note*: A full-color version of this figure appears on the website.

Mistress Quickly: . . . one of them . . . is beaten black and blue.
Falstaff: What tell'st thou me of black and blue? I was beaten myself into all of the colours of the rainbow.
(The Merry Wives of Windsor, IV:5.)

exposure (*12*). It appears that HO-1 is induced via ARE in the same manner as are glutathione transferases (chapter 11).

Hydroxylation disrupts the conjugation of the heme porphyrin π-system, rendering the A and B rings more "pyrrole-like" and susceptible to further oxidation. In subsequent steps, two additional moles of molecular oxygen are consumed and the bridging methene carbon of the porphyrin ring is released as carbon monoxide, CO. This extraordinary reaction is the only metabolic source of carbon monoxide in the body. Indeed, a person's rate of heme catabolism can be determined from the measurement of carbon monoxide in exhaled breath (*13*).

Bilirubin and Jaundice

The product of the heme oxygenase-catalyzed reaction is the blue-green compound *biliverdin*. (Biliverdin is the blue pigment of a robin's egg.) In humans, biliverdin is reduced at the γ-carbon by the action of biliverdin reductase (EC 1.3.1.24) (*14*) to give *bilirubin*. This reduction breaks the conjugated π-system into two halves and shifts the absorbance band to shorter wavelengths: bilirubin is red-orange colored. The catabolic progression from heme to biliverdin to bilirubin can be seen in the changing appearance of a bruise (see sidebar).

Surprisingly, in view of its many hydrogen bond-forming functionalities, bilirubin is very lipophilic and is insoluble in water or methanol. This behavior is due to the formation of strong intramolecular hydrogen bonds, as shown in figure 12-11. Lightner and McDonagh have pointed out that, of the four isomers that would result from heme cleavage at the α-, β-, γ-, or δ-methene bridges, natural bilirubin is the only water-insoluble product (*15*). Bilirubin is toxic at high levels, and cannot be excreted without further conjugative metabolism (see below); birds and reptiles excrete biliverdin directly, without reduction to bilirubin. Why, then, do mammals synthesize bilirubin, which accumulates to levels of 10 μM or higher in the plasma? Bilirubin, like many other lipophilic substances, does not circulate as a free species in plasma, but is bound with high affinity by plasma proteins, especially serum albumin. Polyunsaturated fatty acids, which are particularly prone to autoxidation, are also carried on albumin, and bilirubin acts as an antioxidant, inhibiting this deterioration (*16*).

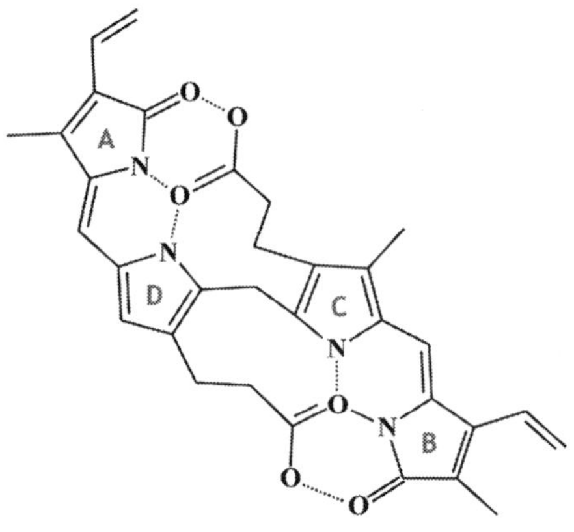

FIGURE 12-11.
Internal hydrogen bonding enhances the lipophilicity of bilirubin.

Recent studies support the idea that this metabolic waste product of heme degradation is an important endogenous antioxidant and may have a protective effect against coronary heart disease (*17–20*). An association between low serum bilirubin and increased risk of coronary heart disease has been observed in several studies. In these studies, serum bilirubin levels $<7\,\mu M$ were associated with increased risk whereas concentrations $>10\,\mu M$ were associated with decreased risk.

Within tissues, the concentration of bilirubin is much lower, below 50 nM. Nevertheless, even these low levels may confer antioxidant protection. As suggested by Solomon Snyder and colleagues (*21*), bilirubin can act catalytically to inhibit oxidative stress: first, it is oxidized to biliverdin, by reactive oxygen species, and then the resulting biliverdin is reduced enzymatically back to bilirubin. Since bilirubin is lipophilic, its antioxidant activity may be particularly protective of biological membranes (*22*).

Excessive accumulation of bilirubin leads to hyperbilirubinemia, the condition known as jaundice. The name is etymologically related to the French *jaune* (yellow), and attests to the characteristic buildup of yellow bilirubin, particularly noticeable in the whites of the eyes. Hyperbilirubinemia is characterized by an elevation either in unconjugated bilirubin alone or in both unconjugated and conjugated bilirubin. Accumulation of bilirubin to plasma levels $>200\,\mu M$ exhausts the binding capacity of serum albumin and leads to bilirubin toxicity. The mechanisms of this toxicity are still only poorly understood, but bilirubin crosses the blood–brain barrier and enters the central nervous system; brain damage (encephalopathy) is the major symptom.

Two ester monoglucuronides (at the C and D ring propionates) of bilirubin are formed, as well as the diglucuronide (figure 12-10). A single enzyme present in hepatocytes, UGT1A1, carries out both glucuronosylation steps. These conjugates are water soluble and readily transported to the kidneys for excretion into the urine; most urinary bilirubin is in the form of the diglucuronide. Approximately 96% of plasma bilirubin is unconjugated. Liver damage, reduced activity of glucose-6-phosphate dehydrogenase (*23*) (which may cause hemolysis), or diminished glucuronic acid conjugation activity (*24*) can result in jaundice.

Inherited defects in the UGT1A1 enzyme can cause significant reduction in the clearance of bilirubin by the liver. These disorders include Crigler–Najjar syndrome and Gilbert's syndrome, which are discussed later in this chapter. Another well-known hyperbilirubinemia syndrome is neonatal jaundice (predominantly from unconjugated bilirubin), which occurs in approximately 50% of newborns during the first five days of life. The human fetus can pass bilirubin transplacentally, relying on the maternal liver and kidneys for glucuronosylation. Newborn infants are suddenly deprived of this resource and have delayed maturation of UGT1A1 expression, with normal activity attained by about three months of age. In some infants (especially premature deliveries), the jaundice becomes severe. A simple and effective treatment is *phototherapy* (*15*). An English nurse first observed that the yellowish skin of jaundiced newborns became bleached upon exposure to sunlight. Indeed, bilirubin is photochemically converted to more soluble and readily excreted products. Phototherapy of jaundiced newborns by exposure to fluorescent light is now routine in maternity wards.

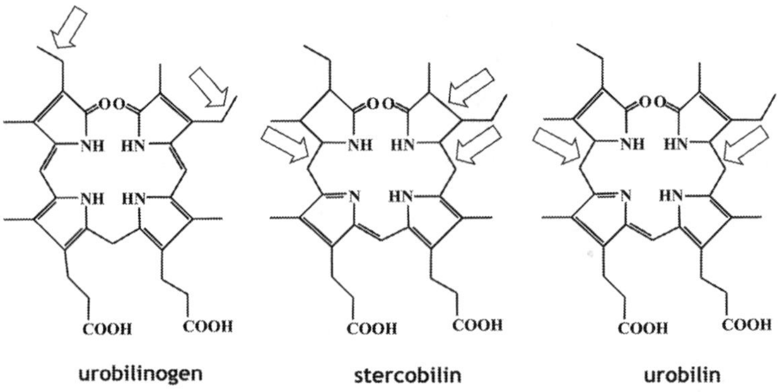

FIGURE 12-12.

Bilirubin reduction; arrows indicate sites of reduction.

The low UDPGT activity in newborns also has implications for drug therapy. The antibacterial drug chloramphenicol is sometimes administered to newborns, for treatment of ampicillin-resistant *Haemophilus influenzae* and other infections. Initially, a dosage regimen based on experience with older children was used. Glucuronide formation is the major metabolic pathway for chloramphenicol elimination. Because newborns have little chloramphenicol glucuronosylation activity, repeated doses of the drug were not cleared from the body, and the drug built up to toxic (in some cases, fatal) levels. It is now recommended that serum levels be monitored when low-birth-weight infants are treated with chloramphenicol (*25*).

Biliary excretion of bilirubin is an important route of elimination; the compound's name reflects its presence in bile. In the intestinal tract, bacterial metabolism releases the glucuronic acid moieties by way of the action of β-glucuronidase, a glucuronide-specific hydrolyzing enzyme. (Human β-glucuronidase also exists but is normally located in the micro-somal and lysosomal fractions, sites that are relatively inaccessible to polar conjugates in cells (*26*).) Presumably, the bacteria are chiefly concerned with liberating sugars, which they can use as foodstuff. But, at the same time, bilirubin is re-formed. In the reducing environment of the intestine, further bacterial metabolism converts bilirubin into stercobilin, a fecal pigment, and urobilinogen (figure 12-12). Urobilinogen, in particular, is readily readsorbed through the intestinal wall, and returns to the blood. This process of conjugation, intestinal hydrolysis, and reabsorption is referred to as *enterohepatic recirculation*. This phenomenon also occurs with many drugs, and prolongs their lifetime in the circulation (*27*). Uro-bilinogen is reoxidized to urobilin in the kidney; urobilin is the major component giving urine its characteristic yellow color. What a diverse family of colored products arises from the heme of our red blood cells!

MORPHINE GLUCURONIDATION

The glucuronosylation pathway is involved in the metabolism of numerous therapeutic drugs, including benzodiazepines (*28*), statins (*29*), neuroleptics, antiepileptic and antineoplastic agents. Among these, opiates are therapeu-tically valuable for the treatment of severe pain, and, of course, they are significant drugs of abuse. Morphine is the major narcotic alkaloid of the

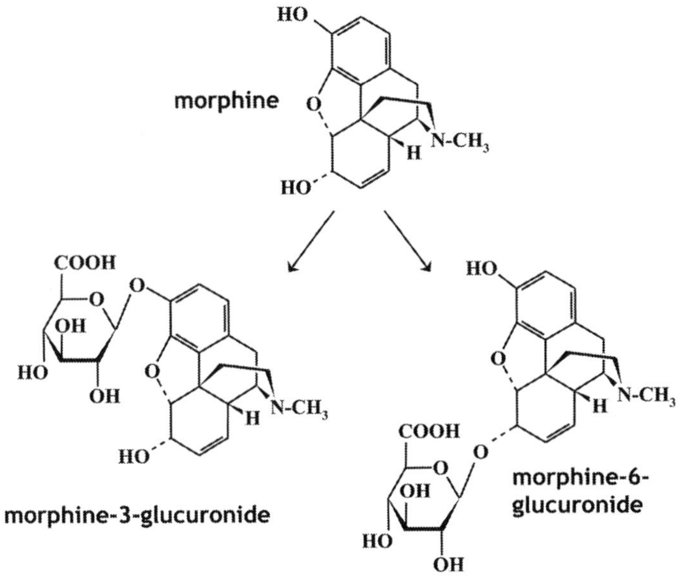

FIGURE 12-13.

Morphine and its glucuronide metabolites.

opium poppy and represents the most widely used opioid throughout the world. Glucuronosylation is an important biotransformation route for morphine. Morphine has two hydroxyl groups (figure 12-13); one is phenolic and the other is secondary aliphatic. Morphine is rapidly metabolized by glucuronide formation at either the 3- or the 6-position. Morphine-3-glucuronide is the major metabolite (*30*). (Synthetic acetylation of both groups, which blocks this route of elimination, yields diacetylmorphine, better known as heroin.) Morphine glucuronosylation represents an exceptional example in regard to the activity of the conjugates formed. Most glucuronosylation reactions yield inactive conjugates. However, morphine-6-glucuronide may possess superior analgesic effect compared to its parent aglycone, morphine (*31*). While lacking analgesic activity, morphine-3-glucuronide is associated with central nervous system toxicity (*32, 33*).

UDP-GLUCURONOSYLTRANSFERASES

Now we turn our attention to the enzymes that catalyze glucuronic acid conjugations, UDP-glucuronosyltransferases (UGTs) (*34–36*). UGT enzyme activity can be measured by incubating an enzyme preparation with appropriate substrate and UDP-glucuronic acid, and monitoring either the formation of the glycoside product or the disappearance of the aglycone substrate. In some cases, the aglycone and glycoside can be separated by organic extraction of the aglycone; either the substrate or product is quantitated by absorbance or fluorescence. In other cases, the glycoside and aglycone are separated chromatographically before quantification. UDP-glucuronic acid radiolabeled in the sugar moiety is available, allowing detection and quantitation of the glycosides by scintillation counting (*37*).

UGTs are integral membrane proteins of the endoplasmic reticulum (ER). UGT proteins are composed of 527–530 amino acid residues. Integral membrane proteins are anchored in the membrane by one or more embedded α-helical segments. These α-helices are, of course, composed largely of hydrophobic residues. Some proteins with a single membrane-spanning helix are oriented with their N-terminus inside the lumen of the ER and C-terminus on the cytoplasmic side (Type I); other proteins have the opposite orientation (Type II) (*38*). Protein topology is determined by primary structure motifs, which interact with the enzymatic machinery responsible for delivery of the protein to the ER and translocation into the membrane in the appropriate orientation. These sequences are not identical among different proteins, but they share certain homologies, or common features, especially with regard to the charge and polarity of the amino acid residues in the sequences.

Proteins destined for the ER usually bear an N-terminal signal sequence. Typically, several polar residues occur near the N-terminus, followed by a dozen or more hydrophobic residues. Since proteins are synthesized from the N-terminal end, the hydrophobic signal sequence extends from the ribosome early in the process of translation. The signal sequence is recognized by a signal recognition particle (SRP) riboprotein complex, which binds to an SRP receptor in the ER membrane. The receptor helps lead the nascent polypeptide chain into the membrane. Polypeptide translation is completed, and, in many cases, the membrane-embedded signal sequence is then cleaved by proteolysis (catalyzed by signal peptidase (*39*)). The new N-terminus of the mature protein is exposed in the lumen. (More extensive discussions of this process are presented in other texts (*40*, figure 27-35). Such cleaved proteins are, therefore, always of Type I, as defined above. All known UGTs fall into this class.

The sequence of human UGT1A1 is shown in figure 12-14. Cleaved signal sequences do not adhere to a simple consensus sequence, but some

```
MAVESQGGRP LVLGLLLCVL GPVVSHAGKI LLIPVDGSHW LSMLGAIQQL 50
           memb. ins. signal

QQRGHEIVVL APDASLYIRD GAFYTLKTYP VPFQREDVKE SFVSLGHNVF 100

ENDSFLQRVI KTYKKIKKDS AMLLSGCSHL LHNKELMASL AESSFDVMLT 150

DPFLPCSPIV AQYLSLPTVF FLHALPCSLE FEATQCPNPF SYVPRPLSSH 200

SDHMTFLQRV KNMLIAFSQN FLCDVVYSPY ATLASEFLQR EVTVQDLLSS 250

ASVWLFRSDF VKDYPRPIMP NMVFVGGINC LHQNPLSQEF EAYINASGEH 300

GIVVFSLGSM VSEIPEKKAM AIADALGKIP QTVLWRYTGT RPSNLANNTI 350

LVKWLPQNDL LGHPMTRAFI THAGSHGVYE SICNGVPMVM MPLFGDQMDN 400
                      UDPGA binding site

AKRMETKGAG VTLNVLEMTS EDLENALKAV INDKSYKENI MRLSSLHKDR 450

PVEPLDLAVF WVEFVMRHKG APHLRPAAHD LTWYQYHSLD VIGFLLAVVL 500
                                              stop-trans.

TVAFITFKCC AYGYRKCLGK KGRVKKAHKS KTH 533
signal                    highly basic region
```

FIGURE 12-14.

Human UGT1A1 protein sequence. Potential N-linked glycosylation sites (NXS or NXT) are indicated (blue). From residue 285 on, the sequence is identical to that of all other proteins of the UGT1A subfamily (common exons). See text for further discussion. *Note*: A full-color version of this figure appears on the website.

of the characteristic features are seen in the UGT1A1 sequence: a basic residue near the amino terminal (arg-9); a highly hydrophobic core of 10 to 15 residues (pro-10 to leu-20); a cleavage site for signal peptidase, with small neutral residues, particularly alanine, at positions −1 and −3 with respect to the cleavage site, located about five residues past the hydrophobic core (ser-his-ala 25-27).

What stops the growing protein chain from passing completely into the lumen of the ER? Another sequence motif, known as the stop-transfer signal or anchor sequence, calls the halt, by remaining embedded in the membrane. The common theme appears to be a hydrophobic (α-helix-forming) stretch, with polar, charged residues on either end, and greater positive charge on the C-terminal end. In the UGT1A1 protein sequence, note the hydrophobicity of the core of the stop-transfer signal (val-ile-gly-phe-leu-leu-ala-val-val-leu-thr-val-ala-phe-ile-thr-phe) and the high density of positively charged (lys and arg) residues near the C-terminal.

No high-resolution crystal structure is available for a UGT enzyme, but a model of the protein can be sketched, based on sequence analysis and physicochemical studies (figure 12-15). The protein is embedded in the ER membrane by the hydrophobic portion of the stop-transfer sequence near the C-terminus. Two domains form the large luminal portion of the protein. A hydrophilic region of highly conserved residues occurs in the vicinity of residues 365–420 of known UGT sequences; this region shows homologies with proteins such as β-galactosidase, pyruvate kinase, xylose transport protein, and pyrophosphatase, proteins that bind nucleotides, sugars, or phosphates. This C-terminal domain contains the UDPGA binding site. The less-conserved N-terminal domain contains the aglycone binding site.

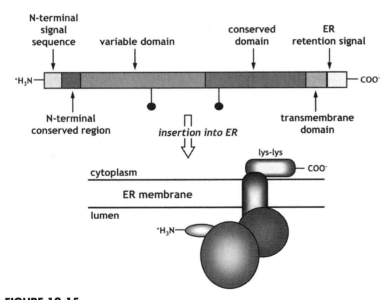

FIGURE 12-15.

Schematic representation of the structural and functional domains in UGTs. (*Adapted from Brierley, C. H.; Burchell, B. Human UDP-glucuronosyltransferases: chemical defence, jaundice and gene therapy.* Bioessays **1993**, *15, 749–754.*) *Note*: A full-color version of this figure appears on the website.

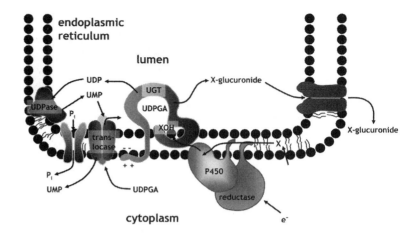

FIGURE 12-16.

Schematic representation of the localization of UGTs in the endoplasmic reticulum, and the transport of their substrates and products. X = aglycone substrate. *Note*: A full-color version of this figure appears on the website.

COMPARTMENTALIZATION OF GLUCURONIDE FORMATION

Glucuronosylation occurs in the lumen of the endoplasmic reticulum (figure 12-16). However, UDPGA is formed in the cytosol, and aglycone substrates (xenobiotics or endogenous substrates, such as bilirubin) reach the ER through the cytosol. This topology implies the existence of multiple transporters. Presumably, the ER membrane must incorporate transporters (channels or carriers) for aglycones (possibly several different transporters corresponding to different classes) and UDPGA. Furthermore, the products of the glucuronosylation reaction must be exported to the cytosol and, in the case of glucuronides, to the bile or bloodstream for excretion. Thus, additional transporters are needed for UMP and phosphate (the products of UDP hydrolysis) and for the polar glucuronides. These carriers include ABC-type (ATP-binding cassette) glucuronide transporters (*41*). Some members of the family, such as ABCB1 (previously called MDR-1) and ABCC2 (previously called MRP-2), act as efflux pumps for hydrophobic drugs (see chapter 9).

FAMILIES OF UDP-GLUCURONOSYLTRANSFERASE ENZYMES

Knowledge about the substrate specificity of UGT enzymes and their tissue expression and regulation has progressed significantly in recent years. As with P450 enzymes, UGTs comprise a large family of related enzymes with partly distinct and partly overlapping enzyme activities and patterns of expression. The molecular genetics of human UGTs are now more clearly understood, with evidence for the existence of more than 26 genes. Eighteen of these genes correspond to functional proteins encoded by two gene families, *UGT1* and *UGT2* (*42a*) (figure 12-17). These families are further divided into three subfamilies, based on their sequence similarities: *UGT1A*, *UGT2A*, and *UGT2B* (figure 12-18). Similar to the nomenclature

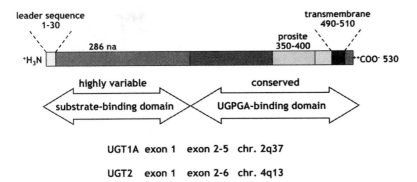

FIGURE 12-17.

Sequence motifs of human UGTs. The high degree of similarity in the carboxyl portions of the UGTs, corresponding to exons 2–5 for UGT1 and exons 2–6 for UGT2Bs, controls the conformational properties that underlie the binding of the cosubstrate UDPGA. A substrate (aglycone) binding pocket is encoded by exon 1 for both the UGT1A and UGT2B enzymes, and a separate UDPGA domain coordinates transfer of glucuronic acid to the aglycone substrate. The UDPGA-binding domain is closely related in all UGTs. *Note*: A full-color version of this figure appears on the website.

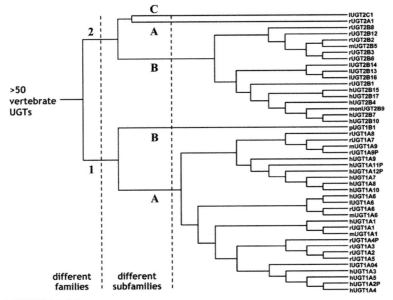

FIGURE 12-18.

Relatedness tree of UGT proteins, showing divergence of the proteins encoded by mammalian UGT genes. h, human; l, rabbit (Lagomorpha); m, mouse; mon, monkey; p, plaice (fish); r, rat.

system for cytochrome P450 enzymes, proteins from the two distinct families are less than 50% identical at the amino acid sequence level; within each family, protein sequences are about 60% identical or more. In humans, the *UGT1* and *UGT2* genes (figure 12-19) and pseudogenes are located on chromosomes 2q37 and 4q13, respectively.

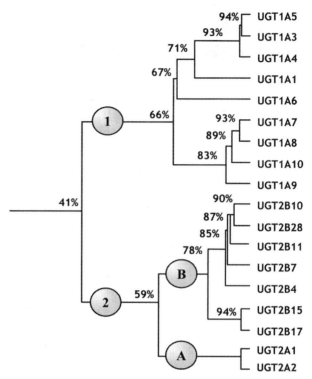

FIGURE 12-19.

Phylogenetic tree for human UGT enzymes. The dendogram shows both UGT families, which share less than 50% identity. Percentage values represent the identity between two groups or single enzymes, at the amino acid level. (Pseudogenes were not analyzed for homology.) The median percentage identity of amino acid sequences between UGTs split by a mode is shown.

UGT1 Gene Family

The chromosomal organization of the *UGT1* gene family (figure 12-20) is remarkable (*42b*). The entire *UGT1* family is derived from a single gene locus (*UGT1*) composed of 17 exons. To synthesize the final protein, only one of 13 different exon-1 sequences on the locus is associated with four downstream exons, common to all UGT1A isoforms. Of the 13 exon-1 sequences, nine code for functional proteins (UGT1A1, UGT1A3–1A10) and four correspond to pseudogenes (p) (UGT1A2p, UGT1A11p, UGT1A12p, and UGT1A13p). The exon-1 sequence of UGT1As codes for the aglycone substrate-binding domain (N-terminal half of the protein), while the four common exons code for the cosubstrate (UDPGA)-binding domain (C-terminal half of the protein). The presence of different substrate-binding domains confers the large substrate specificity and selectivity of UGT1A proteins. The regulatory sequences flanking each of the exon-1 regions are thought to dictate the individual expression profiles of the UGT1A isoforms. Five of the nine UGT1A isoforms were isolated from human liver while the four remaining isoforms have been observed strictly in extrahepatic tissues, mainly in the gastrointestinal tract.

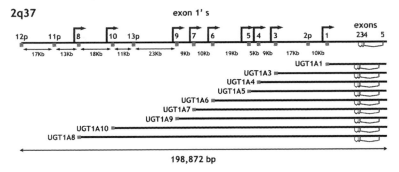

UGT1A1 to UGT1A13: 4 pseudogenes + 9 proteins

▨ exon 1's ■ shared exons

FIGURE 12-20.
Genomic structure of the *UGT1* gene family, based on Genbank accession number AF297093. *Note*: A full-color version of this figure appears on the website. (*Gong, Q. H. et al. Thirteen UDP-glucuronosyltransferase genes are encoded at the human UGT1 gene complex locus.* Pharmacogenetics *2001*, 11, *357–368.*)

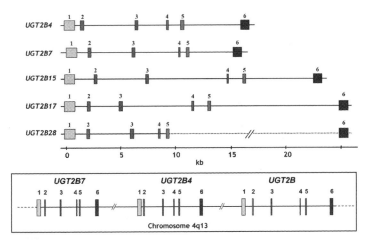

FIGURE 12-21.
Genomic structure of the *UGT2B* genes. Top: the structure of selected human *UGT2B* genes. Bottom: the relative positions of the *UGT2B4*, *UGT2B7*, and *UGT2B15* genes on human chromosome 4q13. *Note*: A full-color version of this figure appears on the website. (*Riedy, M.; Wang, J. Y.; Miller, A. P.; Buckler, A.; Hall, J.; Guida, M. Genomic organization of the UGT2b gene cluster on human chromosome 4q13.* Pharmacogenetics *2000*, 10, *251–260.*)

UGT2 Gene Family

The structures of several *UGT2B* genes have been determined (figure 12-21). Each gene is composed of six exons. Similarly to the UGT1 family, members of the UGT2B subfamily share a high degree of homology in the C-terminal portion of the protein, the highest degree of divergence in sequences being found in the exons 1. However, *UGT2* genes do not share common exons. Two members of the UGT2A subfamily have also been characterized, sharing approximately 70% identity with the UGT2Bs.

The UGT2A subfamily is expressed in the olfactory epithelium. These enzymes may play a major role in termination of odorant signals, by glucuronosylating (and hence, inactivating) hydroxyl-containing odorant molecules, such as eugenol (the scent of cloves) and borneol. This action prevents the odorant from continuing to stimulate the receptor cells (43) and may also protect the brain from exposure to airborne toxicants. However, other functions are presumed to exist, since UGT2A enzymes are also expressed in the liver, small intestine, brain, and fetal lung.

GENETIC UDP-GLUCURONOSYLTRANSFERASE DEFICIENCY CONDITIONS

Genetic defects in the *UGT1* gene complex can have a significant impact on the health of affected individuals. This is especially so for defects in UGT1A1 activity, because of this enzyme's key role in the metabolism of bilirubin. In the most severe cases, known as Crigler–Najjar syndromes, bilirubin glucuronosylation activity is greatly reduced or undetectable. Gilbert's syndrome is a mild form of the disease, with partial activity.

Crigler–Najjar Syndrome

Crigler–Najjar syndrome (also referred to as congenital nonhemolytic jaundice with glucuronosyltransferase deficiency) is a rare autosomal recessive disorder of bilirubin metabolism (44). The syndrome occurs in all population groups and, in some patients, has been associated with consanguinity. Crigler–Najjar syndrome has been divided into two distinct forms, types I and II, based upon the severity of the disease. Type I disease is associated with severe jaundice and neurologic impairment due to kernicterus (bilirubin encephalopathy). Type II disease patients survive into adulthood without neurologic impairment. However, the differential diagnosis of the types is not easy, especially when there is coexisting hemolysis. The administration of phenobarbital, a drug that induces the expression of the *UGT1A1* gene, can help to differentiate between these disorders. The serum bilirubin concentration is reduced by phenobarbital treatment (60 to 120 mg for 14 days) in most patients with type II, but not type I, disease.

The phenotype of Crigler–Najjar syndrome can be caused by a variety of alterations in the sequences of the bilirubin-uridine diphosphate glu-curonosyltransferase (UGT1A1) gene, which is responsible for the conjugation of bilirubin. About 60 rare mutations in the *UGT1A1* gene have been identified, including substitutions, deletions, and insertions. These genetic alterations have been reported throughout the gene, primarily in the coding region, in exon 1 as well as in exons 2–5 (common to all UGT1A proteins). The mutations cause nonsynonymous amino acid changes, frameshifts, or premature truncation of UGT1A1, with consequent complete or partial inactivation of the enzyme. Genetic variations are also present in the promoter region as well as in the introns; the latter may result in the use of a cryptic splice acceptor site. Co-occurrence of different mutations is also frequent. A complete listing of known mutations is available at the UGT website (http://som.flinders.edu.au/FUSA/ClinPharm/UGT/). With this information on the nature of the mutations in the *UGT1A1* gene, a sample of genomic DNA collected from a patient can be used to make a genetic diagnosis.

There are few therapeutic options for these conditions. Phototherapy and phenobarbital treatment have been used in type II cases. Gene therapy has been performed with promising results in an animal model of Crigler–Najjar syndrome (45).

Gilbert's Syndrome

A much more common, but less serious, condition, known as Gilbert's syndrome, is characterized by a mild deficiency in glucuronosylation activity, with elevated levels of plasma bilirubin. About 6–12% of the North American population is believed to be affected (46), but the syndrome is usually asymptomatic (47). The common genetic variant in the *UGT1A1* gene is a dinucleotide repeat polymorphism in the atypical TATA-box region of the *UGT1A1* promoter (48). The common allele (*UGT1A1*1*) consists of six TA repeats in the $A(TA)_nTAA$ motif, while seven TA repeats characterize the variant allele. The presence of the $A(TA)_7TAA$ allele (*UGT1A1*28*) decreases *UGT1A1* gene expression. Homozygous individuals carrying the $A(TA)_7TAA$ allele show significantly higher plasma levels of unconjugated bilirubin, caused by a 30% reduction in *UGT1A1* gene transcription. Other mutations within the coding regions of the *UGT1A1* gene causing the Gilbert's phenotype have been observed in the Japanese population. Clinical conditions associated with *UGT1A1* variants have diverse pathophysiological consequences as well as pharmacological implications (discussed below).

An animal model of inherited UGT deficiency also exists. In 1934 C.H. Gunn, of the Dominion Experimental Fox Ranch, in Prince Edward Island, Canada, observed three yellowish, jaundiced pups among a litter of thirteen borne by a laboratory rat of the Wistar strain. The jaundice was inherited as a recessive Mendelian trait; Gunn wrote that his work gave "new evidence for the single gene theory of a syndrome," and he rightly suspected that a single enzyme was deficient. These animals are the progenitors of a strain now known as the "Gunn rat" (49). In the 1950s the biochemical basis of this mutation was shown to be the absence of bilirubin-UDPGT activity. When the *UGT1A1* gene of the Gunn rat was examined, a −1 base pair frameshift mutation was detected in codon 414; this mutation creates a TGA ("opal") termination codon at codon 416 and the protein is truncated prematurely (50–53).

Feline species also have a very poor capacity for glucuronosylation of phenolic compounds (e.g., acetaminophen (54)), although they can glucuronosylate bilirubin satisfactorily. Consequently, cats tend to excrete drugs as sulfate conjugates rather than as glucuronides. This peculiarity of drug biotransformation has to be considered in veterinary pharmacological practice (55).

PHARMACOGENOMICS OF HUMAN UDP-GLUCURONOSYLTRANSFERASES

Assessing the roles of individual human UGTs in the metabolism of a given xenobiotic remains a difficult task. The lability and difficulty of purification of UGTs (56) long hampered their characterization, but the application of improved biochemical techniques for enzyme purification, and more particularly molecular biological methods, have allowed enormous progress to be made in the last few years. Because of the importance of the glucuronosylation pathway in drug metabolism, the experimental tools necessary for reaction phenotyping UGT substrates are becoming available (57, 58). However, in contrast to the situation with human P450 enzymes, knowledge of "probe" or "selective" substrates for particular human UGTs is still very limited.

As with other drug-metabolizing enzyme pathways, glucuronosylation is subject to large interindividual variations (59). Variability in glucuronosylation capacity towards various molecules can be explained by factors including gender, sex, age, disease, diet, exposure to environmental chemicals, and genetic polymorphisms, including single nucleotide polymorphisms (SNPs). Unlike the rare mutations of the Crigler–Najjar syndromes, only a few genetic variants in UGT genes are found in the general population at a sufficiently high frequency (>1%) to be classified as polymorphisms (46). Polymorphisms are observed in various regions of the genes, including the regulatory and coding sequences, but also in the introns and the 5′ and 3′ untranslated regions. Depending on the nature of the variation and its location within a given gene, the phenotypic consequences may be barely noticeable, or they may alter the function or expression of the protein. The role of genetic factors in determining the variable rates of glucuronosylation of drugs, hormones, tobacco smoke carcinogens, environmental pollutants, and dietary components is still not well understood. Such genetic alterations would potentially modify the glucuronosylation capacity of the individual carrying that polymorphism, as is observed for Crigler–Najjar patients. Knowledge of the genetic mechanisms underlying variability in glucuronosylation capacity is beginning to emerge, but, to date, apart from the UGT1A1 protein and the resulting unconjugated hyperbilirubinemia syndromes, only a few clinically relevant genetic polymorphisms in human UGTs have been described. However, recent work has demonstrated that these genetic variations have physiological, clinical, or pathophysiological implications. Depending on their substrate specificities and locations of expression within the body, some polymorphisms affect glucuronosylation rates and influence the risk that an individual will develop drug-induced toxicity.

Patients affected by Gilbert's syndrome, carriers of the *UGT1A1*28* allele (TA₇) described previously, display lower glucuronosylation rates and altered drug clearance compared to patients with the *wild-type* genotype for a number of therapeutic drugs, including acetaminophen, tolbutamide, and lorazepam. The pharmacogenetic aspects of toxicity to the anticancer drug *irinotecan* (60) are undoubtedly the most pertinent clinical example known to date. Irinotecan (7-ethyl-10-[4-(1-piperidino)-1-piperidino]carbonyloxy camptothecin) is used for the treatment of colorectal cancer. UGT1A1 is primarily involved in the metabolic inactivation of its active metabolite, SN-38. Since UGT1A1 activity is significantly altered by the presence of the *UGT1A1*28* allele linked to Gilbert's syndrome, several recent studies have explored the impact of this polymorphism on the pharmacokinetics and associated toxicity of this drug. Patients with this polymorphism were shown to be approximately seven times more likely to experience severe gastrointestinal or hematological toxicity (61, 62).

The possible impact of UGT polymorphisms on survival and response to therapy still needs to be studied. Potentially, genotyping patients prior to chemotherapy might reduce the incidence of toxic or even life-threatening side effects (see chapter 8).

Recent findings also suggest that metabolic alterations in the glucuronosylation pathway may influence the susceptibility of an individual to toxic or carcinogenic substances. Again, the role of the common *UGT1A1* promoter variant was assessed. UGT1A1 is involved in the inactivation of estradiol and its oxidized metabolites and may help to maintain steady-state levels of steroids in target tissues. Since steroid hormones contribute to the development of endometrial and breast cancers, *UGT1A1* represents a candidate gene in hormonal carcinogenesis. The role of UGT1A1 in estrogen metabolism is also supported by the observation that a Crigler–Najjar patient, deficient in UGT1A1, had a 70% decrease in the hepatic glucuronosylation of estradiol, compared to liver microsomes from healthy subjects. Researchers conducted molecular epidemiological case-control studies (see sidebar on molecular epidemiology, chapter 13) to investigate the association between genetic variability in the *UGT1A1* promoter region and risk of breast and endometrial cancers. Women homozygous for the *UGT1A1*28* allele were shown to have a two-fold increased risk of developing breast cancer but a decreased risk of endometrial cancer, indicating that the lower expression of the UGT1A1 protein caused by this genetic polymorphism may have opposite effects in the uterus and the breast. These observations may be explained by the fact the UGT1A1 protein acts on many estrogen substrates, including estradiol and its catechol estrogen metabolites, both the "protective" 2-hydroxy derivatives and the genotoxic 4-hydroxy catechol estrogens (*63–66*). Thus, the balance between the local formation of catechol estrogens (by cytochrome P450) and their detoxication by UGTs would determine the tissue's exposure to the individual estrogen.

Note

1. For this reason, we prefer not to use the oft-heard expression "metabolic breakdown" of a drug or toxicant. Almost always, the metabolic process is one of biochemical synthesis, not "breakdown": the metabolites are of higher molecular weight than the parent compound. Contrast this pattern with the catabolism of complex energy-rich biomolecules, such as carbohydrates and fats, which are indeed "broken down" to carbon dioxide and water.

References

1. Evans, W. E.; Relling, M. V. Pharmacogenomics: translating functional genomics into rational therapeutics. *Science* **1999**, *286*, 487–491.
2. Hawes, E. M. N$^+$-glucuronidation, a common pathway in human metabolism of drugs with a tertiary amine group. *Drug Metab. Dispos.* **1998**, *26*, 830–837.
3. Abolin, C. R.; Tozer, T. N.; Craig, J. C.; Gruenke, L. D. C-Glucuronidation of the acetylenic moiety of ethchlorvynol in the rabbit. *Science* **1980**, *209*, 703–704.
4. Richter, W. J.; Alt, K. O.; Dieterle, W.; Faigle, J. W.; Kriemler, H. P.; Mory, H.; Winkler, T. C-Glucuronides, a novel type of drug metabolites. *Helv. Chim. Acta* **1975**, *58*, 2512–2517.

5. Dieterle, W.; Faigle, J. W.; Fruh, F.; Mory, H.; Theoblad, W.; Alt, K. O.; Richter, W. J. Metabolism of phenylbutazone in man. *Arzneimittel-forschung* **1976**, *26*, 572–577.

6. Mikkelsen, S. R.; Cortón, E. *Bioanalytical Chemistry*; Wiley-Interscience: Hoboken, NJ, 2004.

7. Jackson, C. J.; Hubbard, J. W.; Midha, K. K. Biosynthesis and characterization of glucuronide metabolites of fluphenazine: 7-hydroxy-fluphenazine glucuronide and fluphenazine glucuronide. *Xenobiotica* **1991**, *21*, 383–393.

8. Kuuranne, T.; Vahermo, M.; Leinonen, A.; Kostianen, R. Electrospray and atmospheric pressure chemical ionization tandem mass spectrometric behavior of eight anabolic steroid glucuronides. *J. Am. Soc. Mass Spectrom.* **2000**, *11*, 722–730.

9. Wijayanti, N.; Katz, N.; Immenschuh, S. Biology of heme in health and disease. *Curr. Med. Chem.* **2004**, *11*, 981–986.

10. Ortiz de Montellano, P. R. The mechanism of heme oxygenase. *Curr. Opin. Chem. Biol.* **2000**, *4*, 221–227.

11. Ewing, J. F.; Maines, M. D. Distribution of constitutive (HO-2) and heat-inducible (HO-1) heme oxygenase isozymes in rat testes: HO-2 displays stage-specific expression in germ cells. *Endocrinology* **1995**, *136*, 2294–2302.

12. Ewing, J. F.; Maines, M. D. Rapid induction of heme oxygenase 1 mRNA and protein by hyperthermia in rat brain: heme oxygenase 2 is not a heat shock protein. *Proc. Natl. Acad. Sci. USA* **1991**, *88*, 5364–5368.

13. Levitt, M. D.; Ellis, C.; Levitt, D. G. Diurnal rhythm of heme turnover assessed by breath carbon monoxide concentration measurements. *J. Lab Clin. Med.* **1994**, *124*, 427–431.

14. Ahmad, Z.; Salim, M.; Maines, M. D. Human biliverdin reductase is a leucine zipper-like DNA-binding protein and functions in transcriptional activation of heme oxygenase-1 by oxidative stress. *J. Biol. Chem.* **2002**, *277*, 9226–9232.

15. Lightner, D. A.; McDonagh, A. F. Molecular mechanisms of photo-therapy for neonatal jaundice. *Acc. Chem. Res.* **1984**, *17*, 417–424.

16. Stocker, R.; Glazer, A. N.; Ames, B. N. Antioxidant activity of albumin-bound bilirubin. *Proc. Natl. Acad. Sci. USA* **1987**, *84*, 5918–5922.

17. Breimer, L. H.; Wannamethee, G.; Ebrahim, S.; Shaper, A. G. Serum bilirubin and risk of ischemic heart disease in middle-aged British men. *Clin. Chem.* **1995**, *41*, 1504–1508.

18. Hopkins, P. N.; Wu, L. L.; Wu, J.; Hunt, S. C.; James, B. C.; Vincent, G. M.; Williams, R. R. Higher plasma homocyst(e)ine and increased susceptibility to adverse effects of low folate in early familial coronary artery disease. *Arterioscler. Thromb. Vasc. Biol.* **1995**, *15*, 1314–1320.

19. Djousse, L.; Levy, D.; Cupples, L. A.; Evans, J. C.; D'Agostino, R. B.; Ellison, R. C. Total serum bilirubin and risk of cardiovascular disease in the Framingham offspring study. *Am. J. Cardiol.* **2001**, *87*, 1196–1200.

20. Bosma, P. J.; van der Meer, I. M.; Bakker, C. T.; Hofman, A.; Paul-Abrahamse, M.; Witteman, J. C. UGT1A1*28 allele and coronary heart disease: the Rotterdam Study. *Clin. Chem.* **2003**, *49*, 1180–1181.

21. Baranano, D. E.; Rao, M.; Ferris, C. D.; Snyder, S. H. Biliverdin reductase: a major physiologic cytoprotectant. *Proc. Natl. Acad. Sci. USA* **2002**, *99*, 16093–16098.

22. Greenberg, D. A. The jaundice of the cell. *Proc. Natl. Acad. Sci. USA* **2002**, *99*, 15837–15839.

23. Kaplan, M.; Renbaum, P.; Levy-Lahad, E.; Hammerman, C.; Lahad, A.; Beutler, E. Gilbert syndrome and glucose-6-phosphate dehydrogenase deficiency: a dose-dependent genetic interaction crucial to neonatal hyperbilirubinemia. *Proc. Natl. Acad. Sci. USA* **1997,** *94,* 12128–12132.

24. Sugatani, J.; Yamakawa, K.; Yoshinari, K.; Machida, T.; Takagi, H.; Mori, M.; Kakizaki, S.; Sueyoshi, T.; Negishi, M.; Miwa, M. Identification of a defect in the UGT1A1 gene promoter and its association with hyperbilirubinemia. *Biochem. Biophys. Res. Commun.* **2002,** *292,* 492–497.

25. Glazer, J. P.; Danish, M. A.; Plotkin, S. A.; Yaffe, S. J. Disposition of chloramphenicol in low birth weight infants. *Pediatrics* **1980,** *66,* 573–578.

26. Miyauchi, S.; Sugiyama, Y.; Iga, T.; Hanano, M. The conjugative metabolism of 4-methylumbelliferone and deconjugation to the parent drug examined by isolated perfused liver and in vitro liver homogenate of rats. *Chem. Pharm. Bull. (Tokyo)* **1989,** *37,* 475–480.

27. Roberts, M. S.; Magnusson, B. M.; Burczynski, F. J.; Weiss, M. Enterohepatic circulation: physiological, pharmacokinetic and clinical implications. *Clin. Pharmacokinet.* **2002,** *41,* 751–790.

28. Court, M. H.; Duan, S. X.; Guillemette, C.; Journault, K.; Krishnaswamy, S.; von Moltke, L. L.; Greenblatt, D. J. Stereoselective conjugation of oxazepam by human UDP-glucuronosyltransferases (UGTs): S-oxazepam is glucuronidated by UGT2B15, while R-oxazepam is glucuronidated by UGT2B7 and UGT1A9. *Drug Metab. Dispos.* **2002,** *30,* 1257–1265.

29. Prueksaritanont, T.; Subramanian, R.; Fang, X.; Ma, B.; Qiu, Y.; Lin, J. H.; Pearson, P. G.; Baillie, T. A. Glucuronidation of statins in animals and humans: a novel mechanism of statin lactonization. *Drug Metab. Dispos.* **2002,** *30,* 505–512.

30. Mulder, G. J. Pharmacological effects of drug conjugates: is morphine 6-glucuronide an exception? *Trends Pharmacol. Sci.* **1992,** *13,* 302–304.

31. Lotsch, J.; Geisslinger, G. Morphine-6-glucuronide: an analgesic of the future? *Clin. Pharmacokinet.* **2001,** *40,* 485–499.

32. Gong, Q.-L.; Hedner, T.; Hedner, J.; Björkman, R.; Nordberg, G. Antinociceptive and ventilatory effects of the morphine metabolites: morphine-6-glucuronide and morphine-3-glucuronide. *Eur. J. Pharmacol.* **1991,** *193,* 47–56.

33. Pasternak, G. W. Incomplete cross tolerance and multiple mu opioid peptide receptors. *Trends Pharmacol. Sci.* **2001,** *22,* 67–70.

34. Tephly, T. R.; Burchell, B. UDP-glucuronosyltransferases: a family of detoxifying enzymes. *Trends Pharmacol. Sci.* **1990,** *11,* 276–279.

35. Brierley, C. H.; Burchell, B. Human UDP-glucuronosyl transferases: chemical defence, jaundice and gene therapy. *Bioessays* **1993,** *15,* 749–754.

36. Burchell, B.; Coughtrie, M. W.; Jansen, P. L. Function and regulation of UDP-glucuronosyltransferase genes in health and liver disease: report of the Seventh International Workshop on Glucuronidation, September 1993, Pitlochry, Scotland. *Hepatology* **1994,** *20,* 1622–1630.

37. Ethell, B. T.; Anderson, G. D.; Beaumont, K.; Rance, D. J.; Burchell, B. A universal radiochemical high-performance liquid chromatographic assay for the determination of UDP-glucuronosyltransferase activity. *Anal. Biochem.* **1998,** *255,* 142–147.

38. Schatz, G.; Dobberstein, B. Common principles of protein translocation across membranes. *Science* **1996,** *271,* 1519–1526.

39. Dalbey, R. E.; von Heijne, G. Signal peptidases in prokaryotes and eukaryotes: a new protease family. *Trends Biochem. Sci.* **1992**, *17*, 474–478.

40. Nelson, D. L.; Cox, M. M. *Lehninger Principles of Biochemistry*; Worth Publishers: New York, 2004.

41. Keppler, D.; Konig, J. Hepatic secretion of conjugated drugs and endogenous substances. *Semin. Liver Dis.* **2000**, *20*, 265–272.

42. (a) Mackenzie, P. I.; Bock, K. W.; Burchell, B.; Guillemette, C.; Ikushiro, S.-I.; Iyanagi, T.; Miners, J. O.; Owens, I. S.; Nebert, D. W. Nomenclature update for the mammalian UDP glycosyltransferase (UGT) gene superfamily. *Pharmacogenet. Genomics* **2005**, *15*, 677–685. (b) Zhang, T.; Haws, P.; Wu, Q. Multiple variable first exons: a mechanism for cell- and tissue-specific gene regulation. *Genome Res.* **2004**, *14*, 79–89.

43. Lazard, D.; Zupko, K.; Poria, Y.; Nef, P.; Lazarovits, J.; Horn, S.; Khen, M.; Lancet, D. Odorant signal termination by olfactory UDP glucuronosyl transferase. *Nature* **1991**, *349*, 790–793.

44. Jansen, P. L. Diagnosis and management of Crigler–Najjar syndrome. *Eur. J. Pediatr.* **1999**, *158* (Suppl. 2), S89–S94.

45. Kren, B. T.; Parashar, B.; Bandyopadhyay, P.; Chowdhury, N. R.; Chowdhury, J. R.; Steer, C. J. Correction of the UDP-glucuronosyl-transferase gene defect in the Gunn rat model of Crigler–Najjar syndrome type I with a chimeric oligonucleotide. *Proc. Natl. Acad. Sci. USA* **1999**, *96*, 10349–10354.

46. Miners, J. O.; McKinnon, R. A.; Mackenzie, P. I. Genetic polymorphisms of UDP-glucuronosyltransferases and their functional significance. *Toxicology* **2002**, *181–182*, 453–456.

47. de Morais, S. M.; Uetrecht, J. P.; Wells, P. G. Decreased glucuronidation and increased bioactivation of acetaminophen in Gilbert's syndrome. *Gastroenterology* **1992**, *102*, 577–586.

48. Burchell, B.; Hume, R. Molecular genetic basis of Gilbert's syndrome. *J. Gastroenterol. Hepatol.* **1999**, *14*, 960–966.

49. Gunn, C. K. Hereditary acholuric jaundice in the rat. *Can. Med. Assoc. J.* **1944**, *50*, 230–237.

50. Iyanagi, T.; Watanabe, T.; Uchiyama, Y. The 3-methylcholanthrene-inducible UDP-glucuronosyltransferase deficiency in the hyperbilirubine-mic rat (Gunn rat) is caused by a −1 frameshift mutation. *J. Biol. Chem.* **1989**, *264*, 21302–21307.

51. Sato, H.; Aono, S.; Kashiwamata, S.; Koiwai, O. Genetic defect of bilirubin UDP-glucuronosyltransferase in the hyperbilirubinemic Gunn rat. *Biochem. Biophys. Res. Commun.* **1991**, *177*, 1161–1164.

52. Iyanagi, T. Molecular basis of multiple UDP-glucuronosyltransferase isoenzyme deficiencies in the hyperbilirubinemic rat (Gunn rat). *J. Biol. Chem.* **1991**, *266*, 24048–24052.

53. Ishii, Y.; Tsuruda, K.; Tanaka, M.; Oguri, K. Purification of a phenobarbital-inducible morphine UDP-glucuronyltransferase isoform, absent from Gunn rat liver. *Arch. Biochem. Biophys.* **1994**, *315*, 345–351.

54. Court, M. H.; Greenblatt, D. J. Molecular basis for deficient acetamino-phen glucuronidation in cats. An interspecies comparison of enzyme kinetics in liver microsomes. *Biochem. Pharmacol.* **1997**, *53*, 1041–1047.

55. Sherding, R. G. *The Cat: Diseases and Clinical Management*; Churchill Livingstone: New York, 1994.

56. Seppen, J.; Jansen, P. L.; Oude Elferink, R. P. Immunoaffinity purification and reconstitution of the human bilirubin/phenol UDP-glucuronosyl-transferase family. *Protein Expr. Purif.* **1995**, *6*, 149–154.

57. Miners, J. O.; Smith, P. A.; Sorich, M. J.; McKinnon, R. A.; Mackenzie, P. I. Predicting human drug glucuronidation parameters: application of in vitro and in silico modeling approaches. *Annu. Rev. Pharmacol. Toxicol.* **2004,** *44,* 1–25.

58. Sorich, M. J.; Miners, J. O.; McKinnon, R. A.; Smith, P. A. Multiple pharmacophores for the investigation of human UDP-glucuronosyltransferase isoform substrate selectivity. *Mol. Pharmacol.* **2004,** *65,* 301–308.

59. Burchell, B. Genetic variation of human UDP-glucuronosyltransferase: implications in disease and drug glucuronidation. *Am. J. Pharmacogenomics* **2003,** *3,* 37–52.

60. Gupta, E.; Lestingi, T. M.; Mick, R.; Ramirez, J.; Vokes, E. E.; Ratain, M. J. Metabolic fate of irinotecan in humans: correlation of glucuronidation with diarrhea. *Cancer Res.* **1994,** *54,* 3723–3725.

61. Guillemette, C. Pharmacogenomics of human UDP-glucuronosyltransferase enzymes. *Pharmacogenomics J.* **2003,** *3,* 136–158.

62. Stoehlmacher, J.; Goekkurt, E.; Lenz, H. J. Pharmacogenetic aspects in treatment of colorectal cancer—an update. *Pharmacogenomics* **2003,** *4,* 767–777.

63. Senafi, S. B.; Clarke, D. J.; Burchell, B. Investigation of the substrate specificity of a cloned expressed human bilirubin UDP-glucuronosyltransferase: UDP-sugar specificity and involvement in steroid and xenobiotic glucuronidation. *Biochem. J.* **1994,** *303,* 233–240.

64. Guillemette, C.; Millikan, R. C.; Newman, B.; Housman, D. E. Genetic polymorphisms in uridine diphospho-glucuronosyltransferase 1A1 and association with breast cancer among African Americans. *Cancer Res.* **2000,** *60,* 950–956.

65. Guillemette, C.; De Vivo, I.; Hankinson, S. E.; Haiman, C. A.; Spiegelman, D.; Housman, D. E.; Hunter, D. J. Association of genetic polymorphisms in UGT1A1 with breast cancer and plasma hormone levels. *Cancer Epidemiol. Biomarkers Prev.* **2001,** *10,* 711–714.

66. Duguay, Y.; McGrath, M.; Lepine, J.; Gagne, J. F.; Hankinson, S. E.; Colditz, G. A.; Hunter, D. J.; Plante, M.; Tetu, B.; Belanger, A.; Guillemette, C.; De Vivo, I. The functional UGT1A1 promoter polymorphism decreases endometrial cancer risk. *Cancer Res.* **2004,** *64,* 1202–1207.

13

▷

Arylamine

N-Acetyltransferase

N-ACETYLATION OF AROMATIC AMINES

N-Acetyltransferase enzymes (NATs) have a limited spectrum of activity: their only substrates are aromatic amines[1] and hydrazines (and some derivatives). Nevertheless, NATs are of much significance in pharmacology and toxicology because these N-containing functional groups are commonly encountered among xenobiotics. NATs are also among the best-studied examples of genetically determined causes of differences in human drug metabolism.

The defining activity of NATs (*1, 2*) is the transfer of acetyl groups from acetyl CoA[2] to an aromatic amine substrate, yielding an aromatic amide (figure 13-1) and free coenzyme A (CoASH). This enzyme activity is formally designated *acetyl CoA: aromatic amine N-acetyltransferase* (EC 2.3.1.5) or NAT.[3] N-Acetylation is an important metabolic route for several widely used drugs (figure 13-2), including sulfonamide antibiotics, such as sulfamethoxazole and sulfamethazine (*3*); the antileprosy drug dapsone; and procainamide (for treatment of cardiac arrhythmia) and its metabolite *p*-aminobenzoic acid (*4*); and hydrazines (figure 13-3) such as the antituberculosis agent isoniazid and the antihypertensive drug hydralazine (*5*). All of these compounds are excreted to a large extent as amides/hydrazides. The natural product caffeine is also metabolized, indirectly, via NAT (see below).

In contrast to most so-called Phase 2 drug metabolism pathways, acetylation does not necessarily increase the water solubility of a xenobiotic substrate. For example, *para*-aminophenol is highly water soluble (as the hydrochloride salt), but its acetylated metabolite, *para*-acetylaminophenol (acetaminophen) is only sparingly water soluble. Also, one should not assume that acetylated metabolites are pharmacologically inactive. Amides may be active per se, and enzymatic deacetylation can occur, that is, the hydrolysis of aromatic amides to aromatic amines. So, for example, monoacetylated dapsone might be usable as a "prodrug," being slowly hydrolyzed to release dapsone (*6, 7*).

Many aromatic amines are chemical carcinogens; these compounds, discussed in chapter 17, are typically polycyclic and much more hydrophobic than most drugs. This class includes several compounds that have

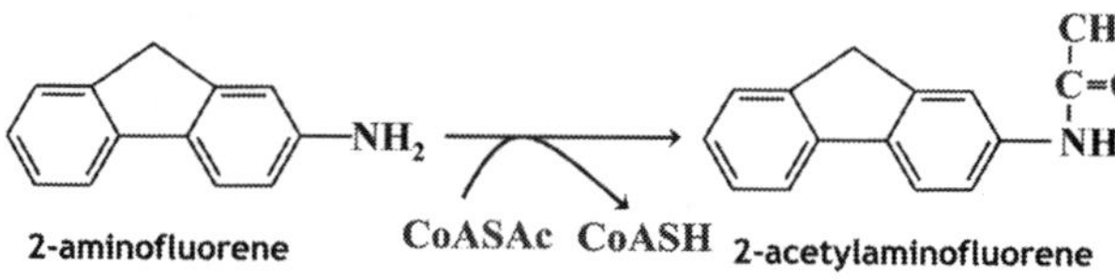

FIGURE 13-1.

NAT-catalyzed reaction; N-acetylation of 2-aminofluorene, a typical substrate.

426

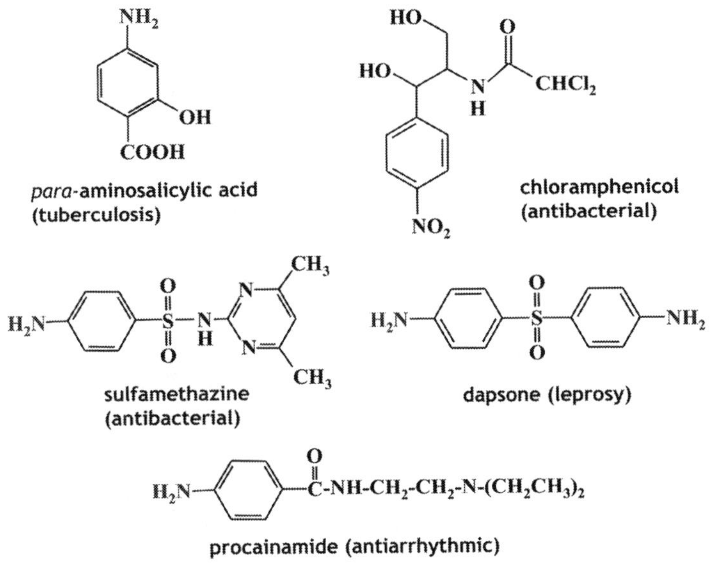

FIGURE 13-2.

Typical aromatic amine drugs and their therapeutic indications.

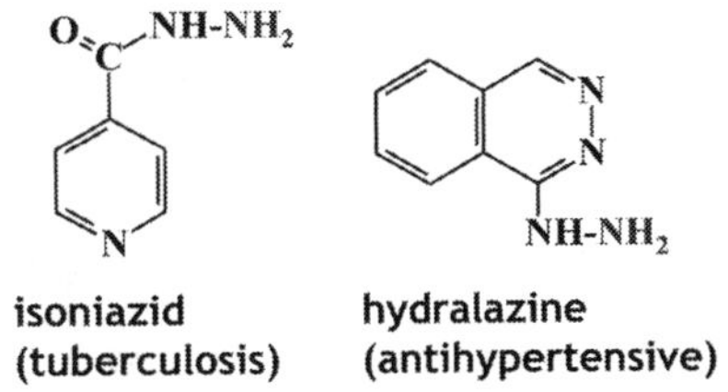

FIGURE 13-3.

Typical hydrazine drugs and their therapeutic indications.

been widely used in industry, as antioxidants and as dyestuff and plastics intermediates (notably benzidine and β-naphthylamine) (2-naphthylamine). Arylamine carcinogens are generally NAT substrates (8).

O-ACETYLTRANSFERASE AND ACETYL CoA-INDEPENDENT ACETYL TRANSFER

NAT enzymes catalyze two additional reactions. Arylhydroxylamines (Ar-NHOH) are products of the P450-catalyzed N-oxidation of aromatic amines (9, 10) or the reduction of nitro compounds. Acetyl groups can be transferred from acetyl CoA to the oxygen atom of arylhydroxylamines (figure 13-4). This activity is classified as *acetyl CoA: N-hydroxyarylamine O-acetyltransferase* (OAT; EC 2.3.1.118). Most NATs also have OAT activity, and we sometimes refer to "NAT/OAT" enzymes.

Acetyl groups may also be transferred intramolecularly. N-Oxidation of arylamides, another P450-catalyzed reaction, generates *arylhydroxamic acids* (figure 13-5). In the acetyl CoA-independent N,O-AT reaction, the acetyl group is transferred from the N atom to the O atom of an arylhydroxamic acid; note that this transfer generates the same product as is formed by the

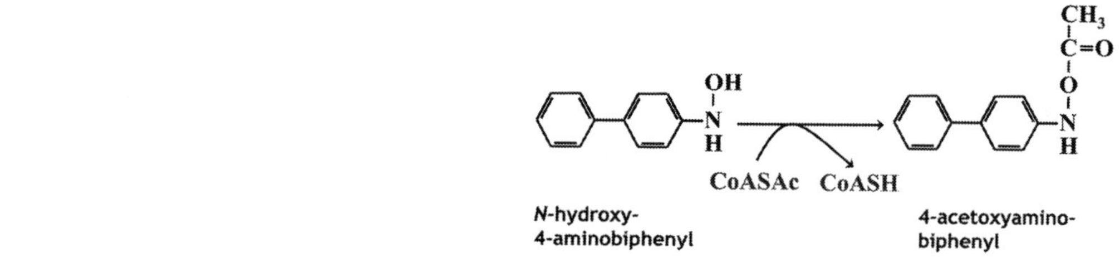

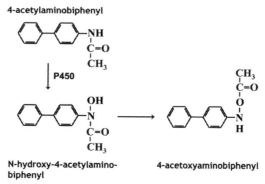

FIGURE 13-4.

OAT-catalyzed reaction: O-acetylation of arylhydroxylamines.

FIGURE 13-5.

P450-catalyzed N-oxidation of arylamides generates arylhydroxamic acids, such as *N*-hydroxyacetylaminobiphenyl, shown here, which are substrates for N,O-AT; note that the N,O-AT-catalyzed reaction is independent of acetyl CoA.

OAT reaction, although from a different class of substrate. The systematic name for this activity is *arylhydroxamic acid* N,O-*acetyltransferase* (EC 2.3.1.56). Both the OAT and N,O-AT reactions are significant processes in the bioactivation of carcinogenic aromatic amines, because the products, *N*-acetoxyarylhydroxylamines, are DNA-reactive electrophiles. We will consider these bioactivation reactions later (chapter 17).

NAT: ASSAY

The conversion of aromatic amines to aromatic amides can be assayed in various ways. For example, the reagent dimethylaminobenzaldehyde (DMAB) reacts with aromatic amines, but not with amides, to form a yellow-colored Schiff base product (*11*) (figure 13-6). Thus, the progress of an NAT-catalyzed reaction can be measured by incubating substrate, enzyme source, and acetyl CoA; removing aliquots from the reaction mix at appropriate time intervals; and adding DMAB to measure, colorimetrically, the amount of substrate remaining. Alternatively, high-performance liquid chromatography (HPLC) can be used to separate and quantitate the amine substrate and amide product. With diamino substrates, such as benzidine (diaminobiphenyl), the colorimetric assay is not applicable, since the first product formed, *N*-acetylbenzidine, also reacts with DMAB. The mono- and diacetylated products can be separated by chromatography (*12*).

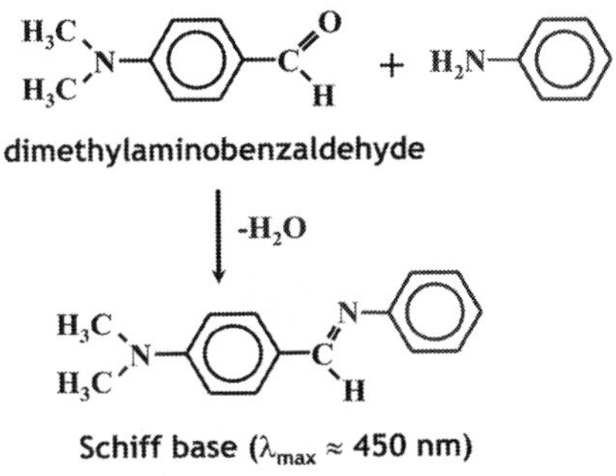

dimethylaminobenzaldehyde

$-H_2O$

Schiff base ($\lambda_{max} \approx 450$ nm)

FIGURE 13-6.

Detection of aromatic amines by formation of a colored Schiff's base product with N,N-dimethylaminobenzaldehyde; this analytical reaction is used in some NAT assays.

OAT: ASSAY

The product of the OAT-catalyzed reaction is an unstable N-acetoxy ester that binds spontaneously to nucleophiles, including DNA. OAT activity can be assayed by incubating a radiolabeled hydroxylamine substrate (such as [³H]-N-OH-aminofluorene), enzyme, acetyl CoA, and high-molecular-weight DNA (e.g., calf thymus DNA). After stopping the reaction, the DNA is recovered and washed free of substrate, and covalent binding to the macromolecule is measured by scintillation counting (13, 14). Since the N,O-AT reaction generates the same reactive intermediate, it can be assayed similarly. However, the radiolabeled substrate used is an aryl-hydroxamic acid, such as [³H]-N-hydroxyacetylaminofluorene, and acetyl CoA is *omitted* from the incubation (15).

NAT: PURIFICATION

Mammalian NATs are cytoplasmic enzymes with molecular masses of about 34 kDa. NATs have been partially purified from liver homogenates of species including chicken, rodents, and humans. Purification of native NATs is often hampered by enzyme instability and by the low abundance of the enzyme proteins, even in tissues where the catalytic activity is relatively high. In human liver, NAT proteins make up less than 1 part in 20,000 of the total cytoplasmic protein, by weight. NAT enzyme was purified about 1000-fold from human liver cytosol, by a series of chromatography steps, including anion exchange, hydroxyapatite, gel filtration, and coenzyme A-Sepharose affinity (16). Recombinant mammalian NAT can be expressed as an active enzyme in E. coli (17, 18) and affinity column methods have been used to purify histidine-tagged or GST-tagged NAT fusion proteins.

▶ **The Discovery of NAT Multiplicity**

An insightful analysis of data obtained from pharmacokinetic studies with rapid and slow acetylator patients, as well as the results of kinetic experiments with partially purified human liver enzymes, prompted J.W. Jenne to conclude that the enzyme responsible for N-acetylation of isoniazid does not have a major role in the N-acetylation of p-aminosalicylic acid (PAS). In 1965 Jenne proposed that two acetylation pathways are available in humans (19). One pathway, which exhibits widely varying interindividual acetylation capacity, was suggested to utilize isoniazid and certain polycyclic aromatic amines as substrates, whereas the other

continues next page

continued from previous page

pathway catalyzes the N-acetylation of PAS and structurally related compounds. Jenne's prescient suggestion was not confirmed until many years later.

In the early 1980s David Hein, a graduate student in Wendell Weber's laboratory at the University of Michigan, initiated NAT purification experiments as part of his investigation of the N-acetylation polymorphism in hamsters. In the Weber laboratory, where most of the preceding NAT purifications had been done with rabbit liver preparations, the customary first step was addition of ammonium sulfate to the liver cytosol. Hein, however, omitted the ammonium sulfate precipitation step and proceeded directly to ion-exchange chromatography. This resulted in the elution of two principal peaks of NAT activity, which led him to conclude that two distinct NAT enzymes were present in hamster liver. In January 1982 Patrick Hanna visited the Weber laboratory, where he discussed the experiments conducted in his laboratory at the University of Minnesota on the self-catalyzed, "mechanism-based" inactivation of hamster hepatic NATs by carcinogenic N-arylhydroxamic acids (20). Hanna believed that his data provided compelling evidence for the presence of at least two NATs in hamster liver. By the end of Hanna's visit, there was agreement on the likelihood of hamster NAT multiplicity. Hein and Weber reported the results at the annual meeting of the American Society for Pharmacology and Experimental Therapeutics in 1982 (21).

In 1985, after overcoming the objection of a reviewer, who believed that one of the peaks of activity was of microsomal origin, Hein, Weber, and co-workers published the first direct evidence for the existence of two NATs in a mammalian tissue (22). Within a year, Smith and Hanna reported the chromatographic resolution of two NATs from hamster intestinal tissue (20). Thanks to the advances made possible by molecular biology, it was soon established that humans and other mammals commonly express more than one functional NAT gene.[4] ◀

BACTERIAL NAT ENZYMES

NAT enzyme activity is found in many species of bacteria. In fact, the first NAT gene to be cloned was that of *Salmonella typhimurium* (23). NAT-minus mutants of *S. typhimurium* are resistant to the toxicity of nitroaromatic mutagens, such as 1,8-dinitropyrene (1,8-DNP). DNP is metabolized to a reactive intermediate by bacterial nitroreduction (to give the arylhydroxylamine), followed by OAT-catalyzed O-acetylation. In the early 1980s DNP-resistant *S. typhimurium* mutants were obtained, by plating bacteria on agar medium containing growth-inhibitory concentrations of 1,8-DNP and isolating rare resistant clones (24). These clones lack NAT activity, cannot bioactivate nitro compounds (25), and are resistant to their toxicity. Takehiko Nohmi and colleagues (23) used this property as the basis of a screen: 1,8-DNP-resistant mutants were transformed with a plasmid library prepared from wild-type (NAT⁺) *S. typhimurium*. Clones were screened for sensitivity to killing by a nitro-aromatic compound, 2-nitrofluorene. Four sensitive clones were obtained and the plasmids in these clones proved to carry the NAT gene. The *S. typhimurium* NAT enzyme has been used in many subsequent mechanistic and structural studies.

E. coli was once thought to lack NAT, because enzyme assays had failed to detect any activity. However, when the *E. coli* genome was completed, a chromosomal sequence highly homologous to the *S. typhimurium* NAT gene was discovered and this proved to encode an active NAT enzyme (26). Like the corresponding *S. typhimurium* mutants, NAT-minus *E. coli* strains (constructed by gene targeting) are resistant to nitroaromatic compounds (27) but have no other discernable growth defects (such as auxotrophies). However, very different findings were obtained in studies of mycobacteria. *Mycobacterium bovis* expresses an NAT enzyme, and deletion of the corresponding gene results in a dramatic reduction in growth rate and changes in the profile of complex lipids elaborated by the bacterium. These findings indicate a role, as yet not defined, for NAT in the biogenesis of membrane lipids by this organism (*28*).

NAT: CATALYTIC MECHANISM

The carbonyl C=O bond of an acetate oxyester is polarized, such that the carbonyl carbon is electrophilic; in the case of a thioester such as acetyl CoA, the electrophilicity of the carbonyl carbon is much greater. The acetylation reaction can be viewed as a nucleophilic displacement on the carbonyl carbon, with the thiolate anion of coenzyme A as the leaving group. *The acetate group is transferred to an active cysteine thiolate residue of the NAT enzyme.* This mechanism was first suggested by biochemical studies of a purified rabbit liver NAT (*29*) and supported by subsequent site-directed mutagenesis experiments, which identified the active-site cysteine residue. Let us consider the biochemical experiment first. Electrophilic reagents such as iodoacetate are often used to alkylate and inactivate the nucleophilic thiol groups of cysteine residues. Wendell Weber and co-workers treated NAT enzyme protein with bromoacetanilide (figure 13-7). This reagent was designed to be an "affinity alkylator": the bromoacyl group is incorporated into a molecule that is a structural analogue of the enzyme's product (acetanilide). The haloacyl group acts as an alkylating agent, and the acetanilide group ensures that the reagent will bind tightly to active site of the enzyme. As the enzyme was titrated with the inhibitor, irreversible loss of enzyme activity was observed, consistent with 1:1 stoichiometric alkylation of the enzyme by the inhibitor (figure 13-8). That is, *each alkylation event inactivates one molecule of enzyme*, presumably by inactivating the active-site cysteine residue.

NAT is a textbook example of a "ping-pong" enzyme mechanism (*30a*, p. 120; *30b*), as illustrated in figure 13-9. In a ping-pong mechanism, a covalent enzyme–substrate intermediate is formed; this intermediate subsequently reacts with the second substrate to complete the reaction cycle. In the case of NAT, the enzyme first attacks acetyl CoA, to form an acyl–enzyme intermediate. The nucleophile (aromatic amine) then attacks the acyl–enzyme, yielding the product amide and the free enzyme. Another characteristic feature of ping-pong mechanisms is that the (apparent) K_M for one substrate (e.g., the arylamine) increases as the concentration of the other substrate (e.g., acetyl CoA) is increased.

Can the acyl–enzyme NAT intermediate be isolated? Weber and colleagues incubated NAT enzyme with [^{3}H]-acetyl CoA in the absence of aromatic amine substrate; the reaction was then stopped by the addition of 1% SDS solution, quickly denaturing the enzyme. Excess radio-labeled acetyl CoA was removed on a gel filtration chromatography

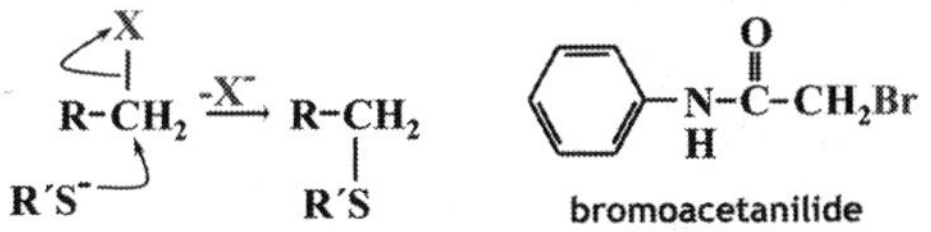

FIGURE 13-7.
Left: alkylation of a thiol group by an electrophilic haloalkane. Right: bromo-acetanilide, an affinity alkylator of NAT.

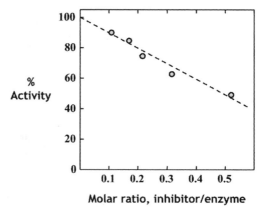

FIGURE 13-8.

Stoichiometry of the covalent inactivation of NAT by bromoacetanilide. Samples of NAT (500 μL; 47 μM) were incubated for 30 min at room temperature after the addition of bromoacetanilide in water (20 μL), to give a final inhibitor concentration of 5, 8, 10, 15, or 25 μM. The incubation mixtures were then measured for remaining NAT activity. (*Data from Andres, H. H.; Klem, A. J.; Schopfer, L. M.; Harrison, J. K.; Weber, W. W. On the active site of liver acetyl-CoA. Arylamine N-acetyltransferase from rapid acetylator rabbits (III/J). J. Biol. Chem. **1988**, 263, 7521–7527.*)

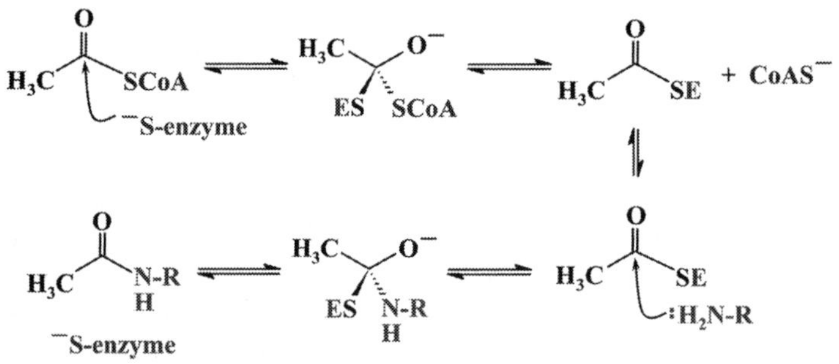

FIGURE 13-9.

Reaction mechanism of NAT. The upper row shows the formation of the covalent acyl-enzyme intermediate; the lower row shows the formation of the amide product. *Note*: A full-color version of this figure appears on the website.

column with a low-molecular-weight cut-off; the coenzyme is retained on the column, while the enzyme passes through. Under these conditions, the ^{3}H acyl–enzyme intermediate could be detected by scintillation counting.

HUMAN NAT POLYMORPHISM

Tuberculosis ("consumption"), a life-threatening lung infection caused by the bacterium *Mycobacterium tuberculosis*, is one of humankind's worst scourges. Until the development of antibiotics, no effective treatment for tuberculosis existed, other than bed rest and fresh air. A compelling account of the horror accompanying a diagnosis of tuberculosis was written by Richard Feynman, whose wife died of the disease in the 1940s

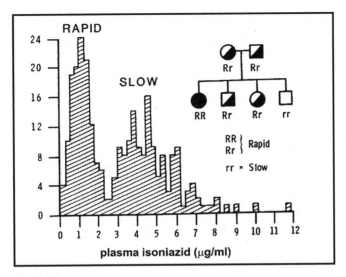

FIGURE 13-10.

Polymorphic metabolism of isoniazid. The inset shows a typical Mendelian pedigree analysis. The vertical axis represents the number of individuals (see text). (*Reproduced from Evans, D. A. P.; Manley, K. A.; McKusick, V. A. Genetic control of isoniazid metabolism in man. Br. Med. J. 1960, 2, 485–491.*)

(*31*, pp. 34ff.). In the early 1950s *isoniazid* (isonicotinic hydrazide) was discovered to be a highly effective treatment for tuberculosis (*32, 33*), transforming the management of the disease in a manner comparable to the later development of protease inhibitors for the control of HIV/AIDS.

Soon after the introduction of isoniazid therapy, clinicians noticed that some patients receiving the drug developed peripheral neuropathy, a toxic response characterized by tingling and numbness in the fingers and toes. (Hepatotoxicity is another serious side effect.) Pharmacokinetic studies of isoniazid elimination were undertaken. Histograms of patients' plasma drug concentrations, following a single oral dose of isoniazid, were discovered to be bimodal: that is, patients are either *rapid* or *slow* eliminators of the drug (figure 13-10). Family pedigree studies verified that this phenotype was an inherited Mendelian trait (*34*) determined by a single autosomal gene, with rapid elimination dominant. This was the first well-characterized example of a pharmacogenetic polymorphism, that is, a genetically determined interindividual difference in drug metabolism. Isoniazid is eliminated from the body largely as *N*-acetylisoniazid. Molecular studies (see below) later revealed that there are two distinct human NAT enzymes. The isoniazid slow elimination phenotype is caused by a reduced rate of isoniazid N-acetylation by liver NAT2. *There is a strong association between the slow acetylator phenotype and the occurrence of isoniazid side effects*, presumably because "normal" dosing regimens lead to the accumulation of the drug to toxic levels in slow excretors. For example, a study in India (*35*) followed more than 1000 tuberculosis patients who were administered "short-course" therapy with rifampicin, isoniazid, streptomycin, and pyrazinamide. Patients were tested for the NAT2 polymorphism by measuring urinary excretion of isoniazid. Hepatitis occurred in 11% of the slow acetylators but only 1% of the rapid acetylators.

Caffeine

Caffeine (1,3,7-trimethylxanthine) is probably the world's most popular natural product, consumed in tea, coffee, and caffeinated soft drinks, as well as in nonprescription pills for combating headache and drowsiness. A cup of tea or coffee can contain 100 mg or more caffeine. The familiar stimulant activity of caffeine is believed to result from its action as an adenosine receptor antagonist (45). Caffeine can be removed from green coffee beans by solvent extraction with methylene chloride. (Since the solvent is volatile, virtually all traces are removed by the subsequent roasting process, which generates much of the characteristic flavor and aroma of coffee. Unfortunately, decaffeination methods remove not only caffeine but also a fraction of the volatile, organic-soluble flavor compounds and their precursors, so decaffeinated coffee tends to be bland-tasting.) Another decaffeination method ("Swiss water process") uses water extraction followed by activated-charcoal filtration. In Germany, supercritical carbon dioxide is used for the extraction.

Caffeine metabolism is highly complex (figure 13-11), involving oxidative N-demethylation at each of the three methyl substituents (catalyzed by P450 1A2 and P450 2E1; see chapter 7) and subsequent biotransformations. ◀

Unfortunately, despite the success of isoniazid therapy, tuberculosis has not been defeated. Even in countries where the disease has become rare among the general population, some groups remain at very high risk, due to poverty and inadequate medical care. Tuberculosis remains far more prevalent among aboriginal (First Nations) peoples in Canada than among nonaboriginals (36). Persons living with HIV/AIDS are very susceptible to tuberculosis (37). Also, isoniazid-resistant strains of the organism have emerged.

Since the discovery of the polymorphic metabolism of isoniazid, many other aromatic amine and hydrazine xenobiotics have been found to show the same behavior. The clinical and toxicological consequences of this variation have also been studied. For example, procainamide therapy for cardiac arrhythmias, and hydralazine treatment for hypertension, occasionally induce *lupus erythematosus* (38), an autoimmune disease characterized by skin rash, erythema (reddening) on the nose and face, and impaired functioning of the heart and lungs. Many drugs, especially aromatic amines and hydrazines, can induce lupus. The NAT2 slow acetylator phenotype is associated with a higher incidence or earlier onset of this adverse drug reaction (39). Drug-induced lupus may be a consequence of oxidative bioactivation of the parent drug, catalyzed by neutrophil myeloperoxidase. One proposed mechanism for drug-induced lupus hypothesizes that the activated form of the drug binds to a particular cellular protein, converting it into an altered form, which induces an autoimmune reaction (40). Presumably, the acetylated form of the drug is not a substrate for oxidation by myeloperoxidase.

Several epidemiological studies have suggested that the NAT2 slow acetylator phenotype is a risk factor for the occurrence of bladder cancer, especially in individuals who are exposed to aromatic amine carcinogens in the workplace (see chapter 17). However, the NAT2–cancer risk correlation remains controversial (41, 42).

In view of the clinical importance of the acetylation polymorphism, protocols have been devised to determine an individual's acetylator phenotype. These methods involve the administration of low doses of "probe drugs," from whose pharmacokinetic profile, or pattern of urinary metabolites, estimates of *N*-acetyltransferase enzyme activity can be made. Isoniazid, sulfamethazine (43), procainamide, and dapsone have been used for this purpose. One of the many biotransformation pathways of caffeine depends on NAT2 activity (figure 13-11). Caffeine (see sidebar) is an excellent probe drug since it is widely consumed, safe, and available without prescription. The test for determining NAT2 acetylator phenotype (figure 13-12) relies on measurement of the ratio of the caffeine metabolites 5-acetylamino-6-formylamino-3-methyluracil (AFMU) and 1-methylxanthine (1X), excreted after administration of a dose of caffeine (44).

NAT: MOLECULAR GENETICS IN HUMANS AND OTHER MAMMALS

Monoclonal antibodies were raised against partially purified chicken liver NAT and used for immunoaffinity purification of the enzyme; amino acid sequences were obtained and, on this basis, oligonucleotide probes

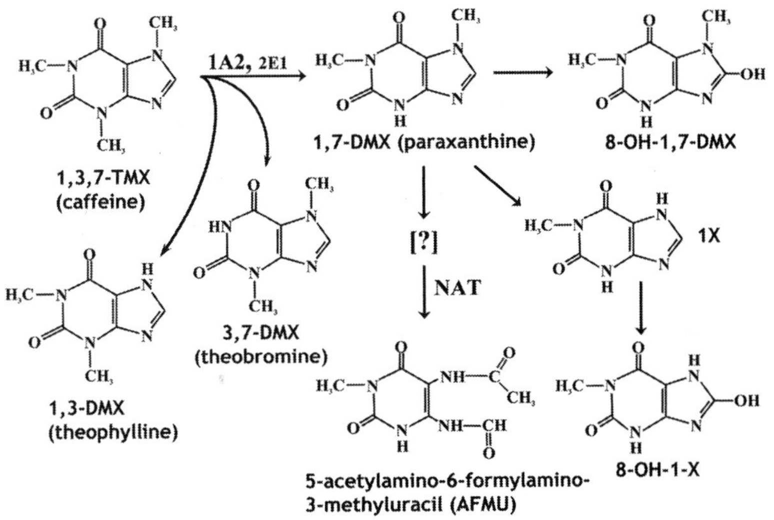

FIGURE 13-11.
Metabolism of caffeine. P450-catalyzed N-demethylation reactions are shown at upper left; additional oxidation and N-demethylation reactions at right. 1,7-Dimethylxanthine (top center) undergoes a ring-opening reaction to produce an intermediate [?] that has not been isolated; its acetylated derivative, 5-acetylamino-6-formyl-amino-3-methyluracil (AFMU), is found as a urinary metabolite of caffeine (see figure 13-12). Even this complex schematic represents only some of the human metabolic pathways of caffeine. See Schneider, H.; Ma, L.; Glatt, H. Extractionless method for the determination of urinary caffeine metabolites using high-performance liquid chromatography coupled with tandem mass spectrometry. *J. Chromatogr. B Analyt. Technol. Biomed. Life Sci.* **2003,** *789,* 227–237 for further discussion.

were synthesized and used to clone the corresponding cDNA (*46*). This achievement made possible the cloning of mammalian NATs, including the human genes (*47*). Two functional NAT genes and one pseudo-gene, each encoded as a single exon, are found in a 2 Mb region of human chromosome 8p22 (*48*). The genes are identified as *AAC1* and *AAC2* and the corresponding proteins are NAT1 and NAT2. Both NAT proteins are 290 amino acids in length, share greater than 80% amino acid sequence identity, and yet display very different substrate selectivities (*49*).

Human NAT2 is the locus of the isoniazid acetylation polymorphism (*50–52*). The molecular basis of the human acetylation polymorphism had remained confusing until the cloning of the NAT genes. Puzzlingly, several aromatic amines (e.g., PABA and PAS) that are highly acetylated, both in vivo and in vitro, showed patterns of interindividual variation unrelated to the isoniazid polymorphism. These substrates were sometimes referred to as "monomorphic" substrates, in contrast to "polymorphic" substrates such as isoniazid. However, we now appreciate that this was a misleading classification; so-called "monomorphic" substrates are metabolized primarily via NAT1. Indeed, both NAT1 and NAT2 show a great deal of genetic polymorphism (see below), and the artificial distinction between "mono-morphic" and "polymorphic" NATs and substrates has been abandoned.

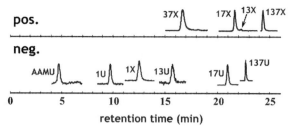

FIGURE 13-12.

HPLC–MS chromatograms of urinary caffeine metabolites in a human volunteer. Metabolites were separated by reversed-phase HPLC with an acetic acid/methanol/2-propanol solvent system and gradient elution. The HPLC system was interfaced with an electrospray source attached to a triple quadrupole mass spectrometer. Multiple reaction monitoring MS–MS was used to obtain specific signals for each analyte. Two HPLC runs (negative ionization and positive ionization) were performed on each sample. Analytes are: 5-acetylamino-6-amino-3-methyluracil (AAMU); 1,3,7-trimethyluric acid (137U); 1,3,7-trimethylxanthine (137X, caffeine); 1,3-dimethyluric acid (13U); 1,3-dimethylxanthine (13X, theophylline); 1,7-dimethyluric acid (17U); 1,7-dimethylxanthine (17X, paraxanthine); 1-methyluric acid (1U); 1-methylxanthine (1X); 3-methyluric acid (3U); 3-methylxanthine (3X); 7-methyluric acid (7U); 7-methylxanthine (7X); and 3,7-dimethylxanthine (37X, theobromine). AAMU is the product of nonenzymatic hydrolysis of 5-acetylamino-6-formylamino-3-methyluracil (AFMU). Samples were run on a urine sample obtained after consumption of coffee. Positive and negative traces refer to the electrospray ionization modes. For each target analyte, only the selected-ion chromatogram in the vicinity of the expected retention time is shown. (*Data kindly provided by Heiko Schneider, German Institute of Human Nutrition, Bergholz-Rehbrücke, Germany.*)

The mouse (*53*) and the rat each have three functional NAT genes rather than two active genes and one pseudogene.[5] The dog is a strikingly exceptional case: domestic dogs and other canids have no NAT genes at all, and do not acetylate aromatic amines (*54, 55*). Cats have NAT1, but not NAT2, and acetylate substrates such as sulfamethazine very poorly (*56*). Confirmation that NAT activity is not essential for mammalian development was obtained by the construction of viable NAT2 knockout (*57*) and NAT1/NAT2 double knockout (*58*) mice.[6]

NAT: STRUCTURE

Chemical modification experiments, discussed earlier, indicated that NAT enzymes possess a catalytically essential cysteine residue. Site-directed mutagenesis studies proved this directly: mutation of a single conserved cysteine residue (Cys68 in human NAT1 and NAT2 (*59*); Cys69 in the salmonella enzyme (*60*)) completely eliminates enzyme activity.

The first crystal structure of an NAT enzyme was published in 2000 (*61*) and the similar *M. tuberculosis* enzyme has also been solved. These structures provided dramatic new insight into NAT biochemistry. The catalytic core of the protein consists of two domains, a helix bundle and a beta barrel (figure 13-13). This architecture resembles that of other

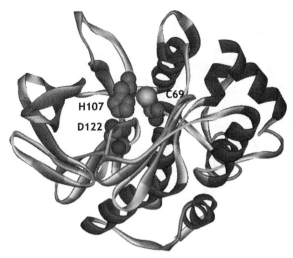

FIGURE 13-13.

Structure of *S. typhimurium* NAT enzyme, showing the catalytic triad residues as space-filling models. Coordinate data file: 1E2T.pdb. *Note*: A full-color version of this figure appears on the website.

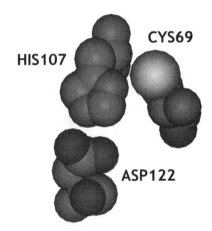

FIGURE 13-14.

Close-up view of the catalytic triad residues of *S. typhimurium* NAT. *Note*: A full-color version of this figure appears on the website.

apparently unrelated enzymes, including *transglutaminase* and the *cysteine proteases*. Transglutaminase (fibrin-stabilizing factor; human blood coagulation factor XIII) (*62*) catalyzes the formation of isopeptide bonds between the side chains of glutamine and lysine residues on fibrin molecules, cross-linking blood fibrin to form the hard clot. Cysteine proteases, such as the plant proteases papain and bromelain, hydrolyze peptide bonds in proteins.

All of these enzymes have a "catalytic triad" of the amino acids Asp (or Asn), His, and Cys (*63*, p. 234). These three conserved residues are distant in the primary structures but close together in the folded proteins. Figure 13-14 shows the NAT catalytic triad and figure 13-15 illustrates the similarity between the protein folding of the catalytic sites of NAT and

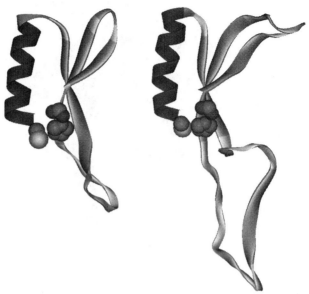

FIGURE 13-15.

Comparison of the catalytic cores of *S. typhimurium* NAT and human trans-glutaminase (structure file 1GGT.pdb). The catalytic triad residue side chains (NAT: Cys69, His107, Asp122; transglutaminase: His373, Cys314, Asp396) are shown as space-filling models. *Note*: A full-color version of this figure appears on the website.

```
                        ⇩                    ⇩               ⇩
S. typh.    RGGYCFELNGLFERA … SLPPRTHRLLLVDV..EDEQWIADVG …
hum NAT1    RGGWCLQVNHLLYWA … ST.GMIHLLLQVTIDGRN..YIVDAG …
hum NAT2    RGGWCLQVNQLLYWA … ST.GMVHLLLQVTIDGRN..YIVDAG …
```

FIGURE 13-16.

The catalytic triad residues are conserved among all known NATs.

transglutaminase. Once the presence of the catalytic triad in the bacterial NAT was appreciated, on the basis of the crystal structure, the same triad was recognized in the primary structure of eukaryotic NATs (figure 13-16).

The role of the Asp (acidic) and His (basic) residues is probably to enhance the acidity of the catalytic cysteine residue, shifting the protonation equilibrium towards the more nucleophilic thiolate anion form. We can see a mechanistic parallel between the cysteine protease, NAT, and transglutaminase reactions (figure 13-17). In each case, *nucleophilic attack of the cysteine residue on a carbonyl carbon* (of the peptide substrate, for the cysteine protease; of acetyl CoA for NAT; of the glutamine side-chain amide, for transglutaminase) *leads to formation of a covalent acyl–enzyme intermediate*. This intermediate is then attacked by a nucleophile: water (cysteine protease), the amino group of an aromatic amine (NAT), or the side-chain ε-amino group of lysine (transglutaminase). In fact, removal of the carboxyl-terminal 11 amino acid residues of *S. typhimurium* NAT results in an enzyme that hydrolyzes acetyl CoA rather than acetylating aromatic amines; that is,

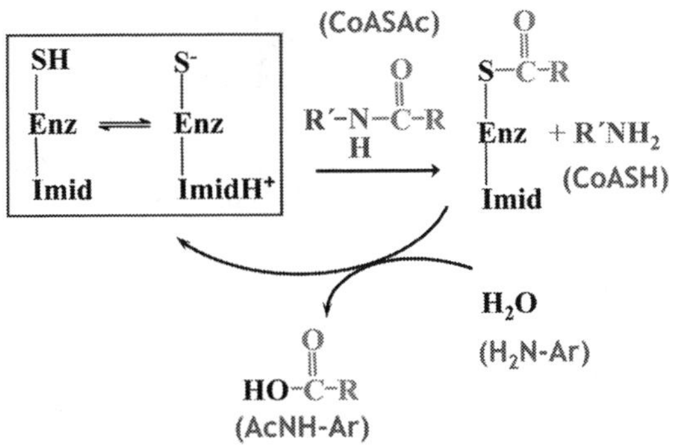

FIGURE 13-17.

Comparison between the reaction mechanisms of NAT and cysteine proteases. *Note*: A full-color version of this figure appears on the website.

the modified enzyme accepts water as the nucleophile, as do cysteine proteases (*64*).

MOLECULAR BASIS OF THE HUMAN NAT POLYMORPHISMS

As more and more individual human NAT sequences have been obtained, an initially simple classification (NAT2 rapid vs. slow) has become very complicated. Dozens of alleles of NAT1 and NAT2 are now catalogued; a complete list is maintained on the NAT internet home page: http:// www.louisville.edu/medschool/pharmacology/NAT.html. Many of these alleles vary from the wild-type sequence at more than one position, and the individual base substitutions are combined in specific haplotypes. For example, seven different NAT2*14 alleles have been identified (NAT2*14A to NAT2*14G); each bears the G to A transition at nucleotide 191 (resulting in the amino acid substitution R64Q), in combination with as many as three additional mutations.

With such extensive polymorphism in the NAT genes, one may well ask how a "wild-type" allele can be designated. In practice, the assignment is rather arbitrary. The alleles NAT1*4 and NAT2*4 are usually considered to be "wild-type" or canonical sequences (a deviation from the usual convention of assigning *1 to the wild-type allele), but these are not necessarily the most common alleles in all population groups.

Nine variant alleles account, together, for more than 98% of those present at the NAT2 locus in the human population (*50*). Since each of these allelic variants contains at least one point mutation that alters a restriction endonuclease recognition sequence, they can be detected by PCR-RFLP tests (*65*). The most common "slow" NAT2 allele is NAT2*5B, which encodes a NAT2 protein with the amino acid substitution I114T. In a yeast recombinant expression system, this substitution resulted in reduced immunoreactive protein and reduced NAT and OAT activities (*66*).

NAT1, although closely related to NAT2 in sequence, shows very different substrate specificity (*67*). NAT1 activity can be measured in blood (neutrophils), using NAT1-selective substrates such as *p*-aminosalicylic acid and *p*-aminobenzoic acid (*68*). The NAT2 polymorphism was discovered much earlier, because of its effect on isoniazid metabolism, but NAT1 is also highly polymorphic (69). The low-activity allele NAT1*14 (substitution R187Q) was found in almost half of the individuals in a Lebanese population (70). Studies of recombinant NAT1 allelic forms expressed in human cells in vitro indicate that the low enzyme activity of NAT1*14 is due to its rapid ubiquitination and proteasomal degradation (71). Interestingly, the same mutations can show up in both NAT1 and NAT2 alleles; for example, the C to T transition at nucleotide position 190, causing the substitution R46W, is found in NAT2*19 and also in NAT1*17. This circumstance may have arisen by a recombination or gene conversion event.

▶ Molecular Epidemiology

Epidemiology is defined as the study of the distribution and determinants of disease in specified populations, with disease prevention as the goal. The science of epidemiology attempts to explain why some people develop disease while others do not. Historically, epidemiology has been used to investigate associations between risk factors and disease outcome. Epidemiology began with the study of infectious diseases. When a cholera outbreak was killing many residents of London, England, Dr. John Snow (1813–1858) went from door to door, asking people with and without the disease whence they obtained their water. After he traced the spread of the disease in one Soho neighborhood back to a specific contaminated well, he removed its pump handle as a public health intervention. (The handle of the infamous "Broad Street pump" is said to remain display in the John Snow pub, near Piccadilly Circus.) John Snow is regarded as the "father of epidemiology."

Today, the most common types of epidemiological investigations are "retrospective case-control" and "prospective cohort" studies. In retrospective case-control studies, people who are newly diagnosed with the disease of interest (the cases) are enrolled into the study, as well as healthy "controls" who are likely to arise from the same source population as the cases. Usually, several hundred individuals in each category are recruited. In most studies, interviews are conducted or surveys completed, with assessment of factors that could be associated with risk of the disease. For cancers, such factors might include diet, smoking, physical activity, medical and reproductive histories, and family history of cancer. The prevalence of these risk factors is then compared between the cases and the controls. Cohort studies collect similar data, but in large populations (thousands) of people who are healthy at the time of entry into the study. These participants are tracked over time and monitored for disease endpoints. Statistical analyses are conducted to look for differences between those who develop the disease and those who remain free from it.

Epidemiology has revealed major risk factors for some cancers: family history (breast cancer), alcohol consumption (esophageal cancer), and smoking (lung cancer). However, even though we know that smoking causes lung cancer, only about one in ten smokers is diagnosed with the disease. Why is this so? Molecular epidemiology has helped to address this question. Individuals differ with regard to relevant biochemical and biological processes, such as carcinogen activation and detoxication, DNA repair, cell cycle control, immune response, and so on, and these differences may influence cancer susceptibility. Molecular epidemiology can be used to identify individuals at greatest risk of disease.

Molecular analysis can be incorporated into epidemiologic studies by collection of blood specimens or, for studies of cancer, retrieval of tumor tissue. To determine the effects of variations in specific genes and enzymes, study participants may be "genotyped" for polymorphisms in the coding or regulatory regions of genes that may be relevant to the diseases and exposures under study. Genetic factors may influence disease risk by acting as modifiers of the relationship between exposure and disease outcome. The effects of specific exposures are expected to be strongest among individuals who are most susceptible to their carcinogenic effects; for example, risk of bladder cancer is probably higher among smokers who have slow N-acetylation genotypes for NAT2 (72). Differences in etiologic pathways may also result in tumors with specific genetic and epigenetic characteristics. Thus, a molecular epidemiologic approach (73) may be used to categorize individuals by susceptible subgroups or by tumor tissue characteristics, so as to refine risk estimates. Biomarkers of environmental exposure may include internal dose, biologically effective dose (e.g., DNA adducts), or early tissue responses. Analysis of these biomarkers may further elucidate disease processes and exposure/disease risk relationships, as shown in figure 13-18.

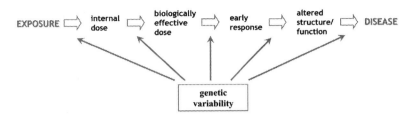

FIGURE 13-18.

Disease processes and exposure/disease risk relationships.

As an example of these approaches, a recent molecular epidemiology investigation will be described (74). There is widespread concern that environmental contaminants, such as the persistent organochlorine compounds (e.g., polychlorinated biphenyls (PCBs) and the insecticide *p,p'*-dichlorodiphenyltrichloroethane, DDT) could contribute to breast cancer risk. However, several studies were designed to test whether serum levels of these organochlorines are higher in breast cancer cases than in controls, and associations with breast cancer were not observed. Because organochlorines induce cytochrome P450 1A1 (chapter 8), and some PCB congeners are metabolized by this enzyme, the investigators proposed to evaluate the role of PCBs in combination with cytochrome P450 1A1 genotypes. About one person in ten carries a P450 1A1 allele encoding a variant enzyme with a valine rather than the wild-type isoleucine at codon 462 (75). This variant allele may be associated with altered P450 enzyme inducibility (76). Several hundred women with breast cancer and controls were enrolled into the study. From each participant, blood samples were drawn and an interview was conducted. Serum samples were analyzed for PCB and DDT levels by gas chromatography. DNA was extracted from the white blood cells ("buffy coat") and genotyping was performed to determine the CYP1A1 gene polymorphism. Cross-tabulations were first performed, using the chi-square statistic for assessment of significance, and then logistic regression models (77) were tested. Breast cancer was the dependent variable and PCB levels (divided into quartiles) and P450 1A1 genotypes were the independent variables. Regression models are used to assess the increase in risk associated with each category of the independent variable. Additional covariates that may confound relationships can be added to the statistical models, to remove their effects from the analysis. In this study, cases were not more likely than controls to have high PCB levels. However, among the women with high PCB levels, there was increased risk of breast cancer associated with the presence of at least one valine allele, compared with women who were homozygous for the (wild-type) isoleucine allele. High PCB levels did not affect risk among the women with the common P450 1A1 genotype and genotype did not increase risk among the women with low PCB levels. This study used biomarkers of internal dose (PCBs) and of susceptibility (P450 1A1). The results show that while an exposure may not be associated with increased risk overall, exposure–risk associations may be discovered among susceptible subgroups.

The realization that exposure effects are likely to be modulated by genetic factors has led to new challenges in epidemiologic design, data analysis, and interpretation. Historically, in epidemiology, associations between risk factors and disease outcomes were evaluated in a relatively straightforward manner, with consideration of possible confounding variables incorporated into multivariate models. However, with our increased understanding of the biochemistry underlying exposure/disease relationships, it is becoming clear that heterogeneity in susceptibility, based on differential metabolism, is likely to alter cancer risk assessment. The use of genotype as a static independent variable in regression models may be a naive approach, however, and future molecular epidemiology studies will need to consider concepts of relationships between genotype and phenotype, target tissue versus hepatic metabolism, enzyme–substrate specificity, and possible exposures that will induce or inhibit the enzymes(s) being evaluated. The incorporation of fundamentals of toxicology, biochemistry, and molecular biology into epidemiological studies will inform the investigation of disease etiology with a new multidisciplinary perspective.[7] ◀

Notes

1. Also referred to as arylamines.

2. Other acyl CoAs (e.g., formyl CoA) may also be minor substrates.

3. NAT should not be confused with unrelated acetyltransferases, such as aralkylamine N-acetyltransferase (EC 2.3.1.87), which catalyzes

acetylation of alkylamino groups in serotonin and other endogenous compounds.

4. Patrick E. Hanna, Medicinal Chemistry and Pharmacology, University of Minnesota; David Hein, Pharmacology and Toxicology, University of Louisville School of Medicine.

5. The nomenclature is confusing, because the rodent (mouse, rat, hamster) NAT most similar to human NAT1, in terms of substrate specificity, is the enzyme denoted as NAT2, and vice versa.

6. The mouse NAT3 gene apparently supports only very slight enzyme activity.

7. Christine B. Ambrosone, Department of Epidemiology, Roswell Park Cancer Institute, Buffalo, N.Y.

References

1. Evans, D. A. N-Acetyltransferase. *Pharmacol. Ther.* **1989**, *42*, 157–234.
2. Sim, E.; Pinter, K.; Mushtaq, A.; Upton, A.; Sandy, J.; Bhakta, S.; Noble, M. Arylamine N-acetyltransferases: a pharmacogenomic approach to drug metabolism and endogenous function. *Biochem. Soc. Trans.* **2003**, *31*, 615–619.
3. Peters, J. H.; Gordon, G. R.; Karat, A. B. Polymorphic acetylation of the antibacterials, sulfamethazine and dapsone, in South Indian subjects. *Am. J. Trop. Med. Hyg.* **1975**, *24*, 641–648.
4. du Souich, P.; Erill, S. Metabolism of procainamide in patients with chronic heart failure, chronic respiratory failure and chronic renal failure. *Eur. J. Clin. Pharmacol.* **1978**, *14*, 21–27.
5. Lemke, L. E.; McQueen, C. A. Acetylation and its role in the mutagenicity of the antihypertensive agent hydralazine. *Drug Metab. Dispos.* **1995**, *23*, 559–565.
6. Pieters, F. A.; Woonink, F.; Zuidema, J. A field trial among leprosy patients in Nigeria with depot injections of dapsone and monoacetyl-dapsone. *Int. J. Lepr. Other Mycobact. Dis.* **1988**, *56*, 10–20.
7. Preuss, C. V.; Svensson, C. K. Arylacetamide deacetylase activity towards monoacetyldapsone. Species comparison, factors that influence activity, and comparison with 2-acetylaminofluorene and p-nitrophenyl acetate hydrolysis. *Biochem. Pharmacol.* **1996**, *51*, 1661–1668.
8. Zenser, T. V.; Lakshmi, V. M.; Rustan, T. D.; Doll, M. A.; Deitz, A. C.; Davis, B. B.; Hein, D. W. Human N-acetylation of benzidine: role of NAT1 and NAT2. *Cancer Res.* **1996**, *56*, 3941–3947.
9. Guengerich, F. P. N-Hydroxyarylamines. *Drug Metab. Rev.* **2002**, *34*, 607–623.
10. Kim, D.; Guengerich, F. P. Cytochrome P450 activation of arylamines and heterocyclic amines. *Annu. Rev. Pharmacol. Toxicol.* **2005**, *45*, 27–49.
11. Andres, H. H.; Klem, A. J.; Szabo, S. M.; Weber, W. W. New spectrophotometric and radiochemical assays for acetyl-CoA: arylamine N-acetyltransferase applicable to a variety of arylamines. *Anal. Biochem.* **1985**, *145*, 367–375.
12. Lakshmi, V. M.; Zenser, T. V.; Goldman, H. D.; Spencer, G. G.; Gupta, R. C.; Hsu, F. F.; Davis, B. B. The role of acetylation in benzidine metabolism and DNA adduct formation in dog and rat liver. *Chem. Res. Toxicol.* **1995**, *8*, 711–720.

13. Flammang, T. J.; Yamazoe, Y.; Guengerich, F. P.; Kadlubar, F. F. The S-acetyl coenzyme A-dependent metabolic activation of the carcinogen N-hydroxy-2-aminofluorene by human liver cytosol and its relationship to the aromatic amine N-acetyltransferase phenotype. *Carcinogenesis* **1987,** *8,* 1967–1970.

14. Boteju, L. W.; Hanna, P. E. Bioactivation of N-hydroxy-2-acetylamino-fluorenes by N,O-acyltransferase: substituent effects on covalent binding to DNA. *Carcinogenesis* **1993,** *14,* 1651–1657.

15. Wick, M. J.; Hanna, P. E. Bioactivation of N-arylhydroxamic acids by rat hepatic N-acetyltransferase. Detection of multiple enzyme forms by mechanism-based inactivation. *Biochem. Pharmacol.* **1990,** *39,* 991–1003.

16. Grant, D. M.; Lottspeich, F.; Meyer, U. A. Evidence for two closely related isozymes of arylamine N-acetyltransferase in human liver. *FEBS Lett.* **1989,** *244,* 203–207.

17. Grant, D. M.; Josephy, P. D.; Lord, H. L.; Morrison, L. D. *Salmonella typhimurium* strains expressing human arylamine N-acetyltransferases: metabolism and mutagenic activation of aromatic amines. *Cancer Res.* **1992,** *52,* 3961–3964.

18. Wang, H.; Vath, G. M.; Kawamura, A.; Bates, C. A.; Sim, E.; Hanna, P. E.; Wagner, C. R. Over-expression, purification, and characterization of recombinant human arylamine *N*-acetyltransferase 1. *Protein J.* **2005,** *24,* 65–77.

19. Jenne, J. W. Partial purification and properties of the isoniazid transacetylase in human liver. Its relationship to the acetylation of p-aminosalicylic acid. *J. Clin. Invest.* **1965,** *44,* 1992–2002.

20. Smith, T. J.; Hanna, P. E. N-Acetyltransferase multiplicity and the bioactivation of N-arylhydroxamic acids by hamster hepatic and intestinal enzymes. *Carcinogenesis* **1986,** *7,* 697–702.

21. Hein, D. W.; Weber, W. W. Separation of genetically determined monomorphic and polymorphic N-acetyltransferase enzymes in the inbred hamster. *The Pharmacologist* **1982,** *24,* 126.

22. Hein, D. W.; Kirlin, W. G.; Ferguson, R. J.; Weber, W. W. Biochemical investigation of the basis for the genetic N-acetylation polymorphism in the inbred hamster. *J. Pharmacol. Exp. Ther.* **1985,** *234,* 358–364.

23. Watanabe, M.; Nohmi, T.; Ishidate, M., Jr. New tester strains of *Salmonella typhimurium* highly sensitive to mutagenic nitroarenes. *Biochem. Biophys. Res. Commun.* **1987,** *147,* 974–979.

24. McCoy, E. C.; Anders, M.; Rosenkranz, H. S. The basis of the insensitivity of *Salmonella typhimurium* strain TA98/1,8-DNP6 to the mutagenic action of nitroarenes. *Mutat. Res.* **1983,** *121,* 17–23.

25. de France, B. F.; Carter, M. H.; Josephy, P. D.; Bryant, D. W.; McCalla, D. R. Metabolism and mutagenesis of benzidine in *Salmonella typhimurium* strains TA98 and TA98/1,8-DNP$_6$. *Mutat. Res.* **1985,** *144,* 159–163.

26. Yamamura, E.; Sayama, M.; Kakikawa, M.; Mori, M.; Taketo, A.; Kodaira, K. Purification and biochemical properties of an N-hydroxy-arylamine O-acetyltransferase from *Escherichia coli. Biochim. Biophys. Acta* **2000,** *1475,* 10–16.

27. Josephy, P. D.; Summerscales, J.; DeBruin, L. S.; Schlaeger, C.; Ho, J. *N*-hydroxyarylamine *O*-acetyltransferase-deficient *Escherichia coli* strains

are resistant to the mutagenicity of nitro compounds. *Biol. Chem.* **2002,** *383,* 977–982.

28. Bhakta, S.; Besra, G. S.; Upton, A. M.; Parish, T.; Sholto-Douglas-Vernon, C.; Gibson, K. J.; Knutton, S.; Gordon, S.; DaSilva, R. P.; Anderton, M. C.; Sim, E. Arylamine *N*-acetyltransferase is required for synthesis of mycolic acids and complex lipids in Mycobacterium bovis BCG and represents a novel drug target. *J. Exp. Med.* **2004,** *199,* 1191–1199.

29. Andres, H. H.; Klem, A. J.; Schopfer, L. M.; Harrison, J. K.; Weber, W. W. On the active site of liver acetyl-CoA. Arylamine *N*-acetyltransferase from rapid acetylator rabbits (III/J). *J. Biol. Chem.* **1988,** *263,* 7521–7527.

30. (a) Fersht, A. *Structure and Mechanism in Protein Science: A Guide to Enzyme Catalysis and Protein Folding*; WH Freeman: New York, 1999. (b) Wang, H.; Liu, L.; Hanna, P. E.; Wagner, C. R. Catalytic mechanism of hamster arylamine *N*-acetyltransferase 2. *Biochemistry* **2005,** *44,* 11295–11306.

31. Feynman, R. P. *What Do You Care What Other People Think?*; Bantam Books: New York, 1989.

32. Weber, W. W. *The Acetylator Genes and Drug Response*; Oxford University Press: New York, 1987.

33. Williamson, J. Tuberculosis revisited or how we nearly conquered tuberculosis. *Scott. Med. J.* **2000,** *45,* 183–185.

34. Evans, D. A. P.; Manley, K. A.; McKusick, V. A. Genetic control of isoniazid metabolism in man. *Br. Med. J.* **1960,** *2,* 485–491.

35. Parthasarathy, R.; Sarma, G. R.; Janardhanam, B.; Ramachandran, P.; Santha, T.; Sivasubramanian, S.; Somasundaram, P. R.; Tripathy, S. P. Hepatic toxicity in South Indian patients during treatment of tuberculosis with short-course regimens containing isoniazid, rifampicin and pyrazinamide. *Tubercle* **1986,** *67,* 99–108.

36. Smeja, C.; Brassard, P. Tuberculosis infection in an Aboriginal (First Nations) population of Canada. *Int. J. Tuberc. Lung Dis.* **2000,** *4,* 925–930.

37. Jones, J. L.; Burwen, D. R.; Fleming, P. L.; Ward, J. W. Tuberculosis among AIDS patients in the United States, 1993. *J. Acquir. Immune. Defic. Syndr. Hum. Retrovirol.* **1996,** *12,* 293–297.

38. Knowles, S.; Shapiro, L.; Shear, N. Reactive metabolites and adverse drug reactions: clinical considerations. *Clin. Rev. Allergy Immunol.* **2003,** *24,* 229–238.

39. Weber, W. W.; Hein, D. W. *N*-Acetylation pharmacogenetics. *Pharmacol. Rev.* **1985,** *37,* 25–79.

40. Jiang, X.; Khursigara, G.; Rubin, R. L. Transformation of lupus-inducing drugs to cytotoxic products by activated neutrophils. *Science* **1994,** *266,* 810–813.

41. Hayes, R. B.; Bi, W.; Rothman, N.; Broly, F.; Caporaso, N.; Feng, P.; You, X.; Yin, S.; Woosley, R. L.; Meyer, U. A. *N*-Acetylation phenotype and genotype and risk of bladder cancer in benzidine-exposed workers. *Carcinogenesis* **1993,** *14,* 675–678.

42. Hirvonen, A. Polymorphic NATs and cancer predisposition. *IARC Sci. Publ.* **1999,** 251–270.

43. Meisel, P.; Arndt, D.; Scheuch, E.; Klebingat, K. J.; Siegmund, W. Prediction of metabolic activity from genotype: the gene-dose effect of *N*-acetyltransferase. *Ther. Drug Monit.* **2001,** *23,* 9–14.

44. Grant, D. M.; Tang, B. K.; Kalow, W. A simple test for acetylator phenotype using caffeine. *Br. J. Clin. Pharmacol.* **1984,** *17,* 459–464.

45. Ribeiro, J. A.; Sebastiao, A. M.; De Mendonca, A. Adenosine receptors in the nervous system: pathophysiological implications. *Prog. Neurobiol.* **2002,** *68,* 377–392.

46. Ohsako, S.; Ohtomi, M.; Sakamoto, Y.; Uyemura, K.; Deguchi, T. Arylamine N-acetyltransferase from chicken liver: II. Cloning of cDNA and expression in Chinese hamster ovary cells. *J. Biol. Chem.* **1988,** *263,* 7534–7538.

47. Ohsako, S.; Deguchi, T. Cloning and expression of cDNAs for polymorphic and monomorphic arylamine N-acetyltransferases from human liver. *J. Biol. Chem.* **1990,** *265,* 4630–4634.

48. Matas, N.; Thygesen, P.; Stacey, M.; Risch, A.; Sim, E. Mapping AAC1, AAC2 and AACP, the genes for arylamine N-acetyltransferases, carcinogen metabolising enzymes on human chromosome 8p22, a region frequently deleted in tumours. *Cytogenet. Cell Genet.* **1997,** *77,* 290–295.

49. Kawamura, A.; Graham, J.; Mushtaq, A.; Tsiftsoglou, S. A.; Vath, G. M.; Hanna, P. E.; Wagner, C. R.; Sim, E. Eukaryotic arylamine N-acetyltransferase. Investigation of substrate specificity by high-throughput screening. *Biochem. Pharmacol.* **2005,** *69,* 347–359.

50. Grant, D. M.; Goodfellow, G. H.; Sugamori, K.; Durette, K. Pharmacogenetics of the human arylamine N-acetyltransferases. *Pharmacology* **2000,** *61,* 204–211.

51. Spielberg, S. P. N-acetyltransferases: pharmacogenetics and clinical consequences of polymorphic drug metabolism. *J. Pharmacokinet. Biopharm.* **1996,** *24,* 509–519.

52. Hein, D. W.; McQueen, C. A.; Grant, D. M.; Goodfellow, G. H.; Kadlubar, F. F.; Weber, W. W. Pharmacogenetics of the arylamine N-acetyltransferases: a symposium in honor of Wendell W. Weber. *Drug Metab. Dispos.* **2000,** *28,* 1425–1432.

53. Fakis, G.; Boukouvala, S.; Buckle, V.; Payton, M.; Denning, C.; Sim, E. Chromosome mapping of the genes for murine arylamine N-acetyltransferases (NATs), enzymes involved in the metabolism of carcinogens: identification of a novel upstream noncoding exon for murine Nat2. *Cytogenet. Cell Genet.* **2000,** *90,* 134–138.

54. Trepanier, L. A.; Ray, K.; Winand, N. J.; Spielberg, S. P.; Cribb, A. E. Cytosolic arylamine N-acetyltransferase (NAT) deficiency in the dog and other canids due to an absence of NAT genes. *Biochem. Pharmacol.* **1997,** *54,* 73–80.

55. Collins, J. M. Inter-species differences in drug properties. *Chem. Biol. Interact.* **2001,** *134,* 237–242.

56. Trepanier, L. A.; Cribb, A. E.; Spielberg, S. P.; Ray, K. Deficiency of cytosolic arylamine N-acetylation in the domestic cat and wild felids caused by the presence of a single NAT1-like gene. *Pharmacogenetics* **1998,** *8,* 169–179.

57. Cornish, V. A.; Pinter, K.; Boukouvala, S.; Johnson, N.; Labrousse, C.; Payton, M.; Priddle, H.; Smith, A. J.; Sim, E. Generation and analysis of mice with a targeted disruption of the arylamine N-acetyltransferase type 2 gene. *Pharmacogenomics J.* **2003,** *3,* 169–177.

58. Sugamori, K. S.; Wong, S.; Gaedigk, A.; Yu, V.; Abramovici, H.; Rozmahel, R.; Grant, D. M. Generation and functional characterization of arylamine N-acetyltransferase Nat1/Nat2 double-knockout mice. *Mol. Pharmacol.* **2003,** *64,* 170–179.

59. Dupret, J. M.; Grant, D. M. Site-directed mutagenesis of recombinant human arylamine N-acetyltransferase expressed in *Escherichia coli*. Evidence for direct involvement of Cys68 in the catalytic mechanism of polymorphic human NAT2. *J. Biol. Chem.* **1992,** *267,* 7381–7385.

60. Watanabe, M.; Igarashi, T.; Kaminuma, T.; Sofuni, T.; Nohmi, T. N-hydroxyarylamine O-acetyltransferase of *Salmonella typhimurium*: proposal for a common catalytic mechanism of arylamine acetyltransferase enzymes. *Environ. Health Perspect.* **1994,** *102* (Suppl. 6), 83–89.

61. Sinclair, J. C.; Sandy, J.; Delgoda, R.; Sim, E.; Noble, M. E. Structure of arylamine N-acetyltransferase reveals a catalytic triad. *Nat. Struct. Biol.* **2000,** *7,* 560–564.

62. Pedersen, L. C.; Yee, V. C.; Bishop, P. D.; Le, T.; I, Teller, D. C.; Stenkamp, R. E. Transglutaminase factor XIII uses proteinase-like catalytic triad to crosslink macromolecules. *Protein Sci.* **1994,** *3,* 1131–1135.

63. Berg, J. M.; Tymoczko, J. L.; Stryer, L. *Biochemistry*; WH Freeman: New York, 2001.

64. Mushtaq, A.; Payton, M.; Sim, E. The COOH terminus of arylamine N-acetyltransferase from *Salmonella typhimurium* controls enzymic activity. *J. Biol. Chem.* **2002,** *277,* 12175–12181.

65. Bell, D. A.; Taylor, J. A.; Butler, M. A.; Stephens, E. A.; Wiest, J.; Brubaker, L. H.; Kadlubar, F. F.; Lucier, G. W. Genotype/phenotype discordance for human arylamine N-acetyltransferase (NAT2) reveals a new slow-acetylator allele common in African-Americans. *Carcinogenesis* **1993,** *14,* 1689–1692.

66. Leff, M. A.; Fretland, A. J.; Doll, M. A.; Hein, D. W. Novel human N-acetyltransferase 2 alleles that differ in mechanism for slow acetylator phenotype. *J. Biol. Chem.* **1999,** *274,* 34519–34522.

67. Goodfellow, G. H.; Dupret, J. M.; Grant, D. M. Identification of amino acids imparting acceptor substrate selectivity to human arylamine acetyltransferases NAT1 and NAT2. *Biochem. J.* **2000,** *348,* 159–166.

68. Cribb, A. E.; Isbrucker, R.; Levatte, T.; Tsui, B.; Gillespie, C. T.; Renton, K. W. Acetylator phenotyping: the urinary caffeine metabolite ratio in slow acetylators correlates with a marker of systemic NAT1 activity. *Pharmacogenetics* **1994,** *4,* 166–170.

69. Bruhn, C.; Brockmoller, J.; Cascorbi, I.; Roots, I.; Borchert, H. H. Correlation between genotype and phenotype of the human arylamine N-acetyltransferase type 1 (NAT1). *Biochem. Pharmacol.* **1999,** *58,* 1759–1764.

70. Dhaini, H. R.; Levy, G. N. Arylamine N-acetyltransferase 1 (NAT1) genotypes in a Lebanese population. *Pharmacogenetics* **2000,** *10,* 79–83.

71. Butcher, N. J.; Arulpragasam, A.; Minchin, R. F. Proteasomal degradation of N-acetyltransferase 1 is prevented by acetylation of the active site cysteine: a mechanism for the slow acetylator phenotype and substrate-dependent down-regulation. *J. Biol. Chem.* **2004,** *279,* 22131–22137.

72. Vineis, P.; Marinelli, D.; Autrup, H.; Brockmoller, J.; Cascorbi, I.; Daly, A. K.; Golka, K.; Okkels, H.; Risch, A.; Rothman, N.; Sim, E.; Taioli, E. Current smoking, occupation, N-acetyltransferase-2 and bladder cancer: a pooled analysis of genotype-based studies. *Cancer Epidemiol. Biomarkers Prev.* **2001,** *10,* 1249–1252.

73. Perera, F. P. Molecular epidemiology: on the path to prevention? *J. Natl. Cancer Inst.* **2000,** *92,* 602–612.

74. Moysich, K. B.; Shields, P. G.; Freudenheim, J. L.; Schisterman, E. F.; Vena, J. E.; Kostyniak, P.; Greizerstein, H.; Marshall, J. R.; Graham, S.; Ambrosone, C. B. Polychlorinated biphenyls, cytochrome P4501A1 polymorphism, and postmenopausal breast cancer risk. *Cancer Epidemiol. Biomarkers Prev.* **1999,** *8*, 41–44.

75. Zhang, Z. Y.; Fasco, M. J.; Huang, L.; Guengerich, F. P.; Kaminsky, L. S. Characterization of purified human recombinant cytochrome P4501A1-Ile462 and -Val462: assessment of a role for the rare allele in carcinogenesis. *Cancer Res.* **1996,** *56*, 3926–3933.

76. Kiyohara, C.; Nakanishi, Y.; Inutsuka, S.; Takayama, K.; Hara, N.; Motohiro, A.; Tanaka, K.; Kono, S.; Hirohata, T. The relationship between CYP1A1 aryl hydrocarbon hydroxylase activity and lung cancer in a Japanese population. *Pharmacogenetics* **1998,** *8*, 315–323.

77. Campillo, C. Standardizing criteria for logistic regression models. *Ann. Intern. Med.* **1993,** *119*, 540–541.

METABOLISM OF PHENOL TO
A SULFATE CONJUGATE

The Hungarian physician Ignaz Semmelweiss is credited with introducing the concept of antisepsis into medical practice, insisting that doctors should wash their hands in between patient examinations (Vienna, 1847), but his radical proposal was not generally accepted. The decisive advance in medical hygiene was made by Joseph Lister at the Glasgow Royal Infirmary in 1867. Lister applied the newly available chemical disinfectant "carbolic acid" (i.e., phenol) to surgical dressings and sprayed it in the hospital wards as an aerosol, thereby much reducing the spread of infections. In 1876 the German organic chemist Eugen Baumann isolated phenyl sulfate from the urine of a patient who had been treated with phenol. Baumann subsequently demonstrated that several other compounds are excreted as sulfates. These were among the first demonstrations of the biotransformation of xenobiotics, coming long before the development of modern concepts of metabolism and enzymology.

Sulfate conjugation is now recognized as a metabolic route for the biotransformation of many endogenous and xenobiotic compounds. The adenosine-containing cofactor PAPS (3'-phosphoadenosine-5'-phosphosulfate) is the universal metabolic donor of sulfate groups.

PAPS

The identity of "activated sulfate," the metabolic donor of sulfate groups, was elucidated by the work of Fritz Lipmann (best known for his development of the concept of ATP as the cell's energy currency; Nobel Prize in Physiology or Medicine 1953) and others, in the late 1950s. 3'-Phosphoadenosine-5'-phosphosulfate is synthesized from ATP and inorganic sulfate (figure 14-1). First, sulfate is activated by linkage to the 5'-phosphate group of adenylate, giving adenylyl sulfate (APS). The free energy change for this reaction is highly positive; even coupling to the subsequent hydrolysis of pyrophosphate is insufficient to drive the overall process forward. Therefore, in a second step, an additional molecule of ATP is used to phosphorylate the 3'-OH of APS, yielding PAPS. This second phosphorylation uses ATP to produce a low energy phosphate ester (3'-phosphate of PAPS), and so is energetically favorable, providing thermodynamic power that drives the previous step to completion. The two steps of PAPS synthesis are catalyzed by the enzymes ATP sulfurylase (EC 2.7.7.4; synthesis of APS) and APS kinase (EC 2.7.1.25; phosphorylation of APS to form PAPS). In mammals, both of these activities are found on a single bifunctional enzyme (*1*). Following the

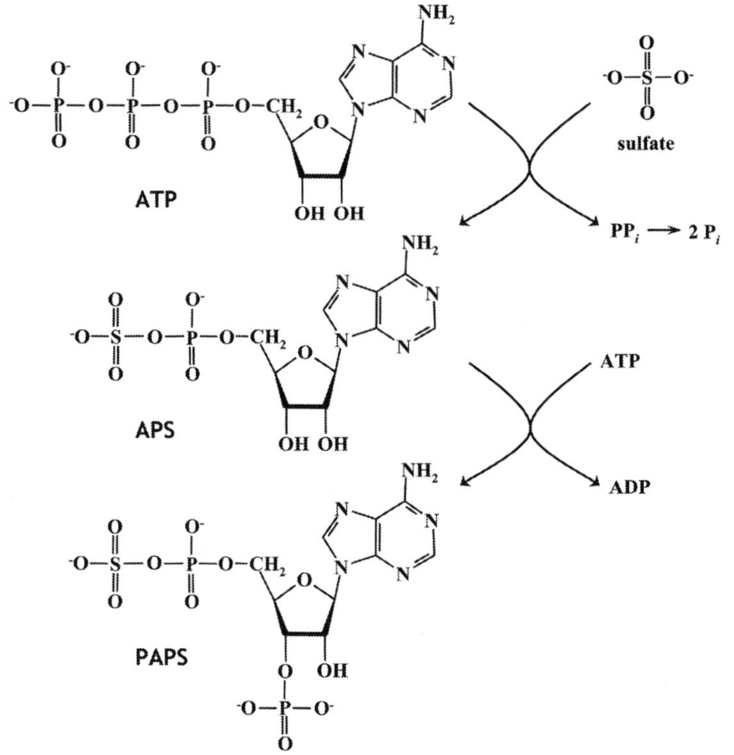

FIGURE 14-1.
PAPS (3′-phosphoadenosine-5′-phosphosulfate) is derived from ATP and inorganic sulfate.

subsequent sulfotransferase-catalyzed transfer of the sulfate moiety to an acceptor, the product 3′-phosphoadenosine-5′-phosphate is cleaved to inorganic phosphate and AMP.

The body's reserves of free sulfate are limited; the serum sulfate concentration in humans is about 0.3 mM. Administration of sulfotransferase substrates, such as acetaminophen, can cause a substantial transient drop in serum sulfate (see chapter 19). The sulfate level is restored by the catabolism of sulfated polysaccharides, such as chondroitin sulfate and keratan sulfate, glycosaminoglycans of the extracellular matrix. *Brachymorphic* (Greek: short-shape) mice have short legs and tails, resulting from defective formation of cartilage glycosaminoglycans. The trait is due to a mutation in the gene for the bifunctional ATP sulfurylase/APS kinase, resulting in reduced formation of PAPS. Brachymorphic mice also have diminished capacity for sulfation of xenobiotics. In humans, a rare inborn error of metabolism, spondyloepimetaphyseal dysplasia, results from mutations in the corresponding gene (2).

▶ Sulfate, Sulfite, Thiosulfate, and Cyanide Toxicity

Bisulfite (HSO_3^-) is used as an antioxidant and food preservative; for example, many wines are treated with bisulfite. Sulfur dioxide (SO_2) is a significant air pollutant in industrialized areas. Both of these species contain sulfur in the +4 oxidation state and, in aqueous solution, exist in equilibrium with sulfite (SO_3^{2-}). In mammals, sulfite is detoxified by oxidation to sulfate, catalyzed by the enzyme sulfite oxidase (EC 1.8.3.1) (figure 14-2).

continues next page

continued from previous page

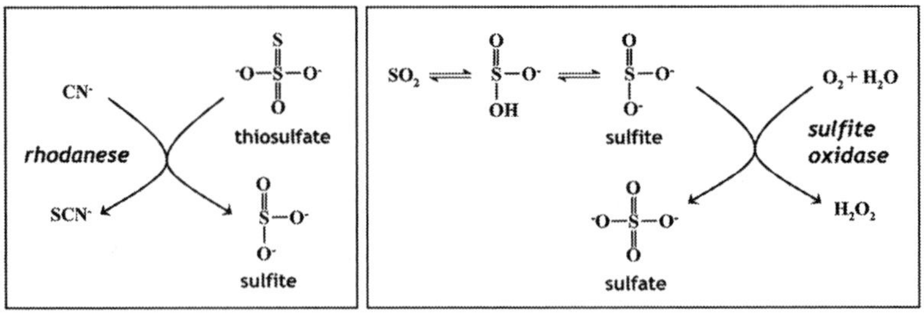

FIGURE 14-2.
Catalytic activities of rhodanese and sulfite oxidase; see text for details.

Thiosulfate (SSO_3^{2-}) plays a key role in detoxication of cyanide. Hydrogen cyanide (HCN) was discovered by the Swedish chemist Scheele in the 18th century—who died from exposure to the gas. The conjugate base of HCN, cyanide ion (CN^-), is a very strong ligand to heme iron; therefore, cyanide is a potent respiratory poison, with a lethal dose of a few milligrams per kilogram body weight. In the late 19th century, the metabolism of sublethal doses of cyanide was studied and the major product excreted was shown to be thiocyanate, SCN^-. This metabolic process, which detoxifies cyanide, is catalyzed by the enzyme *rhodanese* (3). (The enzyme's name derives from "rhodanic acid," an old term for thiocyanate. The unusual suffix "ese" signified an enzyme catalyzing the synthesis of rhodanic acid, as distinct from enzymes effecting the degradation of substrates, such as peptidases. The systematic name for the enzyme is thiosulfate sulfurtransferase (EC 2.8.1.1).) Rhodanese transfers sulfur from various donors to cyanide; the most important donor appears to be thiosulfate. The availability of thiosulfate limits the action of rhodanese; thus, cyanide poisoning can be treated by administration of thiosulfate.

It is unclear whether detoxication of cyanide is the primary physiological role of rhodanese (4). The enzyme's presence in mitochondria suggests a possible link to the respiratory chain, such as the synthesis of iron-sulfur proteins. However, cyanide is released by the hydrolysis of cyanogenic glycosides (5), such as amygdalin, found in apricot pits (figure 14-3). Bitter almonds contain enough amygdalin to produce 250 mg HCN per 100 g seeds. Cassava root, a staple starch crop in Africa, also contains significant amounts of cyanogenic glycosides (6), and the vegetable is traditionally processed by chopping the root under running water, to wash away the cyanogens. (In a tragic incident in March 2005, dozens of children died after eating improperly prepared cassava snacks sold by a street vendor in the town of Mabini, Bohol province, Philippines.) Perhaps, defense against cyanide toxicity has evolved under the evolutionary pressure of exposure to these natural product toxins.

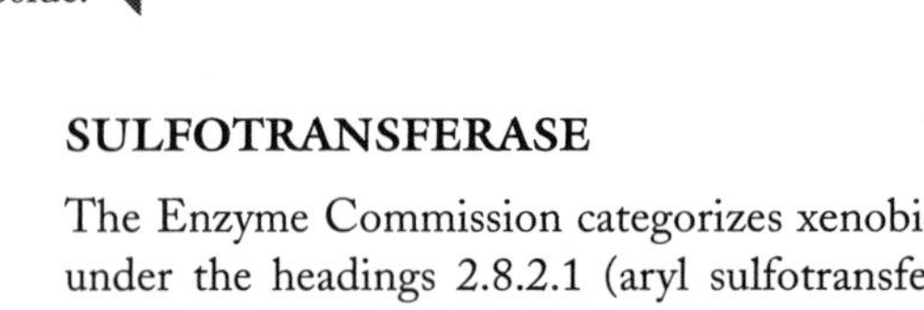

FIGURE 14-3.
Amygdalin, a cyanogenic glucoside. ◀

SULFOTRANSFERASE

The Enzyme Commission categorizes xenobiotic sulfotransferase activities under the headings 2.8.2.1 (aryl sulfotransferase); 2.8.2.2 (alcohol sulfotransferase); and 2.8.2.3 (amine sulfotransferase). Looking at the first two of these reactions, sulfotransferases catalyze the conjugation of aliphatic alcohols and phenols into sulfuric acid esters:

$$R-OH + PAPS \rightarrow R-OSO_3^- + PAP$$

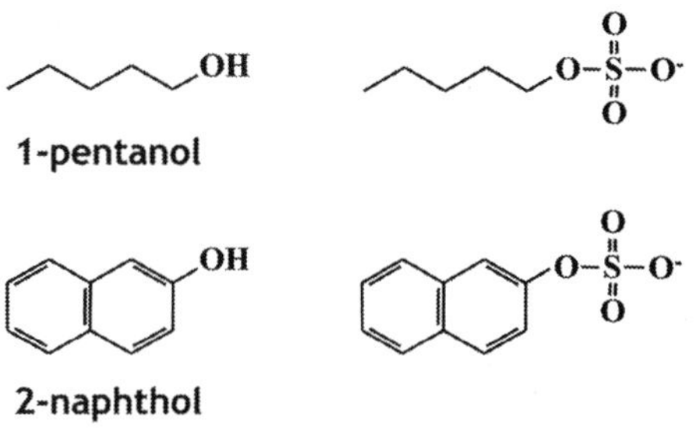

FIGURE 14-4.

Substrates (left) and products (right) of the sulfonation of a typical aliphatic alcohol (top) and phenol (bottom).

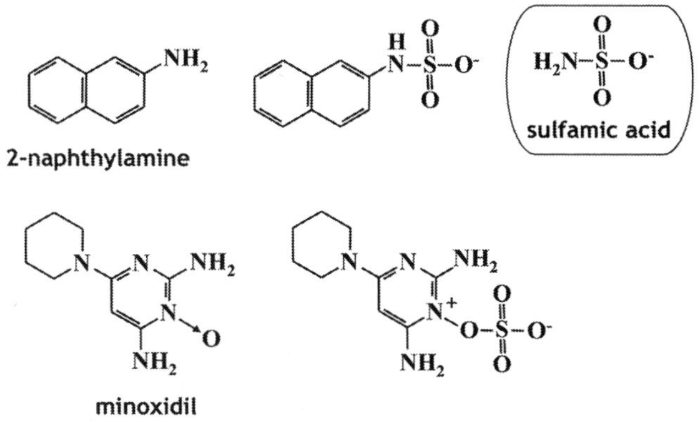

FIGURE 14-5.

Substrates (left) and products (right) of the sulfonation of a typical aromatic amine (top) and of an N-oxide, minoxidil (bottom).

Some authors describe this reaction as "sulfonation"; others prefer to call it "sulfation" (figure 14-4). Regardless of terminology, one should note that the conjugation reaction is a transfer of SO_3^-, breaking an S–O bond in one sulfate (PAPS) and forming an S–O bond in another (the alkyl sulfate product). (This reaction should not be confused with the formation of a C–S bond by the reaction of an aromatic compound (e.g., benzene) with sulfuric acid[1] a synthetic method that is also called "sulfonation.") The third process, EC 2.8.2.3, is the sulfonation of amines to give *sulfamates*, R–$NHSO_3^-$ (alkyl or aryl derivatives of *sulfamic acid*, $H_2NSO_3^-$; figure 14-5).

SULFOTRANSFERASE: ASSAYS

Fritz Lipmann, the discoverer of PAPS, developed a simple colorimetric assay for sulfotransferase activity in the 1950s. With some organic sulfates, the cationic dye methylene blue (see chapter 1) forms an ion pair that can be extracted into organic solvents and quantitated by absorbance. This assay has been used, for example, to guide the purification of a recombinant rat hydroxysteroid sulfotransferase (7). Reaction mixtures containing PAPS, dehydroepiandrosterone, and enzyme were incubated at 37°C. After addition of methylene blue solution, the incubations were stopped by addition of chloroform to extract the ion pair complex of sulfated dehydroepiandrosterone and methylene blue, and the absorbance of the chloroform layer was determined at 651 nm. This assay is only applicable to very hydrophobic alcohol substrates, such as steroids, because other ion pairs are too polar to be extracted.

Thin-layer chromatography or high-performance liquid chromatography (HPLC) can be used to separate sulfated products from substrates (8), providing the basis of a more general sulfotransferase assay. Since [^{35}S]-PAPS is commercially available, scintillation counting can be used for very sensitive quantitation of the labeled product.

The barium salts of PAPS and inorganic sulfate are insoluble, but many substrates give sulfate esters that are not precipitated by Ba^{2+}. This observation provides a straightforward assay for sulfotransferase activity, using [^{35}S]-PAPS. Radioactivity remaining in solution after treatment with Ba^{2+} is determined by scintillation counting (9).

Many of the early reports on N-sulfonation reactions used 2-naphthylamine as substrate. However, a meticulous study (10) using HPLC analysis revealed that commercial batches of 2-naphthylamine contain about 1% 2-naphthol impurity. The contaminating 2-naphthol is a much better substrate than 2-naphthylamine itself, so earlier assays of "2-naphthylamine sulfotransferase" activity were probably measuring mainly 2-naphthol sulfotransferase activity (O-sulfonation). HPLC purification of the substrate allows genuine 2-naphthylamine sulfotransferase activity to be detected. This case illustrates the importance of using highly purified substrates: even a small amount of contaminant can mask (or even masquerade as!) the desired activity.

SULFOTRANSFERASES: PURIFICATION

Several sulfotransferases have been obtained in partially pure or homogeneous form (11, 12). Purification methods typically involve ion exchange and gel filtration chromatography steps. Purification by affinity chromatography has also been accomplished. The agarose-based matrix Affi-Gel Blue (Bio-Rad) incorporates the ligand *Cibacron blue*, a dye that binds many nucleotide-requiring enzymes; this matrix was used in the purification of a rat hepatic aryl sulfotransferase (13). Hirshey and Falany (14) used ATP-agarose for purification of a minoxidil sulfotransferase; the enzyme was eluted with PAPS-containing buffer. The same group also successfully used adenosine 3',5'-diphosphate-agarose (i.e., a column bearing the PAP product of the sulfotransferase reaction) for purification of a steroid sulfotransferase (15). Recombinant human sulfotransferases have been successfully expressed as GST fusions, followed by purification on glutathione-Sepharose affinity columns and subsequent proteolytic cleavage of the GST domain, giving highly purified preparations (16).

SULFOTRANSFERASES: SPECIES DISTRIBUTION

Sulfotransferase activity has been observed in all vertebrate classes examined, including fish, amphibians, and birds. Plant sulfotransferases act on natural products such as jasmonates (17, 18). There are very few reports of insect sulfotransferase. However, an insect enzyme catalyzing a step in retinoid biotransformation is clearly a close relative of the xenobiotic sulfotransferases (19). Bacterial enzymes (arylsulfate sulfotransferases) catalyze the transfer of sulfate groups from donors such as p-nitrophenyl sulfate to acceptors such as phenol and naphthol (20), but bacterial PAPS-dependent sulfotransferases have not been observed.

HUMAN SULFOTRANSFERASE ENZYMES

Cloning of a cDNA encoding a sulfotransferase enzyme was accomplished in 1989 (21), by screening a rat liver cDNA expression library with a rabbit antiserum raised against purified hydroxysteroid sulfotransferase. Subsequently, many human sulfotransferases were cloned (22) and the completion of the human genome project establishes the existence of ten human sulfotransferase genes. Unfortunately, nonsystematic (and even contradictory) nomenclature has been applied to the xenobiotic sulfotransferases, making the research literature frustratingly difficult to follow. A sequence-based nomenclature system for xenobiotic sulfotransferase genes has recently been established (23). The sulfotransferase terminology was modeled on that of the P450 genes, with the designation SULT followed by a numeric-alphabetic-numeric classification of family, subfamily, and gene. The human SULT genes/enzymes are listed in table 14-1, following the currently recommended (but still not entirely standardized) nomenclature. Some typical substrates of the human sulfotransferases are also indicated. However, the unraveling of the relationships between the specific SULT genes/enzymes and enzyme activities for particular substrates is still a work in progress, much less well delineated than for the human P450 enzymes. There is much overlap of enzyme activities. For example, seven different SULT enzymes were reported to have catechol estrogen sulfonation activity (24); and sulfonation of the thyroid hormone 3,3′,5-triiodothyronine (figure 14-6) is associated primarily with SULT1B1, but forms 1A1 and 1E1 also contribute (25).

Thermal stability has been used to differentiate human sulfotransferases. Richard Weinshilboum and colleagues found that human blood platelet phenol sulfotransferase activity could be separated into thermostable and thermolabile (heat-sensitive) fractions, as shown in figure 14-7. The thermostable and thermolabile activities are associated mainly with SULT1A1 and SULT1A3, respectively.

STEROID SULFOTRANSFERASES

Sulfotransferases play important roles in the metabolism of endogenous lipophilic compounds, notably steroid hormones and bile salts. M.W. Coughtrie (27) points out that in humans, several classes of hormones and neurotransmitters, including catecholamines, estrogens, and thyroid hormones, circulate mainly as sulfate conjugates. (This is not necessarily the case in rats or mice, which may be poor models for the physiology of human sulfate conjugation.) Steroid sulfonation occurs in the liver and in organs that are targets of steroid hormone action, such as adrenal glands, testis, ovary, and uterus. Many milligrams of steroid hormone metabolites are excreted daily by humans, largely in the form of urinary sulfate and

TABLE 14-1.

Human Sulfotransferase Genes and Enzymes

ENZYME	TYPICAL SUBSTRATES	CHR.	EXPRESSION AND OTHER FEATURES
SULT1A1	4-Nitrophenol	16	Liver, GI tract; "thermostable phenol sulfotransferase 1"
SULT1A2			"Thermostable phenol sulfotransferase 2"; not expressed?
SULT1A3	Dopamine		GI tract, platelets; "thermolabile phenol sulfotransferase"
SULT1B1	3,3′,5′-Triiodothyronine	4	Liver, GI tract; "thyroid hormone sulfotransferase"; "hST1B2"
SULT1C2	4-Nitrophenol	2	Fetal lung and kidney
SULT1C4			
SULT1E1	17-β-Estradiol	4	Liver; fetal liver, lung, kidney
SULT2A1	Dehydroepiandrosterone	19	Liver and adrenals
SULT2B1			Skin, prostate; two splicing variants are known (2B1a, 2B1b)
SULT4A1	Unknown	22	Brain

*"Chr." indicates the chromosomal location of the SULT gene. SULT1 and SULT2 are regarded as the "phenol sulfotransferase" and "hydroxysteroid sulfotransferase" families, respectively, although this should not be regarded as a definitive classification of their substrate specificities. SULT forms 1C2 and 1C4 were, until recently, identified as forms 1C1 and 1C2, respectively. Crystal structures have been published for forms 1A1, 1A3, 1E1, and 2A1. (Adapted from Adjei, A. A.; Weinshilboum, R. M. Catecholestrogen sulfation: possible role in carcinogenesis. Biochem. Biophys. Res. Commun. **2002**, 292, 402–408; Glatt, H. Sulfotransferases in the bioactivation of xenobiotics. Chem. Biol. Interact. **2000**, 129, 141–170; Coughtrie, M. W. Sulfation through the looking glass: recent advances in sulfotransferase research for the curious. Pharmacogenomics J. **2002**, 2, 297–308.) See also (28).*

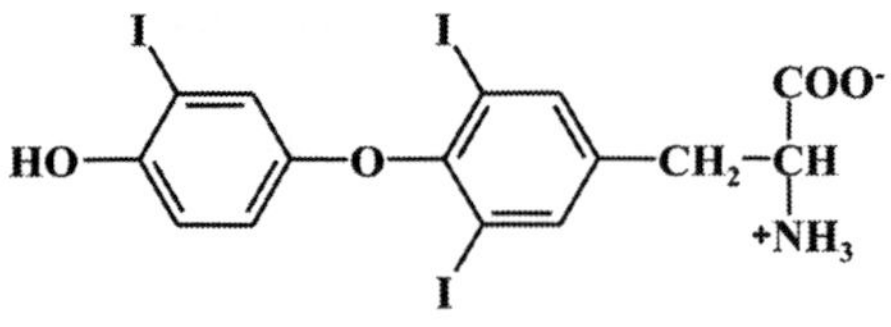

**3,3′,5-triiodothyronine
(thyroid hormone T$_3$)**

FIGURE 14-6.

3,3′,5-Triiodothyronine.

glucuronide conjugates (29). Multiple sites within the steroid ring system can bear hydroxyl groups; probably all of these sites are subject to sulfonation. Dihydroxy steroids can form disulfates, and mixed sulfate–glucuronide conjugates have also been identified (e.g., pregnanediol 3-sulfate 20-glucuronide).

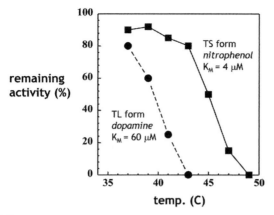

FIGURE 14-7.

Thermolabile and thermostable phenol sulfotransferase activity in human platelets. Homogenates of pooled platelets, obtained from ten subjects, were preincubated at the indicated temperature for 15 min. Phenol sulfotransferase activity was then assayed with either dopamine or *para*-nitrophenol as substrate, as noted. (*Data from Weinshilboum, R. Sulfotransferase pharmacogenetics.* Pharmacol. Ther. **1990**, 45, 93–107; Aksoy, I. A.; Weinshilboum, R. M. Human thermolabile phenol sulfotransferase gene (STM): molecular cloning and structural characterization. Biochem. Biophys. Res. Commun. **1995**, 208, 786–795.)

Some steroid sulfates are transported into cells, via specific carriers, and then subjected to further metabolism, including transformation of the steroid nucleus of the sulfate conjugate (steroid sulfate interconversion). Steroid *sulfatases*, which hydrolyze the sulfates and release the unconjugated steroids, are also known. Within the cell, steroid sulfates are mainly bound to the protein *ligandin* (glutathione transferase; see chapter 10). They are transported in the serum, bound to serum albumin and other proteins (including steroid-binding proteins) and are excreted in the urine or feces. The male sex hormone testosterone is a substrate for both glucuronidation and sulfonation, at the 17β-hydroxyl group. Estrogen (female sex hormone) steroids, such as estradiol and estrone, are characterized by an aromatic "A" ring, the absence of C-19, and a phenolic hydroxyl group at the 3-position. Estrogens are synthesized from testosterone in the ovaries, via the action of the P450 enzyme *aromatase*. Estrogen sulfotransferases, which catalyze sulfonation of the phenolic (3-position) hydroxyl, are found in liver, mammary gland, uterus, and other tissues.

Polychlorinated biphenyls (PCBs; see chapter 8) are widespread and persistent organic pollutants. Many studies have indicated that PCBs act as *endocrine disruptors*, mimicking the action of estrogen in experimental animals. However, neither PCBs nor their hydroxylated (P450-mediated) metabolites show high affinities for binding to the estrogen receptor, which appears to rule out the most obvious explanation for their estrogenic effects. Recently, however, hydroxylated PCBs were discovered to be very potent inhibitors of human estrogen sulfotransferases (*30*). This raises the intriguing possibility that PCBs act as endocrine disruptors because their metabolites inhibit estrogen metabolism, thereby increasing the levels of active estrogens in tissues.

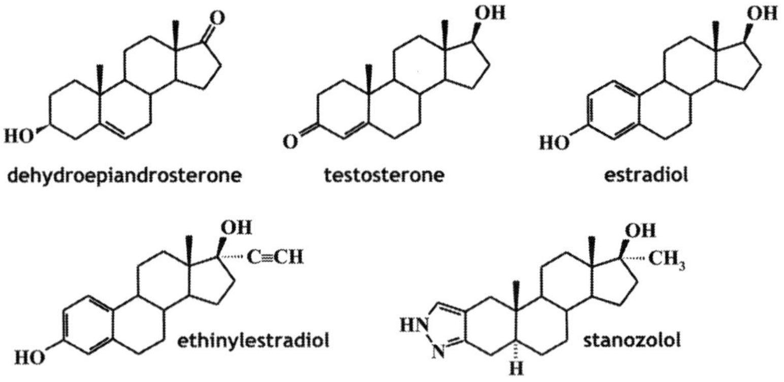

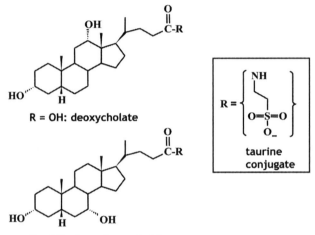

FIGURE 14-8.
Selected natural and synthetic steroid sulfotransferase substrates.

FIGURE 14-9.
Typical bile salts.

SULFONATION OF STEROID DRUGS AND CONTRACEPTIVES

Many steroid derivatives are used medicinally (figure 14-8). Ethinylestradiol is a common oral contraceptive; stanozolol is an anabolic steroid abused by athletes (*31*). These synthetic steroids are metabolized by P450-catalyzed hydroxylation and are also sulfated extensively (*32*). Knockout of the mouse SULT 1E1 gene resulted in reduced fertility, due to placental thrombosis (*33*).

BILE SALT SULFOTRANSFERASES

The major metabolic fate of cholesterol, quantitatively, is its conversion to *bile salts* (bile acids) such as *deoxycholic acid* (Greek χολή, "bile") and *chenodeoxycholic acid* (figure 14-9). The biosynthesis of bile salts begins with P450-catalyzed 7α- or 27α-hydroxylation of cholesterol, followed by further P450-catalyzed transformations (*34*). Bile salts are secreted by the liver, stored in the gall bladder, and then released into the intestines (especially after lipid-rich meals), where they emulsify dietary lipids and assist their digestion and absorption. This detergent action of bile salts is a consequence of their amphipathic structures, which incorporate both hydrophobic and hydrophilic (anionic) moieties.

The liver conjugates bile salts in several ways. The side chain C-24 carboxylate group of cholic acid can be linked by an amide bond to the amino groups of either glycine or *taurine* (cysteamine sulfonic acid). The 3α-hydroxyl group of cholic acid can also be sulfated.

As much as 50 g of bile salt is secreted daily by the adult human liver, mainly as glycine and taurine conjugates. Almost all of this material is reabsorbed by the intestine, much of it following hydrolysis of the glycine and taurine conjugates by the action of intestinal bacteria. This is another example of *enterohepatic recirculation* (also discussed in the context of glucuronidation). *This efficient reabsorption of bile salts is required to conserve the body pool of these compounds, which totals only a few grams.* Without this "recycling system," the absorption of dietary lipids would require the excretion of a comparable amount of lipid material, in the form of bile salts. In fact, less than 1 g of bile salts is excreted in the feces daily.

Under normal circumstances, very little of the bile salt pool is conjugated to sulfate. However, *cholestasis* (impairment of the flow of bile) can result from injury, disease (liver cirrhosis), chemical toxicity, or biliary atresia (obstruction of the bile ducts). This condition leads to accumulation of bile salts (and also bilirubin) in the tissues. Elevated circulating levels of these detergent molecules are acutely toxic. Under these conditions, bile salt sulfonation increases; the sulfates are efficiently cleared by the kidney and excreted in the urine. In effect, sulfonation is a back-up system for the detoxication of bile salts (*35*).

SULFOTRANSFERASES: STRUCTURE AND MECHANISM

Most xenobiotic sulfotransferases are cytosolic enzymes of about 300 amino acid residues, lacking prosthetic groups. Many, but not all, sulfotransferases associate to form homodimers (or intrafamily heterodimers) (*36*). Another group of sulfotransferases acts on large endogenous substrates such as glucosaminoglycans and heparin; these are larger, membrane-bound Golgi complex enzymes and will not be discussed here.

Since 1997, crystal structures have been published for four human sulfotransferases (*37–39*). All of the enzymes are single-domain globular proteins with similar tertiary structures (figure 14-10) and well-conserved PAPS binding sites. Most of the protein is α-helical, but a five-parallel-strand β-sheet region forms much of the active site (figure 14-11). A conserved histidine residue (His108 in SULT1A1) in the active site is of key importance; mutation of this histidine to other residues—even to arginine or lysine—abolishes or greatly reduces catalytic activity (*37*). A catalytic mechanism in which histidine acts as a base catalyst is shown in figure 14-12. The histidine imidazole ring deprotonates the alcohol substrate to give a more reactive alkoxide (or phenolate) anion and the negatively charged alkoxide oxygen then attacks the sulfur atom of PAPS to form the sulfate product and PAP.

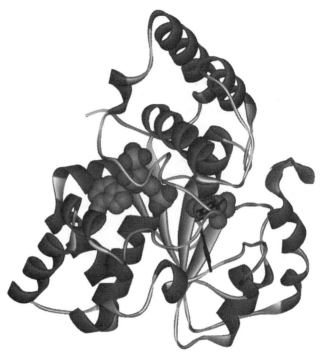

FIGURE 14-10.

Tertiary structure of human phenol sulfotransferase SULT1A1 (structure file: 1LS6.pdb). PAP (product) is shown as a space-filling model, CPK colors. The active-site histidine residue (H108) is shown as a space-filling model, pink. Two molecules of substrate *p*-nitrophenol are visible (black stick models). *Note*: A full-color version of this figure appears on the website. (*Gamage, N. U.; Duggleby, R. G.; Barnett, A. C.; Tresillian, M.; Latham, C. F.; Liyou, N. E.; McManus, M. E.; Martin, J. L. Structure of a human carcinogen-converting enzyme, SULT1A1. Structural and kinetic implications of substrate inhibition.* J. Biol. Chem. **2003**, *278, 7655–7662.*)

PAPS is bound by interactions with polar residues, including conserved serine and lysine residues. The xenobiotic substrate is held in a deep and very hydrophobic pocket, whose properties must substantially dictate xenobiotic substrate specificity. Figure 14-13 shows the constellation of aromatic (Phe and Tyr) residues surrounding the nitrophenol substrate in sulfotransferase 1A1. The hydrophobic pocket of this enzyme is large enough to bind two molecules of *p*-nitrophenol, one situated in "catalytic position," with its phenolic –OH hydrogen bonded to the catalytic histidine, and the other bound at an adjacent site. SULT1E1 binds one molecule of estradiol in a similarly hydrophobic pocket (*40*).

SULFOTRANSFERASE-CATALYZED METABOLIC ACTIVATION REACTIONS

Sulfate conjugation is implicated in the metabolic activation of several classes of toxicants (*26*). Aryl hydroxylamines (R–N(H)–OH) and hydroxamic acids (R–N(Ac)–OH) are sulfonated to give compounds of formula R–N(H)OSO$_3^-$ or R–N(Ac)OSO$_3^-$, respectively (*N-sulfonoxy* or

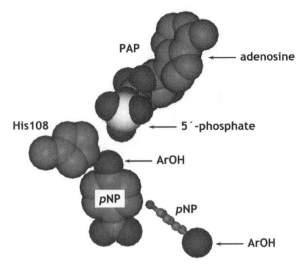

FIGURE 14-11.

Active site of human phenol sulfotransferase SULT1A1 (coordinate file: 1LS6.pdb). PAP (product), the active-site histidine residue (H108), and two molecules of substrate *p*-nitrophenol are shown as space-filling models. The substrate molecule seen perpendicular to the aromatic ring is bound by a hydrogen bond to the catalytic site histidine imidazole ring; the substrate molecule seen edge-on (ball-and-stick model) is not activated for catalysis. *Note*: A full-color version of this figure appears on the website.

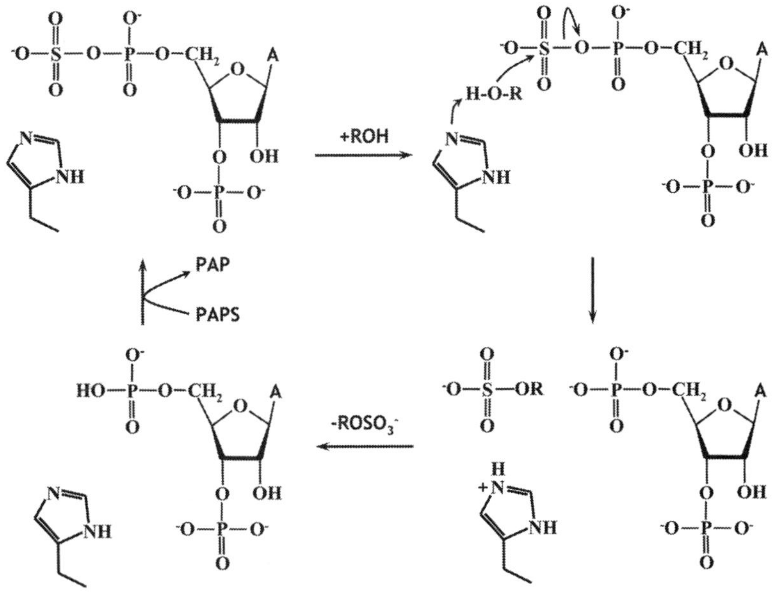

FIGURE 14-12.

Catalytic mechanism of sulfotransferase. Upper left: PAPS and the active-site histidine residue. Upper right: histidine imidazole abstracts −OH proton of alcohol substrate; nucleophilic attack of alkoxide anion on PAPS sulfate sulfur. Lower right: products are formed. Lower left: histidine imidazole protonates PAP leaving group phosphate.

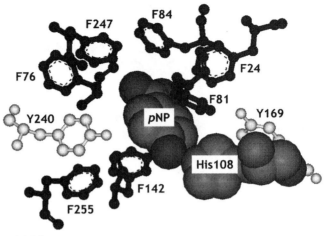

FIGURE 14-13.

Active site of human phenol sulfotransferase SULT1A1 (coordinate file: 1LS6.pdb). The active-site histidine residue (H108) and substrate *p*-nitrophenol are shown as space-filling models. Adjacent aromatic amino acid residues are shown as ball-and-stick models, colored yellow (Tyr) or blue (Phe). *Note*: A full-color version of this figure appears on the website.

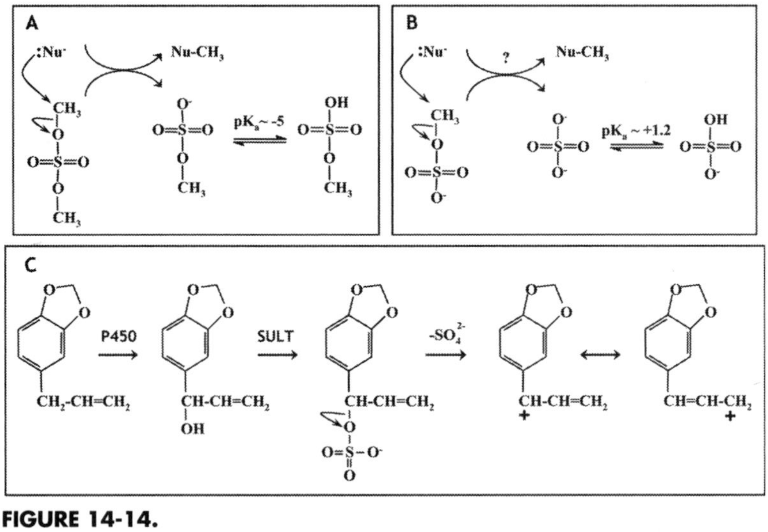

FIGURE 14-14.

PAPS-dependent metabolic activation of safrole. See text for details.

N-sulfonatoöxy compounds) (*41*). These compounds are reactive metabolites in aromatic amine carcinogenesis (*42, 43*): they generate nitrenium ions by heterolytic loss of sulfate. This metabolic activation process is also considered in chapter 17. Here, we discuss several other instances of sulfate-dependent activation.

Safrole is a constituent of natural flavorings such as sassafras and cinnamon oils; it is a rodent hepatocarcinogen when administered at high doses in the diet. Elizabeth Cavert Miller and James Miller and co-workers at the University of Wisconsin investigated the metabolic activation of safrole (*44*) and proposed the mechanism shown in figure 14-14. Safrole is hydroxylated at the benzylic carbon, in a typical P450-catalyzed reaction (see chapter 7); the resulting $1'$-hydroxy metabolite is a substrate for sulfonation. Why is the resulting sulfate a reactive intermediate? To understand this, we need to consider the chemistry of sulfuric acid esters.

Alkyl *di*esters of sulfuric acid, such as dimethyl sulfate (figure 14-14A), are potent alkylating agents, frequently used in organic synthesis. S_N2 reaction with a nucleophile (such as an alcohol or thiol) releases an alkyl sulfate ion; since this ion is the conjugate base of a very strong acid (comparable in strength to sulfuric acid), it is an excellent leaving group. In contrast, with an alkyl *mono*ester of sulfuric acid, such as dodecyl sulfate (figure 14-14B), the leaving group would be SO_4^{2-} ion; this ion is the conjugate base of an alkyl bisulfate ion, which is very much weaker. Therefore, typical alkyl sulfates are *not* electrophilic alkylating agents. However, the safrole metabolite (figure 14-14C) presents a special case. The heterolytic loss of SO_4^{2-} from this sulfate ester should be particularly facile, since it results in a highly resonance-stabilized allylic cation. The genotoxic effects of safrole and its DNA binding in rat hepatocytes are inhibited by coadministration of pentachlorophenol, an inhibitor of sulfotransferase, consistent with the postulated mechanism of activation by sulfate conjugation (*45*).

Hansruedi Glatt and colleagues have shown that benzylic alcohols of polycyclic aromatic hydrocarbons can also be activated by sulfotransferases (*26, 46*). The mechanism is analogous to that for safrole, with heterolytic loss of SO_4^{2-} generating a resonance-stabilized electrophilic cation (figure 14-15). Theta class GST enzymes can inactivate such sulfate esters (chapter 10).

The pyrimidine *N*-oxide drug *minoxidil* was originally introduced as an antihypertensive agent (vasodilator). During clinical trials, minoxidil was observed to promote facial hair growth in female patients and to be effective at reversing *alopecia* (hair loss). Minoxidil is metabolized to an N,O-sulfate ester (figure 14-5), and the sulfate appears to be the active form of the drug (*47, 48*). The sulfate is pharmacologically active in vitro (e.g., it induces relaxation of smooth muscle vasculature), although the parent

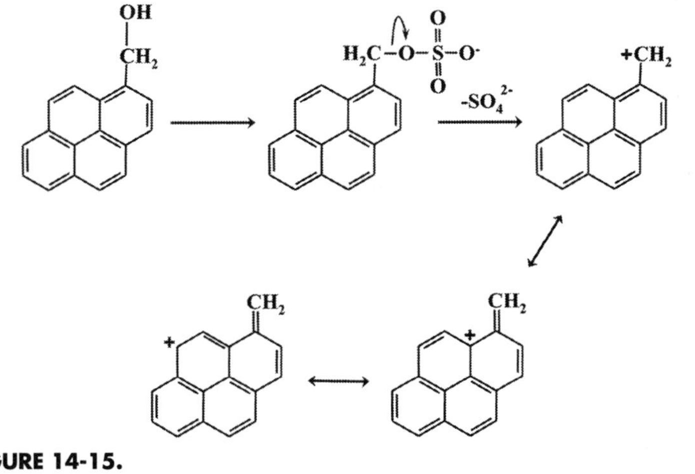

FIGURE 14-15.
PAPS-dependent metabolic activation of a polycyclic aromatic hydrocarbon benzylic alcohol (1-hydroxymethylpyrene).

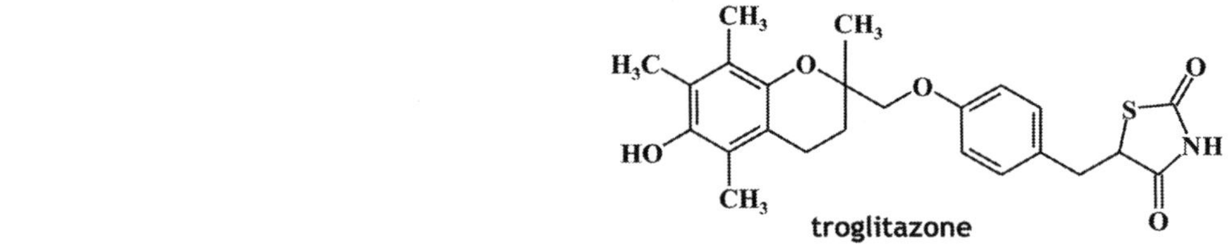

FIGURE 14-16.
Troglitazone.

compound is not. Minoxidil sulfate is more soluble in organic solvents than in water, probably because of its zwitterionic character. This unusual lipophilicity of the sulfate may account for its ability to be taken up by cells and exert pharmacological effects (*49, 50*).

The thiazolidinedione drug *troglitazone* (figure 14-16), a PPARγ agonist (see chapter 8), was marketed in 1997 as a treatment for type II diabetes (*51*), but was withdrawn in 2000, due to instances of fatal hepatotoxicity. Toxicological studies in rats revealed that the drug reduced bile flow and increased the plasma concentration of bile salts, indicating a cholestatic toxicity. Troglitazone is sulfated much more readily by male rats than by female rats, but male rats are more—not less—sensitive to troglitazone toxicity. The sulfate metabolite is a potent inhibitor of the bile salt export pump in the hepatocyte plasma membrane, whereas the parent drug is much less inhibitory. These results are consistent with the view that troglitazone sulfate is a toxic metabolite of troglitazone (*52*). (In addition, troglitazone is activated by CYP3A4 to give GSH-reactive metabolites, which may also contribute to the drug's hepatoxicity (*53*).) Troglitazone has been replaced by the drugs rosiglitazone and pioglitazone, which do not have such serious hepatotoxic side effects (*54*).

PHARMACOGENETICS

As mentioned earlier, blood platelets express both a "thermolabile" dopamine sulfotransferase (SULT1A3) and a "thermostable" *p*-nitrophenol sulfotransferase (SULT1A1). However, subsequent studies by Weinshilboum and colleagues showed that the supposedly "thermostable" enzyme SULT1A1 displays thermolability in some individuals, and this observation led to the identification of a genetic polymorphism affecting SULT1A1. A common allelic variant, SULT1A1*2, bearing the amino acid substitution R213H, shows substantially reduced expression/activity in blood platelets. Explorations of the polymorphisms of this and other human sulfotransferases, and their possible functional consequences, are in progress.

Note

1. $C_6H_6 + H_2SO_4 \rightarrow C_6H_5-SO_3H + H_2O$.

References

1. Kurima, K.; Warman, M. L.; Krishnan, S.; Domowicz, M.; Krueger, R. C., Jr.; Deyrup, A.; Schwartz, N. B. A member of a family of sulfate-activating enzymes causes murine brachymorphism. *Proc. Natl. Acad. Sci. USA* **1998**, *95*, 8681–8685.

2. ul Haque, M. F.; King, L. M.; Krakow, D.; Cantor, R. M.; Rusiniak, M. E.; Swank, R. T.; Superti-Furga, A.; Haque, S.; Abbas, H.; Ahmad, W.; Ahmad, M.; Cohn, D. H. Mutations in orthologous genes in human spondyloepimetaphyseal dysplasia and the brachymorphic mouse. *Nat. Genet.* **1998**, *20*, 157–162.

3. Bordo, D.; Bork, P. The rhodanese/Cdc25 phosphatase super-family. Sequence–structure–function relations. *EMBO Rep.* **2002**, *3*, 741–746.

4. Aminlari, M.; Vaseghi, T.; Kargar, M. A. The cyanide-metabolizing enzyme rhodanese in different parts of the respiratory systems of sheep and dog. *Toxicol. Appl. Pharmacol.* **1994**, *124*, 67–71.

5. Vetter, J. Plant cyanogenic glycosides. *Toxicon* **2000**, *38*, 11–36.

6. Yeoh, H. H.; Sun, F. Assessing cyanogen content in cassava-based food using the enzyme-dipstick method. *Food Chem. Toxicol.* **2001**, *39*, 649–653.

7. Sheng, J. J.; Duffel, M. W. Bacterial expression, purification, and characterization of rat hydroxysteroid sulfotransferase STa. *Protein Expr. Purif.* **2001**, *21*, 235–242.

8. Honma, W.; Kamiyama, Y.; Yoshinari, K.; Sasano, H.; Shimada, M.; Nagata, K.; Yamazoe, Y. Enzymatic characterization and interspecies difference of phenol sulfotransferases, ST1A forms. *Drug Metab. Dispos.* **2001**, *29*, 274–281.

9. Toth, L. A.; Kao, G.; Elchisak, M. A. Factors influencing the recovery of dopamine sulfate in the assay of phenol sulfotransferase. *Life Sci.* **1987**, *40*, 473–480.

10. Hernandez, J. S.; Powers, S. P.; Weinshilboum, R. M. Human liver aryl-amine N-sulfotransferase activity. Thermostable phenol sulfotransferase catalyzes the N-sulfation of 2-naphthylamine. *Drug Metab. Dispos.* **1991**, *19*, 1071–1079.

11. Falany, C. N. Molecular enzymology of human liver cytosolic sulfo-transferases. *Trends Pharmacol. Sci.* **1991**, *12*, 255–259.

12. Weinshilboum, R. M.; Otterness, D. Sulfotransferase enzymes. In *Handbook of Experimental Pharmacology, Vol. 112, Conjugation–Deconjugation Reactions in Drug Metabolism and Toxicity*; Kauffman, F. C., Ed.; Springer: Berlin, 1994; pp. 45–78.

13. Mangold, B. L.; Erickson, J.; Lohr, C.; McCann, D. J.; Mangold, J. B. Self-catalyzed irreversible inactivation of rat hepatic aryl sulfotrans-ferase IV by N-hydroxy-2-acetylaminofluorene. *Carcinogenesis* **1990**, *11*, 1563–1567.

14. Hirshey, S. J.; Falany, C. N. Purification and characterization of rat liver minoxidil sulphotransferase. *Biochem. J.* **1990**, *270*, 721–728.

15. Radominska, A.; Comer, K. A.; Zimniak, P.; Falany, J.; Iscan, M.; Falany, C. N. Human liver steroid sulphotransferase sulphates bile acids. *Biochem. J.* **1990**, *272*, 597–604.

16. Sakakibara, Y.; Takami, Y.; Nakayama, T.; Suiko, M.; Liu, M. C. Localization and functional analysis of the substrate specificity/catalytic domains of human M-form and P-form phenol sulfotransferases. *J. Biol. Chem.* **1998**, *273*, 6242–6247.

17. Varin, L.; Marsolais, F.; Richard, M.; Rouleau, M. Sulfation and sulfotransferases: 6. Biochemistry and molecular biology of plant sulfotransferases. *FASEB J.* **1997**, *11*, 517–525.

18. Gidda, S. K.; Miersch, O.; Levitin, A.; Schmidt, J.; Wasternack, C.; Varin, L. Biochemical and molecular characterization of a hydroxyjasmonate

sulfotransferase from *Arabidopsis thaliana*. *J. Biol. Chem.* **2003**, *278*, 17895–17900.

19. Vakiani, E.; Luz, J. G.; Buck, J. Substrate specificity and kinetic mechanism of the insect sulfotransferase, retinol dehydratase. *J. Biol. Chem.* **1998**, *273*, 35381–35387.

20. Kang, J. W.; Kwon, A. R.; Kim, D. H.; Choi, E. C. Cloning and sequencing of the *astA* gene encoding arylsulfate sulfotransferase from *Salmonella typhimurium*. *Biol. Pharm. Bull.* **2001**, *24*, 570–574.

21. Ogura, K.; Kajita, J.; Narihata, H.; Watabe, T.; Ozawa, S.; Nagata, K.; Yamazoe, Y.; Kato, R. Cloning and sequence analysis of a rat liver cDNA encoding hydroxysteroid sulfotransferase. *Biochem. Biophys. Res. Commun.* **1989**, *165*, 168–174.

22. Dooley, T. P. Molecular biology of the human phenol sulfotransferase gene family. *J. Exp. Zool.* **1998**, *282*, 223–230.

23. Weinshilboum, R. M.; Otterness, D. M.; Aksoy, I. A.; Wood, T. C.; Her, C.; Raftogianis, R. B. Sulfation and sulfotransferases: 1. Sulfotransferase molecular biology: cDNAs and genes. *FASEB J.* **1997**, *11*, 3–14.

24. Adjei, A. A.; Weinshilboum, R. M. Catecholestrogen sulfation: possible role in carcinogenesis. *Biochem. Biophys. Res. Commun.* **2002**, *292*, 402–408.

25. Li, X.; Clemens, D. L.; Cole, J. R.; Anderson, R. J. Characterization of human liver thermostable phenol sulfotransferase (SULT1A1) allozymes with 3,3′,5-triiodothyronine as the substrate. *J. Endocrinol.* **2001**, *171*, 525–532.

26. Glatt, H. Sulfotransferases in the bioactivation of xenobiotics. *Chem. Biol. Interact.* **2000**, *129*, 141–170.

27. Coughtrie, M. W. Sulfation through the looking glass: recent advances in sulfotransferase research for the curious. *Pharmacogenomics J.* **2002**, *2*, 297–308.

28. Blanchard, R. L.; Freimuth, R. R.; Buck, J.; Weinshilboum, R. M.; Coughtrie, M. W. A proposed nomenclature system for the cytosolic sulfotransferase (SULT) superfamily. *Pharmacogenetics* **2004**, *14*, 199–211.

29. Raftogianis, R.; Creveling, C.; Weinshilboum, R.; Weisz, J. Estrogen metabolism by conjugation. *J. Natl. Cancer Inst. Monogr.* **2000**, 113–124.

30. Kester, M. H.; Bulduk, S.; Tibboel, D.; Meinl, W.; Glatt, H.; Falany, C. N.; Coughtrie, M. W.; Bergman, A.; Safe, S. H.; Kuiper, G. G.; Schuur, A. G.; Brouwer, A.; Visser, T. J. Potent inhibition of estrogen sulfotransferase by hydroxylated PCB metabolites: a novel pathway explaining the estrogenic activity of PCBs. *Endocrinology* **2000**, *141*, 1897–1900.

31. Huenerbein, A.; Sipoli Marques, M. A.; Pereira, A. S.; Aquino Neto, F. R. Improvement in steroid screening for doping control with special emphasis on stanozolol. *J. Chromatogr. A* **2003**, *985*, 375–386.

32. Schanzer, W.; Opfermann, G.; Donike, M. Metabolism of stanozolol: identification and synthesis of urinary metabolites. *J. Steroid Biochem.* **1990**, *36*, 153–174.

33. Tong, M. H.; Jiang, H.; Liu, P.; Lawson, J. A.; Brass, L. F.; Song, W. C. Spontaneous fetal loss caused by placental thrombosis in estrogen sulfotransferase-deficient mice. *Nat. Med.* **2005**, *11*, 153–159.

34. Javitt, N. B. Cholesterol, hydroxycholesterols, and bile acids. *Biochem. Biophys. Res. Commun.* **2002**, *292*, 1147–1153.

35. Cowen, A. E.; Korman, M. G.; Hofmann, A. F.; Cass, O. W. Metabolism of lithocholate in healthy man: I. Biotransformation and biliary excretion

of intravenously administered lithocholate, lithocholylglycine, and their sulfates. *Gastroenterology* **1975**, *69*, 59–66.

36. Kiehlbauch, C. C.; Lam, Y. F.; Ringer, D. P. Homodimeric and heterodimeric aryl sulfotransferases catalyze the sulfuric acid esterification of N-hydroxy-2-acetylaminofluorene. *J. Biol. Chem.* **1995**, *270*, 18941–18947.

37. Kakuta, Y.; Petrotchenko, E. V.; Pedersen, L. C.; Negishi, M. The sulfuryl transfer mechanism. Crystal structure of a vanadate complex of estrogen sulfotransferase and mutational analysis. *J. Biol. Chem.* **1998**, *273*, 27325–27330.

38. Negishi, M.; Pedersen, L. G.; Petrotchenko, E.; Shevtsov, S.; Gorokhov, A.; Kakuta, Y.; Pedersen, L. C. Structure and function of sulfotransferases. *Arch. Biochem. Biophys.* **2001**, *390*, 149–157.

39. Gamage, N. U.; Duggleby, R. G.; Barnett, A. C.; Tresillian, M.; Latham, C. F.; Liyou, N. E.; McManus, M. E.; Martin, J. L. Structure of a human carcinogen-converting enzyme, SULT1A1. Structural and kinetic implications of substrate inhibition. *J. Biol. Chem.* **2003**, *278*, 7655–7662.

40. Kakuta, Y.; Pedersen, L. G.; Carter, C. W.; Negishi, M.; Pedersen, L. C. Crystal structure of estrogen sulphotransferase. *Nat. Struct. Biol.* **1997**, *4*, 904–908.

41. Yoshinari, K.; Nagata, K.; Ogino, M.; Fujita, K.; Shiraga, T.; Iwasaki, K.; Hata, T.; Yamazoe, Y. Molecular cloning and expression of an amine sulfotransferase cDNA: a new gene family of cytosolic sulfotransferases in mammals. *J. Biochem. (Tokyo)* **1998**, *123*, 479–486.

42. Gilissen, R. A.; Bamforth, K. J.; Stavenuiter, J. F.; Coughtrie, M. W.; Meerman, J. H. Sulfation of aromatic hydroxamic acids and hydroxylamines by multiple forms of human liver sulfotransferases. *Carcinogenesis* **1994**, *15*, 39–45.

43. Glatt, H. Sulfation and sulfotransferases 4: bioactivation of mutagens via sulfation. *FASEB J.* **1997**, *11*, 314–321.

44. Miller, J. A.; Miller, E. C. The metabolic activation and nucleic acid adducts of naturally-occurring carcinogens: recent results with ethyl carbamate and the spice flavors safrole and estragole. *Br. J. Cancer* **1983**, *48*, 1–15.

45. Daimon, H.; Sawada, S.; Asakura, S.; Sagami, F. Inhibition of sulfotransferase affecting in vivo genotoxicity and DNA adducts induced by safrole in rat liver. *Teratog. Carcinog. Mutagen.* **1997**, *17*, 327–337.

46. Glatt, H.; Pauly, K.; Czich, A.; Falany, J. L.; Falany, C. N. Activation of benzylic alcohols to mutagens by rat and human sulfotransferases expressed in *Escherichia coli*. *Eur. J. Pharmacol.* **1995**, *293*, 173–181.

47. Buhl, A. E.; Waldon, D. J.; Baker, C. A.; Johnson, G. A. Minoxidil sulfate is the active metabolite that stimulates hair follicles. *J. Invest. Dermatol.* **1990**, *95*, 553–557.

48. Anderson, R. J.; Kudlacek, P. E.; Clemens, D. L. Sulfation of minoxidil by multiple human cytosolic sulfotransferases. *Chem. Biol. Interact.* **1998**, *109*, 53–67.

49. Mulder, G. J. Pharmacological effects of drug conjugates: is morphine 6-glucuronide an exception? *Trends Pharmacol. Sci.* **1992**, *13*, 302–304.

50. Dooley, T. P. Molecular biology of the human cytosolic sulfotransferase gene superfamily implicated in the bioactivation of minoxidil and cholesterol in skin. *Exp. Dermatol.* **1999**, *8*, 328–329.

51. Stumvoll, M.; Haring, H. U. Glitazones: clinical effects and molecular mechanisms. *Ann. Med.* **2002**, *34*, 217–224.

52. Funk, C.; Pantze, M.; Jehle, L.; Ponelle, C.; Scheuermann, G.; Lazendic, M.; Gasser, R. Troglitazone-induced intrahepatic cholestasis by an interference with the hepatobiliary export of bile acids in male and female rats. Correlation with the gender difference in troglitazone sulfate formation and the inhibition of the canalicular bile salt export pump (Bsep) by troglitazone and troglitazone sulfate. *Toxicology* **2001**, *167*, 83–98.

53. Kassahun, K.; Pearson, P. G.; Tang, W.; McIntosh, I.; Leung, K.; Elmore, C.; Dean, D.; Wang, R.; Doss, G.; Baillie, T. A. Studies on the metabolism of troglitazone to reactive intermediates in vitro and in vivo. Evidence for novel biotransformation pathways involving quinone methide formation and thiazolidinedione ring scission. *Chem. Res. Toxicol.* **2001**, *14*, 62–70.

54. Lebovitz, H. E. Differentiating members of the thiazolidinedione class: a focus on safety. *Diabetes Metab. Res. Rev.* **2002**, *18* (Suppl. 2), S23–S29.

Part Three

▷

Molecular

Principles

Applied

to

Specific

Toxicants

ALKYLATING AGENTS

The subject of alkylating agents has far-reaching implications, ranging from the finest human achievements in medicine to the most dastardly war crimes. In this chapter we recount the history of alkylating agents and describe their chemistry, in the context of biochemical toxicology.

Alkylation refers to the attachment of an alkyl group to a lone pair of electrons on a C, N, O, S, or other atom in an organic molecule. (We use the terms methylation, ethylation, etc., for transfer of specific alkyl groups.) Compounds that can effect such reactions (figure 15-1) are called *alkylating agents*. In effect, the alkylating agent transfers a carbocation (R^+) to the nucleophile. Alcohols, amines, thiols, and other nucleophilic functionalities are ubiquitous in biological molecules. An organic chemist might carry out a methylation with an agent such as methyl iodide:

$$CH_3CH_2OH + ICH_3 \rightarrow CH_3CH_2OCH_3 + HI$$

We may distinguish between "direct-acting" alkylating agents, such as methyl iodide, and "indirect-acting" compounds, such as dialkylnitrosamines, which are metabolized to alkylating agents (e.g., by cytochrome P450-catalyzed oxidation). Alkylating agents are valuable reagents in synthetic chemistry, and they also encompass many classes of toxicologically important compounds that damage proteins (causing acute toxicity), DNA (causing mutations and killing proliferating cells), and other critical target molecules.

MUSTARD GAS

The synthetic chemistry is straightforward: mix the simplest alkene, ethylene, with sulfur chloride, S_2Cl_2. Probably, the first chemist to attempt this reaction was the Belgian Cesar-Mansuet Despretz, in the 1820s, although he did not characterize the product. The reaction was reproduced multiple times, during the 19th century, as organic chemistry developed into a mature science. The product, eventually identified as bis(2-chloroethyl) sulfide (figure 15-2), possessed a smell reminiscent of garlic or mustard. Chemists also noticed its vesicant (blistering) action on the skin, and some scientists abandoned this line of research rather than deal with the hazard. Alternative syntheses were developed and pure bis(2-chloroethyl) sulfide was a well-known compound to organic chemists before the end of the 19th century, acquiring the common name of "mustard gas" (although, at room temperature, it is actually a slightly volatile liquid, rather than a gas). The term "mustard" is now used generically to refer to any powerful alkylating agent in which a chlorine

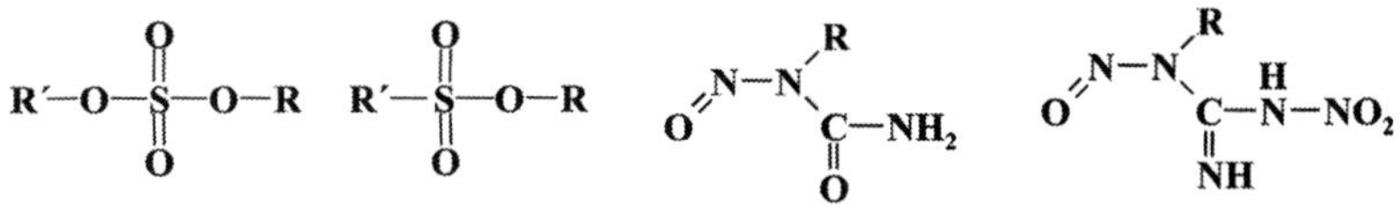

dialkyl sulfate   alkyl alkane   N-alkylnitrosourea   N-alkyl-N'-nitro-
               sulfonate   N-nitrosoguanidine

FIGURE 15-1.

Some typical alkylating agents.

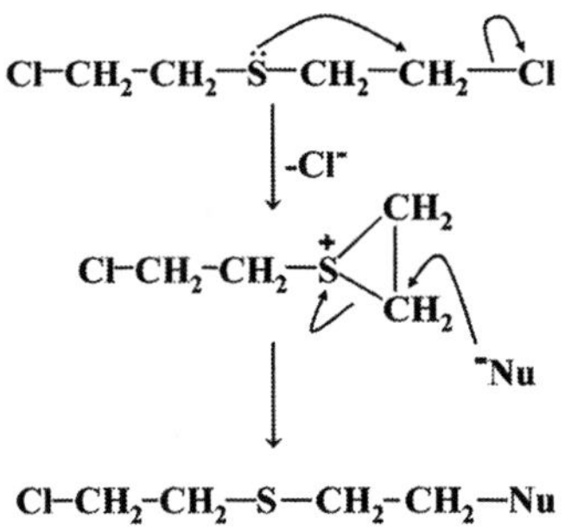

FIGURE 15-2.

Chemistry of mustard gas; see text.

leaving group is combined with an electron-rich sulfur or nitrogen atom, as discussed below.

CHEMICAL WARFARE

World War I began in August 1914. Generals trained in the military tactics of the cavalry age led their armies into the age of total war. The campaign quickly turned into a murderous war of attrition. German and Allied armies faced each other along extended front lines of trenches, protected by barbed wire, minefields, machine guns, and artillery. They were trapped in an apparent stalemate, with casualties threatening to climb beyond any nation's endurance. In the spring of 1915 the German command opted to use a new and terrifying weapon in the Second Battle of Ypres (Belgium). They moved thousands of cylinders of chlorine gas into position on the front line, waited for the wind to blow in the direction of the enemy, and then opened the valves. Dense clouds of chlorine were blown into the trenches, causing terrible casualties among the French, Algerian, and Canadian soldiers (1). The era of chemical warfare had begun.

Chlorine was cheap and readily produced, but more severely incapacitating agents were demanded. Mustard gas immediately attacks the eyes and skin, and severe exposure rapidly causes lethal lung damage (2, 3). The German army introduced mustard gas into battle at Ypres in July 1917 and, shortly afterwards, against the Russians. Both the British and French armies adopted the use of mustard gas, in retaliation, but their production capacity lagged behind that of the Germans, and the war ended (November 1918) before they had much opportunity to deploy it. The British used

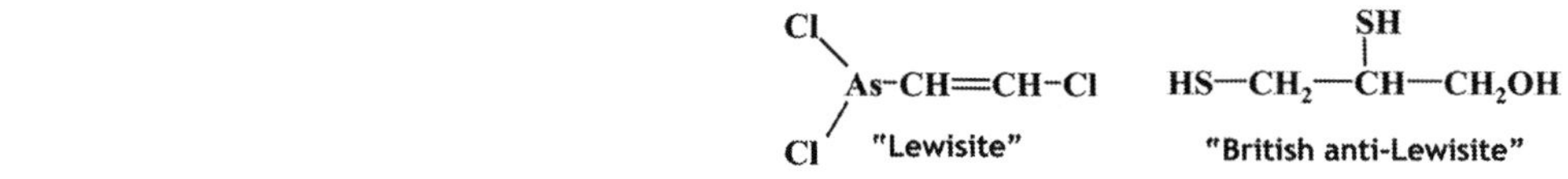

$$\begin{array}{c} Cl \\ \diagdown \\ \diagup \\ Cl \end{array} As\text{-}CH\text{=}CH\text{-}Cl \qquad HS\text{—}CH_2\text{—}\overset{\overset{\displaystyle SH}{|}}{CH}\text{—}CH_2OH$$

"Lewisite"   "British anti-Lewisite"

FIGURE 15-3.

Lewisite and British anti-Lewisite.

phosgene ($COCl_2$) gas, along with chlorine ("white star" agent) in the battle of the Somme, in 1916.

"Lewisite," named after its American discoverer, is dichloro (2-chlorovinyl) arsine (figure 15-3). Lewisite was not ready in time to be used in World War I, but was produced and stockpiled by many countries afterwards (4). During World War II, intensive research on countermeasures to chemical warfare led to the development of "British anti-Lewisite" (2,3-dimercaptopropanol), a thiol agent which could be used to inactivate lewisite (5).

Mustard gas has been a menace in many conflicts since World War I, and continues to be a threat, despite the signing (from 1925) of treaties banning chemical warfare. It was used by the Italian army in Ethiopia in 1935 and by the Japanese army occupying China during World War II. Mustard gas was available to both sides in the European theater, during World War II, but was never actually used. (Reportedly, Hitler was reluctant to do so, because he himself had been gassed, as a soldier in World War I). Ironically, the only Allied victims of mustard gas during the war were poisoned by *American* mustard gas. The US ship *John Harvey*, carrying tons of the agent, was docked in the harbor of Bari, on the Adriatic coast of Italy, when a massive German bomber raid ("the second Pearl Harbor") struck the port on December 2, 1943. The *John Harvey* was one of many ships sunk, and hundreds of casualties resulted from exposure to its mustard gas, released into the water of the harbor. Mustard gas was reportedly used by both sides during the bloody war between Iraq and Iran (1983–1988) and against Kurdish towns in northern Iraq by the regime of Saddam Hussein (figure 15-4) (6).

THE CHEMICAL REACTIVITY OF MUSTARDS

Alkylating agents are electrophiles that attack nucleophilic sites, and "mustards," such as bis(2-chloroethyl) sulfide, are especially reactive electrophiles. The mechanism accounting for this reactivity is the "neighboring group effect," also called "anchimeric assistance." The presence of a lone pair of electrons on the central sulfur atom of the mustard facilitates the loss of Cl^- and enhances the electrophilicity of the molecule (figure 15-2). Mustard gas reacts avidly with water, to give the corresponding alcohol and hydrochloric acid.

ALKYLATING AGENTS AS CHEMICAL MUTAGENS

Mustard gas was the first known chemical mutagen. The U.S. geneticist Hermann J. Müller had discovered the mutagenic action of X-rays on *Drosophila* in 1927 (see chapter 5). During World War II, he suggested to Charlotte Auerbach (7), at the Institute of Animal Genetics, Edinburgh,

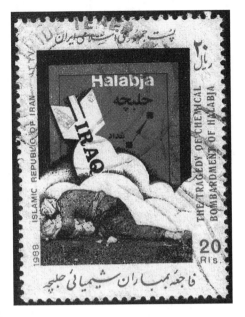

FIGURE 15-4.

Iranian postage stamp (1988) commemorating the chemical attack on Halabja, Iraq. *Note*: A full-color version of this figure appears on the website.

Scotland, that mustard gas might also be mutagenic, since its action on animals produced lesions reminiscent of those resulting from X-ray exposure. Auerbach soon demonstrated that mustard gas potently induced sex-linked recessive lethal mutations in drosophila (*8*) (see chapter 4). Because of the possibility that mustard gas would be used in the war, her findings were suppressed until 1946. With the development of short-term assays for chemical mutagens, such as the Ames test, all of the alkylating agents discussed here were found to be mutagenic (*9*).

DNA DAMAGE INDUCED BY ALKYLATING AGENTS

Alkylating agents react with all four DNA bases, especially guanine, at multiple sites (*10*) (figure 15-5). The sizes of the stars in this figure indicate, approximately, the relative proportion of alkylation that occurs

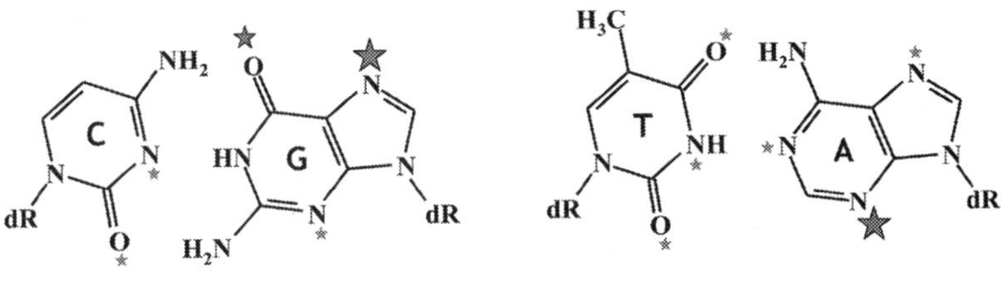

FIGURE 15-5.

Sites of alkylation of DNA bases; sizes of stars indicate approximate relative extent of reaction at each site.

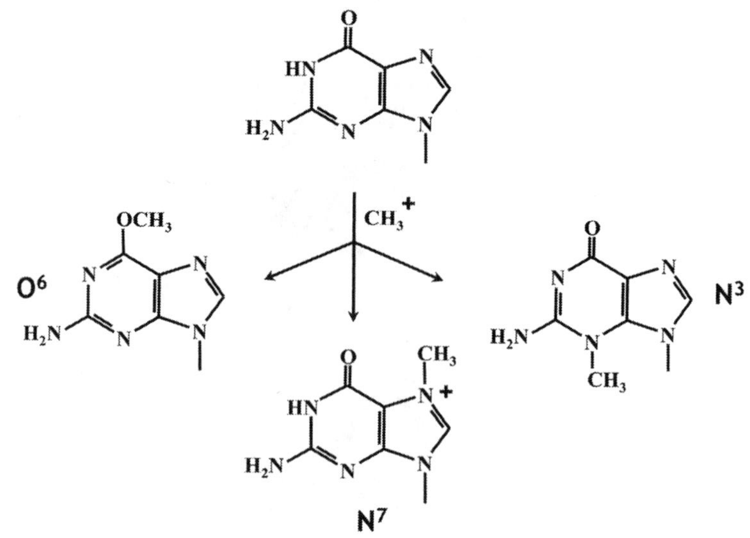

FIGURE 15-6.

Major products of guanine methylation.

at each site. Guanine N-7 is much the most reactive position (*11*), although most of the oxygen and nitrogen atoms, both within the rings and exocyclic, are alkylated to some extent (*12, 13*). Guanine N7 adduction by alkylating agents also labilizes the glycosylic bond and induces apurinic sites (*14*). (This reaction is exploited in the chemical cleavage method for DNA sequencing developed by Maxam and Gilbert (*15*).)

REPAIR OF DNA ALKYLATION DAMAGE

The O^6 position of guanine is a major site of DNA alkylation. The enzyme O^6-methylguanine DNA methyltransferase (MGMT; methylated-DNA-protein-cysteine S-methyltransferase; EC 2.1.1.63) (*16–18*) repairs guanine residues bearing methyl (and some other alkyl) substituents on the O^6 position (figure 15-6) by transferring the alkyl group to a cysteine residue in the enzyme active site (*19*). In the process, the guanine residue is returned to its intact state, and the enzyme is irreversibly inactivated: instead of acting as a catalyst, this unusual "enzyme" is actually a "once-only" reagent, or "suicide enzyme," rather than a true catalyst. The presence of such an enzyme (in organisms ranging from bacteria to humans (*20*)) indicates that alkylation has presented a challenge to cells throughout evolutionary history; the cost to the cell of "sacrificing" one molecule of protein, per alkylguanosine residue repaired, testifies to the biological importance of removal of this lesion.

E. coli has two MGMT proteins, encoded by the *ada* and *ogt* genes (*21–23*), and mutants lacking these proteins are extremely sensitive to alkylating agent toxicity. Ames test *Salmonella typhimurium* strains possess orthologous MGMT genes and the mutagenicity of alkylating agents is very much greater in mutant strains lacking these activities (*24*) (figure 15-7).

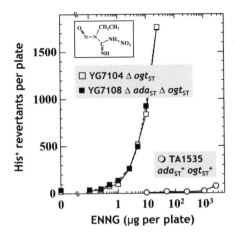

FIGURE 15-7.

Ames mutagenicity assay (see chapter 4) data for the alkylating mutagen ENNG (*N*-ethyl-*N'*-nitro-*N*-nitrosoguanidine; structure shown in inset). Three *S. typhimurium* strains were tested. Strain TA1535 (open circles) is one of original strains developed by Ames et al.; detects base-substitution mutations. Strain TA1535 has two active (wild-type) O^6-methylguanine DNA methyltransferase enzymes, OGT and ADA. Strain YG7104 is a null mutant for the gene encoding the OGT enzyme, and strain YG7108 is a null mutant for the genes encoding both the OGT and ADA enzymes. (*Data kindly provided by Masami Yamada and Takehiko Nohmi, NIHS, Tokyo.*)

Damage to normal cells limits the doses of alkylating agents that can be used in cancer therapy. Knockout mice lacking MGMT activity are more susceptible to these agents (*25*). Many researchers are studying the role of the human MGMT in alkylating agent toxicity, with a view to improving cancer chemotherapy either by sensitizing the tumor cells or protecting the normal cells (*18, 26–28*).

Recently, a very different mechanism for direct-reversal repair of alkylated bases was discovered. The gene *alkB* was identified in 1983 as an *E. coli* gene required for resistance to alkylating agents, but the catalytic mechanism of AlkB protein remained unknown. In 2002 Tomas Lindahl and colleagues (*29*) and Erling Seeberg and colleagues (*30*) independently determined that AlkB is a dioxygenase enzyme. AlkB repairs 1-methyladenine and 3-methylcytosine bases in DNA by catalyzing the oxygen- and 2-oxoglutarate-dependent hydroxylation of the methyl groups of these bases, releasing the methyl carbon as formaldehyde and regenerating the normal base. Two AlkB-homologue dioxygenases exist in humans (*31*).

THE MUTATIONAL FINGERPRINT OF ALKYLATING AGENTS

A strong mutational "fingerprint" (see chapter 4) is exhibited by alkylating agents: the induction of G:C → A:T transitions. This mutation accounts for up to 98% of the base substitutions induced by *N*-methyl-*N'*-nitro-*N*-nitrosoguanidine (MNNG) or ethyl methane sulfonate (EMS) in the

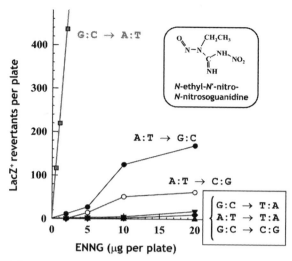

FIGURE 15-8.

Mutational specificity of *N*-ethyl-*N'*-nitro-*N*-nitrosoguanidine (ENNG) in the *E. coli lacZ* reversion assay. (*Data from Ohta, T.; Watanabe-Akanuma, M.; Tokishita, S.; Shiga, Y.; Yamagata, H. Development of new tester strains derived from* E. coli *WP2uvrA for the determination of mutational specificity.* Mutat. Res. *1998, 413, 219–225.*)

E. coli lacI gene (*32*). The same mutagenic specificity is apparent in the *lacZ* reversion assay (*33*), as shown for the ethylating agent *N*-ethyl-*N'*-nitro-*N*-nitrosoguanidine (figure 15-8).

O^6-Alkylguanine, the most significant premutagenic DNA lesion generated by alkylating agents, tends to template thymine rather than cytosine during replication, fixing G:C → A:T transitions (figure 15-9). An early explanation of this characteristic templating error was that the alkylated guanine forms a more stable hydrogen bonded base pair with thymine than it does with cytosine. X-ray crystallographic studies (*34*) of double-stranded oligodeoxynucleotides incorporating O^6-methylguanine at specific sites opposite T showed that such base pairing can occur with approximately Watson–Crick geometry (figure 15-10). However, further X-ray (*35*) and NMR (*36*) studies showed that O^6-alkylguanine can also form a "wobble" base pair[1] with cytosine, which is at least as strong as the O^6-alkylguanine–T interaction (*36*). The geometry of the wobble base pair is different from that of standard Watson–Crick pairing: the N1 nitrogen of the purine ring has slipped away from the N3 nitrogen of the pyrimidine, instead bonding with cytosine's exocyclic amino group (figure 15-10). The O^6-alkylguanine–T interaction, although weaker, adopts the standard Watson–Crick geometry, and this factor probably favors the misincorporation of thymine. As we discussed in chapter 3, the steric fit of the template base and the incoming base is the criterion that DNA polymerase uses to select dNTPs, rather than the hydrogen bonding interaction per se (*37*). The propensity of DNA polymerases to insert T rather than C opposite O^6-alkylguanine has been demonstrated directly by kinetic studies (*38–40*).

```
                    G:C ─────┐
                     │       │
                     ↓       │
                 O⁶-MeG:C    │
                   ↙   ↘     │
   ┌── O⁶-MeG:T    G:C       │
   │        │                │
   │        ↓                │
   │       G:T               │
   │        │                │
   │        ↓                │
   └──────→ A:T ←────────────┘
```

FIGURE 15-9.

Postulated mechanism of alkylating agent-induced G:C → A:T transition. The overall process is represented by the long curved arrow at right: a G:C base pair is replaced by an A:T base pair. The mutational mechanism is believed to begin with modification of a guanine base by the methylating agent, yielding an O⁶-methylguanine adduct. If unrepaired, at the time of replication, the adduct G may template a thymine base (T) rather than the normal C. (No mutation occurs in the other daughter duplex, because the undamaged C on the complementary strand acts as a template for a G.) At the next replication, the T will template an A, fixing (i.e.; making permanent) the transition mutation (curved arrow at left). Alternatively (vertical arrows) the methylated G base of the mispaired O⁶-methylguanine:T pair may be repaired (methyltransferase) to give a normal G mispaired to T, and this mispair can lead to a transition mutation.

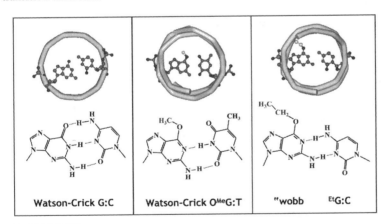

| Watson-Crick G:C | Watson-Crick OᴹᵉG:T | "wobb   ᴱᵗG:C |

FIGURE 15-10.

Base pairing of O⁶-alkylguanine residues. Left: a standard Watson–Crick G:C base pair; center: base pairing of O⁶-methylguanine with thymine in pseudo-Watson–Crick geometry; right: "wobble" base pairing of O⁶-ethylguanine with cytosine. The O⁶-methyl and O⁶-ethyl carbon atoms are shown in yellow. All views are along the helix axis. Crystal coordinates for the structures of the O⁶-methylguanine-containing and O⁶-ethylguanine-containing oligonucleotides are taken from 1D27.pdb and 1D85.pdb. Bottom: interpretive schemes. *Note*: A full-color version of this figure appears on the website. (*1D27.pdb: Leonard, G. A.; Thomson, J.; Watson, W. P.; Brown, T. High-resolution structure of a mutagenic lesion in DNA. Proc. Natl. Acad. Sci. USA* **1990**, *87, 9573–9576; 1D85.pdb: Sriram, M.; van der Marel, G. A.; Roelen, H. L.; van Boom, J. H.; Wang, A. H. Structural consequences of a carcinogenic alkylation lesion on DNA: effect of O6-ethylguanine on the molecular structure of the d(CGC[e6G]AATTCGCG)-netropsin complex. Biochemistry* **1992**, *31, 11823–11834.*)

Mammalian cell mutation assays can yield very different results from those obtained in bacteria. N-Ethyl-N-nitrosourea (ENU) induces mutations primarily at A:T base pairs in the mouse (*41, 42*). This difference may be due to much more effective repair of O^6-ethylguanine lesions relative to alkylated thymine residues (O^4-ethyl- and O^2-ethylthymidine adducts) in the mammal.

ALKYLATING AGENTS AND CANCER CHEMOTHERAPY

Mustard gas was studied as a chemotherapeutic agent against experimental rat tumors in the 1930s, but its acute toxicity precluded clinical use. The systematic development of mustard analogues as cancer chemotherapeutic agents began with the studies of Louis Goodman and Alfred Gilman (perhaps best known as coauthors of the textbook *The Pharmacological Basis of Therapeutics*) at Yale University during World War II. Their research was funded by the military, which wanted antidotes to chemical warfare agents, but Goodman and Gilman had sufficient latitude that they were able to explore chemotherapeutic applications as well. The nitrogen mustard methyl-bis(2-chloroethyl)amine was first tested as an anticancer agent in mice, and then administered to cancer patients, on an experimental basis, in December 1942. These efforts marked the beginning of modern chemotherapy for cancer (*43*). Many other nitrogen mustard derivatives, including melphalan and chlorambucil, were later developed as anticancer drugs.

Nitrosoureas were recognized as therapeutically useful alkylating agents as a result of the program of random screening by the USA National Cancer Institute, which identified the activity of N-methyl-N-nitrosourea (MNU). The chemical decomposition of nitrosoureas to generate electrophilic species is illustrated in figure 15-11. The strong alkylating agent, $R-N\!=\!N^+$, rapidly binds to a hard nucleophile, such as a heteroatom in DNA. Further drug development led to more satisfactory therapeutic alkylating agents, bis-1,3-(2-chloroethyl)-1-nitrosourea (BCNU) and other 1-(2-chloroethyl)-1-nitrosoureas (*44*) (figure 15-12). DNA is rapidly 2-chloroethylated, and the chlorine can subsequently (slowly) be replaced by a heteroatom from the adjacent strand, resulting in DNA cross-linking and inhibition of cell division. Nitrosoureas are also commonly used in experimental toxicology and mutation research. BCNU is an inhibitor

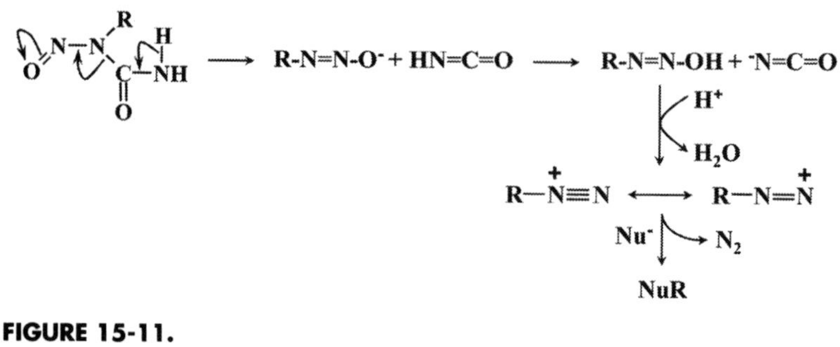

FIGURE 15-11.

The mechanism of alkylation of nucleophiles (Nu^-) by an alkylnitrosourea.

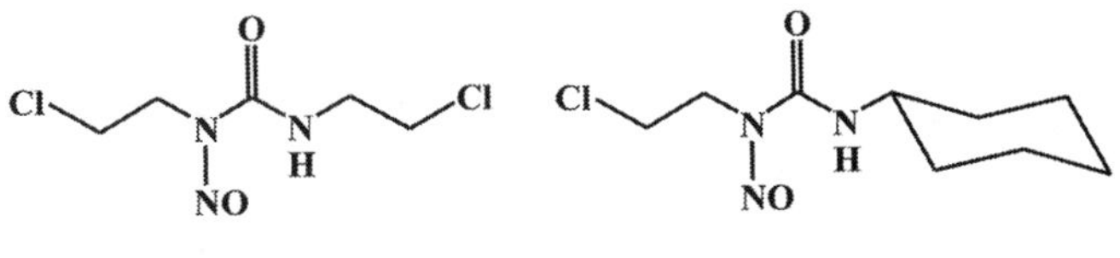

BCNU
***bis*-1,3-(2-chloroethyl)-**
1-nitrosourea

CCNU
1-(2-chloroethyl)-3-cyclohexyl-
1-nitrosourea

FIGURE 15-12.
Left: BCNU (bis-1,3-(2-chloroethyl)-1-nitrosourea); right: CCNU (1-(2-chloroethyl)-3-cyclohexyl-1-nitrosourea).

of glutathione-disulfide reductase (*45, 46*). *N*-Ethyl-*N*-nitrosourea (ENU) is a potent experimental mutagen in vitro and in vivo (e.g., (*47, 48*)).

GSTs AND TUMOR RESISTANCE TO CYTOSTATIC DRUGS

Alkylating agents have found important applications in therapeutic regimens, especially for the treatment of cancer and for immunosuppression (in preparation for tissue transplantations). These drugs include the nitrosoureas (BCNU, CCNU) and the nitrogen mustards (melphalan, chlorambucil, cyclophosphamide, and iphosphamide). However, the treatment is associated with adverse side effects on nontargeted tissues, and this severe toxicity limits the efficacy of the agents.

The idea of engineering enzymes for protection of normal sensitive tissues against alkylating drugs has been attempted for MGMT, as discussed above, and moved forward to glutathione transferases (GSTs; see chapter 10) (*49, 50*). Wild-type GSTs are not very efficient catalysts for the degradation of alkylating drugs, and improved variants are desirable. GSTs with adequate catalytic efficiency could be administered to patients by two alternative modes. One approach is ex vivo GST-gene transfer to stem cells of the bone marrow, which could then be transplanted to the patient. Another mode is topical administration of the purified recombinant GST protein to sensitive tissues.

FORMATION OF SULFUR MUSTARDS BY GSH CONJUGATION OF HALOALKANES

1,2-Dibromoethane (ethylene dibromide; EDB; figure 15-13) is a volatile compound used as a fumigant and insecticide, and as an additive in leaded gasoline. EDB is acutely nephrotoxic in human poisonings. In 1982 the National Toxicology Program, USA, reported that long-term inhalation exposure to EDB was carcinogenic to mice and rats. Ulf Rannug and colleagues discovered that the related mutagen 1,2-dichloroethane is activated by GSH conjugation (*51*) and the detailed mechanism of activation and DNA modification of dihaloalkanes has been elucidated by Fred Guengerich and colleagues, Vanderbilt University, Tennessee (*52, 53*). Remarkably, a "lethal synthesis" reaction occurs, in which GSH conjugation generates an alkylating agent with mustard characteristics. The reaction

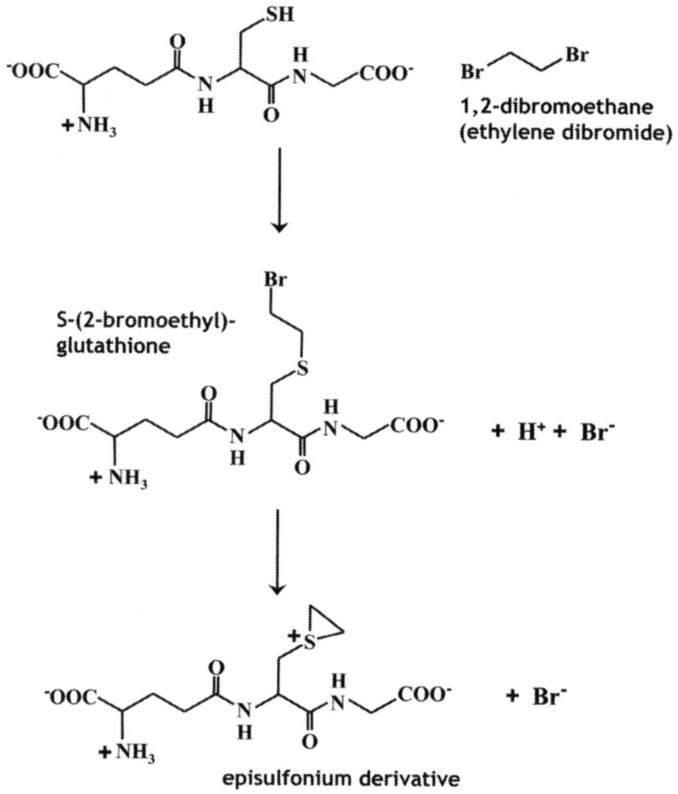

FIGURE 15-13.

GSH-dependent activation of ethylene dibromide (see text for details).

between GSH and vicinal dihaloalkanes such as EDB, catalyzed by GSTs, forms *S*-(2-haloethyl) conjugates:

$$GSH + BrCH_2CH_2Br \rightarrow GSCH_2CH_2Br + H^+ + Br^-$$

The GSH conjugate of EDB is a sulfur "half-mustard," having one halogenated group, rather than two, as in mustard gas. Such conjugates undergo cyclization (figure 15-13), giving rise to strongly electrophilic episulfonium ions, which can react with deoxyguanosine residues in DNA, cross-linking GSH to DNA via an ethylene bridge. EDB-derived DNA adducts have been isolated and structurally characterized (*54*).

FORMATION OF ALKYLATING AGENTS BY THE ACTION OF CYSTEINE CONJUGATE β-LYASE

1,1,2-Trichloroethylene was previously used as an industrial solvent for the extraction of oil from soybean meal. The protein-rich residue was used as cattle feed, until the discovery that it induced lethal aplastic anemia in the animals. The toxic agent was isolated and characterized (*55*) as *S*-(1,2-dichlorovinyl)-L-cysteine (DCVC), formed by the reaction of the solvent with cysteine residues of the soy protein (figure 15-14). DCVC is also a potent nephrotoxin in rodents.

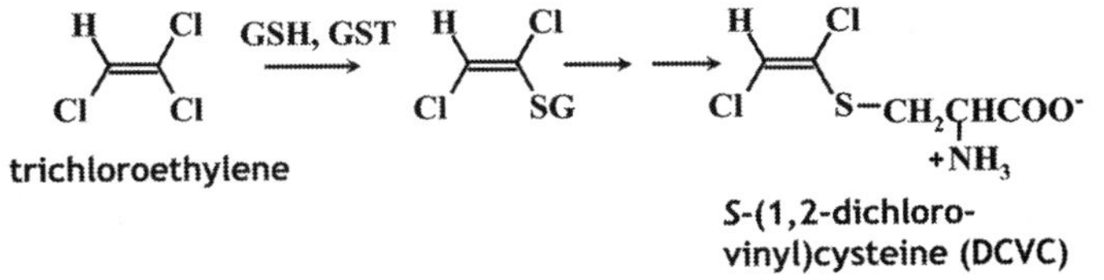

FIGURE 15-14.
GSH-dependent activation of 1,1,2-trichloroethylene (see text for details).

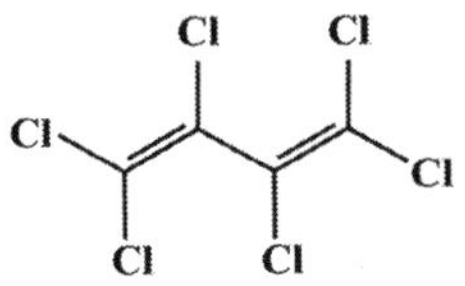

FIGURE 15-15.
Hexachlorobutadiene.

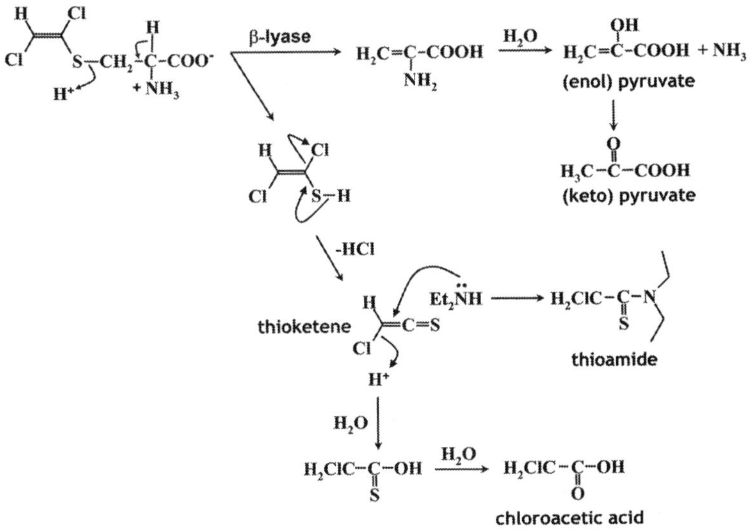

FIGURE 15-16.
Cysteine conjugate β-lyase-dependent activation of haloalkene S-conjugates (see text for details).

Chlorinated alkenes, such as the solvents 1,1,2-trichloroethylene and hexachloro-1,3-butadiene (56) (figure 15-15), are conjugated with GSH; the hepatic membrane-bound MGST1 catalyzes the conjugation. The action of γ-glutamyltranspeptidase and dipeptidase (the metabolic pathway leading to mercapturic acids) catalyzes the formation of the corresponding cysteine S-conjugates. However, rather than simply being N-acetylated and excreted as mercapturic acids (see chapter 9), the cysteine conjugate is a substrate for the kidney enzyme *cysteine conjugate β-lyase*. Several forms of this enzyme have been identified (57); most of them are pyridoxal phosphate-dependent transaminases, notably glutamine-phenylpyruvate transaminase, EC 2.6.1.64 (58). In the case of haloalkene S-conjugates, catalysis by this enzyme leads to the formation of reactive intermediates (59), as illustrated in figure 15-16 (60). The primary product of the lyase reaction is a thiol, which, in the present case, undergoes elimination of HCl to give a *thioketene* (or, possibly, a closely related species). Thioketenes, like the oxygen analogues, ketenes, are strongly electrophilic agents and react with DNA to form covalent adducts (*61*).

Note

1. In "wobble" base pairs, the relative positions of the paired bases slip slightly away from the standard Watson–Crick geometry, allowing nonstandard pairings, such as G:U. Wobble pairing was invoked by Crick (1966) to explain unusual base pairings in codon–anticodon (tRNA) interactions, and have since been observed in various nonstandard DNA structures.

References

1. Cook, T. *No Place to Run: The Canadian Corps and Gas Warfare in the First World War*; University of British Columbia Press: Vancouver, Canada, 1999.

2. Dacre, J. C.; Goldman, M. Toxicology and pharmacology of the chemical warfare agent sulfur mustard. *Pharmacol. Rev.* **1996**, *48*, 289–326.

3. Borak, J.; Sidell, F. R. Agents of chemical warfare: sulfur mustard. *Ann. Emerg. Med.* **1992**, *21*, 303–308.

4. Goldman, M.; Dacre, J. C. Lewisite: its chemistry, toxicology, and biological effects. *Rev. Environ. Contam. Toxicol.* **1989**, *110*, 75–115.

5. Vilensky, J. A.; Redman, K. British anti-Lewisite (dimercaprol): an amazing history. *Ann. Emerg. Med.* **2003**, *41*, 378–383.

6. Hawrami, S. A.; Ibrahim, N. Experiencing chemical warfare: two physicians tell their story of Halabja in Northern Iraq. *Can. J Rural Med.* **2004**, *9*, 178–181.

7. Kilbey, B. J. In memoriam Charlotte Auerbach, FRS (1899–1994). *Mutat. Res.* **1995**, *327*, 1–4.

8. Sobels, F. H. Charlotte Auerbach and chemical mutagenesis. *Mutat. Res.* **1975**, *29*, 171–180.

9. Elespuru, R. K.; Stupar, L. L.; Gordon, J. A. Discrimination of mutagenic intermediates derived from alkylating agents by mutational patterns generated in *Escherichia coli. Carcinogenesis* **1991**, *12*, 1161–1167.

10. Singer, B. Alkylation, mutagenesis and repair. *Mutat. Res.* **1990**, *233*, 289–290.

11. Gates, K. S.; Nooner, T.; Dutta, S. Biologically relevant chemical reactions of N7-alkylguanine residues in DNA. *Chem. Res. Toxicol.* **2004**, *17*, 839–856.

12. Singer, B. All oxygens in nucleic acids react with carcinogenic ethylating agents. *Nature* **1976**, *264*, 333–339.

13. Bodell, W. J.; Singer, B. Influence of hydrogen bonding in DNA and polynucleotides on reaction of nitrogens and oxygens toward ethylnitrosourea. *Biochemistry* **1979**, *18*, 2860–2863.

14. Singer, B. In vivo formation and persistence of modified nucleosides resulting from alkylating agents. *Environ. Health Perspect.* **1985**, *62*, 41–48.

15. Maxam, A. M.; Gilbert, W. A new method for sequencing DNA. *Proc. Natl. Acad. Sci. USA* **1977**, *74*, 560–564.

16. Demple, B. Self-methylation by suicide DNA repair enzymes. In *Protein Methylation*; Paik, W. K., Kim, S., Eds.; CRC Press: Boca Raton, FL, 1990; pp. 285–304.

17. Pegg, A. E. Repair of O^6-alkylguanine by alkyltransferases. *Mutat. Res.* **2000**, *462*, 83–100.

18. Gerson, S. L. MGMT: its role in cancer aetiology and cancer therapeutics. *Nat. Rev. Cancer* **2004**, *4*, 296–307.

19. Daniels, D. S.; Mol, C. D.; Arvai, A. S.; Kanugula, S.; Pegg, A. E.; Tainer, J. A. Active and alkylated human AGT structures: a novel zinc site, inhibitor and extrahelical base binding. *EMBO J.* **2000**, *19*, 1719–1730.

20. Tano, K.; Shiota, S.; Collier, J.; Foote, R. S.; Mitra, S. Isolation and structural characterization of a cDNA clone encoding the human DNA repair protein for O^6-alkylguanine. *Proc. Natl. Acad. Sci. USA* **1990**, *87*, 686–690.

21. Rebeck, G. W.; Coons, S.; Carroll, P.; Samson, L. A second DNA methyltransferase repair enzyme in *Escherichia coli*. *Proc. Natl. Acad. Sci. USA* **1988**, *85*, 3039–3043.

22. Rebeck, G. W.; Samson, L. Increased spontaneous mutation and alkylation sensitivity of *Escherichia coli* strains lacking the *ogt* O^6-methylguanine DNA repair methyltransferase. *J. Bacteriol.* **1991**, *173*, 2068–2076.

23. Samson, L. The suicidal DNA repair methyltransferases of microbes. *Mol. Microbiol.* **1992**, *6*, 825–831.

24. Yamada, M.; Sedgwick, B.; Sofuni, T.; Nohmi, T. Construction and characterization of mutants of *Salmonella typhimurium* deficient in DNA repair of O^6-methylguanine. *J. Bacteriol.* **1995**, *177*, 1511–1519.

25. Shiraishi, A.; Sakumi, K.; Sekiguchi, M. Increased susceptibility to chemotherapeutic alkylating agents of mice deficient in DNA repair methyltransferase. *Carcinogenesis* **2000**, *21*, 1879–1883.

26. Hobin, D. A.; Fairbairn, L. J. Genetic chemoprotection with mutant O^6-alkylguanine-DNA-alkyltransferases. *Curr. Gene Ther.* **2002**, *2*, 1–8.

27. Pegg, A. E.; Dolan, M. E.; Moschel, R. C. Structure, function, and inhibition of O^6-alkylguanine-DNA alkyltransferase. *Prog. Nucleic Acid Res. Mol. Biol.* **1995**, *51*, 167–223.

28. Davis, B. M.; Encell, L. P.; Zielske, S. P.; Christians, F. C.; Liu, L.; Friebert, S. E.; Loeb, L. A.; Gerson, S. L. Applied molecular evolution of O^6-benzylguanine-resistant DNA alkyltransferases in human hematopoietic cells. *Proc. Natl. Acad. Sci. USA* **2001**, *98*, 4950–4954.

29. Trewick, S. C.; Henshaw, T. F.; Hausinger, R. P.; Lindahl, T.; Sedgwick, B. Oxidative demethylation by *Escherichia coli* AlkB directly reverts DNA base damage. *Nature* **2002**, *419*, 174–178.

30. Falnes, P. O.; Johansen, R. F.; Seeberg, E. AlkB-mediated oxidative demethylation reverses DNA damage in *Escherichia coli*. *Nature* **2002**, *419*, 178–182.

31. Duncan, T.; Trewick, S. C.; Koivisto, P.; Bates, P. A.; Lindahl, T.; Sedgwick, B. Reversal of DNA alkylation damage by two human dioxygenases. *Proc. Natl. Acad. Sci. USA* **2002**, *99*, 16660–16665.

32. Horsfall, M. J.; Gordon, A. J.; Burns, P. A.; Zielenska, M.; van der Vliet, G. M.; Glickman, B. W. Mutational specificity of alkylating agents and the influence of DNA repair. *Environ. Mol. Mutagen.* **1990**, *15*, 107–122.

33. Ohta, T.; Watanabe-Akanuma, M.; Tokishita, S.; Shiga, Y.; Yamagata, H. Development of new tester strains derived from *E. coli* WP2*uvrA* for the determination of mutational specificity. *Mutat. Res.* **1998**, *413*, 219–225.

34. Leonard, G. A.; Thomson, J.; Watson, W. P.; Brown, T. High-resolution structure of a mutagenic lesion in DNA. *Proc. Natl. Acad. Sci. USA* **1990**, *87*, 9573–9576.

35. Sriram, M.; van der Marel, G. A.; Roelen, H. L.; van Boom, J. H.; Wang, A.-H. Structural consequences of a carcinogenic alkylation lesion on DNA: effect of O^6-ethylguanine on the molecular structure of the d(CGC[e6G]AATTCGCG)-netropsin complex. *Biochemistry* **1992**, *31*, 11823–11834.

36. Patel, D. J.; Shapiro, L.; Kozlowski, S. A.; Gaffney, B. L.; Jones, R. A. Structural studies of the O^6meG.T interaction in the d(C-G-T-G-A-A-T-T-C-O^6meG-C-G) duplex. *Biochemistry* **1986**, *25*, 1036–1042.

37. Kuchta, R. D.; Benkovic, P.; Benkovic, S. J. Kinetic mechanism whereby DNA polymerase I (Klenow) replicates DNA with high fidelity. *Biochemistry* **1988**, *27*, 6716–6725.

38. Tan, H. B.; Swann, P. F.; Chance, E. M. Kinetic analysis of the coding properties of O^6-methylguanine in DNA: the crucial role of the conformation of the phosphodiester bond. *Biochemistry* **1994**, *33*, 5335–5346.

39. Woodside, A. M.; Guengerich, F. P. Effect of the O^6 substituent on misincorporation kinetics catalyzed by DNA polymerases at O^6-methylguanine and O^6-benzylguanine. *Biochemistry* **2002**, *41*, 1027–1038.

40. Swann, P. F. Why do O^6-alkylguanine and O^4-alkylthymine miscode? The relationship between the structure of DNA containing O^6-alkylguanine and O^4-alkylthymine and the mutagenic properties of these bases. *Mutat. Res.* **1990**, *233*, 81–94.

41. Walker, V. E.; Gorelick, N. J.; Andrews, J. L.; Craft, T. R.; deBoer, J. G.; Glickman, B. W.; Skopek, T. R. Frequency and spectrum of ethylnitrosourea-induced mutation at the hprt and lacI loci in splenic lymphocytes of exposed lacI transgenic mice. *Cancer Res.* **1996**, *56*, 4654–4661.

42. Dobrovolsky, V. N.; Chen, T.; Heflich, R. H. Molecular analysis of in vivo mutations induced by N-ethyl-N-nitrosourea in the autosomal Tk and the X-linked Hprt genes of mouse lymphocytes. *Environ. Mol. Mutagen.* **1999**, *34*, 30–38.

43. Einhorn, J. Nitrogen mustard: the origin of chemotherapy for cancer. *Int. J Radiat. Oncol. Biol. Phys.* **1985**, *11*, 1375–1378.

44. Izbicka, E.; Tolcher, A. W. Development of novel alkylating drugs as anticancer agents. *Curr. Opin. Investig. Drugs* **2004**, *5*, 587–591.

45. Frischer, H.; Ahmad, T. Severe generalized glutathione reductase deficiency after antitumor chemotherapy with BCNU (1,3-bis(chloroethyl)-1-nitrosourea). *J. Lab. Clin. Med.* **1977**, *89*, 1080–1091.

46. Babson, J. R.; Reed, D. J. Inactivation of glutathione reductase by 2-chloroethyl nitrosourea-derived isocyanates. *Biochem. Biophys. Res. Commun.* **1978**, *83*, 754–762.

47. Burkhart, J. G.; Malling, H. V. Mutagenesis and transgenic systems: perspective from the mutagen, N-ethyl-N-nitrosourea. *Environ. Mol. Mutagen.* **1993**, *22*, 1–6.

48. Srivastava, A. K.; Mohan, S.; Wergedal, J. E.; Baylink, D. J. A genomewide screening of N-ethyl-N-nitrosourea-mutagenized mice for musculoskeletal phenotypes. *Bone* **2003**, *33*, 179–191.

49. Gulick, A. M.; Fahl, W. E. Forced evolution of glutathione S-transferase to create a more efficient drug detoxication enzyme. *Proc. Natl. Acad. Sci. USA* **1995**, *92*, 8140–7144.

50. Mannervik, B.; Etahadieh, M.; Fernandez, E.; Gustafsson, A.; Hansson, L. O.; Hubatsch, I.; Jemth, P.; Johansson, A.-S.; Larsson, A.-K.; Nilsson, L. O.; Olin, B.; Ridderström, M.; Stenberg, G.; Tronstad, L.; Widersten, M. Novel natural substrates and novel isoenzymes of glutathione transferase. *Clin. Chem. Enzymol. Commun.* **2000**, *8*, 189–202.

51. Rannug, U.; Sundvall, A.; Ramel, C. The mutagenic effect of 1,2-dichloroethane on *Salmonella typhimurium*: I. Activation through conjugation with glutathion in vitro. *Chem. Biol. Interact.* **1978**, *20*, 1–16.

52. Guengerich, F. P. Activation of dihaloalkanes by thiol-dependent mechanisms. *J. Biochem. Mol. Biol.* **2003**, *36*, 20–27.

53. Guengerich, F. P. Principles of covalent binding of reactive metabolites and examples of activation of bis-electrophiles by conjugation. *Arch. Biochem. Biophys.* **2005**, *433*, 369–378.

54. Kim, M. S.; Guengerich, F. P. Synthesis of oligonucleotides containing the ethylene dibromide-derived DNA adducts S-[2-(N^7-guanyl)ethyl]-glutathione, S-[2-(N^2-guanyl)ethyl]glutathione, and S-[2-(O^6-guanyl)ethyl]glutathione at a single site. *Chem. Res. Toxicol.* **1997**, *10*, 1133–1143.

55. McKinney, L. L.; Picken, J. C., Jr.; Weakley, F. B.; Eldridge, A. C.; Campbell, R. E.; Cowan, J. C.; Biester, H. E. Possible toxic factor of trichloroethylene-extracted soybean oil meal. *J. Am. Chem. Soc.* **1959**, *81*, 909–915.

56. Dekant, W.; Vamvakas, S.; Anders, M. W. Bioactivation of hexachlorobutadiene by glutathione conjugation. *Food Chem. Toxicol.* **1990**, *28*, 285–293.

57. Commandeur, J. N.; Andreadou, I.; Rooseboom, M.; Out, M.; de Leur, L. J.; Groot, E.; Vermeulen, N. P. Bioactivation of selenocysteine Se-conjugates by a highly purified rat renal cysteine conjugate β-lyase/glutamine transaminase K. *J. Pharmacol. Exp. Ther.* **2000**, *294*, 753–761.

58. Lash, L. H.; Nelson, R. M.; Van Dyke, R. A.; Anders, M. W. Purification and characterization of human kidney cytosolic cysteine conjugate beta-lyase activity. *Drug Metab. Dispos.* **1990**, *18*, 50–54.

59. Anders, M. W. Glutathione-dependent bioactivation of haloalkanes and haloalkenes. *Drug Metab. Rev.* **2004**, *36*, 583–594.

60. Patel, N.; Birner, G.; Dekant, W.; Anders, M. W. Glutathione-dependent biosynthesis and bioactivation of S-(1,2-dichlorovinyl)glutathione and S-(1,2-dichlorovinyl)-L-cysteine, the glutathione and cysteine S-conjugates of dichloroacetylene, in rat tissues and subcellular fractions. *Drug Metab. Dispos.* **1994**, *22*, 143–147.

61. Muller, M.; Birner, G.; Dekant, W. Reactivity of haloketenes and halothioketenes with nucleobases: chemical characterization of reaction products. *Chem. Res. Toxicol.* **1998**, *11*, 454–463.

16

Oxidative Stress in the Erythrocyte: Congenital and Xenobiotic-Induced Methemoglobinemia

THE ERYTHROCYTE

The erythrocyte (red blood cell), regarded by early microscopists as almost devoid of interest, is actually a "tiny dynamo" of biochemical activity (*1*). Erythrocytes are easily obtained, and, because of their high buoyant density, they can be isolated free of other blood cells by differential centrifugation. Mature human erythrocytes are relatively simple cells, in that they do not contain nuclei or other organelles. (Erythrocytes are derived from nucleated precursor cells in the bone marrow. Immature erythrocytes, known as *reticulocytes*, comprise about 1% of the circulating red cell population; these cells still contain ribosomes and synthesize hemoglobin. The ribosomes are lost as the reticulocyte matures into the erythrocyte.) Probably no other human cell type is as well characterized as the red blood cell, and cataloguing of the erythrocyte's enzymes and metabolites is now so comprehensive that detailed computer simulations have been constructed (*2*). Nevertheless, we are far from exhausting the list of questions about erythrocyte biochemistry (*3*).

The erythrocyte probably encounters higher oxygen tensions than any other cell in the body, other than the cells of the lung, and is particularly sensitive to oxidative stress (*4*). Most drugs and toxicants are distributed throughout the body via the blood, and so the erythrocyte cannot avoid exposure to xenobiotics. Drug-induced toxic effects on the erythrocyte will be discussed later in this chapter. Damage to erythrocytes can result in hemolysis (release of hemoglobin into the blood plasma), anemia, and kidney damage (*5*). The severity of a hemolytic response to a drug or environmental chemical can range from mild to life-threatening. Since analysis of blood biochemistry is a routine component of medical diagnosis, many inborn errors of metabolism that affect the blood, and especially the erythrocyte, are known. These "natural experiments" have provided important clues to the metabolic roles of individual enzymes.

Since the mature erythrocyte is nonnucleated, protein synthesis cannot be carried out, and so protein damage inevitably results in loss of cell function. The human erythrocyte circulates for a few months, at most, before being removed in the spleen and recycled. Hemolytic anemia does not necessarily involve direct lysis of erythrocytes in the circulating blood. Commonly, hematocrit (red blood cell content) drops because of the premature uptake of the damaged red cells into the spleen. However, when the hemolytic injury is severe, the spleen becomes engorged and the Kupffer cells of liver become active. Plasma hemoglobin levels rise precipitously, due to "spill" from the spleen and liver (and probably also due to some direct lysis of the damaged red cells within the blood stream). Hemoglobinuria and kidney damage result. Such a massive hemolytic response can occur; for example, certain highly susceptible individuals who ingest raw fava beans may lose almost half their circulating red cell mass within a day or two. This condition, termed favism, is discussed later in this chapter.

Hemoglobin, the oxygen-carrying component of the erythrocyte, constitutes more than 90% of the cell's total protein; not surprisingly, then, hemoglobin is a critical target of oxidative damage, as explored in this chapter. Besides hemoglobin, other erythrocyte proteins, including enzymes, and the cell membrane are also potential targets for oxidative damage (7).

The membrane of the erythrocyte is composed primarily of phospholipids and proteins; it combines great mechanical strength, required to remain intact throughout its traverse of the circulatory system, with the fluidity required to maintain the rheological properties of the blood. One of the most extraordinary properties of the red blood cell is its capacity to undergo repetitive deformation/reformation. The diameter of a human red cell is about 10 μm, actually larger than the width of many arterioles and venules. To traverse the vasculature, the red cell must deform its discoidal shape and become elongated while in these narrow passageways; yet, on emerging, it must immediately snap back to a biconcave disc shape, in order to flow smoothly in the major vessels, where turbulence would rapidly lead to blood clots and death. Since the mean circulation time of a red cell in a human is about eight seconds, this deformation/reformation must be performed several times per minute, throughout the cell's three-month lifetime. This resilience is made possible by the cytoskeletal protein meshwork that lies just under the lipid membrane. The "beams" of this meshwork are formed from two proteins, known as spectrins, plus ancillary proteins that anchor the protein grid to two transmembrane proteins, glycophorin and "band 3". To deform, the meshwork must be detached from the anchors and transmembrane proteins. This is thought to occur passively as the red cell enters a confining space. Reformation is thought to be an active process, requiring ATP. While the precise mechanism of deformation/reformation is not known, it is clear that the "spontaneous" deformation is not random; the points of attachment must remain in proximity, such that reattachment can occur rapidly. Damage to red blood cell membrane lipids or proteins may also lead to inactivation of the Na^+/K^+ ATPase (Na^+/K^+ pump), which regulates ionic composition and cell volume (6).

HEMOGLOBIN AND METHEMOGLOBINEMIA

Native hemoglobin contains ferrous (Fe^{2+}) heme iron; ferric (Fe^{3+}) heme, the usual oxidation state of most other heme proteins, is ineffective as an oxygen carrier. The oxygen-carrying capacity of hemoglobin is due to the ability of the ferrous iron in the heme prosthetic group to coordinate molecular oxygen:

$$Fe^{2+} + O_2 \rightleftharpoons Fe^{2+} \bullet O_2 \text{ (fast)}$$

(For simplicity, in this and subsequent equations, we will indicate only the iron and oxygen, not the heme or apoprotein. The center dot between the iron ion and the oxygen molecule denotes the bound complex.) When oxygen binds to the ferrous iron of hemoglobin, the heme switches from the high-spin to the low-spin state (see chapter 7) but does not *undergo complete electron transfer*. Nevertheless, dissociation into methemoglobin and superoxide does occur at an appreciable rate:

$$Fe^{2+} + O_2 \rightleftharpoons Fe^{2+}{\bullet}O_2 \text{ (fast)} \rightarrow Fe^{3+} + O_2^{\bullet-} \text{ (slow)}$$

Such dissociation converts a fraction of our hemoglobin to the ferric form (*7*). Ferric hemoglobin (i.e., at least one of the four heme groups oxidized) is known as *methemoglobin* (pronounced with a hard "t"; the Greek prefix *met-* means beyond, as in *metaphysics*). Enzyme systems are required to effect the reduction of methemoglobin, as we discuss later. In a healthy individual, about 1% of total hemoglobin is present as methemoglobin. The packing of the heme group inside the globin protein makes reversible oxygen binding possible; free heme is rapidly and irreversibly oxidized to the Fe^{3+} state. Elevated methemoglobin in the blood is known as *methemoglobinemia*. Thus, the cost of the red cell's work of delivering oxygen to the tissues is the constant low-level production of superoxide radical. The red cell's defense against oxidative stress comprises an array of enzymes (superoxide dismutase, catalase, glutathione peroxidase, glutathione reductase, glucose-6-phosphate dehydrogenase) that is discussed in more detail later in this chapter. Only when the rate of reactive oxygen species formation is markedly enhanced, or when the natural defenses are compromised, does toxicity ensue. One may refer to the normal steady-state production of superoxide and methemoglobin as "oxidant pressure" and to excessive production as "oxidant (or oxidative) stress."

The oxygen transport capacity of the blood is far in excess of the minimum level needed to sustain vital functions, so even a much greater level of methemoglobin (up to about 20%) may be asymptomatic. Since methemoglobin is dark blue in color, methemoglobinemia becomes apparent as *cyanosis* (blue skin coloration) at levels of about 15%. Around 50%, seizures and coma may ensue. Methemoglobinemia becomes life-threatening due to impairment of oxygen transport at levels of about 75%. Methemoglobinemia should not be confused with *hypoxia*, in which the hemoglobin lacks bound oxygen but remains in the ferrous state, or *anemia*, in which the red cell content of the blood is reduced.

Hemoglobin is a tetramer with subunit composition $\alpha_2\beta_2$. The binding of oxygen by hemoglobin is highly cooperative; the entire tetramer undergoes a cooperative conformational shift from the "tight," low-oxygen-affinity form into the "relaxed," high-oxygen-affinity form (*8*, p. 271). The presence of even a single ferric monomer subunit in a hemoglobin molecule greatly reduces the oxygen affinity and oxygen-carrying capacity of the entire tetramer.

Many different circumstances can cause methemoglobinemia, and we consider three of these causes in more detail: chemical toxicity (*9–11*), inherited abnormal hemoglobin, and inherited defects in the enzyme systems that maintain hemoglobin in the reduced state.

Since the absorbance spectrum of the heme group is substantially shifted by the binding of axial ligands, the spectrum of hemoglobin also exhibits characteristic changes (*7*). These shifts allow the detection and quantitation of the binding of ligands (e.g., oxygen, carbon monoxide, cyanide) to hemoglobin, or its oxidation to methemoglobin. Figure 16-1 lists the

Hb form	λ_{max} (nm)	
	β band	α band
Fe^{2+} (deoxy)	-	555
$Fe^{2+} O_2$	541	577
$Fe^{2+} CO$	540	569
Fe^{3+} (pH 6.4)	500	630
$Fe^{3+} CN^-$	-	540

FIGURE 16-1.
Wavelength maxima (λ_{max}) of characteristic absorption bands of various hemoglobin states.

wavelength maxima of the characteristic α and β visible-light absorption bands of these hemoglobin states.

HEMOGLOBIN AUTOXIDATION

The simplest interpretation of the mechanism of hemoglobin autoxidation (i.e., spontaneous oxidation to the ferric form by molecular oxygen) is one-electron transfer from dioxygen to iron:

$$Fe^{2+}O_2 \rightarrow Fe^{3+} + O_2^{\bullet-}$$

However, this is not the whole story; the detailed mechanism of hemoglobin autoxidation is the subject of ongoing research (*12*). In a model system (i.e., pure hemoglobin), superoxide generated by the autoxidation may spontaneously dismutate to hydrogen peroxide, which may then react with additional molecules of oxyhemoglobin (*13*):

$$Fe^{2+}O_2 + H_2O_2 + H^+ \rightarrow [Fe^{4+}OH^-] + O_2 + H_2O$$

where the product is a transient ferryl (+4 oxidation state) heme; followed by

$$[Fe^{4+}OH^-] + Fe^{2+}O_2 + H^+ \rightarrow 2Fe^{3+} + O_2 + H_2O$$

The sum of these two reactions is

$$2Fe^{2+}O_2 + H_2O_2 + 2H^+ \rightarrow 2Fe^{3+} + 2O_2 + 2H_2O$$

Thus, oxyhemoglobin acts as an antioxidant, decomposing hydrogen peroxide to oxygen and water, with concomitant formation of methemoglobin. In the erythrocyte, superoxide dismutase and catalase (or glutathione peroxidase) would also convert superoxide to oxygen and water. Superoxide itself may react with oxyhemoglobin (*14*):

$$Fe^{2+}\bullet O_2 + O_2^{\bullet-} + 2H^+ \rightarrow Fe^{3+} + O_2 + H_2O_2$$

In this reaction, a reducing agent (superoxide) generates methemoglobin and hydrogen peroxide, unleashing the oxidizing power of the hemoglobin-bound oxygen molecule. This demonstrates that *a reducing species can cause oxidative stress*. This mechanism underlies the apparently paradoxical induction of methemoglobinemia by reducing agents such as nitrite (*15*). Methemoglobinemia induced by toxicant exposures is considered at the end of this chapter.

METHEMOGLOBIN REDUCTION AND CONGENITAL METHEMOGLOBINEMIA

Congenital methemoglobinemia is caused by mutations in one of two types of gene: inherited amino acid substitutions in one of the hemoglobin polypeptide chains (hemoglobinopathies), or inherited defects in one of the enzymes that act to maintain hemoglobin in the reduced state. Typically, the hemoglobinopathies are inherited in a dominant fashion. One variant β allele (i.e., a heterozygote) will give rise to about 50% abnormal hemoglobin β chains. Since each hemoglobin tetramer contains two β subunits, about three-quarters of hemoglobin molecules will be abnormal. Homozygous defective hemoglobins are usually lethal. Enzyme defects causing methemoglobinemia are usually recessive, since even 50% enzyme activity, in heterozygotes, suffices to maintain methemoglobin at a level below that which causes disease.

Hemoglobin Variants

Adult hemoglobin (16) ($\alpha_2\beta_2$) is encoded by the α-globin gene on chromosome 16 and the β-globin gene on chromosome 11. In fact, most human have two very closely linked, identical α-globin genes, $\alpha1$ and $\alpha2$ (17). Variations in the numbers of globin genes, some of which are associated with hemoglobinopathies (thalassemias) are common (18), presumably due to facile duplication or deletion events that add or remove copies. Hundreds of variant forms of hemoglobin α and β chains have been discovered, mainly by the analysis of human blood samples by electrophoresis. The "Online Mendelian Inheritance in Man" database at NIH, USA (http://www.ncbi.nlm.nih.gov/entrez) currently lists 208 ($\alpha1$) and 59 ($\alpha2$) variants of the α chain and 516 variants of the β chain. "Hemoglobin M" variants are those in which the ferric state dominates, "freezing" the protein in the "T" state. "Hemoglobin M" variants are usually amino acid substitutions of the proximal (iron-bound) histidine F8 or the distal histidine E7. Examples include hemoglobin M Boston (α chain E7 his $\rightarrow$ tyr); hemoglobin M Iwate (α chain F8 his $\rightarrow$ tyr); hemoglobin M Saskatoon (β chain E7 his $\rightarrow$ tyr); hemoglobin M Bicetre (β chain E7 his $\rightarrow$ pro). (Each hemoglobin variant is named after the location where it was first identified.) Hemoglobin M Iwate was identified in Iwate prefecture, Honshu, Japan, where the inherited "lavender-blue" phenotype has been recorded since the 18th century.

Metabolic Reduction of Methemoglobin

Autoxidation of hemoglobin is unavoidable, even in the absence of xenobiotic stress, and hemoglobin protein cannot be replaced by the red cell. Methemoglobin must be reduced enzymatically back to the ferrous state and the superoxide/hydrogen peroxide flux generated by autoxidation must be detoxified. Both of these metabolic challenges require reducing power.

The red blood cell relies almost exclusively on blood glucose for energy. It has no mitochondria, and, therefore, cannot utilize the Krebs cycle or oxidative phosphorylation. Glucose is catabolized by glycolysis (Embden–Meyerhof pathway) to pyruvate or by the hexose monophosphate shunt pathway.

Glycolysis (glucose to lactate) is a redox-balanced process; overall, glucose is simply split into two three-carbon fragments. The cofactor

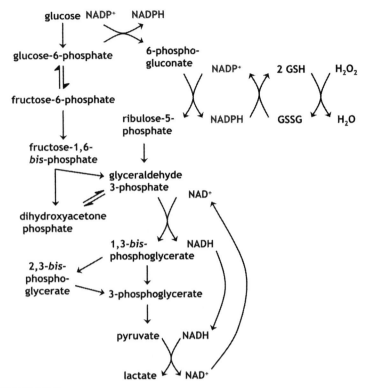

FIGURE 16-2.

Pathways of glucose catabolism in the erythrocyte.

NAD^+ required by glyceraldehyde-3-phosphate dehydrogenase is replaced by lactate dehydrogenase (figure 16-2). However, if an alternative route for regeneration of NAD^+ from NADH is available, then glycolysis can terminate at pyruvate. The reduction of methemoglobin provides such an avenue: NADH is the main source of reducing equivalents for regeneration of ferrous hemoglobin from methemoglobin.

Inherited Methemoglobinemia Due to Enzyme Defects

The study of congenital methemoglobinemia led to the first identification of a specific enzyme defect in a human inherited disease, in the late 1940s (*19*). Quentin Gibson has recently recalled the unusual circumstances that culminated in this landmark discovery (*20*):

> It all started with Dr. Deeny, a general practitioner in Banbridge, a town...some 20 miles from Belfast...Looking out of his window one morning, he saw an obviously blue man walking by; so at the end of his office hours, he called in at the local police station and asked who the blue man might be, learning that there were actually two similarly blue brothers.

Dr. Deeny was convinced of the benefits of vitamin C (ascorbate), and so he decided to try treating the "blue brothers" with it:

> He approached the brothers and offered to turn them pink, starting with Fred Martin and keeping Russell as a control. Fred's cyanosis was barely detectable after a month on 0.2 g ascorbic acid daily...At

this point, Professor Henry Barcroft, professor of Physiology in the medical school, was called in.... The diagnosis [of methemoglobinemia] was clinched by observing the 630 nm band of methemoglobin... and its disappearance after treatment with dithionite or cyanide... I knew that methylene blue had a potent effect in accelerating methemoglobin reduction and happened to wonder whether it would work in vitro.... I ... begged a sample of blood from one of the cases to try methylene blue. It did indeed work, with very rapid oxygen uptake as the methemoglobin level became reduced...

This research established that the cyanotic brothers from Banbridge had normal hemoglobin but were defective in an enzyme required to keep hemoglobin in the reduced state. Reducing agents such as ascorbate (taken orally) or dithionite (in the in vitro experiment) converted the methemoglobin back to the ferrous state. Methylene blue, as we discuss later, activates a "dormant" alternative metabolic pathway for methemoglobin reduction.

NADH-Dependent Reduction of Methemoglobin

Further biochemical studies clarified the nature of the enzyme system responsible for methemoglobin reduction. In 1959 NADH was shown to support reduction of methemoglobin in a cell-free system (21). This research, too, was provoked by investigations of methemoglobinemic patients. E.M. Scott, a physician working for the Public Health Service in Anchorage, Alaska, found that congenital methemoglobinemia was very prevalent among native people in that region. By this time, it was clear that congenital methemoglobinemia resulted from defects either in hemoglobin or in the methemoglobin reduction system, and Scott knew that his patients fell into the second category. Scott and his co-worker Isabelle Griffith used blood samples from these individuals in their experiments (21). Today, methemoglobin reductase activity could be assayed directly, by monitoring the NADH-dependent reduction of methemoglobin. However, in those days, spectrophotometers were rare (especially in Alaska!). Also, the presence of other light-absorbing species in a crude red blood cell hemolysate (osmotically ruptured cells) would have interfered with such a measurement. Therefore, a simple colorimetric assay was devised. The artificial electron acceptor dichloroindophenol (DCIP; figure 16-3) is purple in its oxidized form and colorless in the reduced "leuco" form. DCIP rapidly redox-equilibrates with the hemoglobin/methemoglobin couple,

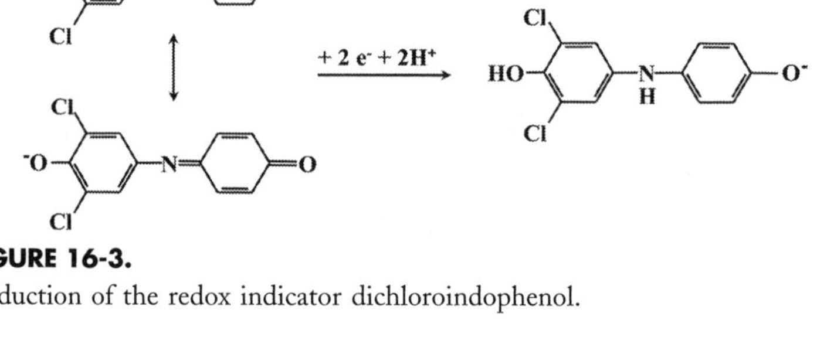

FIGURE 16-3.
Reduction of the redox indicator dichloroindophenol.

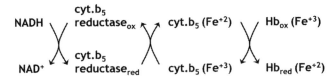

FIGURE 16-4.

NADH-dependent reduction of methemoglobin.

so reduction of DCIP can be used to monitor methemoglobin reduction. Nitrite-treated hemolyzate from normal individuals catalyzed the NADH-dependent reduction of DCIP but nitrite-treated hemolyzate from persons with congenital methemoglobinemia did not do so. This result established the role of NADH as the source of reducing power for methemoglobin reduction (figure 16-4).

Cytochrome b_5 and Cytochrome b_5 Reductase

Donald Hultquist and colleagues at the University of Michigan were studying erythrocyte redox enzymes, and discovered the presence of both a b-type cytochrome (cytochrome b_5) and a flavoenzyme that could reduce it. They found that a reconstituted system of the cytochrome plus the flavoenzyme catalyzes the NADH-dependent reduction of methemoglobin in vitro (22). The erythrocyte enzyme that accepts electrons from NADH was therefore renamed as NADH-cytochrome b_5 reductase (EC 1.6.2.2), rather than "diaphorase," the generic term for flavoenzymes capable of reducing dyes. Reducing equivalents from NADH are carried through an electron transport chain, via the flavoprotein (NADH-cytochrome b_5 reductase) and the cytochrome (b_5), to methemoglobin.

A spectroscopically similar cytochrome b_5 was already known to be involved in the hepatic microsomal electron transfer system responsible for the synthesis of unsaturated fatty acids (8, pp. 626–627). In that system, too, electrons are transferred from NADH to cytochrome b_5 via a flavoprotein. However, these enzymes are integral membrane proteins of the endoplasmic reticulum; in contrast, erythrocyte cytochrome b_5 and cytochrome b_5 reductase are cytosolic.

In 1975 a severe form of NADH-cytochrome b_5 reductase deficiency was discovered (23). In this "type II" or "generalized" deficiency, patients are not only cyanotic but also suffer severe neurological problems and mental retardation. This form of the disease affects both methemoglobin reduction and the microsomal fatty acid desaturase in other tissues and cells (e.g., leukocytes), indicating that both activities are encoded by the same gene. The erythrocyte NADH-cytochrome b_5 reductase enzyme (24) is a 275 amino acid polypeptide (figure 16-5); the microsomal enzyme has an additional 25 amino acid residue N-terminal membrane-binding signal sequence (see chapter 12). The human gene for NADH-cytochrome b_5 reductase is located on chromosome 22. The mature hepatic message contains all nine exons, but in the reticulocyte only exons 2–9 are present, accounting for the absence of the N-terminal 25 amino acids (25). The transcriptional mechanisms responsible for the alternative splicing of the gene are still being sorted out (26). More than 30 different mutations in the gene have been reported, affecting almost every exon (25). The most drastic, such as frameshifts, result in Type II disease (27). Almost six

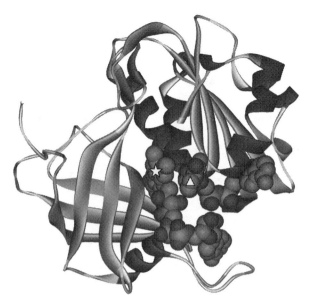

FIGURE 16-5.
Structure of rat cytochrome b_5 reductase. The FAD and NAD^+ cofactors are shown as space-filling models. The isoalloxazine ring of FAD is indicated by the star and the pyridine ring of NAD^+ is indicated by the triangle. Structure file: 1IB0.pdb. *Note*: A full-color version of this figure appears on the website.

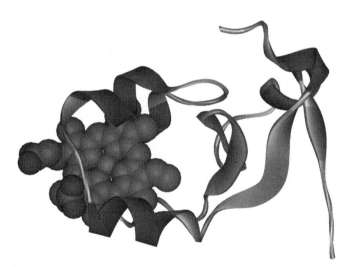

FIGURE 16-6.
Crystal structure of cytochrome b_5 (93-residue heme-binding core of the bovine enzyme, oxidized state). The heme is shown as a space-filling model. Structure file: 1CYO.pdb. *Note*: A full-color version of this figure appears on the website.

decades after he strolled past Dr. Deeny's office window, Fred Martin donated a blood sample and researchers used DNA sequencing to identify the mutations in each of his alleles for cytochrome b_5 reductase (*25*).

In the case of cytochrome b_5 (figure 16-6), once again, a single gene encodes both the membrane-bound hepatic microsomal (endoplasmic reticulum) form (134 residues) and the soluble erythrocyte form (98 residues) (*28*). The microsomal protein has a C-terminal membrane-binding "tail" that is absent in the reticulocyte form of the enzyme (*29*). Mutations in the gene for cytochrome b_5 (chromosome 18) also cause congenital methemoglobinemia. The first such case was reported from Israel in 1986 (*30*). This finding proves that cytochrome b_5 is indeed required for efficient reduction of methemoglobin. Cytochrome b_5 mutations are much less commonly reported than mutations in cytochrome b_5 reductase, perhaps because they are so likely to be lethal.

NADPH-Dependent Methemoglobin Reduction

About 5% of the flux of glucose catabolism in the red blood cell occurs via the pentose phosphate pathway. The oxidative steps of the pathway, catalyzed by the enzymes glucose-6-phosphate dehydrogenase (G6PDH; EC 1.1.1.49) and 6-phosphogluconate dehydrogenase (*8*, pp. 563 ff.), generate NADPH, and this is the only source of NADPH in the erythrocyte. In the red cell, the pentose phosphate pathway operates primarily to generate NADPH; the carbohydrate product of the oxidative reactions, ribulose-5-phosphate, is converted to fructose-6-phosphate and glyceraldehyde-3-phosphate, which re-enter the glycolytic pathway to pyruvate.

The major sink for red cell NADPH is the reduction of hydrogen peroxide via the action of catalase and glutathione peroxidase (*31*). However, an NADPH-dependent pathway for methemoglobin reduction also exists. This activity is usually "dormant," but the treatment of red cells with certain redox-active dyes stimulates this pathway, by facilitating intermolecular electron transfer processes. The best-known agent (first used by Warburg in 1930) is *methylene blue* (figure 16-7). Methylene blue can penetrate the erythrocyte membrane, and, as mentioned above, is used clinically for the treatment of methemoglobinemia. The enzyme that catalyzes NADPH-dependent reduction of methemoglobin in the presence of methylene blue (figure 16-8) had been referred to generically as

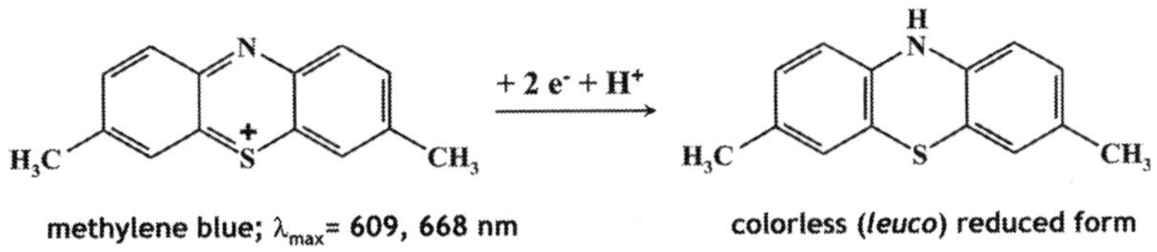

FIGURE 16-7.
Methylene blue, oxidized and reduced forms.

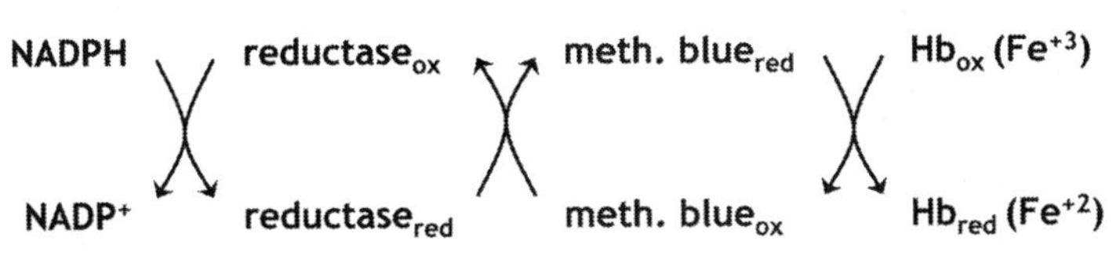

FIGURE 16-8.
The "dormant" NADPH-dependent pathway of methemoglobin reduction, which is activated by methylene blue. The flavoenzyme reductase, now identified as biliverdin reductase, has previously been given generic designations, such as "flavin reductase."

▶ The Blue Fugates of Kentucky

Congenitally methemoglobinemic population groups have arisen in many parts of the world, especially in isolated and inbred communities. One of the best-known instances is that of the "blue people of Troublesome Creek" and Madison Cawein, the doctor who came to treat them in the 1960s (34). The story was recounted by journalist Cathy Trost in 1982 (35):

> Martin Fugate was a French orphan who emigrated to Kentucky in 1820 . . . No mention of his skin color is made in the early histories of the area, but family lore has it that Martin himself was blue . . . Martin Fugate managed to find and marry a woman who carried the same recessive gene . . . Of their seven children, four were reported to be blue. The clan kept multiplying. Fugates married other Fugates. Sometimes they married first cousins. And they married the people who lived closest to them, the Combses, Smiths, Ritchies, and Stacys . . . They're known simply as the "blue people" in the hills and hollows around Troublesome and Ball Creeks. Most lived to their 80s and 90s without serious illness . . . For some, though, there was a pain not seen in lab tests. That was the pain of being blue in a world that is mostly shades of white to black . . . Madison Cawein began hearing rumors about the blue people when he went to work at the University of Kentucky's Lexington medical clinic in 1960 . . . Cawein drew "lots of blood" from the Ritchies and hurried back to his lab. He tested first for abnormal hemoglobin, but the results were negative. Stumped, the doctor turned to the medical literature for a clue . . . It wasn't until he came across E. M. Scott's 1960 report . . . that the answer [NADH-cytochrome b₅ reductase deficiency] began to emerge . . . Cawein packed his black bag and rounded up Nurse Pendergrass . . . They went over to Patrick and Rachel Ritchie's house and injected each of them with 100 mg of methylene blue. "Within a few minutes the blue color was gone from their skin," the doctor said . . . "They changed colors!" remembered Pendergrass. "It was really something exciting to see." The doctor gave each blue family a supply of methylene blue tablets to take as a daily pill. The drug's effects are temporary, as methylene blue is normally excreted in the urine. One day, one of the older mountain men cornered the doctor. "I can see that old blue running out of my skin," he confided. ◀

"diaphorase" or "flavin reductase." Hultquist and colleagues purified an NADPH-methylene blue reductase from bovine erythrocytes (*32*); the protein proved to be identical to a previously identified "green heme-binding" protein, and was subsequently identified as biliverdin reductase, an enzyme of heme catabolism (*33*). It seems likely that the ability of this protein to catalyze methemoglobin reduction via the redox carrier methylene blue may be adventitious, but it is certainly useful clinically.

Glucose-6-phosphate Dehydrogenase Deficiency

Glucose-6-phosphate dehydrogenase (G6PDH) is the first of the two pentose phosphate pathway enzymes that generate NADPH for the reduction of hydrogen peroxide in red blood cells. G6PDH deficiency is probably the most common "genetic disease" (perhaps better described simply as a genetic polymorphism) in the world, affecting · at least 400 million people (*36–38*). More than 80 polymorphic gene variants are present at frequencies of greater than 1% in the population, making this one of the most polymorphic human genetic loci known. Diminished G6PDH enzyme activity predisposes individuals to drug-induced hemolytic anemia and protects against the malaria parasite (*39*), as we discuss later in this chapter. Impairment of NADPH generation results in depletion of GSH and diminished ability to scavenge superoxide and hydrogen peroxide. Erythrocyte catalase contains bound NADPH that protects the enzyme against peroxide-induced inactivation. Reduced catalase activity in G6PDH-deficient cells contributes to their hypersensitivity to oxidants (*40*).

The gene encoding G6PDH is located on the long arm of the X-chromosome, so the phenotype is sex-linked. G6PDH deficiency in females provides a textbook illustration of the phenomenon of X-chromosome *mosaicism*. During development of the female embryo, one X-chromosome in each cell is inactivated. As a consequence, the blood of female heterozygotes contains two distinct populations of red cells, with either deficient or normal levels of G6PDH (*41*). Since the G6PDH-deficient cells are sensitive to hemolysis, such individuals often show clinical symptoms of the deficiency. Males have only one X-chromosome, and are, therefore, hemizygous. More than 10% of the male African-American population is G6PDH type A(−): the enzyme is destabilized and older red cells have very little activity. Another prevalent variant is found mainly in populations living near the Mediterranean Sea, including Sephardic Jews (*42*). These individuals are usually asymptomatic, but exposure to oxidant drugs can trigger severe hemolysis.

MECHANISMS OF METHEMOGLOBIN INDUCTION BY XENOBIOTICS

Nitrite-Induced Methemoglobinemia

The stoichiometry of nitrite-induced methemoglobin formation can be represented as:

$$4Fe^{2+}O_2 + 4NO_2^- + 4H^+ \rightarrow 4Fe^{3+} + 4NO_3^- + O_2 + 2H_2O$$

Both nitrite and hemoglobin are oxidized in this reaction; the oxidant is molecular oxygen. The kinetics of the process are characterized by an initial lag phase and a subsequent autocatalytic phase (*43, 44*).

Sodium nitrite ($NaNO_2$) is commonly used as a meat preservative (*45, 46*) and excessive dietary exposure to nitrite can result in acquired methemoglobinemia. An outbreak of methemoglobinemia in Dublin, Ireland, was traced to a butcher's careless application of nitrite to pork at a level almost 100 times above the legal limit (*47*). One man who had eaten the pickled pork became cyanotic and was brought to the emergency room unconscious; his methemoglobin level reached 66%, but he soon recovered after injection of methylene blue.

Nitrate (NO_3^-) salts are very important fertilizers and can contaminate ground water in agricultural areas (*48*). Nitrate can be reduced to nitrite by intestinal microflora, resulting in risk of methemoglobinemia. For example, a recent clinical account from the farm state of Wisconsin, USA (*49*) reports several cases of methemoglobinemia in infants whose formula had been prepared with water from nitrate-contaminated wells.

Phenylhydrazine; Heinz Bodies

Phenylhydrazine (phenyl–NH–NH$_2$) was used in the experimental induction of methemoglobinemia as early as the 19th century. In 1890 the German physician Robert Heinz noted that red cells from guinea pigs treated with acetylphenylhydrazine acquired an unusual appearance under the microscope: the cells accumulated a number of very dense granules, now known as *Heinz bodies*. These granules are aggregates composed of degraded, insoluble pigments derived from hemoglobin oxidation. Methemoglobinemia does not necessarily lead to Heinz body accumulation, but many agents cause both effects. Heinz bodies interfere with red cell fluidity and function, and mark the cell for repair or elimination by the spleen. (Heinz bodies are commonly observed in the red blood cells of healthy cats; the basis of this peculiarity is still obscure (50).)

MALARIA AND OXIDATIVE STRESS

Malaria is an infection by protozoa of the genus *Plasmodium*. Malaria is one of the most widespread parasitic diseases in the world. More than 200 million people suffer from its effects and at least one million die each year. Most of these people live in the tropical countries of Africa, South America, and Asia, although malaria was once endemic as far north as Canada and even Siberia (51).

The parasite undergoes sexual development in the anopheles mosquito (figure 16-9) and malaria is transmitted to humans by its bite. Several different species of parasite are known, and produce characteristic forms of the disease. Infections with *Plasmodium falciparum*, the most debilitating species, are often fatal; *Plasmodium vivax* disease is usually less severe. The parasite undergoes a complex life cycle, multiplying in both the human liver and the erythrocyte. As with other parasitic diseases, chemotherapy is difficult. The similarity between the metabolism of the parasite and that of the human host can frustrate the design of selective chemical agents.

Several lines of evidence support the view that oxidative stress can play a significant role in the treatment of malaria; nevertheless, the connection cannot yet be considered proven (52, 53). In tissue culture, the malaria parasite grows best at low partial pressures of oxygen (about 2%). Indeed, laboratory culture of the parasite was difficult until this oxygen sensitivity was appreciated. The metabolic basis of this sensitivity is unclear, but it may be related to the parasite's difficulty dealing with the heme released by catabolism of hemoglobin. The malaria parasite is also sensitive to pro-oxidant drugs, such as phenylhydrazine, divicine, alloxan, and the Chinese traditional medicine qinghaosu (artemisinin (54)). Many antimalarial drugs induce red cell oxidative stress, methemoglobinemia, glutathione depletion, and even hemolysis. These drugs act, at least in part, by placing increased oxidative stress on the parasite.

Many variant hemoglobins (e.g., thalassemias and hemoglobin S, which causes sickle cell anemia) and inherited deficiencies of erythrocyte metabolism (e.g., G6PDH deficiency) are common in the regions of the world where malaria is endemic, as was first pointed out by J.B.S. Haldane (55). Haldane suggested that these alleles persist because the heterozygotes (carriers) are relatively resistant to malaria infection. Malaria is such a common and serious disease that it may be one of the strongest selective pressures on the human population in these regions. Recent molecular genetic studies support this interpretation (56, 57). Experimental studies have shown that the malaria parasite's growth is impeded in G6PdH-deficient red blood cells (58, 59) (reviewed in (39)).

Favism

Favism (60) is acute hemolytic anemia that occurs after ingestion of the Mediterranean broad bean (*Vicia faba*). This bean is a common foodstuff in Italy, Greece, and Middle Eastern countries. Only certain individuals are sensitive, and G6PDH deficiency is an important (but not the only)

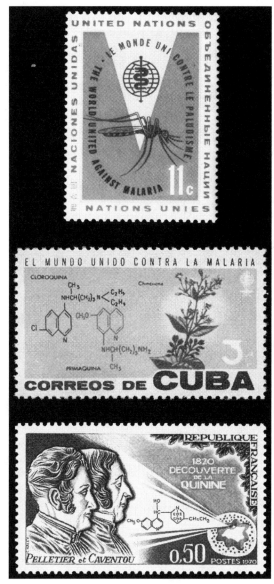

FIGURE 16-9.

The world united against malaria (1962); United Nations stamp showing anopheles mosquito; Cuban stamp showing cinchona plant and chemical formulae for chloroquine and primaquine; French stamp showing chemical formula for quinine. *Note*: A full-color version of this figure appears on the website. (*Cuban and French stamp images kindly provided by Stanford Shulman, M.D.; Chief, Division of Infectious Diseases, Children's Memorial Hospital, Chicago.*)

contributing factor. It is said that the mathematician Pythagoras advised his followers not to eat fava beans—perhaps an indication that this condition was already appreciated in antiquity. The main active constituents of the fava bean are believed to be the glycosides *vicine* and *convicine*. Bacteria in the gut hydrolyze these glycosides to the active aglycones divicine and isouramil (*61*) (figure 16-10).

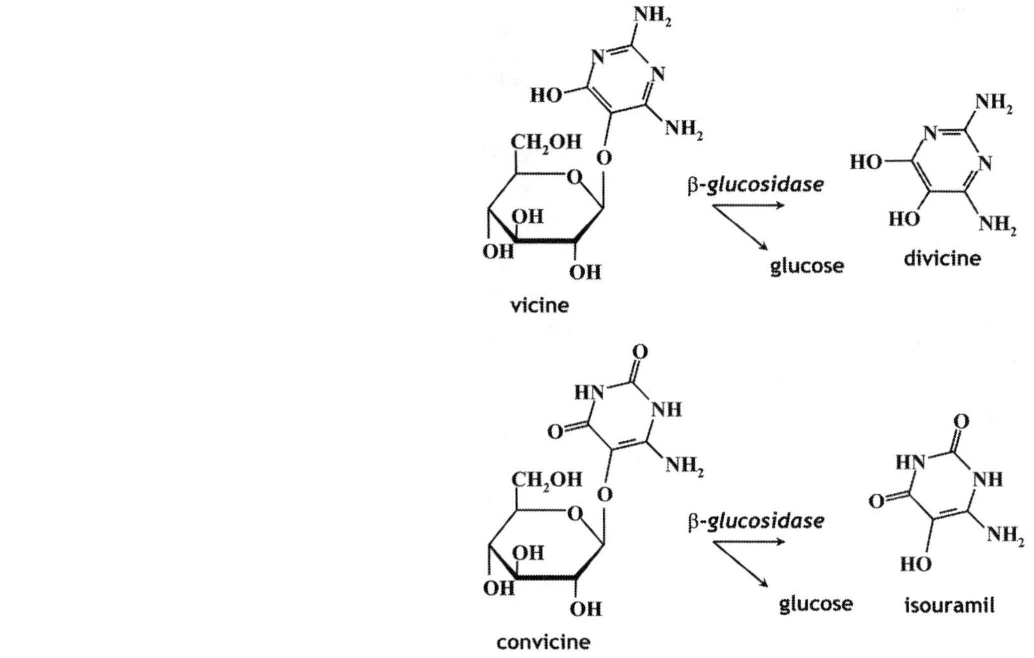

FIGURE 16-10.

Hydrolysis of glycosides.

Since G6PDH-deficient individuals are particularly susceptible to favism, the local diet should have selected against, rather than for, this enzyme deficiency. But the predilection for eating fava beans may have been driven by the same selective pressure: malaria. Vicine probably has some antimalarial activity and "a staple diet of fava beans may have been the equivalent of a regular intake of prophylactic doses of antimalarial drugs over many generations" (62).

Development of Quinoline Antimalarial Drugs

Malaria was a major impediment to the expansion of European colonial empires into tropical countries in Africa, South America, and Asia. Native people in South America knew that the bark of the indigenous cinchona tree could be brewed to make a tea that alleviated the symptoms of the disease. The Spanish colonialists quickly appreciated the value of this remedy, which became known in Europe as "Jesuit tea" and they were desperate to prevent acquisition of the plant by competing European powers. The struggle for control of the secret of the cinchona tree is described in a recent best-selling book (63). The active ingredient of cinchona bark is the alkaloid quinine (figure 16-11). (As mentioned in chapter 17, this is the compound that William Henry Perkin was attempting to synthesize when he accidentally discovered mauveine.)

In a historical echo of the colonial wars of the 16th century, malaria again became a crucial factor in warfare in the 20th century, when allied troops fought in the Pacific theater of World War II and again in the Korean War. The USA began an enormous screening and testing program, aimed at finding substances that could combat mosquitoes (the insecticide

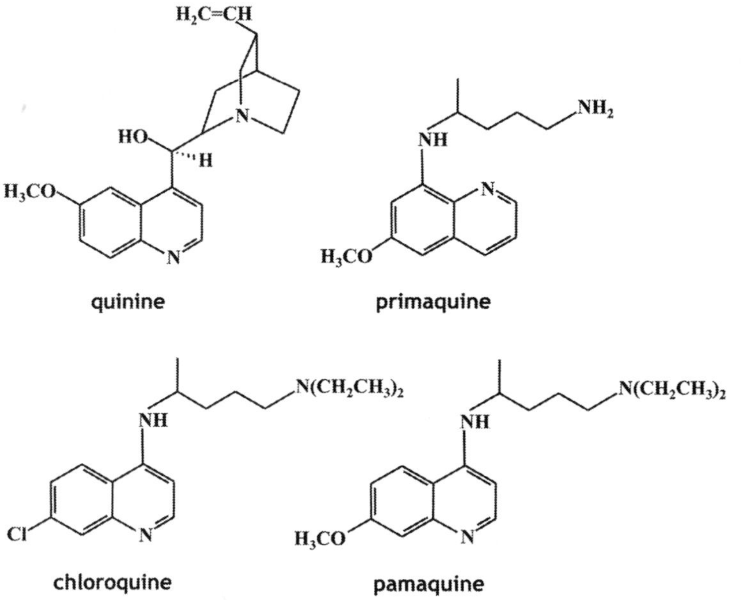

FIGURE 16-11.

The natural product quinine, and some synthetic quinoline antimalarial drugs.

dichlorodiphenyl-trichloroethane, DDT, and the mosquito repellant *N,N*-diethyl-*m*-toluamide, DEET (*64*)) and treat malaria. These efforts led to the development of the quinoline antimalarial agents, drugs that remain in wide use today (*65*):

> Clinical investigations having as their primary aim the finding of new and better anti-malarial drugs...were greatly expanded after the fall of the Dutch East Indies, the source of 90% of the world's quinine, in the spring of 1942...[T]he first phase of investigation...led to the correct use of quinacrine (Atabrine)...[which] had a spectacular effect on the malaria rate in troops during World War II...The upshot of these investigations was a rediscovery of the usefulness of the 4-aminoquinolines and the development of...chloroquine...which was used most successfully as a suppressive agent in Korea...Over 14,000 drugs were explored in all and about 100 reached the clinical level. The third phase of World War II investigations was begun...when it was found that drugs having suppressive effect far greater than Atabrine or quinine still did not cause radical cure, that is, did not prevent relapses in vivax infections. The new orientation began with the re-testing of...pamaquine. Pamaquine, an 8-aminoquinoline, had previously been found to have curative properties by British investigators but had proved too toxic for practical use. Final investigations...led to the demonstration of the clinical usefulness of several analogues of pamaquine— pentaquine in 1946, isopentaquine in 1948 and finally primaquine in 1950—as successively more effective curative anti-malarial agents in vivax infections...[1]

When U.S. soldiers were administered the drug *primaquine*, as a routine antimalarial prophylactic, during the war in Korea, primaquine sensitivity manifesting as hemolytic anemia became a serious issue (http://history.amedd.army.mil/booksdocs/KOREA/recad2/ch5-2.htm). This side effect occurred mainly in personnel of black African or Mediterranean backgrounds: the culprit was G6PDH deficiency (66). The research that established the connection between the enzyme deficiency and the drug toxicity was carried out under the aegis of the U.S. Army, and relied on the participation of inmates of the Stateville Penitentiary near Chicago, who acted both as experimental subjects and as research assistants. The history of this enterprise has been related by Beutler (1) and by Harkness (67).

Antimalarial Drugs: Mechanisms of Action

Despite the long history and importance of quinoline antimalarial drugs (68), neither their mechanism of action nor their mechanism of toxicity (69) is definitively understood. Quite possibly, multiple molecular mechanisms contribute. We have already mentioned evidence that both the antiparasitic and toxic effects involve the imposition of oxidative stress, affecting both the parasite and the host. This idea is widely held although still disputed (70).

Another lead (71) was provided by a recent "proteomic" analysis (72). In this study, primaquine was covalently linked to Sepharose, to form an affinity column. Human red blood cell lysate was then passed over this column; bound proteins were eluted with 5 mM primaquine and resolved by electrophoresis on SDS-polyacrylamide gels. The proteins were digested with trypsin, in the gels, and then identified by mass spectrometry and comparison to genome-derived databases of human proteins. Two proteins were found to bind to the primaquine column with high affinity, one of which was *quinone reductase 2* (EC 1.6.99.2). This enzyme proved to be potently inhibited by quinoline drugs (73).

How could this inhibitory effect contribute to the antimalarial action effectiveness of quinoline drugs? One possibility returns us to the oxidative stress hypothesis. Quinones can undergo redox cycling (see chapter 1), that is, one-electron reduction to semiquinones, which reduce oxygen to superoxide, regenerating the quinone. This redox cycling can generate oxidative stress that kills the parasite (74). Quinone reductases are flavoenzymes that catalyze two-electron transfers from reduced pyridines to quinones, reducing them to hydroquinones (75–77) without the formation of semiquinone radical intermediates. That is, quinone reductases detoxify quinones. Inhibition of quinone reductase 2 could therefore enhance oxidative stress due to ambient quinones.

Very different mechanisms of quinoline antimalarial drug action have also been proposed. The parasite, growing within the erythrocyte, degrades hemoglobin in its digestive vacuole and thereby releases free heme. This heme is sequestered by polymerization within the vacuole. Chloroquine blocks this polymerization and the resulting accumulation of free heme may kill the parasite (78–80).

PRIMAQUINE: MECHANISMS OF TOXICITY

When primaquine is incubated in vitro with erythrocytes, neither methemoglobin formation nor hemolysis (the toxicities that arise in some patients) occurs. This indicates that the toxicity is due to metabolites (presumably formed in the liver) rather than the parent compound.

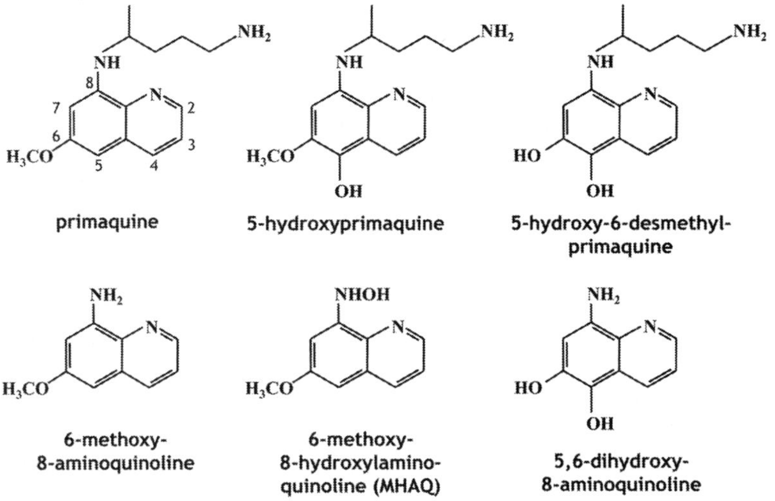

FIGURE 16-12.

Selected metabolites of primaquine.

Identification of a critical metabolite is complicated by the large number of known or postulated metabolites of primaquine. At least three chemically distinct redox-cycling metabolite pairs (figure 16-12) may be formed: aminophenol/quinoneimine pair (5-hydroxyprimaquine and its oxidation product); hydroxylamine/nitroso pair (6-methoxy-8-hydroxylamino-quinoline and its oxidation product); and hydroquinone/quinone pair (5-hydroxy-6-desmethylprimaquine and its oxidation product). Each of these pairs may undergo redox cycling and generate reactive oxygen species within the red cell.

Jeannette Vásquez-Vivar and Ohara Augusto (*81*) demonstrated that, in the presence of NADPH and a catalyst, 5-hydroxyprimaquine can generate hydrogen peroxide. Subsequent studies by Augusto and colleagues (*82, 83*) documented the ability of this metabolite, when incubated with red cells, to generate methemoglobin, oxidize GSH, and activate the hexose monophosphate shunt. Recent studies by David Jollow, David McMillan, and colleagues (*84*) have confirmed that the prooxidant cellular effects of this putative human metabolite occur at hemolytic concentrations. A standard human clinical test was adapted for measurement of red cell life span in rats (*85, 86*). Radioactive $^{51}Cr^{6+}$ (Na$_2$CrO$_4$) is added to isolated rat erythrocytes. The Cr(VI) ion is taken up by the cells and reduced (chiefly by GSH) to Cr(III), which binds tightly to hemoglobin and other molecules within the cell. The radiolabeled erythrocytes are transfused back into a rat. Subsequently, blood samples are withdrawn and radioactivity is counted with a gamma counter. As damaged (and nondamaged senescent) red cells are removed by the spleen, blood radioactivity decreases. For toxicity studies, the washed and labeled rat red cells are incubated in vitro with various concentrations of the test compound for two hours and the cells are then washed and returned to isologous rats. The direct-acting hemolytic capacity of the test compound is determined by the extent to which the lifespan of the treated cells is reduced. The fate of the damaged cells (uptake into the spleen vs. lysis in the vasculature) is determined by measurement of radioactivity in the spleen (whole cell uptake) as compared to uptake into the liver (mostly fragments and other cellular debris). Lysis can also be measured by determination of hemoglobin release into the incubation medium.

Using this technique, 5-hydroxyprimaquine was found to be a direct-acting hemolytic agent with an EC_{50} of about 40 mM. When GSH was extensively depleted from the red cells (by titration with diethylmaleate) prior to exposure to 5-hydroxyprimaquine, the potency of this putative metabolite was increased by a factor of greater than five. Loss of GSH is a characteristic of older G6PDH-deficient red cells and is a major factor in the relative inability of such cells to detoxify reactive oxygen species via the action of glutathione peroxidase. The GSH-depleted (G6PDH-normal) rat red cell is thus an experimental model for the human G6PDH-deficient red cell.

Jollow and colleagues have also synthesized and tested 6-methoxy-8-hydroxylaminoquinoline (MHAQ) (87–89). Previous studies from this group had shown that 6-methoxy-8-aminoquinoline, a known human metabolite of primaquine, is oxidized to MHAQ by human liver fractions. Thus, MHAQ is likely also to be a human metabolite of primaquine. When ^{51}Cr-labeled erythrocytes were incubated for two hours with MHAQ in vitro, followed by intravenous administration to rats, there was a concentration-dependent reduction in the survival of the tagged cells. Hemoglobin was not released into the incubation mixture, indicating that direct lysis does not occur under these conditions. At hemolytic concentrations, MHAQ induced methemoglobin formation, oxidation of gluta-thione, and generation of •OH radicals (as measured by spin-trapping) in erythrocyte suspensions in vitro. Prior depletion of red cell GSH, used as a surrogate for G6PDH deficiency, caused a marked potentiation in the hemolytic activity of MHAQ. Thus, MHAQ is a direct-acting hemolytic agent and can produce an oxidant stress within the red cell. These results suggest that MHAQ could be an important contributor to the hemotoxicity of primaquine.

Another potential human metabolite is 5-hydroxy-6-desmethyl-primaquine (90), structurally analogous to naphthoquinones such as menadione, a known hemolytic agent (91). 5-Hydroxy-6-desmethylprima-quine has the capacity to redox cycle and generate reactive oxygen species and hence it must also be considered a possible contributor to primaquine-induced hemolytic anemia. Determining the relative importance of each of these systems to the parent drug's toxicity is difficult. To make such an assessment, we need (at least) to know the relative potencies of each metabolite and how much of each is produced in the liver. One can assess their potencies using the in vitro exposure/in vivo ^{51}Cr-tagged life-span technique. Determination of metabolite production in the liver is difficult, because the compounds are unstable in the presence of blood and will not survive transit to the kidney; hence, excretion into the urine is unlikely. Furthermore, there will be interactions among the various metabolites. For example, 5-hydroxyprimaquine is very potent with respect to depleting reduced glutathione from the red cell, an effect that greatly enhances the hemolytic activity of MHAQ. Consequently, it is probably unrealistic to expect, in the case of primaquine, that the toxicity of the parent compound can be ascribed entirely to the action of a single metabolite.

Note

1. A.S. Alving, Clinical treatment of malaria, in Medical Science Pubn. #4, Recent Advances in Medicine and Surgery Based on Professional Medical Experiences in Japan and Korea 1950–1953, Vol. 2, U.S. Army Medical Service Graduate School, Walter Reed Army Medical Center, Washington, D.C.

References

1. Beutler, E. The red cell: a tiny dynamo. In *Blood, Pure and Eloquent*; Wintrobe, M. M., Ed.; McGraw-Hill: New York, 1980; pp. 141–168.

2. Kauffman, K. J.; Pajerowski, J. D.; Jamshidi, N.; Palsson, B. O.; Edwards, J. S. Description and analysis of metabolic connectivity and dynamics in the human red blood cell. *Biophys. J.* **2002,** *83*, 646–662.

3. Greenwalt, T. J. Red but not dead: not a hapless sac of hemoglobin. *Immunol. Invest.* **1995,** *24*, 3–21.

4. Jollow, D. J.; McMillan, D. C. Oxidative stress, glucose-6-phosphate dehydrogenase and the red cell. *Adv. Exp. Med. Biol.* **2001,** *500*, 595–605.

5. Ucar, K. Clinical presentation and management of hemolytic anemias. *Oncology (Huntingt.)* **2002,** *16*, 163–170.

6. Siems, W.; Capuozzo, E.; Lucano, A.; Salerno, C.; Crifo, C. High sensitivity of plasma membrane ion transport ATPases from human neutrophils towards 4-hydroxy-2,3-trans-nonenal. *Life Sci.* **2003,** *73*, 2583–2590.

7. Winterbourn, C. C. Oxidative reactions of hemoglobin. *Methods Enzymol.* **1990,** *186*, 265–272.

8. Berg, J. M.; Tymoczko, J. L.; Stryer, L. *Biochemistry*; WH Freeman: New York, 2001.

9. Coleman, M. D.; Coleman, N. A. Drug-induced methaemoglobinaemia. Treatment issues. *Drug Saf.* **1996,** *14*, 394–405.

10. Bradberry, S. M. Occupational methaemoglobinaemia. Mechanisms of production, features, diagnosis and management including the use of methylene blue. *Toxicol. Rev.* **2003,** *22*, 13–27.

11. Hall, A. H.; Kulig, K. W.; Rumack, B. H. Drug- and chemical-induced methaemoglobinaemia. Clinical features and management. *Med. Toxicol.* **1986,** *1*, 253–260.

12. Shikama, K. The molecular mechanism of autoxidation for myoglobin and hemoglobin: a venerable puzzle. *Chem. Rev.* **1998,** *98*, 1357–1374.

13. Giulivi, C.; Davies, K. J. A novel antioxidant role for hemoglobin. The comproportionation of ferrylhemoglobin with oxyhemoglobin. *J. Biol. Chem.* **1990,** *265*, 19453–19460.

14. Watkins, J. A.; Kawanishi, S.; Caughey, W. S. Autoxidation reactions of hemoglobin A free from other red cell components: a minimal mechanism. *Biochem. Biophys. Res. Commun.* **1985,** *132*, 742–748.

15. Castro, C. E.; Wade, R. S.; Belser, N. O. Conversion of oxyhemoglobin to methemoglobin by organic and inorganic reductants. *Biochemistry* **1978,** *17*, 225–231.

16. Dickerson, R. E.; Geis, I. *Hemoglobin: Structure, Function, Evolution, and Pathology*; Benjamin-Cummings: Menlo Park, 1983.

17. Higgs, D. R.; Vickers, M. A.; Wilkie, A. O.; Pretorius, I. M.; Jarman, A. P.; Weatherall, D. J. A review of the molecular genetics of the human α-globin gene cluster. *Blood* **1989,** *73*, 1081–1104.

18. Akerman, B. R.; Fujiwara, T. M.; Lancaster, G. A.; Morgan, K.; Scriver, C. R. Identification of deletion and triple α-globin gene haplotypes

in the Montreal β-thalassemia screening program: implications for genetic medicine. *Am. J. Med. Genet.* **1990,** *36,* 76–84.

19. Gibson, Q. The reduction of methemoglobin in red blood cells and studies on the cause of idiopathic methemoglobinemia. *Biochem. J.* **1948,** *42,* 13–23.

20. Gibson, Q. Introduction: congenital methemoglobinemia revisited. *Blood* **2002,** *100,* 3445–3446.

21. Scott, E. M.; Griffith, I. V. The enzymic defect of hereditary methemoglobinemia: diaphorase. *Biochim. Biophys. Acta* **1959,** *34,* 584–586.

22. Hultquist, D. E.; Passon, P. G. Catalysis of methaemoglobin reduction by erythrocyte cytochrome b$_5$ and cytochrome b$_5$ reductase. *Nat. New Biol.* **1971,** *229,* 252–254.

23. Leroux, A.; Junien, C.; Kaplan, J.; Bamberger, J. Generalised deficiency of cytochrome b$_5$ reductase in congenital methaemoglobinaemia with mental retardation. *Nature* **1975,** *258,* 619–620.

24. Bewley, M. C.; Marohnic, C. C.; Barber, M. J. The structure and biochemistry of NADH-dependent cytochrome b$_5$ reductase are now consistent. *Biochemistry* **2001,** *40,* 13574–13582.

25. Percy, M. J.; Gillespie, M. J.; Savage, G.; Hughes, A. E.; McMullin, M. F.; Lappin, T. R. Familial idiopathic methemoglobinemia revisited: original cases reveal 2 novel mutations in NADH-cytochrome b$_5$ reductase. *Blood* **2002,** *100,* 3447–3449.

26. Leroux, A.; Mota, V. L.; Kahn, A. Transcriptional and translational mechanisms of cytochrome b$_5$ reductase isoenzyme generation in humans. *Biochem. J.* **2001,** *355,* 529–535.

27. Vieira, L. M.; Kaplan, J. C.; Kahn, A.; Leroux, A. Four new mutations in the NADH-cytochrome b$_5$ reductase gene from patients with recessive congenital methemoglobinemia type II. *Blood* **1995,** *85,* 2254–2262.

28. Giordano, S. J.; Steggles, A. W. The human liver and reticulocyte cytochrome b$_5$ mRNAs are products from a single gene. *Biochem. Biophys. Res. Commun.* **1991,** *178,* 38–44.

29. Kaderbhai, M. A.; Morgan, R.; Kaderbhai, N. N. The membrane-interactive tail of cytochrome b$_5$ can function as a stop-transfer sequence in concert with a signal sequence to give inversion of protein topology in the endoplasmic reticulum. *Arch. Biochem. Biophys.* **2003,** *412,* 259–266.

30. Hegesh, E.; Hegesh, J.; Kaftory, A. Congenital methemoglobinemia with a deficiency of cytochrome b$_5$. *N. Engl. J. Med.* **1986,** *314,* 757–761.

31. Gaetani, G. F.; Rapezzi, D.; Mangerini, R.; Racchi, O.; Rolfo, M.; Ferraris, A. M. Exposure of erythrocytes to methylene blue shows the active role of catalase in removing hydrogen peroxide. *Br. J. Haematol.* **2002,** *119,* 833–838.

32. Xu, F.; Quandt, K. S.; Hultquist, D. E. Characterization of NADPH-dependent methemoglobin reductase as a heme-binding protein present in erythrocytes and liver. *Proc. Natl. Acad. Sci. USA* **1992,** *89,* 2130–2134.

33. Shalloe, F.; Elliott, G.; Ennis, O.; Mantle, T. J. Evidence that biliverdin-IX beta reductase and flavin reductase are identical. *Biochem. J.* **1996,** *316,* 385–387.

34. Cawein, M.; Behlen, C. H.; Lappat, E. J.; Cohn, J. E. Hereditary diaphorase deficiency and methemoglobinemia. *Arch. Intern. Med.* **1964,** *113,* 578–585.

35. Trost, C. The blue people of Troublesome Creek. *Science 82,* **1982,** 35–39.

36. Senozan, N. M.; Thielman, C. A. Glucose-6-phosphate dehydrogenase deficiency, an inherited ailment that affects 100 million people. *J. Chem. Educ.* **1991**, *68*, 7–10.

37. Vulliamy, T.; Mason, P.; Luzzatto, L. The molecular basis of glucose-6-phosphate dehydrogenase deficiency. *Trends Genet.* **1992**, *8*, 138–143.

38. Beutler, E.; Vulliamy, T.; Luzzatto, L. Hematologically important mutations: glucose-6-phosphate dehydrogenase. *Blood Cells Mol. Dis.* **1996**, *22*, 49–56.

39. Ruwende, C.; Hill, A. Glucose-6-phosphate dehydrogenase deficiency and malaria. *J. Mol. Med.* **1998**, *76*, 581–588.

40. Scott, M. D.; Wagner, T. C.; Chiu, D. T. Decreased catalase activity is the underlying mechanism of oxidant susceptibility in glucose-6-phosphate dehydrogenase-deficient erythrocytes. *Biochim. Biophys. Acta* **1993**, *1181*, 163–168.

41. Gandini, E.; Gartler, S. M. Glucose-6-phosphate dehydrogenase mosaicism for studying the development of blood cell precursors. *Nature* **1969**, *224*, 599–600.

42. Kaplan, M.; Vreman, H. J.; Hammerman, C.; Leiter, C.; Abramov, A.; Stevenson, D. K. Contribution of haemolysis to jaundice in Sephardic Jewish glucose-6-phosphate dehydrogenase deficient neonates. *Br. J. Haematol.* **1996**, *93*, 822–827.

43. Spagnuolo, C.; Rinelli, P.; Coletta, M.; Chiancone, E.; Ascoli, F. Oxidation reaction of human oxyhemoglobin with nitrite: a reexamination. *Biochim. Biophys. Acta* **1987**, *911*, 59–65.

44. Lissi, E. Autocatalytic oxidation of hemoglobin by nitrite: a possible mechanism. *Free Radic. Biol. Med.* **1998**, *24*, 1535–1536.

45. Cammack, R.; Joannou, C. L.; Cui, X. Y.; Torres, M. C.; Maraj, S. R.; Hughes, M. N. Nitrite and nitrosyl compounds in food preservation. *Biochim. Biophys. Acta* **1999**, *1411*, 475–488.

46. Gladwin, M. T. Haldane, hot dogs, halitosis, and hypoxic vasodilation: the emerging biology of the nitrite anion. *J. Clin. Invest.* **2004**, *113*, 19–21.

47. Walley, T.; Flanagan, M. Nitrite-induced methaemoglobinaemia. *Postgrad. Med. J.* **1987**, *63*, 643–644.

48. Fan, A. M.; Steinberg, V. E. Health implications of nitrate and nitrite in drinking water: an update on methemoglobinemia occurrence and reproductive and developmental toxicity. *Regul. Toxicol. Pharmacol.* **1996**, *23*, 35–43.

49. Knobeloch, L.; Proctor, M. Eight blue babies. *WMJ* **2001**, *100*, 43–47.

50. Christopher, M. M.; White, J. G.; Eaton, J. W. Erythrocyte pathology and mechanisms of Heinz body-mediated hemolysis in cats. *Vet. Pathol.* **1990**, *27*, 299–310.

51. Miller, L. H.; Greenwood, B. Malaria: a shadow over Africa. *Science* **2002**, *298*, 121–122.

52. Clark, I. A.; Chaudhri, G.; Cowden, W. B. Some roles of free radicals in malaria. *Free Radic. Biol. Med.* **1989**, *6*, 315–321.

53. Hunt, N. H.; Stocker, R. Oxidative stress and the redox status of malaria-infected erythrocytes. *Blood Cells* **1990**, *16*, 499–526.

54. Wu, Y. How might qinghaosu (artemisinin) and related compounds kill the intraerythrocytic malaria parasite? A chemist's view. *Acc. Chem. Res.* **2002**, *35*, 255–259.

55. Lederberg, J. J.B.S. Haldane (1949) on infectious disease and evolution. *Genetics* **1999**, *153*, 1–3.

56. Sabeti, P. C.; Reich, D. E.; Higgins, J. M.; Levine, H. Z.; Richter, D. J.; Schaffner, S. F.; Gabriel, S. B.; Platko, J. V.; Patterson, N. J.; McDonald, G. J.; Ackerman, H. C.; Campbell, S. J.; Altshuler, D.; Cooper, R.; Kwiatkowski, D.; Ward, R.; Lander, E. S. Detecting recent positive selection in the human genome from haplotype structure. *Nature* **2002,** *419*, 832–837.

57. Tishkoff, S. A.; Varkonyi, R.; Cahinhinan, N.; Abbes, S.; Argyropoulos, G.; Destro-Bisol, G.; Drousiotou, A.; Dangerfield, B.; Lefranc, G.; Loiselet, J.; Piro, A.; Stoneking, M.; Tagarelli, A.; Tagarelli, G.; Touma, E. H.; Williams, S. M.; Clark, A. G. Haplotype diversity and linkage disequilibrium at human G6PD: recent origin of alleles that confer malarial resistance. *Science* **2001,** *293*, 455–462.

58. Friedman, M. J. Oxidant damage mediates variant red cell resistance to malaria. *Nature* **1979,** *280*, 245–247.

59. Roth, E. F., Jr.; Raventos-Suarez, C.; Rinaldi, A.; Nagel, R. L. Glucose-6-phosphate dehydrogenase deficiency inhibits in vitro growth of *Plasmodium falciparum. Proc. Natl. Acad. Sci. USA* **1983,** *80*, 298–299.

60. Arese, P.; Turrini, F.; Fasler, S.; Lutz, H. U. Recent advances in the biochemistry of favism. *Biomed. Biochim. Acta* **1990,** *49*, S284–S288.

61. Chevion, M.; Navok, T.; Glaser, G.; Mager, J. The chemistry of favism-inducing compounds. The properties of isouramil and divicine and their reaction with glutathione. *Eur. J. Biochem.* **1982,** *127*, 405–409.

62. Clark, I. A.; Cowden, W. B. Antimalarials. In *Oxidative Stress*; Sies, H., Ed.; Academic Press: New York, 1985; pp. 131–149.

63. Rocco, F. *The Miraculous Fever Tree, Malaria and the Quest for a Cure That Changed the World*, Harper-Collins: New York, 2003.

64. Mafong, E. A.; Kaplan, L. A. Insect repellents. What really works? *Postgrad. Med.* **1997,** *102*, 63, 68–69, 74.

65. Baird, J. K.; Fryauff, D. J.; Hoffman, S. L. Primaquine for prevention of malaria in travelers. *Clin. Infect. Dis.* **2003,** *37*, 1659–1667.

66. Alving, A. S.; Carson, P. E.; Flanagan, C. L.; Ickes, C. E. Enzymatic deficiency in primaquine-sensitive erythrocytes. *Science* **1956,** *124*, 484–485.

67. Harkness, J. M. Nuremberg and the issue of wartime experiments on U.S. prisoners. The Green Committee. *JAMA* **1996,** *276*, 1672–1675.

68. O'Neill, P. M.; Bray, P. G.; Hawley, S. R.; Ward, S. A.; Park, B. K. 4-Aminoquinolines: past, present, and future: a chemical perspective. *Pharmacol. Ther.* **1998,** *77*, 29–58.

69. Taylor, W. R.; White, N. J. Antimalarial drug toxicity: a review. *Drug Saf.* **2004,** *27*, 25–61.

70. Monti, D.; Basilico, N.; Parapini, S.; Pasini, E.; Olliaro, P.; Taramelli, D. Does chloroquine really act through oxidative stress? *FEBS Lett.* **2002,** *522*, 3–5.

71. Petri, W. A., Jr. Can a proteomics strategy be used to identify the anti-malarial activity of chloroquine? *Trends Pharmacol. Sci.* **2003,** *24*, 210–212.

72. Graves, P. R.; Kwiek, J. J.; Fadden, P.; Ray, R.; Hardeman, K.; Coley, A. M.; Foley, M.; Haystead, T. A. Discovery of novel targets of quinoline drugs in the human purine binding proteome. *Mol. Pharmacol.* **2002,** *62*, 1364–1372.

73. Kwiek, J. J.; Haystead, T. A.; Rudolph, J. Kinetic mechanism of quinone oxidoreductase 2 and its inhibition by the antimalarial quinolines. *Biochemistry* **2004,** *43*, 4538–4547.

74. Molina Portela, M. P.; Fernandez Villamil, S. H.; Perissinotti, L. J.; Stoppani, A. O. Redox cycling of *o*-naphthoquinones in trypanosomatids. Superoxide and hydrogen peroxide production. *Biochem. Pharmacol.* **1996,** *52,* 1875–1882.

75. Foster, C. E.; Bianchet, M. A.; Talalay, P.; Faig, M.; Amzel, L. M. Structures of mammalian cytosolic quinone reductases. *Free Radic. Biol. Med.* **2000,** *29,* 241–245.

76. Dinkova-Kostova, A. T.; Talalay, P. Persuasive evidence that quinone reductase type 1 (DT diaphorase) protects cells against the toxicity of electrophiles and reactive forms of oxygen. *Free Radic. Biol. Med.* **2000,** *29,* 231–240.

77. Bianchet, M. A.; Foster, C.; Faig, M.; Talalay, P.; Amzel, L. M. Structure and mechanism of cytosolic quinone reductases. *Biochem. Soc. Trans.* **1999,** *27,* 610–615.

78. Famin, O.; Ginsburg, H. Differential effects of 4-aminoquinoline-containing antimalarial drugs on hemoglobin digestion in *Plasmodium falciparum*-infected erythrocytes. *Biochem. Pharmacol.* **2002,** *63,* 393–398.

79. Sullivan, D. J., Jr.; Matile, H.; Ridley, R. G.; Goldberg, D. E. A common mechanism for blockade of heme polymerization by antimalarial quinolines. *J. Biol. Chem.* **1998,** *273,* 31103–31107.

80. Sullivan, D. J.; Jr.; Gluzman, I. Y.; Russell, D. G.; Goldberg, D. E. On the molecular mechanism of chloroquine's antimalarial action. *Proc. Natl. Acad. Sci. USA* **1996,** *93,* 11865–11870.

81. Vasquez-Vivar, J.; Augusto, O. Hydroxylated metabolites of the anti-malarial drug primaquine. Oxidation and redox cycling. *J. Biol. Chem.* **1992,** *267,* 6848–6854.

82. da Silva Morais, M.; Augusto, O. Peroxidation of the antimalarial drug primaquine: characterization of a benzidine-like metabolite with methaemoglobin-forming activity. *Xenobiotica* **1993,** *23,* 133–139.

83. Vasquez-Vivar, J.; Augusto, O. Oxidative activity of primaquine metab-olites on rat erythrocytes in vitro and in vivo. *Biochem. Pharmacol.* **1994,** *47,* 309–316.

84. Bowman, Z. S.; Oatis, J. E., Jr.; Whelan, J. L.; Jollow, D. J.; McMillan, D. C. Primaquine-induced hemolytic anemia: susceptibility of normal versus glutathione-depleted rat erythrocytes to 5-hydroxyprimaquine. *J. Pharmacol. Exp. Ther.* **2004,** *309,* 79–85.

85. Aaseth, J.; Alexander, J.; Norseth, T. Uptake of ^{51}Cr-chromate by human erythrocytes: a role of glutathione. *Acta Pharmacol. Toxicol. (Copenh.)* **1982,** *50,* 310–315.

86. Cavill, I. Red cell lifespan estimation by ^{51}Cr labelling. *Br. J. Haematol.* **2002,** *117,* 997.

87. Bolchoz, L. J.; Budinsky, R. A.; McMillan, D. C.; Jollow, D. J. Primaquine-induced hemolytic anemia: formation and hemotoxicity of the arylhydroxylamine metabolite 6-methoxy-8-hydroxylaminoquinoline. *J. Pharmacol. Exp. Ther.* **2001,** *297,* 509–515.

88. Bolchoz, L. J.; Gelasco, A. K.; Jollow, D. J.; McMillan, D. C. Primaquine-induced hemolytic anemia: formation of free radicals in rat erythrocytes exposed to 6-methoxy-8-hydroxylaminoquinoline. *J. Pharmacol. Exp. Ther.* **2002,** *303,* 1121–1129.

89. Bolchoz, L. J.; Morrow, J. D.; Jollow, D. J.; McMillan, D. C. Primaquine-induced hemolytic anemia: effect of 6-methoxy-8-hydroxylaminoquinoline on rat erythrocyte sulfhydryl status, membrane lipids, cytoskeletal proteins, and morphology. *J. Pharmacol. Exp. Ther.* **2002,** *303,* 141–148.

90. Thompson, S. F.; Fraser, I. M.; Strother, A.; Bull, B. S. Change of deformability and Heinz body formation in G6PD-deficient erythrocytes treated with 5-hydroxy-6-desmethylprimaquine. *Blood Cells* **1989,** *15,* 443–452.

91. Chung, S. M.; Lee, J. Y.; Lee, M. Y.; Bae, O. N.; Chung, J. H. Adverse consequences of erythrocyte exposure to menadione: involvement of reactive oxygen species generation in plasma. *J. Toxicol. Environ. Health A* **2001,** *63,* 617–629.

17

$\triangleright$

Aromatic

Amines

and

Related

Toxic

Compounds

AROMATIC AND HETEROCYCLIC AMINES

Aromatic amines are compounds of structural formula Ar–NH$_2$, where Ar represents a homoaromatic or heteroaromatic ring. (We can distinguish the latter class as "heterocyclic amines.") Aromatic amines are the most chemically reduced members of a larger class of N-aryl compounds: hydroxylamines, nitroso compounds,[1] and nitro compounds (figure 17-1). Redox enzymes catalyze their interconversions, as we discuss below, so any consideration of aromatic amine toxicology also encompasses these related N-aryl compounds. We have already encountered aromatic amines as substrates for P450, NAT, and SULT enzymes. In this chapter, we consider the toxicology of aromatic amines and their bioactivation by redox and conjugating enzymes (*1, 2*).

SYNTHETIC DYES

In 1856 the 18-year-old Englishman William Henry Perkin, working in his home laboratory, decided to attempt the total synthesis of quinine (*3*). Quinine, an alkaloid natural product extracted from the bark of South American cinchona trees, was the only effective treatment for malaria (see chapter 16)—and malaria was perhaps the biggest obstacle to the expansion of the British empire. Perkin never came close to synthesizing quinine, but, nevertheless, he made a celebrated discovery. He took a crude sample of aniline, the simplest aromatic amine, which had been discovered 30 years earlier, and oxidized it with nitric and sulfuric acids. The product was a purple-colored phenazine dye. (The impure starting material also contained toluidines, which were essential for the formation of this product.) Perkin quickly recognized the value of this dye, which he named *mauveine* (figure 17-2). Perkin obtained a patent and embarked on the industrial-scale production of mauveine, the first important synthetic dye. By age 36, already a very rich man, he retired from industry to devote his time to basic research in chemistry.

Benzidine-Based Dyes

The aromatic diamine benzidine (figure 17-3) was synthesized in 1845 by the acid-catalyzed "benzidine rearrangement" of hydrazobenzene. In 1860 Johann Peter Griess discovered the *diazotization* reaction: treatment of primary aromatic amines with nitrous acid (HNO$_2$) yields reactive diazonium salts, key electrophilic intermediates in aromatic chemistry, which can readily couple with nucleophiles, and be replaced by hydroxyl, halogen, or other functionalities (figure 17-4). The German chemist Böttiger applied this chemistry to benzidine and synthesized Congo red,[2] the first benzidine-based azo dye, in 1884 (figure 17-5). Extended

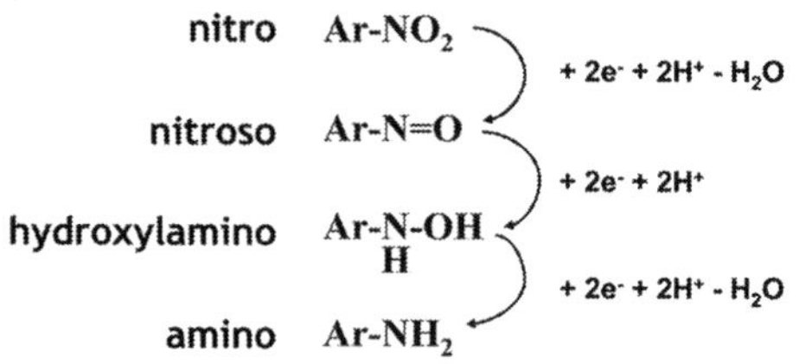

nitro $Ar\text{-}NO_2$

$+2e^- + 2H^+ - H_2O$

nitroso $Ar\text{-}N{=}O$

$+2e^- + 2H^+$

hydroxylamino $Ar\text{-}\underset{H}{N}\text{-}OH$

$+2e^- + 2H^+ - H_2O$

amino $Ar\text{-}NH_2$

FIGURE 17-1.
N-Aryl compounds.

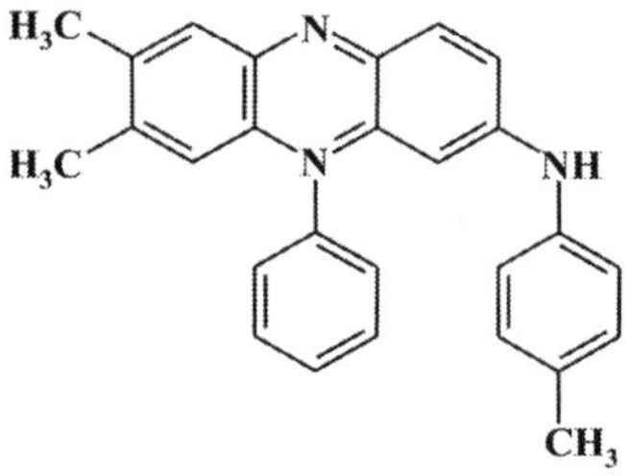

FIGURE 17-2.
Mauveine.

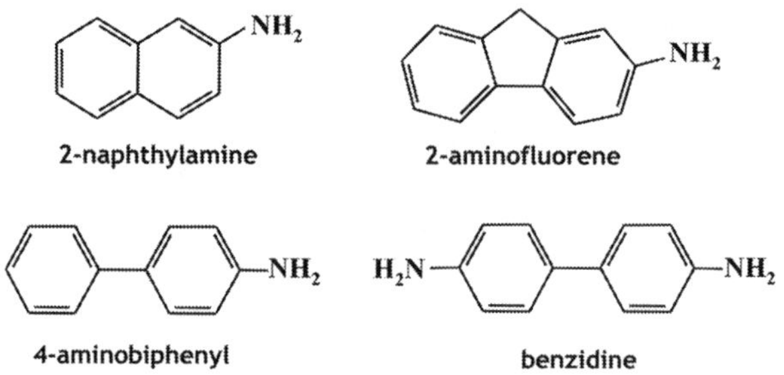

2-naphthylamine   2-aminofluorene

4-aminobiphenyl   benzidine

FIGURE 17-3.
Aromatic amines.

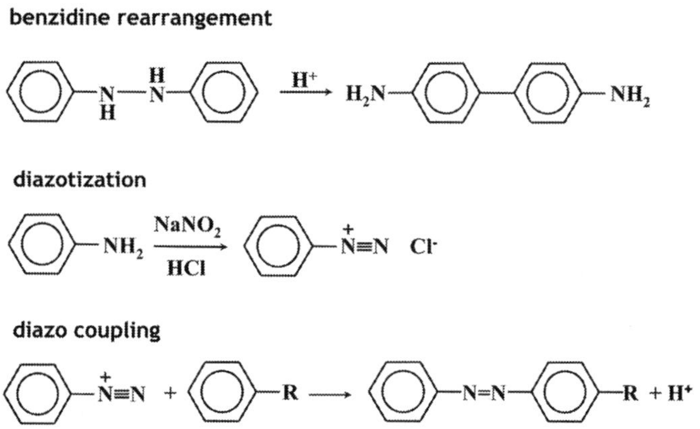

benzidine rearrangement

diazotization

diazo coupling

FIGURE 17-4.
Benzidine rearrangement, diazotization, and diazo coupling.

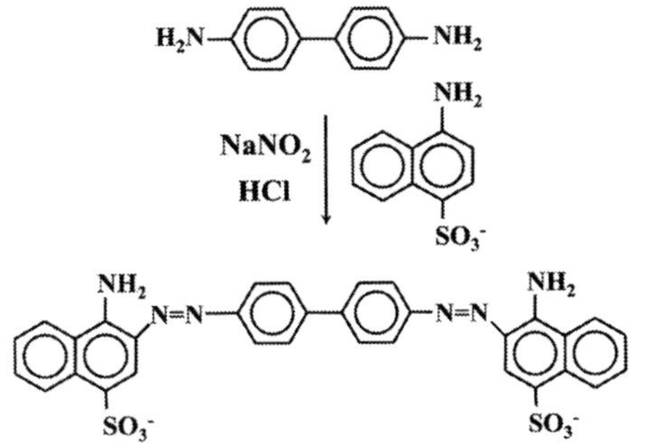

FIGURE 17-5.
Synthesis of Congo Red.

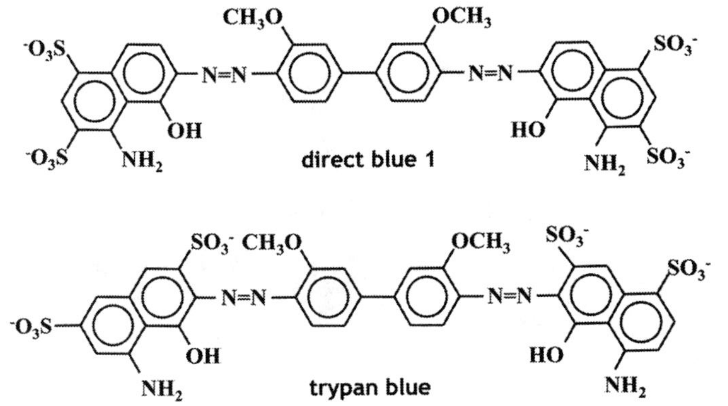

FIGURE 17-6.
Azo dyes.

conjugated systems, linked by azo chromophores, make these compounds intensely colored, and Congo red proved to be an excellent dye for cotton. By varying the substituents on the benzidine moiety and by choosing appropriate naphthylamine or naphthol coupling components, useful synthetic dyes in a range of colors could be prepared (figure 17-6). By the 1890s, which became known as the "mauve decade," inexpensive synthetic textile dyes had displaced natural dyes, such as indigo, and the chemical industry was flourishing. Production of benzidine-based dyes for use on textiles, leather, paper, and so on, grew rapidly, first in Germany, then in England and the United States.

"Aniline Cancer"

At the age of 26, Dr. Ludwig Rehn (figure 17-7) secured an appointment as company physician at the Hoechst dyestuff factory in the town of Griesheim, near Frankfurt-am-Main, Germany. Rehn was startled by the frequency with which Hoechst employees presented with urinary bladder cancer,[3] usually a rare tumor. He realized that the disease was occurring in factory workers employed in the production of fuchsin dye from aniline, and by the 1880s he was bringing the attention of other doctors to a condition he described as "aniline cancer" (although benzidine and naphthylamine, rather than aniline itself, would later prove to be the cause).

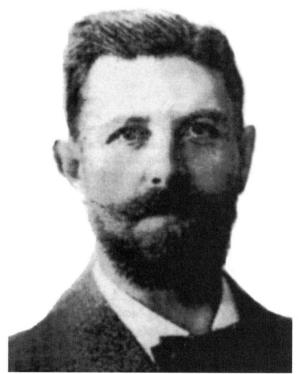

FIGURE 17-7.
Dr. Ludwig Rehn (1849–1930).

In 1895 he published his observations[4] (*4*), writing that "It is...very striking...that the majority of the tumors occur around the ureters... One can imagine that materials are present in solution in the urine (formed by the kidneys), which evoke tumor formation by chemical irritation."

Occupational Exposure to Aromatic Amines

Benzidine was produced in vast cauldrons, and factory workers scoured out the vats by hand, after each batch was prepared. Very large quantities of these compounds were ingested, by breathing the dust, through the skin, or by contamination of hands, clothing, food, and so on. Within 15 years, Rehn had observed more than 50 cases of bladder cancer among chemical industry workers in the Frankfurt area. However, despite the accumulating evidence, little was done to protect chemical industry workers in Europe and the United States until the post-World War II era. The most important improvement was "captive synthesis": benzidine is produced, diazotized, and coupled to form the dye, in sealed production units.

Many subsequent epidemiological studies confirmed the link between occupational exposure to benzidine and bladder cancer incidence (*5–8*). For example, Japanese workers employed in benzidine manufacture developed bladder cancer at a rate more than 60-fold higher than that of nonexposed controls (*7*). The occupational hazard has gradually abated, with improvements in manufacturing practices and workplace hygiene. However, benzidine manufacture, prohibited in North America and Europe since the 1970s, continues in several developing countries (9, 10); the consequences of these exposures are all too predictable. Benzidine congeners such as dichlorobenzidine are still widely used in dye manufacture and some of these compounds are more potent mutagens than is benzidine itself (11).

Hundreds of benzidine congener-based azo dyes are still used, in printing inks, textiles, paints and enamels, and other applications. The benzidine-based dyes are, of course, not aromatic amines, but azo compounds. Residual benzidine congener, per se, may be present in the dyes. If ingested, the dyes can be metabolized to liberate the aromatic amines. Ingested benzidine-based azo dyes are reduced to the parent benzidine congener by the action of azoreductase enzymes of gut bacteria (12); animals fed the benzidine dyes Direct Black 38 and Direct Brown 95 excrete benzidine and its metabolites (13). These observations indicate that dye users, not just persons involved in dye manufacture, may be at risk. Increased incidence of bladder cancer has been reported among Japanese kimono painters (who used benzidine-based dyes, and "pointed" brushes with their mouths) and among artistic painters in the United States (14).

The two isomers of naphthylamine (1- and 2-, also known as α- and β-, respectively) have also been used on an industrial scale, as antioxidants for rubber production and chemical intermediates for dye and herbicide production. (Although the commercial articles were sold as "1-naphthylamine" and "2-naphthylamine," each contained a significant percentage of the other isomer, as well as the corresponding naphthol isomer; many biological studies used impure preparations, and should be interpreted cautiously.) By the 1950s, it became apparent that 2-naphthylamine as well as benzidine was a significant occupational bladder carcinogen; production of 2-naphthylamine in the United States was finally halted in 1972 (15).

AROMATIC AMINE AND NITROHETEROCYCLIC DRUGS

Many aromatic amines and nitro compounds are mutagens and rodent carcinogens, as we have seen. Nevertheless, these functional groups are also found in many drugs (see chapter 13). Compared to carcinogens such as aminobiphenyl or aminofluorene, aromatic amine drugs are usually more polar; monocyclic rather than polycyclic; more heavily functionalized; and more rapidly excreted. Consequently, they are unlikely to be potent carcinogens, but cancer risks associated with aromatic amine drugs have been suggested. Acetaminophen (para-acetylaminophenol; Tylenol®) is a common analgesic. Heavy use of phenacetin, the ethyl ether of acetylaminophenol, is associated with renal cancer (16, 17) (see chapter 19). Aromatic amines or nitro compounds used as antibiotics include chloramphenicol; nitrofurans; "sulfa" drugs, such as sulfamethazine; and antiprotozoal agents; and dapsone (used to treat leprosy). Metronidazole (1-[2-hydroxyethyl]-2-methyl-5-nitroimidazole; Flagyl™) is a commonly prescribed antibiotic treatment for protozoal and anaerobic bacterial infections, including giardiasis, trichomoniasis, and amebiasis (18). It is probably a rodent carcinogen but there is no clear evidence for carcinogenicity in humans (19).

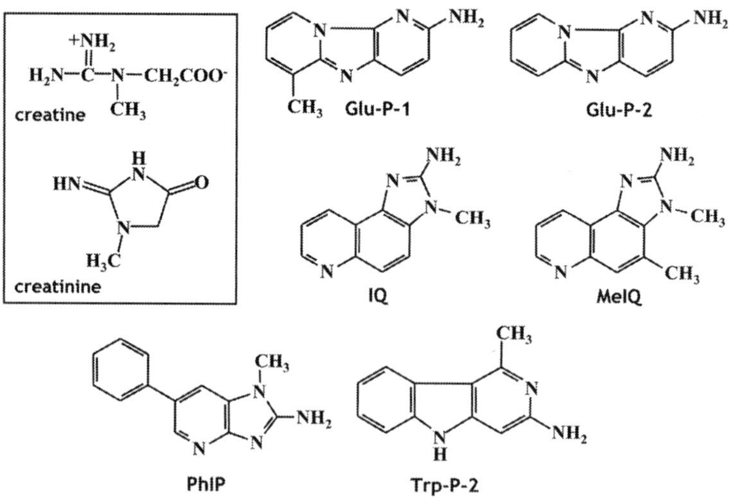

FIGURE 17-8.

Heterocyclic amine food pyrolysis products. Glu-P-l, 2-amino-6-methyl-dipyrido[1,2-a:3′,2′-d]imidazole; Glu-P-2, 2-amino-dipyrido[1,2-a:3′,2′-d] imidazole; IQ, 2-amino-3-methylimidazo[4,5-f]quinoline; MeIQ, 2-amino-3,4-dimethylimidazo[4,5-f]quinoline; PhIP, 2-amino-1-methyl-6-phenyl-imidazo[4,5-b]pyridine; Trp-P-2, 3-amino-1-methyl-5H-pyrido[4,3-b]indole.

FOOD PYROLYSIS PRODUCTS

As we discussed in chapter 4, the Ames assay is particularly sensitive to the mutagenicity of aromatic amines and nitroaromatics. Several new classes of mutagens have been discovered by testing environmental samples for mutagenicity in the Ames test. In 1976 Takashi Sugimura, of the National Cancer Centre, Tokyo, and his colleagues reported the presence of high mutagenic activity in the charred portion of grilled fish and meat (20, 21). Using mutagenicity as a bioassay, several highly active compounds were isolated from pyrolyzed foods; they proved to be previously unknown polycyclic heterocyclic amines (figure 17-8).

Mutagenic pyrolysis products are formed by complex, poorly understood reactions occurring at high temperatures (200–300°C) during grilling; the main precursors are probably amino acids and creatine (22). (Creatine, in its phosphorylated form, creatine phosphate, is an important energy storage molecule in muscles. Spontaneous cyclization of creatine phosphate, releasing inorganic phosphate, yields creatinine. The heterocyclic amine mutagens are only formed in muscle meats, because other meats or vegetables do not contain large concentrations of creatine.) Heterocyclic amines include some of the most potent mutagens known; they are also carcinogenic in rodents. For example, MeIQ causes tumors in the liver and forestomach of mice and in the Zymbal's gland, oral cavity, colon, skin, and mammary gland of rats (23–25).

PhIP was characterized by James Felton and colleagues in 1986 (26). It is found in cooked beef, pork, and chicken at levels up to many parts per billion. Higher cooking temperatures generate larger amounts of the mutagen. PhIP is the most abundant heterocyclic amine in meat cooked under typical grilling conditions, and dietary intakes by meat-eating individuals may be of the order of 100 ng per day (27). Epidemiological studies have suggested that consumption of well-done meat is associated with increased cancer risk at several common sites, including breast (28), colon, and possibly prostate, pancreas, and bladder. The consumption of cooked-meat mutagens can be greatly reduced without adopting a vegetarian diet, by measures such as cooking to "medium-rare" rather than "well-done" conditions, scraping charred residues from the surface of barbecued meats, and using marinades or sauces to prevent charring. All of these modifications are compatible with safe preparation of meat, in terms of killing contaminating microorganisms, so dietary avoidance of heterocyclic amines is a sensible precaution that may afford important benefits at no risk.

OXIDATIVE HAIR DYES

Permanent hair dyes are formulations of oxidizable compounds, mainly substituted anilines, which are mixed with hydrogen peroxide (oxidant) and applied to the hair. High-molecular-weight, insoluble, colored products are generated within the hair shaft. Compounds used in hair dyes include phenylenediamines (1,2-, 1,3-, and 1,4-diaminobenzene), 2,4-diamino-toluene (until its use was banned in 1971), anisidine isomers (1,2- and 1,4-aminotoluene), 4-nitro-1,3-diaminobenzene, and so on (29).

Some of the aromatic amine components used in hair dyes have proved to be mutagens. Ames and colleagues discovered, in 1975, that many hair dye chemicals are mutagenic, and the *oxidation* of hair dye formulations with hydrogen peroxide generates new mutagenic products (30, 31). Recent epidemiological studies have indicated an increased risk of bladder cancer among women who use permanent hair dyes (32).

CIGARETTE SMOKE

The risk of bladder cancer among persons occupationally exposed to aromatic amines is huge, as discussed above. However, the total number of such exposed individuals is small. Considering the whole population, far and away the most important environmental risk factor for bladder cancer in both men (33) and women (34) is cigarette smoking. Both mainstream and sidestream cigarette smoke contain a plethora of substituted anilines at levels of many micrograms per cigarette (35). Polycyclic aromatic amines such as aminobiphenyl and naphthylamine are also present (36). 4-Aminobiphenyl-derived DNA adducts have been detected (by the ^{32}P postlabeling technique) in the bladder epithelium of cigarette smokers (37). 4-Aminobiphenyl binds covalently to blood proteins, including serum albumin and hemoglobin (38). Figure 17-9 illustrates the mechanism that is believed to account for this binding. 4-Aminobiphenyl is N-oxidized to the hydroxylamine, which is further oxidized to the nitroso product by interaction with heme iron in oxyhemoglobin. The nitrosobiphenyl reacts with the hemoglobin polypeptide (particularly at cysteine 93 of the β chain) to form a covalent sulfinamide[5] adduct (39). Mild hydrolysis of the adducted hemoglobin releases free 4-aminobiphenyl, which provides a sensitive biomarker of exposure. Levels of hemoglobin-4-aminobiphenyl

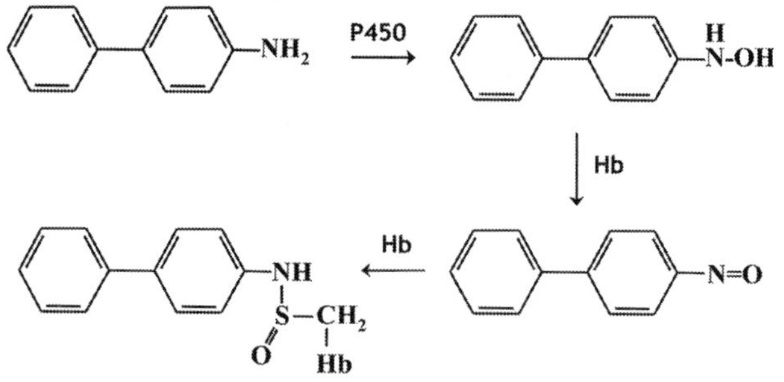

FIGURE 17-9.
Oxidation of 4-aminobiphenyl to a hemoglobin adduct.

adducts are about five times higher in smokers than in nonsmokers, and the decline in the level of the adducts can be observed over the course of a few months, once cigarette smokers quit the habit (*40*). Although aromatic amines are only one of many classes of carcinogens in cigarette smoke, they are the most likely causative agent of smoking-related bladder cancer.

NITRO COMPOUNDS AND NITROREDUCTASES

Nitro compounds are activated by reduction and aromatic amines are activated by oxidation. Both processes can generate hydroxylamino- and nitroso-aromatics and related reactive intermediates. Nitro compounds are best known as explosives (trinitrotoluene, TNT), but many also have antimicrobial activity, as mentioned above. Furylfuramide (2-(2-furyl)-3-(5-nitro-2-furyl)acrylamide), for example, was used as a food preservative in Japan, but was banned when it was found to be a rodent carcinogen (*41*). Many nitroaromatic compounds are mutagens (*42*). As was mentioned in chapter 4, mutagenicity was detected in carbon black photocopier toners in 1980, and 1,8- and 1,6-dinitropyrene proved to be responsible. Although photocopier toner is now free of dinitropyrenes, they remain important environmental contaminants. 1-Nitropyrenenitropyrene, 2-nitrofluoranthene, and other nitro polycyclic aromatic hydrocarbons, including dinitropyrenes, are ubiquitous combustion byproducts, produced especially by diesel and aircraft engines (*43*).

Nitroreductases are the enzymes that catalyze reduction of nitroaromatics. Nitroreductase activity is often associated with redox enzymes that were named on the basis of a different metabolic process. "Diaphorase" is the traditional name for flavoenzymes that catalyze the reduction of various indicator dyes (such as dichloroindophenol) using NADH or NADPH as electron donors. The systematic name for these enzymes is NAD(P)H dehydrogenase (EC 1.6.99.2). One such enzyme was found to be equally active with either NADH or NADPH (cofactors that were then called DPNH and TPNH, respectively).[6] In view of this very unusual lack of selectivity, the enzyme was named "DT-diaphorase" (*44a*). The enzyme is probably best known as "quinone reductase" (*44b*), but it also reduces nitroaromatics, including dinitropyrenes (*45*). Xanthine oxidase (EC 1.1.3.22) (*46*), which catalyzes the oxidation of xanthine to hypoxanthine and uric acid, is another mammalian enzyme with nitroreductase activity

(*47*). Nitroreductases are also found in bacteria (*48, 49*). The activity of these bacterial enzymes is required for the activation of nitroaromatic compounds in mutagenicity assays such as the Ames test (*50*), as discussed in chapter 4.

STRUCTURE–ACTIVITY RELATIONSHIPS

Many researchers have tried to establish systematic rules that can predict carcinogenic/mutagenic potency of aromatic amines based on their chemical structures. A few generalizations are apparent even on a cursory analysis of the literature. All of the potent aromatic amine carcinogens are polycyclic structures (at least two aromatic rings). None of the aniline derivatives are *potent* carcinogens, although some are positive at high doses and the most potent compounds (such as the nitropyrenes and the food pyrolysis products) have three or more aromatic rings, in fused structures. Halogenation usually increases activity. The *para principle* is an empirical rule stating that the most active congeners in extended aromatic structures, such as biphenyl, terphenyl, and fluorene, have amino groups in the *para* positions; for example, 2-aminofluorene is more potent than 3-aminofluorene; 4,4′-diaminobiphenyl (*para*-benzidine) is more potent than 2,2′-diaminobiphenyl (*ortho*-benzidine). Hydrophobicity is usually a strong indicator of potency, and some of the rules cited above, such as the greater activity of polycyclic structures, may be a consequence of this effect.

At a more sophisticated level of analysis, we can try to make numerical correlations between chemical structure and toxic activity, establishing so-called QSAR (quantitative structure–activity relations) (*51, 52*). Such rules are usually formulated as linear combinations of chemical parameters, each weighted by a numerical coefficient. The chemical parameters may include molar mass, lipophilicity (e.g., octanol–water partition coefficient), ionic properties (e.g., pK_a or dipole moment), and quantum mechanical parameters such as LUMO (lowest unoccupied molecular orbital) energy, which are indicators of reactivity. The numerical weighting coefficients are then estimated by regression analysis of the biological data. Another approach is to use a computerized "pattern-recognition" approach, which searches for chemical substructures (recognizable functional groups or other patterns of bonded atoms) that correlate with activity (*53*).

Let us sound a warning, however, to those who expect that computers rather than humans will alert us to potential mutagens and carcinogens. Anyone who has read to this point understands that most carcinogens require metabolic activation. One compound may give rise to a broad spectrum of metabolites with different properties and toxicities, a spectrum that will be different from one cell, tissue, or species to another. Metabolite profiles are almost impossible to predict, since they depend not only on the structures of the toxic substances but also on the structures of the enzymes that act on them. Any analysis that looks only at the parent compounds—the compounds for which activity data have been obtained—and ignores their metabolism, can give, at best, an indirect indication of the chemical factors affecting biological activity.

We should also remember the adage from computer science: garbage in = garbage out. There is little point in doing precise QSAR calculations based on imprecise or questionable biological data. QSAR can be effective in guiding drug design (*54*), where the biological response is simply the inhibitory IC_{50} of a series of test compounds acting against a specific target enzyme in vitro. But reducing complex biological responses to simple numerical potencies is fraught with danger. There is no consensus as to how to express carcinogenic potency, especially when the routes and schedules of administration of test substance differ. And just how should we compare the potency of an agent that induces mammary tumors (for example) to that of an agent that induces liver tumors? Even calculating the activity of a mutagen in, say, the Ames test can be problematical, since dose–responses are often nonlinear. When QSAR analyses combine data from different laboratories, or even from different assay systems, misleading results may be inevitable.

METABOLIC ACTIVATION

Even before the development of short-term assays such as the Ames test, it was apparent that aromatic amines per se did not react directly with macromolecules. Aromatic amines are generally negative in mutagenicity assays unless a metabolic activation system, such as hepatic S9, is supplied.

Considering the industrial importance of many aromatic amines, it is odd that some of the pioneering studies on aromatic amine metabolism focused on a compound of little environmental significance: 2-acetylamino-fluorene (2-AAF). The related aromatic amine 2-aminofluorene was patented in 1938 by the U.S. Department of Agriculture, for possible use as an insecticide, but its development was abandoned when 2-AAF was found to be a rodent carcinogen (*55*).

John and Elizabeth Weisburger at the National Cancer Institute, USA, studied the metabolism of 2-AAF by the rat and detected hydroxylated metabolites such as 7-hydroxy-2-AAF. As we have seen (chapter 7), aromatic hydroxylation is a common P450-catalyzed reaction. A crucial advance in understanding the metabolic activation of aromatic amines came from the work of Elizabeth Cavert Miller (*56*) and James Miller (*57*) at the McCardle Laboratory for Cancer Research, University of Wisconsin-Madison (figure 17-10). (We have also mentioned the pioneering work of Miller and Miller and their students in several other chapters, including discoveries related to cytochrome P450 induction, covalent binding of xenobiotics to macromolecules, and the metabolic activation of PAH carcinogens.) The Millers observed that, following prolonged (months) administration of 2-AAF to rats, a new metabolite was observed in the urine. This compound was identified as *N*-hydroxy-2-AAF (figure 17-11), an *arylhydroxamic acid;* its isolation was the first demonstration of metabolic N-hydroxylation (*58*). We now know that this is a characteristic P450 1 family[7] activity, as discussed in chapter 7.

2-AAF N-hydroxylation was the first example of the activation of a carcinogen to a metabolite with increased activity. When synthetic *N*-hydroxy-2-AAF was administered to rats in the diet, it was found to be a more potent carcinogen than 2-AAF (*60*). Furthermore, the aryl-hydroxamic acid, administered intraperitoneally, induced tumors *at the injection site*, whereas 2-AAF never did so. This striking result suggested

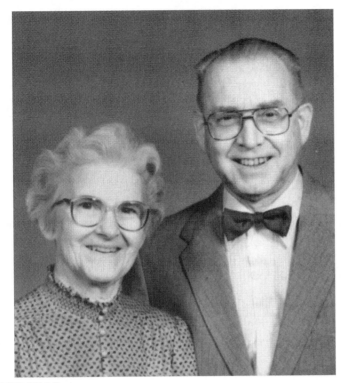

FIGURE 17-10.
Elizabeth Cavert Miller (1920–1987) and James A. Miller (1915–2000), pioneer investigators of the metabolism of chemical carcinogens to reactive electrophiles. (*Photo from* Cancer Res. ***2001***, 61, *3847–3848 and* Chem. Res. Toxicol. ***2001***, 14, *335–337.*)

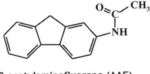

2-acetylaminofluorene (AAF)

P450-catalyzed
N-oxidation
(CYP1A2)

P450-catalyzed
C-oxidation

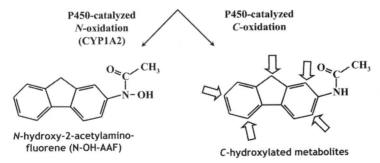

N-hydroxy-2-acetylamino-
fluorene (N-OH-AAF)

C-hydroxylated metabolites

FIGURE 17-11.
P450-catalyzed N- and C-hydroxylation of 2-acetylaminofluorene.

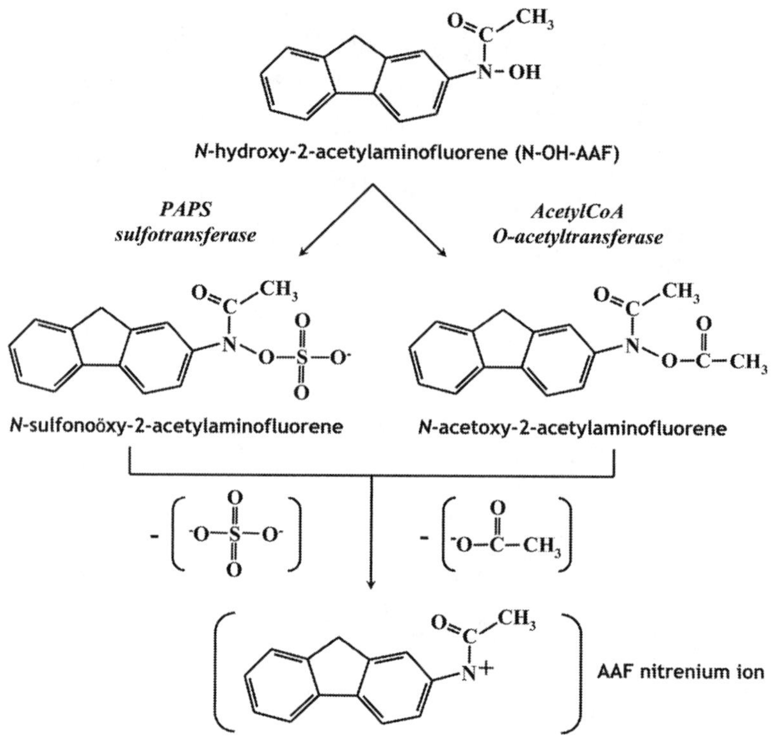

FIGURE 17-12.

Activation of *N*-hydroxy-2-acetylaminofluorene by acetate or sulfate conjugation.

that the metabolite did not require further hepatic activation, but was active locally.

N-Hydroxy-2-AAF, like benzo[*a*]pyrene 7,8-dihydrodiol, is a proximate carcinogen that requires further activation to generate the ultimate DNA-reactive species. Multiple pathways have been discovered; some of these generate an acetylated (AAF-type) reactive intermediate, while others generate a reactive intermediate that does not carry an acetate group (AF-type). These two classes of reactive species result in acetylated or nonacetylated DNA adducts, respectively.

N-Hydroxy-2-AAF can be conjugated by O-acetylation (see chapter 13) or O-sulfonation (see chapter 14) (*61*), producing *N*-acetoxyacetylamino-fluorene (*62*) or *N*-sulfonoöxy-2-acetylaminofluorene (*63*), respectively (figure 17-12). These esters are very reactive compounds, but they are sufficiently stable, at least at low temperatures, to be chemically synthesized and isolated. In both cases, conjugation yields metabolites that incorporate good *leaving groups*. Acetate anion and sulfate dianion are much better leaving groups than is hydroxide ion. Consequently, the esters undergo facile heterolytic cleavage to generate $RN^+(Ac)$, a *nitrenium ion* reactive intermediate. Nitrenium ions (*64*) are six-electron cations, nitrogen-centered electrophiles analogous to carbenium ions. Like those species, they are reactive, short-lived electrophiles (*65*). DNA adducts that are consistent with the intermediacy of nitrenium ions have been identified in many studies of aromatic amine activation (*66*).

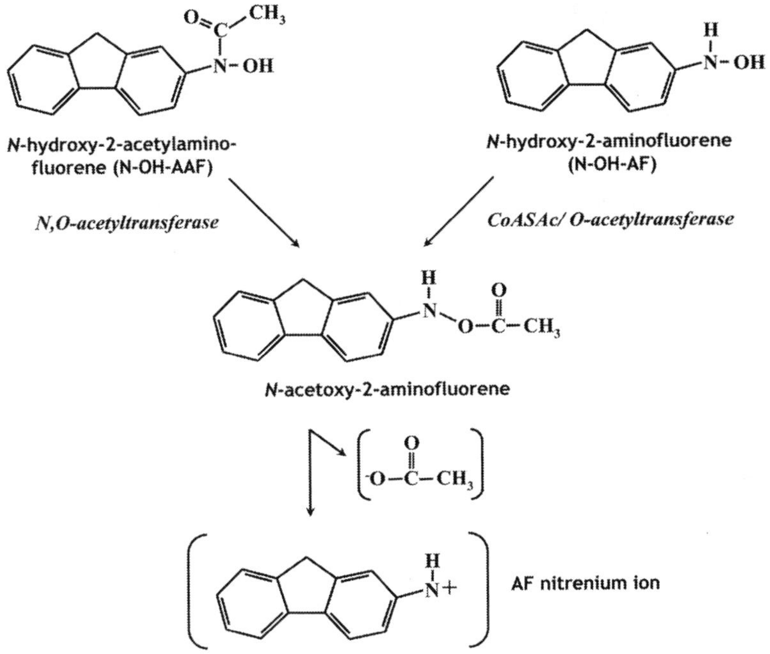

FIGURE 17-13.

Further pathways of activation of *N*-hydroxy-2-acetylaminofluorene and *N*-hydroxy-2-aminofluorene.

Another activation route for *N*-hydroxy-2-AAF is the *intramolecular* transfer of the acetyl moiety from the N to the O atom (N,O-acetyltransfer, see chapter 13 (*67*)). This transformation (figure 17-13) yields the highly reactive *N*-acetoxy-2-aminofluorene; loss of acetate anion from this intermediate yields the arylnitrenium ion (RN⁺H).

Reactive N-acetoxy esters such as *N*-acetoxy-2-aminofluorene can also be formed via *N*-arylhydroxylamines (*68*). One route for generation of *N*-arylhydroxylamines is the enzyme-catalyzed *deacetylation* of arylhydroxamic acids (*69*). This reaction is catalyzed by a microsomal deacetylase enzyme (*70, 71*) that also catalyzes the hydrolysis of arylamides to arylamines (*72*); in effect, the enzyme reverses the action of the arylamine *N*-acetyltransferases described in chapter 13. Recent studies suggest that the physiological role of this enzyme is as a lipase, that is, an enzyme catalyzing the hydrolysis of triacylglycerols (*73*).

Another route to *N*-arylhydroxylamines is the P450-catalyzed N-oxidation of aromatic amines (*74*); P450 family 1 members catalyze this oxidation reaction (*75*), as mentioned in chapter 7. *N*-Arylhydroxylamines can be metabolized to reactive esters by O-acetylation (chapter 13) or sulfate conjugation (chapter 14).

GUANINE C8 ADDUCTS OF AROMATIC AMINES: MECHANISM OF FORMATION

The characteristic DNA lesions formed from aromatic amines and nitro-aromatic compounds (including the heterocyclic amine food pyrolysis products (*76*)) are *adducts at the C8 carbon atoms of deoxyguanosine residues*.

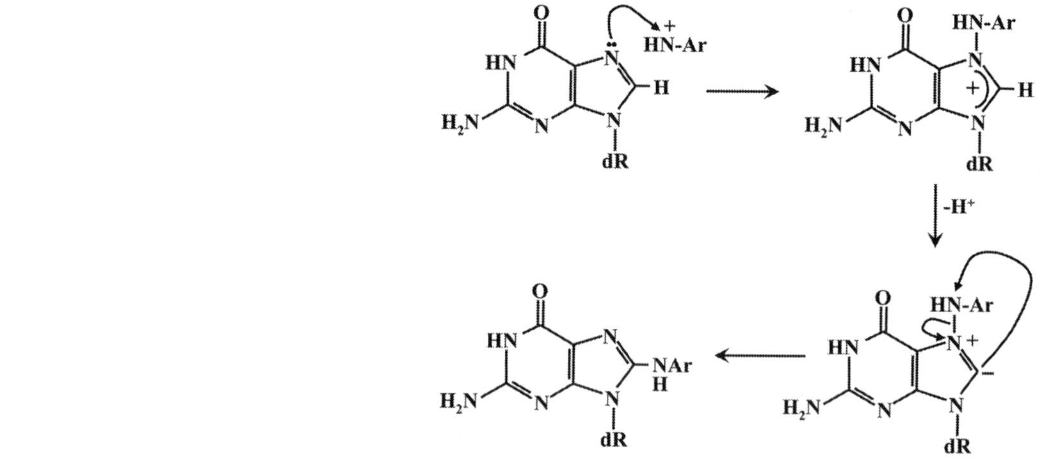

FIGURE 17-14.

Postulated mechanism for formation of guanine C8 adducts of arylamines; see text.

This site specificity seems odd, since the C8 position is not a particularly nucleophilic site on DNA, but a chemical explanation has been offered by the work of Humphreys et al. (77). In their experiments, C8,N9-dimethylguanine, rather than guanine itself, was used as the target. The unstable N-acetoxyaminofluorene was generated in vitro by the acetylation of N-hydroxy-2-aminofluorene. With the C8 position of the base blocked by methylation, aminofluorene added *at the N7 nitrogen atom instead.* Based on this evidence, it was proposed that, in the case of regular DNA guanine residues, the initial site of reaction is also at N7, forming an N7 adduct that rearranges to give the characteristic C8 adduct (figure 17-14). This rearrangement is analogous to the Stevens 1,2-rearrangement of ylides[8] (78), except that the migrating substituent is Ar–NH– rather than Ar–CH$_2$–group. The initial N7 adduct is an imidazolium (purine) cation, and the C8 proton of this adduct is acidic. Loss of the C8 proton gives a species with ylide character, which rearranges to form the C8 adduct, as indicated in figure 17-14. Whether this rearrangement mechanism accounts for the C8 specificity of activated aromatic amines remains controversial, however, and some researchers believe that direct interaction of the nitrenium ion with the C8 carbon atom is more likely (79).

GUANINE C8 ADDUCTS OF AROMATIC AMINES: EFFECTS ON DNA STRUCTURE

How do aromatic amine C8 guanine adducts modify the conformation of DNA? Structural analysis may help to explain why these adducts frequently induce mutations when damaged template strands are "read" by DNA polymerases. These questions can now be addressed experimentally. To do so, we need to prepare defined DNA oligonucleotides bearing covalent adducts on specific bases. This can be accomplished either by preparing 3'-phosphoramidite derivatives of modified bases, which are then incorporated into oligonucleotides by standard solid-phase synthesis chemistry (80); or by treating an oligonucleotide with a reactive species such as an N-acetoxyarylamine, and then purifying an adducted product to homogeneity, usually by HPLC. The latter method is simplified if the target oligonucleotide contains, for example, only a single G residue, since N-acetoxyarylamines preferentially modify guanine bases (81). For structural studies, duplex DNA can be formed by annealing modified oligonucleotides with (unadducted) complementary single strands.

NMR methods (82) have been especially useful for the analysis of the conformations of such modified DNA molecules. NMR is used to solve the structure of the molecule in solution, so crystallization is not required. An example of this approach is a recent study of the conformation of a synthetic double-stranded DNA carrying a PhIP-C8-deoxyguanosine adduct on one strand (83). In the predominant conformation (figure 17-15), the PhIP moiety of the guanosine adduct is intercalated into the core of the DNA helix, causing local denaturation of the normal Watson–Crick structure and significant bending of the axis of the double helix. This structure illustrates a common feature of bulky carcinogen adducts: planar hydrophobic moieties, such as polycyclic aromatic hydrocarbons and aromatic amines, prefer to reside in the hydrophobic core of the DNA double helix, stacked with the adjacent bases. The intercalated adduct occupies the position normally belonging to the DNA base, thereby forcing

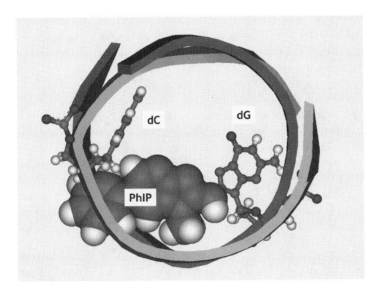

FIGURE 17-15.
Structure of PhIP-C8-deoxyguanosine adduct in a defined DNA oligo-nucleotide duplex; coordinate file: 1HZ0.pdb (structure 1). The view is along the helix axis. The adducted deoxyguanosine nucleoside (dG) and its (normally base-paired) deoxycytidine (dC) partner are shown as stick models. The PhIP moiety of the dG adduct is shown as a space-filling model. Note the intercalation of the PhIP moiety into the position normally occupied by a base, and the displacement of the dC base, almost at right angles to its usual Watson–Crick orientation. *Note*: A full-color version of this figure appears on the website. (*Brown, K.; Hingerty, B. E.; Guenther, E. A.; Krishnan, V. V.; Broyde, S.; Turteltaub, K. W.; Cosman, M. Solution structure of the 2-amino-1-methyl-6-phenylimidazo[4,5-b]pyridine C8-deoxyguanosine adduct in duplex DNA.* Proc. Natl. Acad. Sci. USA **2001**, 98, 8507–8512.)

the base into an unusual conformation, for example, parallel rather than perpendicular to the helix axis, or flipped outside of the helix core altogether.

ORGAN SPECIFICITY IN AROMATIC AMINE CARCINOGENESIS

Finally, let us return to an observation made at the beginning of this chapter—and at the beginning of the study of aromatic amine carcinogenesis. The characteristic human tumor induced by benzidine (and probably by most aromatic amines) is urinary bladder carcinoma.[9] Why? Even today, we cannot give a complete explanation, but Rehn's 19th-century suggestion still seems like the right idea: "materials... present in solution in the urine..." are responsible.

Many common human cancers are carcinomas, that is, cancers that occur in epithelial tissues, the linings that cover the surfaces where the body contacts the "external" environment. These sites include the skin, oral cavity, trachea, lung, esophagus, stomach, colon, mammary gland (ducts), bladder, and so on. In some cases, there seems to be an obvious relationship between a causative agent and the target tissue; for example, ultraviolet light striking exposed skin surfaces, cigarette smoke inhaled into the lungs, snuff or betel quid held against the mucous membranes of the mouth. So, we need to ask how aromatic amine metabolites might reach the bladder. There are two possible routes: through the circulatory system or via the urine, produced in the kidneys. The circulation reaches every organ, so it seems an unlikely explanation for a bladder-specific effect. But the bladder specifically accumulates urine, containing xenobiotic conjugates that are destined for excretion. Several routes can be envisaged for such urinary metabolites to damage the bladder epithelium, and it is still unclear which of these possibilities is the most important (figure 17-16). One scheme postulates that benzidine is acetylated, oxidized, and glucuronidated in the liver. The glucuronide is transported via the kidneys to the urine and stored in the bladder lumen. There (particularly if the urine is acidic, as is usually the case), the N-glucuronide may hydrolyze, releasing N-hydroxy-N'-acetylbenzidine. This metabolite may act directly as an

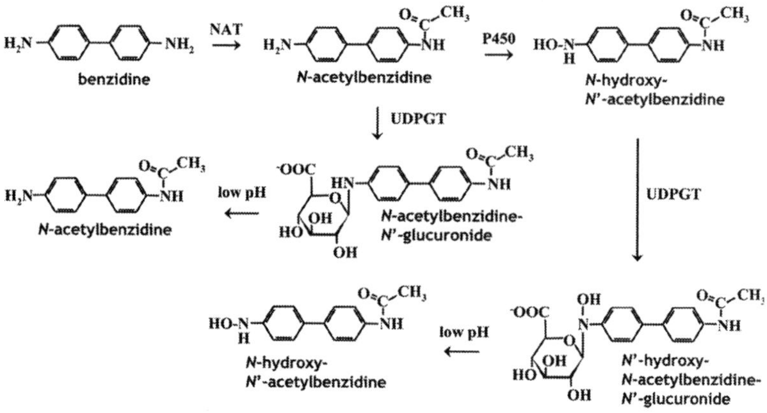

FIGURE 17-16.
Potential pathways for activation of benzidine to a bladder carcinogen; see text.

electrophile or may be further activated (perhaps by *O*-acetyltransferase activity in the bladder epithelium). Another proposal (*86*) is that benzidine is transported to the urine as a glucuronide, following acetylation, but without prior N-oxidation; hydrolyzed in the bladder lumen; and the liberated *N*-acetylbenzidine is activated by peroxidase enzymes (such as prostaglandin synthase (*87*)).

Notes

1. That is, aryl C-nitroso compounds, which should not be confused with alkyl N-nitroso compounds, discussed in chapter 7.

2. Why "Congo" red? At this time, the European imperial powers were meeting in Berlin to divide up the newly "discovered" territories of the Congo river basin. Africa represented everything new, exotic, and mysterious.

3. Why should the bladder be the target organ? This question is discussed in the final section of this chapter.

4. Rehn went on to become professor of surgery at Frankfurt University; he is now remembered chiefly for his suture of the right heart ventricle of a stabbing victim (1886), regarded as the first successful cardiac surgery.

5. A sulfinamide (RSON(H)R′) can be regarded as the product of condensation of a sulfinic acid (RSO_2H) and an amine (R′–NH_2).

6. The old (pre-1960s) names for NADH and NADPH were diphosphopyridine and triphosphopyridine nucleotide, respectively, hence "D" and "T."

7. P450 1A2 has long been regarded as the major enzyme catalyzing aromatic amine N-hydroxylation, but studies with 1A2-null mice (*59*) have brought this assumption into question; P450 1B1 or other enzymes may actually be more important.

8. An ylide is an organic species in which a negatively charged carbon atom is stabilized by an adjacent positively charged heteroatom.

9. Benzidine is also a bladder carcinogen in dogs (*84*). Nevertheless, aromatic amines can act at other sites: in humans, breast and colon cancer may also be induced, as mentioned earlier; in mice, liver tumors are commonly observed (*85*).

References

1. Vineis, P.; Pirastu, R. Aromatic amines and cancer. *Cancer Causes Control* **1997**, *8*, 346–355.

2. Weisburger, J. H. Comments on the history and importance of aromatic and heterocyclic amines in public health. *Mutat. Res.* **2002**, *506–507*, 9–20.

3. Garfield, S. *Mauve: How One Man Invented a Color That Changed the World*; W. W. Norton: New York, 2001.

4. Dietrich, H.; Dietrich, B. Ludwig Rehn (1849–1930): pioneering findings on the aetiology of bladder tumours. *World J. Urol.* **2001**, *19*, 151–153.

5. Cartwright, R. A. Historical and modern epidemiological studies on populations exposed to N-substituted aryl compounds. *Environ. Health Perspect.* **1983**, *49*, 13–19.

6. Choudhary, G. Human health perspectives on environmental exposure to benzidine: a review. *Chemosphere* **1996**, *32*, 267–291.

7. Naito, S.; Tanaka, K.; Koga, H.; Kotoh, S.; Hirohata, T.; Kumazawa, J. Cancer occurrence among dyestuff workers exposed to aromatic amines. A long term follow-up study. *Cancer* **1995**, *76*, 1445–1452.

8. Littlefield, N. A.; Nelson, C. J.; Gaylor, D. W. Benzidine dihydrochloride: risk assessment. *Fundam. Appl. Toxicol.* **1984**, *4*, 69–80.

9. Michaels, D. When science isn't enough: Wilhelm Hueper, Robert A. M. Case, and the limits of scientific evidence in preventing occupational bladder cancer. *Int. J. Occup. Environ. Health* **1995**, *1*, 278–288.

10. Dewan, A.; Jani, J. P.; Shah, K. S.; Kashyap, S. K. Urinary excretion of benzidine in relation to the acetylator status of occupationally exposed subjects. *Hum. Toxicol.* **1986**, *5*, 95–97.

11. Savard, S.; Josephy, P. D. Synthesis and mutagenicity of 3,3′-dihalogenated benzidines. *Carcinogenesis* **1986**, *7*, 1239–1241.

12. Chung, K. T.; Stevens, S. E., Jr.; Cerniglia, C. E. The reduction of azo dyes by the intestinal microflora. *Crit. Rev. Microbiol.* **1992**, *18*, 175–190.

13. Nony, C. R.; Bowman, M. C.; Cairns, T.; Lowry, L. K.; Tolos, W. P. Metabolism studies of an azo dye and pigment in the hamster based on analysis of the urine for potentially carcinogenic aromatic amine metabolites. *J. Anal. Toxicol.* **1980**, *4*, 132–140.

14. Miller, B. A.; Silverman, D. T.; Hoover, R. N.; Blair, A. Cancer risk among artistic painters. *Am. J. Ind. Med.* **1986**, *9*, 281–287.

15. Cassidy, L. D.; Youk, A. O.; Marsh, G. M. The Drake Health Registry Study: cause-specific mortality experience of workers potentially exposed to beta-naphthylamine. *Am. J. Ind. Med.* **2003**, *44*, 282–290.

16. Hinson, J. A. Reactive metabolites of phenacetin and acetaminophen: a review. *Environ. Health Perspect.* **1983**, *49*, 71–79.

17. Gago-Dominguez, M.; Yuan, J. M.; Castelao, J. E.; Ross, R. K.; Yu, M. C. Regular use of analgesics is a risk factor for renal cell carcinoma. *Br. J. Cancer* **1999**, *81*, 542–548.

18. Raether, W.; Hanel, H. Nitroheterocyclic drugs with broad spectrum activity. *Parasitol. Res.* **2003**, *90* (Suppl. 1), S19–S39.

19. Bendesky, A.; Menendez, D.; Ostrosky-Wegman, P. Is metronidazole carcinogenic? *Mutat. Res.* **2002**, *511*, 133–144.

20. Sugimura, T. Studies on environmental chemical carcinogenesis in Japan. *Science* **1986**, *233*, 312–318.

21. Ohgaki, H.; Takayama, S.; Sugimura, T. Carcinogenicities of heterocyclic amines in cooked food. *Mutat. Res.* **1991**, *259*, 399–410.

22. Jagerstad, M.; Skog, K.; Grivas, S.; Olsson, K. Formation of heterocyclic amines using model systems. *Mutat. Res.* **1991**, *259*, 219–233.

23. Layton, D. W.; Bogen, K. T.; Knize, M. G.; Hatch, F. T.; Johnson, V. M.; Felton, J. S. Cancer risk of heterocyclic amines in cooked foods: an analysis and implications for research. *Carcinogenesis* **1995**, *16*, 39–52.

24. Turesky, R. J. Heterocyclic aromatic amine metabolism, DNA adduct formation, mutagenesis, and carcinogenesis. *Drug Metab. Rev.* **2002**, *34*, 625–650.

25. Sugimura, T. Food and cancer. *Toxicology* **2002**, *181–182*, 17–21.

26. Felton, J. S.; Knize, M. G.; Shen, N. H.; Lewis, P. R.; Andresen, B. D.; Happe, J.; Hatch, F. T. The isolation and identification of a new mutagen from fried ground beef: 2-amino-1-methyl-6-phenylimidazo[4,5-b]pyridine (PhIP). *Carcinogenesis* **1986**, *7*, 1081–1086.

27. Sinha, R.; Kulldorff, M.; Chow, W. H.; Denobile, J.; Rothman, N. Dietary intake of heterocyclic amines, meat-derived mutagenic activity, and risk

of colorectal adenomas. *Cancer Epidemiol. Biomarkers Prev.* **2001,** *10,* 559–562.

28. Zheng, W.; Gustafson, D. R.; Sinha, R.; Cerhan, J. R.; Moore, D.; Hong, C. P.; Anderson, K. E.; Kushi, L. H.; Sellers, T. A.; Folsom, A. R. Well-done meat intake and the risk of breast cancer. *J. Natl. Cancer Inst.* **1998,** *90,* 1724–1729.

29. Marzulli, F. N.; Green, S.; Maibach, H. I. Hair dye toxicity: a review. *J. Environ. Pathol. Toxicol.* **1978,** *1,* 509–530.

30. Ames, B. N.; Kammen, H. O.; Yamasaki, E. Hair dyes are mutagenic: identification of a variety of mutagenic ingredients. *Proc. Natl. Acad. Sci. USA* **1975,** *72,* 2423–2427.

31. Watanabe, T.; Hirayama, T.; Fukui, S. Mutagenicity of commercial hair dyes and detection of 2,7-diaminophenazine. *Mutat. Res.* **1990,** *244,* 303–308.

32. Yu, M. C.; Skipper, P. L.; Tannenbaum, S. R.; Chan, K. K.; Ross, R. K. Arylamine exposures and bladder cancer risk. *Mutat. Res.* **2002,** *506–507,* 21–28.

33. Brennan, P.; Bogillot, O.; Cordier, S.; Greiser, E.; Schill, W.; Vineis, P.; Lopez-Abente, G.; Tzonou, A.; Chang-Claude, J.; Bolm-Audorff, U.; Jockel, K. H.; Donato, F.; Serra, C.; Wahrendorf, J.; Hours, M.; T'Mannetje, A.; Kogevinas, M.; Boffetta, P. Cigarette smoking and bladder cancer in men: a pooled analysis of 11 case-control studies. *Int. J. Cancer* **2000,** *86,* 289–294.

34. Tripathi, A.; Folsom, A. R.; Anderson, K. E. Risk factors for urinary bladder carcinoma in postmenopausal women. The Iowa Women's Health Study. *Cancer* **2002,** *95,* 2316–2323.

35. Luceri, F.; Pieraccini, G.; Moneti, G.; Dolara, P. Primary aromatic amines from side-stream cigarette smoke are common contaminants of indoor air. *Toxicol. Ind. Health* **1993,** *9,* 405–413.

36. Smith, C. J.; Livingston, S. D.; Doolittle, D. J. An international literature survey of "IARC Group I carcinogens" reported in mainstream cigarette smoke. *Food Chem. Toxicol.* **1997,** *35,* 1107–1130.

37. Talaska, G.; al Juburi, A. Z.; Kadlubar, F. F. Smoking related carcinogen-DNA adducts in biopsy samples of human urinary bladder: identification of N-(deoxyguanosin-8-yl)-4-aminobiphenyl as a major adduct. *Proc. Natl. Acad. Sci. USA* **1991,** *88,* 5350–5354.

38. Sabbioni, G.; Jones, C. R. Biomonitoring of arylamines and nitroarenes. *Biomarkers* **2002,** *7,* 347–421.

39. Ringe, D.; Turesky, R. J.; Skipper, P. L.; Tannenbaum, S. R. Structure of the single stable hemoglobin adduct formed by 4-aminobiphenyl in vivo. *Chem. Res. Toxicol.* **1988,** *1,* 22–24.

40. Maclure, M.; Bryant, M. S.; Skipper, P. L.; Tannenbaum, S. R. Decline of the hemoglobin adduct of 4-aminobiphenyl during withdrawal from smoking. *Cancer Res.* **1990,** *50,* 181–184.

41. Takayama, S.; Kuwabara, N. Carcinogenic activity of 2-(2-furyl)-3-(5-nitro-2-furyl)-acrylamide, a food additive, in mice and rats. *Cancer Lett.* **1977,** *3,* 115–120.

42. Rosenkranz, H. S.; Mermelstein, R. Mutagenicity and genotoxicity of nitroarenes. All nitro-containing chemicals were not created equal. *Mutat. Res.* **1983,** *114,* 217–267.

43. Bamford, H. A.; Bezabeh, D. Z.; Schantz, S.; Wise, S. A.; Baker, J. E. Determination and comparison of nitrated-polycyclic aromatic

hydrocarbons measured in air and diesel particulate reference materials. *Chemosphere* **2003**, *50*, 575–587.

44. (a) Ernster, L. DT diaphorase. *Methods Enzymol.* **1967**, *10*, 309–317. (b) Bianchet, M. A.; Foster, C.; Faig, M.; Talalay, P.; Amzel, L. M. Structure and mechanism of cytosolic quinone reductases. *Biochem. Soc. Trans.* **1999**, *27*, 610–615.

45. Hajos, A. K.; Winston, G. W. Dinitropyrene nitroreductase activity of purified NAD(P)H-quinone oxidoreductase: role in rat liver cytosol and induction by Aroclor-1254 pretreatment. *Carcinogenesis* **1991**, *12*, 697–702.

46. Ueda, O.; Kitamura, S.; Ohashi, K.; Sugihara, K.; Ohta, S. Xanthine oxidase-catalyzed metabolism of 2-nitrofluorene, a carcinogenic air pollutant, in rat skin. *Drug Metab. Dispos.* **2003**, *31*, 367–372.

47. Enroth, C.; Eger, B. T.; Okamoto, K.; Nishino, T.; Nishino, T.; Pai, E. F. Crystal structures of bovine milk xanthine dehydrogenase and xanthine oxidase: structure-based mechanism of conversion. *Proc. Natl. Acad. Sci. USA* **2000**, *97*, 10723–10728.

48. Lovering, A. L.; Hyde, E. I.; Searle, P. F.; White, S. A. The structure of *Escherichia coli* nitroreductase complexed with nicotinic acid: three crystal forms at 1.7 A, 1.8 A and 2.4 A resolution. *J. Mol. Biol.* **2001**, *309*, 203–213.

49. Nokhbeh, M. R.; Boroumandi, S.; Pokorny, N.; Koziarz, P.; Paterson, E. S.; Lambert, I. B. Identification and characterization of SnrA, an inducible oxygen-insensitive nitroreductase in *Salmonella enterica* serovar Typhimurium TA1535. *Mutat. Res.* **2002**, *508*, 59–70.

50. Yamada, M.; Espinosa-Aguirre, J. J.; Watanabe, M.; Matsui, K.; Sofuni, T.; Nohmi, T. Targeted disruption of the gene encoding the classical nitroreductase enzyme in *Salmonella typhimurium* Ames test strains TA1535 and TA1538. *Mutat. Res.* **1997**, *375*, 9–17.

51. Benigni, R., Ed. *Quantitative Structure–Activity Relationship: QSAR Models of Mutagens and Carcinogens*; CRC Press: Boca Raton, FL, 2003.

52. Debnath, A. K.; Debnath, G.; Shusterman, A. J.; Hansch, C. A QSAR investigation of the role of hydrophobicity in regulating mutagenicity in the Ames test: 1. Mutagenicity of aromatic and heteroaromatic amines in *Salmonella typhimurium* TA98 and TA100. *Environ. Mol. Mutagen.* **1992**, *19*, 37–52.

53. Cunningham, A. R.; Klopman, G.; Rosenkranz, H. S. Identification of structural features and associated mechanisms of action for carcinogens in rats. *Mutat. Res.* **1998**, *405*, 9–27.

54. Perkins, R.; Fang, H.; Tong, W.; Welsh, W. J. Quantitative structure–activity relationship methods: perspectives on drug discovery and toxicology. *Environ. Toxicol. Chem.* **2003**, *22*, 1666–1679.

55. Wilson, R. H.; DeEds, F.; Cox, A. J. The toxicity and carcinogenic activity of 2-acetaminofluorene. *Cancer Res.* **1941**, *1*, 608.

56. Miller, J. A. The metabolism of xenobiotics to reactive electrophiles in chemical carcinogenesis and mutagenesis: a collaboration with Elizabeth Cavert Miller and our associates. *Drug Metab. Rev.* **1998**, *30*, 645–674.

57. Kadlubar, F. F. In memoriam: James A. Miller (1915–2000). *Chem. Res. Toxicol.* **2001**, *14*, 335–337.

58. Cramer, J. W.; Miller, J. A.; Miller, E. C. N-Hydroxylation: a new metabolic reaction observed in the rat with the carcinogen 2-acetylaminofluorene. *J. Biol. Chem.* **1960**, *235*, 885–888.

59. Tsuneoka, Y.; Dalton, T. P.; Miller, M. L.; Clay, C. D.; Shertzer, H. G.; Talaska, G.; Medvedovic, M.; Nebert, D. W. 4-Aminobiphenyl-induced liver and urinary bladder DNA adduct formation in Cyp1a2$^{(-/-)}$ and Cyp1a2$^{(+/+)}$ mice. *J. Natl. Cancer Inst.* **2003,** *95,* 1227–1237.

60. Miller, E. C.; Miller, J. A.; Hartmann, H. A. N-Hydroxy-2-acetylamino-fluorene: a metabolite of 2-acetylaminofluorene with increased carcino-genic activity in the rat. *Cancer Res.* **1961,** *21,* 815–831.

61. Wu, S. G.; Straub, K. D. Purification and characterization of N-hydroxy-2-acetylaminofluorene sulfotransferase from rat liver. *J. Biol. Chem.* **1976,** *251,* 6529–6536.

62. Van Roy, F. P.; Moyer, G. H.; Austin, G. E. A novel method for the small scale synthesis of N-acetoxy-2-acetylaminofluorene and its adducts. *Cancer Lett.* **1981,** *12,* 147–152.

63. Smith, B. A.; Springfield, J. R.; Gutmann, H. R. Solvolysis and metabolic degradation, by rat liver, of the ultimate carcinogen, N-sulfonoxy-2-acetylaminofluorene. *Mol. Pharmacol.* **1987,** *31,* 438–445.

64. Ford, G. P.; Herman, P. S. Relative stabilities of nitrenium ions derived from polycyclic aromatic amines. Relationship to mutagenicity. *Chem. Biol. Interact.* **1992,** *81,* 1–18.

65. Novak, M.; Toth, K.; Rajagopal, S.; Brooks, M.; Hott, L. L.; Moslener, M. Reactivity and selectivity of the N-acetyl-Glu-P-1, N-acetyl-Glu-P-2, N-acetyl-MeIQx, and N-acetyl-IQx nitrenium ions: comparison to carbo-cyclic N-arylnitrenium ions. *J. Am. Chem. Soc.* **2002,** *124,* 7972–7981.

66. Bol, S. A.; de Groot, A. J.; Tijdens, R. B.; Meerman, J. H.; Mullenders, L. H.; van Zeeland, A. A. Electrochemical detection and quantification of the acetylated and deacetylated C8-deoxyguanosine DNA adducts induced by 2-acetylaminofluorene. *Anal. Biochem.* **1997,** *251,* 24–31.

67. Land, S. J.; Zukowski, K.; Lee, M. S.; Debiec-Rychter, M.; King, C. M.; Wang, C. Y. Metabolism of aromatic amines: relationships of N-acetylation, O-acetylation, N,O-acetyltransfer and deacetylation in human liver and urinary bladder. *Carcinogenesis* **1989,** *10,* 727–731.

68. Guengerich, F. P. N-Hydroxyarylamines. *Drug Metab. Rev.* **2002,** *34,* 607–623.

69. Lai, C. C.; Miller, E. C.; Miller, J. A.; Liem, A. The essential role of microsomal deacetylase activity in the metabolic activation, DNA-(deoxyguanosin-8-yl)-2-aminofluorene adduct formation and initiation of liver tumors by N-hydroxy-2-acetylaminofluorene in the livers of infant male B6C3F1 mice. *Carcinogenesis* **1988,** *9,* 1295–1302.

70. Probst, M. R.; Jeno, P.; Meyer, U. A. Purification and characterization of a human liver arylacetamide deacetylase. *Biochem. Biophys. Res. Commun.* **1991,** *177,* 453–459.

71. Probst, M. R.; Beer, M.; Beer, D.; Jeno, P.; Meyer, U. A.; Gasser, R. Human liver arylacetamide deacetylase. Molecular cloning of a novel esterase involved in the metabolic activation of arylamine carcinogens with high sequence similarity to hormone-sensitive lipase. *J. Biol. Chem.* **1994,** *269,* 21650–21656.

72. Kudo, S.; Umehara, K.; Hosokawa, M.; Miyamoto, G.; Chiba, K.; Satoh, T. Phenacetin deacetylase activity in human liver microsomes: distribution, kinetics, and chemical inhibition and stimulation. *J. Pharmacol. Exp. Ther.* **2000,** *294,* 80–88.

73. Trickett, J. I.; Patel, D. D.; Knight, B. L.; Saggerson, E. D.; Gibbons, G. F.; Pease, R. J. Characterization of the rodent genes for arylacetamide

deacetylase, a putative microsomal lipase, and evidence for transcriptional regulation. *J. Biol. Chem.* **2001**, *276*, 39522–39532.

74. Kim, D.; Guengerich, F. P. Cytochrome P450 activation of arylamines and heterocyclic amines. *Annu. Rev. Pharmacol. Toxicol.* **2005**, *45*, 27–49.

75. Josephy, P. D.; Batty, S. M.; Boverhof, D. R. Recombinant human P450 forms 1A1, 1A2, and 1B1 catalyze the bioactivation of heterocyclic amine mutagens in *Escherichia coli lacZ* strains. *Environ. Mol. Mutagen.* **2001**, *38*, 12–18.

76. Schut, H. A.; Snyderwine, E. G. DNA adducts of heterocyclic amine food mutagens: implications for mutagenesis and carcinogenesis. *Carcinogenesis* **1999**, *20*, 353–368.

77. Humphreys, W. G.; Kadlubar, F. F.; Guengerich, F. P. Mechanism of C8 alkylation of guanine residues by activated arylamines: evidence for initial adduct formation at the N7 position. *Proc. Natl. Acad. Sci. USA* **1992**, *89*, 8278–8282.

78. Ollis, W. D.; Rey, M.; Sutherland, I. O. Base catalyzed rearrangements involving ylide intermediates: 15. The mechanism of the Stevens [1,2] rearrangement. *J. Chem. Soc., Perkin Trans. I* **1983**, 1009–1027.

79. McClelland, R. A.; Ahmad, A.; Dicks, A. P.; Licence, V. E. Spectroscopic characterization of the initial C8 intermediate in the reaction of the 2-fluorenylnitrenium ion with 2′-deoxyguanosine. *J. Am. Chem. Soc.* **2002**, *121*, 3303–3310.

80. Chenna, A.; Singer, B. Large scale synthesis of *p*-benzoquinone-2′-deoxycytidine and *p*-benzoquinone-2′-deoxyadenosine adducts and their site-specific incorporation into DNA oligonucleotides. *Chem. Res. Toxicol.* **1995**, *8*, 865–874.

81. Brown, K.; Guenther, E. A.; Dingley, K. H.; Cosman, M.; Harvey, C. A.; Shields, S. J.; Turteltaub, K. W. Synthesis and spectroscopic characterization of site-specific 2-amino-1-methyl-6-phenylimidazo[4,5-*b*]pyridine oligodeoxyribonucleotide adducts. *Nucleic Acids Res.* **2001**, *29*, 1951–1959.

82. Berg, J. M.; Tymoczko, J. L.; Stryer, L. *Biochemistry*; W. H. Freeman: New York, 2001.

83. Brown, K.; Hingerty, B. E.; Guenther, E. A.; Krishnan, V. V.; Broyde, S.; Turteltaub, K. W.; Cosman, M. Solution structure of the 2-amino-1-methyl-6-phenylimidazo[4,5-*b*]pyridine C8-deoxyguanosine adduct in duplex DNA. *Proc. Natl. Acad. Sci. USA* **2001**, *98*, 8507–8512.

84. Whysner, J.; Verna, L.; Williams, G. M. Benzidine mechanistic data and risk assessment: species- and organ-specific metabolic activation. *Pharmacol. Ther.* **1996**, *71*, 107–126.

85. Schieferstein, G. J.; Littlefield, N. A.; Gaylor, D. W.; Sheldon, W. G.; Burger, G. T. Carcinogenesis of 4-aminobiphenyl in BALB/cStCrlfC3Hf/Nctr mice. *Eur. J. Cancer Clin. Oncol.* **1985**, *21*, 865–873.

86. Zenser, T. V.; Lakshmi, V. M.; Hsu, F. F.; Davis, B. B. Metabolism of N-acetylbenzidine and initiation of bladder cancer. *Mutat. Res.* **2002**, *506–507*, 29–40.

87. Flammang, T. J.; Yamazoe, Y.; Benson, R. W.; Roberts, D. W.; Potter, D. W.; Chu, D. Z.; Lang, N. P.; Kadlubar, F. F. Arachidonic acid-dependent peroxidative activation of carcinogenic arylamines by extra-hepatic human tissue microsomes. *Cancer Res.* **1989**, *49*, 1977–1982.

THE "SOOTY WART"

Coal was the first fossil fuel of the industrial age. In the years following the Great Fire of London (1666), coal replaced wood as the major fuel for residential heating in English towns and cities. Coal furnace chimneys accumulate combustible soot, posing a serious risk of chimney fires, unless the narrow flues are cleaned out by a sweep. The task of sweeping sooty chimneys, often in stifling summer heat, fell to small children: they were suited to the task, because they were small enough to fit into the confined workspace. Children as young as five, from poor families, worked under conditions amounting to slavery. This appalling abuse prompted Parliament, in 1788, to enact one of the first bills regulating employment standards: the minimum age of sweeps was raised to eight, and the common practice of forcing children to go up chimneys that were actually *on fire* was prohibited!

> "This here boy, sir, wot the parish wants to 'prentis," said Mr. Gamfield.
> "Aye, my man," said the gentleman in the white waistcoat, with a condescending smile. "What of him?"
> "If the parish vould like him to learn a light pleasant trade, in a good 'spectable chimbley-sweepin' bisness," said Mr. Gamfield, "I wants a 'prentis, and I'm ready to take him."...
> "It's a nasty trade," said Mr. Limbkins, when Gamfield had again stated his wish.
> "Young boys have been smothered in chimneys before now," said another gentleman.
> "That's acause they damped the straw afore they lit it in the chimbley to make 'em come down again," said Gamfield; "that's all smoke, and no blaze; veras smoke ain't o' no use at all in makin' a boy come down, for it only sinds him to sleep, and that's wot he likes. Boys is wery obstinit, and wery lazy, gen'lmen, and there's nothink like a good hot blaze to make 'em come down vith a run. It's humane, too, gen'lmen, acause, even if they've stuck in the chimbley, roastin' their feet makes 'em struggle to hextricate theirselves."...
> At length...Mr. Limbkins said: "We have considered your proposition, and we don't approve of it."...
> Charles Dickens, *Oliver Twist* (1837), chapter III.

In 1775 the eminent surgeon Sir John Percivall Pott[1] (1714–1788; figure 18-1) observed, in his *Chirurgical Works*, that scrotal cancer was extraordinarily common among chimney sweeps in London. This report was the first published description of an occupational cancer. Several aspects

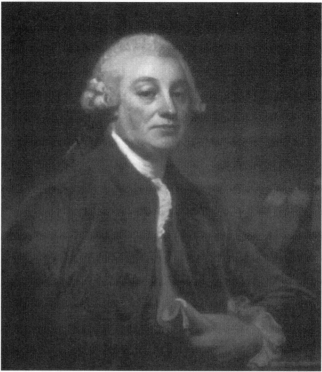

FIGURE 18-1.

Sir John Percivall Pott; portrait by George Romney, RA. (*Image kindly provided by Tina Craig, deputy head of library and information services, Royal College of Surgeons of England; from the RCS collection.*)

of the disease are worth noting, since they were repeated in many subsequent instances of occupational carcinogenesis. First, the disease was hardly ever seen among the general population. Second, the workers suffered repeated exposure to the causative agent (coal soot) at very high levels, extended over years of employment (if they survived the many other life-threatening dangers of the job). Third, the cancer was *site-specific*; since the site affected was a rare one, the connection between the exposure and the disease could be perceived by an insightful clinical observer. Indeed, the link was understood by the sweeps themselves, well before Pott's published findings; they called it the "sooty wart." Despite the gradual improvement in working conditions and general hygiene, the disease was still prevalent among chimney sweeps in Victorian times.

BENZO[*a*]PYRENE: THE COAL TAR CARCINOGEN

Coal can be pyrolyzed in the absence of air, supported by the oxygen present in the coal; the product is *coke*. Subsequent distillation yields coal gas (methane and other light hydrocarbons), light oil, naphthalene, and other industrial products. The heavy black residue the process leaves behind is called "coal tar." Millions of tons of this material are produced annually in many industrialized countries. Coal tar can be further processed to yield creosote, asphalt, and pitch, used in paving and roofing. Skin cancer and scrotal cancer were reported among workers in coal tar plants and paraffin factories in Germany and England, beginning in the 1880s. Could the association between exposure to coal tar and cancer be demonstrated experimentally? Which particular chemicals in coal tar and soot were the cause of the disease? An animal model was needed to address these questions. Several attempts to induce tumors in animals by treatment with materials such as soot and paraffin were unsuccessful. Finally, in 1915, Katsusaburo Yamagiwa (1863–1930), in Tokyo, applied coal tar to the inside skin of rabbits' ears, and persisted with the treatment protocol, three times a week, for three months. Towards the end of this period, the rabbits developed proliferative lesions (papillomas), and, eventually, malignant carcinomas. Coal tar was also shown to cause skin cancer in mice: a much smaller animal, easier to maintain in the laboratory. These achievements mark the beginning of the science of experimental chemical carcinogenesis and provided a bioassay that could be used to guide the purification of the active constituents of complex mixtures.

The search for the active component of coal tar was undertaken by Sir Ernest Kennaway and colleagues, in England (1). The mouse skin papilloma bioassay was the decisive guide. Two approaches were attempted simultaneously: synthesizing and testing new compounds, and painstakingly fractionating the coal tar, retaining the fractions with biological activity. By 1922 Kennaway had determined that the active compound had a high boiling point and contained no detectable nitrogen or sulfur (2). This evidence was consistent with the possibility that the active agent was a polycyclic aromatic hydrocarbon (PAH), such as anthracene, but PAH chemistry was largely an unexplored field of organic chemistry at that time.

By 1929 Cook and Kennaway had synthesized dozens of new PAHs and had more than 100 mouse skin painting experiments underway. A positive "hit" was finally obtained with the synthetic compound[2] in 1930. For the first time, a single pure chemical had been shown to induce cancer in animals. The demonstration of the carcinogenicity of this PAH facilitated the isolation of the coal tar carcinogen. In particular, the observed intense fluorescence of dibenz[a,h]anthracene led the research group to focus their attention on the fluorescent polycyclic components of coal tar.

Two *tons* (thousands of kilograms) of pitch were distilled and extracted with various organic solvents; fractions were tested on mice. By a tedious process of sequential extractions and crystallizations, increasingly active fractions were purified. After two years of these heroic labors, a 7 g sample of yellow crystals with very high biological activity was obtained. By 1933 this potent coal tar carcinogen had been identified as the PAH benzo[a]pyrene. The research trail pioneered by Yamagiwa and Ichikawa had culminated in the successful identification of an environmental carcinogen.

Benzo[a]pyrene is just one of many carcinogenic PAH compounds (figure 18-2). The study of PAHs is now a well-developed branch of organic chemistry (3). Hundreds of PAH compounds and their derivatives have been synthesized and studied. Much of this research has been stimulated by the toxicological importance of PAHs, although some applications for PAHs in spectroscopy, semiconductors, and other fields have been developed.

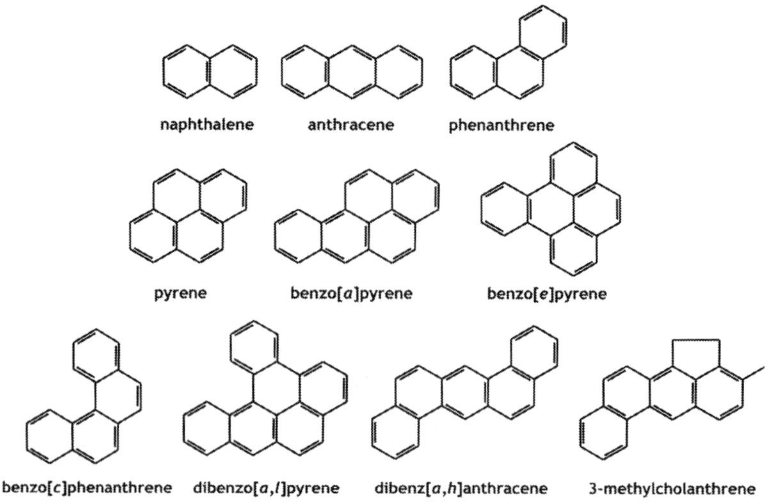

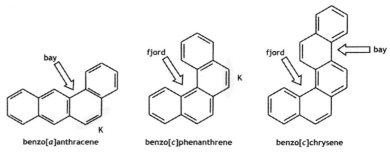

FIGURE 18-2.
Polycyclic aromatic hydrocarbons.

FIGURE 18-3.
Bay and fjord regions of PAHs. *Note*: A full-color version of this figure appears on the website.

BAY AND FJORD REGIONS

Special terminology has been adopted to describe the arrangements of the benzene rings in PAHs. The term *bay region* refers to the relatively hindered "inner corner" region in phenanthrene and compounds that contain a phenanthrene substructure, such as chrysene and benzo[*a*]pyrene (figure 18-3). We only use the term bay region when this structure has a terminal ring on one side. As we will see below, metabolic oxidation of this terminal ring is a crucial step in bioactivation of PAHs. When the bay region is even more hindered (figure 18-3), we refer to a *fjord region*. (Fjords are the narrow ocean inlets familiar from the coastlines of Norway or British Columbia.)

POLYCYCLIC AROMATIC HYDROCARBONS IN THE ENVIRONMENT

Analytical methods, especially gas chromatography–mass spectrometry (GC-MS), have been used to characterize the complex PAH mixtures present in coal tar and other combustion products. Coal is no longer

TABLE 18-1.

Concentrations of PAHs in Dust (Respirable Particulate Matter) Sampled in a Diesel Bus Depot in Lausanne, Switzerland (*4*)

COMPOUND	GC-MS ANALYSIS (ng/m^3)	COMPOUND	GC-MS ANALYSIS (ng/m^3)
Benz[*a*]anthracene	0.57	Indeno[1,2,3-*c,d*]pyrene	0.95
5-Methylchrysene	0.06	Dibenz[*a,h*]anthracene	0.08
Benzo[*b*]fluoranthene	0.78	Dibenzo[*a,l*]pyrene	0.07
Benzo[*k*]fluoranthene	0.3	Dibenzo[*a,e*]pyrene	0.1
Benzo[*j*]fluoranthene	0.47	Dibenzo[*a,i*]pyrene	0.06
Benzo[*a*]pyrene	1.09	Dibenzo[*a,h*]pyrene	0.01

commonly used for home heating in the developed world but coal-fired generating stations still supply about half of the electric power production in North America. These stations are major sources of air pollution, including PAHs. Gasoline and diesel exhaust also contain PAHs, because combustion of hydrocarbon fuel to carbon dioxide and water is never complete. Table 18-1 shows some of the PAH constituents that adhere to the particulate exhaust emitted by diesel bus engines. Many of these PAHs are known or suspect carcinogens.

"Fjord" regions of PAHs, as noted above, are the very highly hindered regions found in molecules such as dibenzo[*a,l*]pyrene (also called dibenzo[*def,p*]chrysene) and benzo[*c*]chrysene (which has both bay and fjord regions) (figure 18-3). Although the fjord region PAHs are generally larger and less environmentally prevalent than the bay region PAHs (such as benzo[*a*]pyrene), they are exceptionally potent mutagens and carcinogens (*5*). Dibenzo[*a,l*]pyrene, in particular, is the most potent PAH carcinogen yet discovered (*6*). Some fjord region PAHs are found in the environment. Sauvain and colleagues measured various PAH compounds in diesel particulate, by GC-MS, and found that dibenzo[*a,l*]pyrene was present at levels of about 1 μg/g total particulate, roughly one-fifth of the level of benzo[*a*]pyrene (*7*). Seidel and colleagues have analyzed cigarette smoke condensate by GC-MS and determined the presence of dibenzo[*a,l*]pyrene at a level of about 0.1 ng per cigarette, roughly 1% of the level of benzo[*a*]pyrene (*8*).

MOLECULAR ORBITAL THEORY OF POLYCYCLIC AROMATIC HYDROCARBONS

Understanding the toxicology of PAHs presents an intriguing challenge: while some compounds are potent carcinogens (e.g., benzo[*a*]pyrene), close analogues may be inactive (e.g., benzo[*e*]pyrene; figure 18-2). PAHs are particularly amenable to theoretical analysis, because of their structural simplicity. Many attempts have been made to develop a theoretical framework for predicting the biological activity of these compounds. Early efforts in this regard (from the 1950s) were limited to the analysis of the molecular structures of the parent PAHs, because the importance of

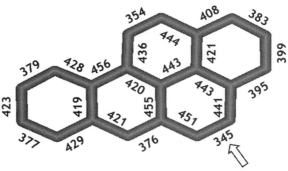

FIGURE 18-4.

Bond lengths in benzo[*a*]pyrene, determined by X-ray crystallography. The three-digit number adjacent to each bond is the fractional part of the length in ångstrom units, that is, 395 represents a bond length of 1.395 Å.

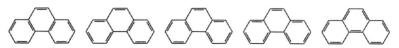

FIGURE 18-5.

Resonance hybrid structures of anthracene. Note that four of the five structures have a double bond at the uppermost (K-region) C–C bond.

metabolic activation was not yet appreciated, but theoretical methods can also provide insight into the chemical properties of activated metabolites.

In the case of benzene, all C–C bonds are equivalent, by symmetry, and, not surprisingly, have a bond length (1.39 Å) part way between that of a typical single bond (1.54 Å) and double bond (1.33 Å). *This symmetry is broken in fused PAHs.* Figure 18-4 shows the bond lengths for benzo[*a*]pyrene, as determined by X-ray crystallography (*9, 10*). We can see the effects of asymmetry on the chemistry of fused PAHs by simple evaluation of resonance hybrid structures; quantum mechanical analysis bears out these general features. If we consider the five possible structures of phenanthrene, we see that the 9,10 carbon–carbon bond, isolated from the biphenyl substructure of the remainder of the molecule, bears a double bond in four of the five (figure 18-5). Consequently, this bond is particularly "alkene-like" in its reactivity. The same consideration applies to the 4,5 and 9,10 carbon–carbon bonds of pyrene (figure 18-2). *This region of high π-electron density is known as the K-region*, following the notation introduced by Alberte and Bernard Pullman, who pioneered the theoretical study of the chemistry of PAHs in the 1950s.

Structural analysis by crystallography confirms the double-bond character of the K-region: the K-region bonds of pyrene, for example, have a bond length of only 1.34 Å, almost the same as that of a typical alkene. The K-region bonds are especially reactive. For example, oxidation of phenanthrene with CrO_3 gives the red-orange product 9,10-phenanthrenequinone; catalytic hydrogenation gives 9,10-dihydrophenanthrene; both reactions are entirely regiospecific (figure 18-6). Oxidation with hypochlorite or *meta*-chloroperoxybenzoic acid gives the K-region arene oxides (*11*). The K-region is also a major site of metabolic oxidation.

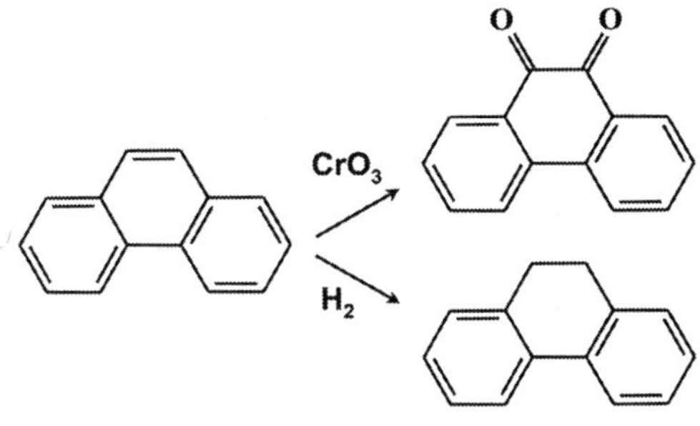

FIGURE 18-6.
Oxidation and catalytic hydrogenation of phenanthrene.

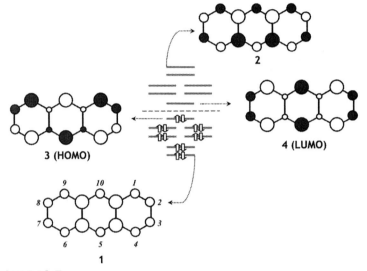

FIGURE 18-7.
Molecular orbitals for anthracene. *Note*: A full-color version of this figure appears on the website.

A rigorous theoretical study of the chemistry of PAHs (or any other molecules, for that matter) must be based on quantum mechanical principles. In this section, the elements of the molecular orbital analysis of PAH structures are presented in a nonmathematical way. We will see that quantum mechanical analysis can readily explain some of the typical features of the chemical behavior of these molecules.

Molecular orbital theory describes the electronic structure of molecules in terms of molecular orbitals constructed from linear combinations of atomic orbitals. As in the simpler case of homonuclear diatomic molecules (*12*), we can construct a manifold of molecular orbitals for a given molecule; each molecular orbital has a defined energy. In the molecular electronic ground state, electrons fill the molecular orbitals in order, from the lowest energy upwards. Each orbital accommodates two electrons, with opposite spins.

In the case of PAHs (*13*), these π molecular orbitals are delocalized over the entire conjugated framework. The molecular orbitals at lowest energy have the greatest amount of bonding character. Figure 18-7 shows four of the 14 π molecular orbitals for anthracene. In these sketches, the molecule is viewed from the top. The contribution of each 2p atomic orbital to the molecular orbital is illustrated by the size of the circle (representing the top lobe of the 2p orbital). Shaded and unshaded lobes have opposite phases; that is, the shading represents the sign of the atomic orbital's contribution to the molecular orbital wavefunction.

MO1 shows phase agreement (π bonding) between every neighboring pair of carbon atoms. As a result, MO1 is the lowest-energy π molecular orbital. The second molecular orbital illustrated (MO2) shows phase *disagreements* between every pair of neighbors; hence, MO2 is at the top of the energy spectrum. In fact, this molecular orbital is just the same as the first, but with each of the phase agreements reversed: MO2 is just as *antibonding* as MO1 is bonding. Hence, these two molecular orbitals are referred to as "paired." It can be shown that, for π systems containing no odd-numbered rings, *all* the molecular orbitals are paired, at a simple level of quantum mechanical approximation (Hückel theory). Each pair of molecular orbitals straddles the midpoint of the energy spectrum and has the same magnitudes of atomic orbital contributions, but with phases reversed at every other carbon.

The third molecular orbital (MO3) in figure 18-7 shows both phase agreements and disagreements between neighbors. MO3 lies just below the midpoint of the energy spectrum, and has a partner (MO4) just *above* the midpoint. It is easily seen that the MO4 can be constructed from MO3 by reversing the phase of every second atomic orbital.

Each carbon atom in the conjugated system uses three of its valence electrons for covalent bonding to its three neighbors (either carbon or hydrogen atoms), through σ bonds. This leaves one electron for contribution to the π system. Anthracene, with 14 conjugated carbons, has 14 π electrons distributed among the 14 π molecular orbitals. These electrons are placed pairwise, with opposite spins, in the seven lowest-energy molecular orbitals. As a result, any hydrocarbon (without odd-numbered rings) has all the π molecular orbitals in the lower half of the energy spectrum filled and all the molecular orbitals above the energy midpoint empty, in its ground electronic state.

Some correlation is observed between those atoms whose atomic orbital coefficients are most prominent contributors to a molecular orbital and that molecular orbital's position in the energy spectrum. Thus, the carbon atoms at the ring fusion sites (which are the atoms with the largest number of carbon neighbors) dominate in the lowest energy molecular orbital and its partner. This arises because these are just the positions from which a π atomic orbital can achieve the most bonding (or antibonding) character, due to the larger number of carbon neighbors. Less well-connected carbons tend to be dominant in the molecular orbitals nearer the center of the energy spectrum. These characteristics can be seen in the anthracene molecular orbitals (figure 18-7).

The correlation of molecular orbital energy with atomic orbital dominance is important, because molecular orbital theory uses these two factors in predicting the relative reactivities of different sites in PAHs. A frequently used shortcut in reactivity predictions is to focus only on the highest occupied molecular orbital (HOMO). (Often, the atomic orbitals dominating the HOMO turn out to be the same ones dominating the whole set of molecular orbitals near the energy midpoint.) The partner of this molecular orbital is the lowest unfilled molecular orbital (LUMO). Focusing on these orbitals as a key to understanding chemical reactivity is the basis of the *frontier molecular orbital* approach.

An effective way to predict the sites where a molecule is more likely to respond to *electrophilic* attack is to identify the sites that dominate the HOMO. These are atoms having a relatively large amount of π electronic charge density that is not being used very effectively for bonding. (That is why the molecular orbital energies are high.) Conversely, a nucleophilic reaction is likely to occur preferentially at an atom that is prominent in the LUMO. This allows the nucleophile to connect its Lewis-base electron pair charge density to an atom that can accept it. But, for PAHs, the HOMO and LUMO are paired; hence, they are dominated by the same atoms. *So, molecular orbital theory predicts that the same sites should be favored for either electrophilic or nucleophilic reactions.*

We can already see that molecular orbital theory will predict the most reactive sites of PAHs to be carbons having two, rather than three, nearest-neighbor carbons. This because the three-neighbor carbons dominate the π molecular orbitals away from the spectral center (i.e., above the LUMO or below the HOMO), leaving the two-neighbor carbons to dominate the π molecular orbitals around the spectral center.

But there are many such two-neighbor carbons. Anthracene has three distinct types (positions 1, 2, and 10). Understanding PAH metabolism requires knowing the relative reactivities of such sites. Inspection of the HOMO, LUMO pair shown in figure 18-7 leads us to predict a reactivity order of $10 > 1 > 2$, and this agrees with experiment.

In general, PAHs show greater reactivity at carbons that are one bond (α) rather than two bonds (β) away from a fusion site. There is a simple molecular orbital-based explanation for this trend (*14*). A molecular orbital having its energy right at the midpoint of the spectrum (called a nonbonding molecular orbital) is characterized by an atomic orbital pattern where every second carbon π atomic orbital has a zero coefficient. The "wavelength" of the envelope of these atomic orbitals is four carbon–carbon bond lengths. The HOMO in a PAH lies somewhat below the energy midpoint, and, hence, has a wavelength slightly longer than this (typically closer to five bond lengths). This gives us a wavelength estimate for a HOMO. We also have a boundary condition, namely that the *atomic orbital contribution at a fusion site tends to be small* (having been preferentially used up in lowest/highest energy molecular orbitals). If we draw an envelope wave having wavelength equal to five C–C bonds, and place a node at one fusion atom, we find that the resulting wave "dictates" an atomic orbital coefficient that is considerably larger at the carbon one bond from the node than at the carbon two bonds from the node (figure 18-8). *This implies that carbons one bond from a fusion site should be more reactive than those two bonds away.* PAHs sometimes show this pattern very clearly in their HOMO/LUMO pair, as in anthracene. In other cases, the connection pattern of the hydrocarbon leads to conflicts that cause this behavior to be spread among several of the higher-energy occupied molecular orbitals. This tends to disguise the cause, but does not alter the general effect: α *carbons are more reactive for electrophilic or nucleophilic reactions than are* β *carbons.* In anthracene, carbon atom 10 is α to *two* fusion sites: such atoms tend to be especially reactive.

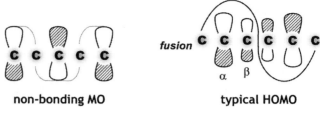

non-bonding MO | typical HOMO

FIGURE 18-8.

Envelope wave having wavelength of five C–C bonds.

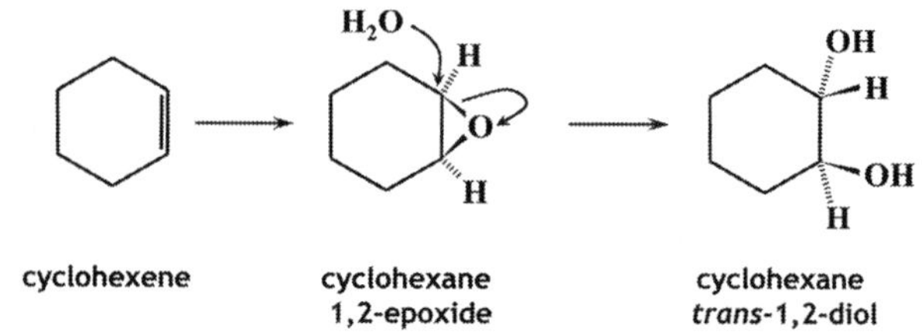

cyclohexene | cyclohexane 1,2-epoxide | cyclohexane *trans*-1,2-diol

FIGURE 18-9.

Formation of a dihydrodiol metabolite by epoxidation of an alkene followed by hydrolysis of the epoxide.

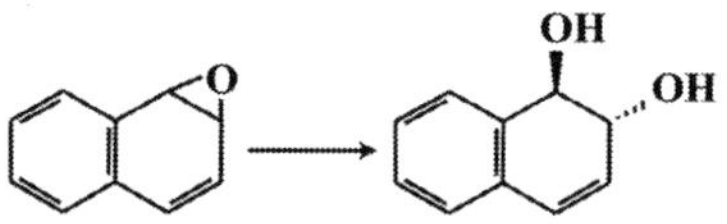

FIGURE 18-10.

Formation of dihydrodiol metabolite of naphthalene by hydrolysis of the arene oxide.

ARENE OXIDES

The formation of epoxides by P450-catalyzed oxidation of olefins and aromatic compounds was discussed in chapter 7. As early as 1950 (before the discovery of monooxygenase reactions), Eric Boyland pointed out that epoxides were possible intermediates in the metabolism of PAHs (*15*). *trans*-Dihydrodiols had already been isolated as metabolites of small PAHs, such as naphthalene and phenanthrene, and Boyland suggested that *epoxides were the probable precursors to dihydrodiols.* Most epoxides are highly reactive, because of the strained three-membered ring structure. Aliphatic epoxides react with nucleophiles such as water: hydrolysis proceeds by an S_N2 attack of hydroxide (or water) on the three-membered ring, resulting in stereochemical (Walden) inversion. So, for example, the epoxidation and hydrolysis of cyclohexene (figure 18-9) gives *trans*-cyclohexane-1,2-diol. PAH dihydrodiols might arise in the same manner (figure 18-10). At the time of Boyland's suggestion, arene oxides (the aromatic analogues of olefinic epoxides) were completely unknown. However, with the development of the chemistry of arene oxides (discussed in chapter 7) and the biochemistry of P450-dependent oxidations, Boyland's idea was shown to be correct and led to swift progress in understanding the toxicity of PAHs.

POLYCYCLIC AROMATIC HYDROCARBONS: METABOLISM AND BIOACTIVATION

In the early 1950s Elizabeth Cavert Miller determined that a metabolite of benzo[a]pyrene reacts with the proteins in mouse skin (16). Benzo[a]pyrene was painted onto the skin of the animals, and the skin proteins were isolated. Unmetabolized benzo[a]pyrene was extracted with organic solvents. The purified protein residue left after extraction was fluorescent, and the fluorescence spectrum resembled that of benzo[a]pyrene. Clearly, some reactive metabolite (or metabolites) of the parent hydrocarbon became bound to the protein and this binding was too strong to be disrupted even by exhaustive washings: it was apparently covalent in nature.

Miller referred to the then-unknown reactive metabolite as the *ultimate carcinogen* and asserted that covalent binding was the key step in bioactivation of PAH carcinogens. Studies by Miller and Miller on the covalent binding of carcinogenic aminoazo dyes reached similar conclusions, and they suggested that metabolic activation followed by covalent binding might be a general paradigm for chemical carcinogenesis. (Previous theories of PAH carcinogenesis had been based on very different concepts, such as the postulated biological activities of PAHs as analogues of steroid hormones.) The Millers' concept of metabolic activation to reactive intermediates has since been verified and extended to other classes of chemical carcinogens, including aromatic amines and nitrosamines.

In 1961 Heidelberger (17) and Davenport demonstrated that ^{14}C-labeled dibenz[a,h]anthracene painted onto mouse skin became bound to nucleic acids. DNA was isolated from the skin tissue and freed from contaminating protein and RNA by digestion with proteases and ribonuclease, and covalent binding to DNA was observed. Brookes and Lawley compared the extent of DNA binding by a series of ^{3}H-labeled PAHs, and reported that the extent of binding correlated with carcinogenic potency (18). This was consistent with the hypothesis that *covalent binding to DNA is a prerequisite for chemical carcinogenesis.*

K-REGION EPOXIDE METABOLITES OF POLYCYCLIC AROMATIC HYDROCARBONS

Following Boyland's suggestion that epoxides could be intermediates in PAH metabolism, PAHs such as 7,12-dimethylbenz[a]anthracene were shown indeed to be metabolized to K-region epoxides (arene oxides) (21, 22). When cells were treated with K-region epoxide metabolites of PAHs, covalent DNA adducts were formed (23). This result agreed with the postulate that carcinogens are metabolized to reactive intermediates, as had been advanced by Elizabeth Cavert Miller and James Miller. Before continuing our discussion of PAHs, we consider the formation and metabolism of epoxides.

Metabolism of Epoxides

Arene oxides (see above and discussion in chapter 7) and dihydrodiol epoxides (see below) are particular classes of epoxides. Epoxides arise whenever oxygen atoms are added across double bonds, either by the action of enzymes or in uncatalyzed oxidation processes. Epoxides are commonly observed as P450-dependent metabolites of olefins, as mentioned in

▶ **PAH–DNA Binding In Vivo**

Although DNA is a biologically important target for covalent binding, it is only present in small amounts in the cell. The composition of liver tissue, for example, is approximately 70% water, 20% protein, 5% lipid, 1% RNA, and only 0.2% DNA, by weight. *The fraction of administered dose of a carcinogen that is metabolized to DNA adducts is exceedingly small.* Indeed, direct measurement of this DNA binding by tracing the in vivo fate of radiolabeled carcinogens is so difficult that it is not often attempted. Stowers and Anderson administered ^{3}H-labeled benzo[a]pyrene orally to mice (19), at a dose of about 25 µmol per mouse. The recovery of DNA adducts in the liver tissue was less than 10 pmol per mg DNA. Since 1 g of liver tissue contains about 2 mg DNA, this corresponds to about 20 pmol hepatic DNA adducts per mouse. Thus, only about 1 part per million of the administered dose is recovered as hepatic DNA adducts. Similar levels of DNA binding were found in other tissues. Protein specific binding levels were much higher (about 300 pmol per mg protein) and total protein mass is about 100 times greater than DNA mass. *Protein binding is much greater than DNA binding in vivo.* Most studies of DNA adduct formation in vivo are conducted using ultrasensitive assays such as ^{32}P-postlabeling (20) or immunoassay (19), as discussed in chapter 2. ◀

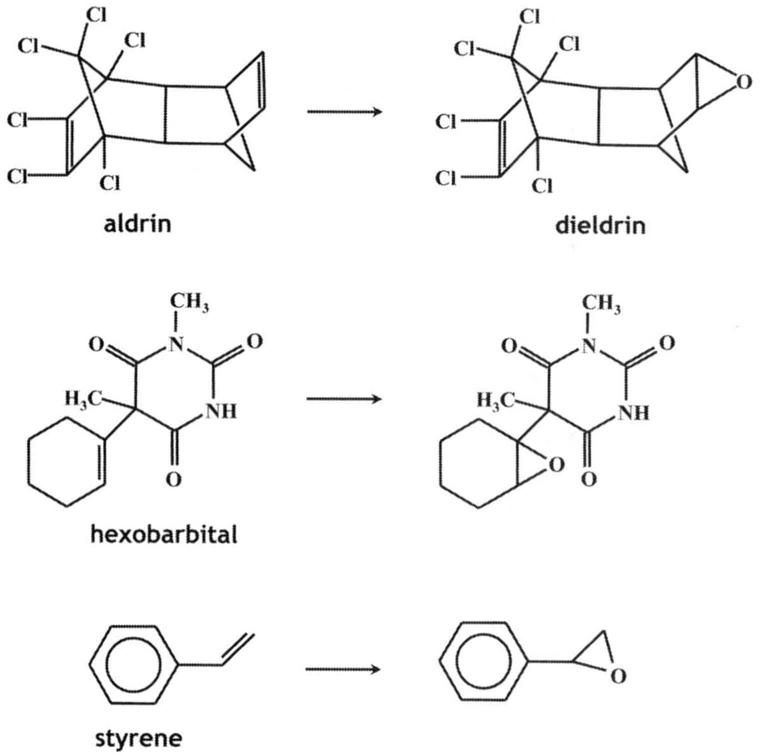

aldrin → dieldrin

hexobarbital

styrene

FIGURE 18-11.

Some P450-catalyzed alkene epoxidation reactions.

chapter 7. Xenobiotic precursors of epoxides include the insecticide aldrin (*24*); the sedative hexobarbital; and the plastics monomer styrene, which was discussed in chapter 11 (*25*) (figure 18-11). As already noted, epoxides are electrophilic species that react with nucleophiles, including water and GSH (figure 18-12); GSH conjugation of epoxides was discussed in chapter 9.

EPOXIDE HYDROLASE

The hydrolysis of epoxides to give *trans* diols is catalyzed by a family of enzymes called *epoxide hydrolases* (*26, 27*) (EC 3.3.2.3). (Previously, this enzyme has been called *epoxide hydrase* or *epoxide hydratase*.) The delineation of the human epoxide hydrolases is perhaps not yet complete, but it appears that at least five such enzymes exist (*28*). The crystal structure of a soluble epoxide hydrolase was solved in 1999 (*29*). Microsomal epoxide hydrolase (*30*) is a membrane-bond enzyme, a monomeric protein of 455 amino acid residues. Its substrates include many xenobiotic epoxides, such as PAH metabolites and the epoxide metabolites of benzene, 1,3-butadiene, and aflatoxin B_1.

Soluble (cytosolic) epoxide hydrolase (*31, 32*) metabolizes some xenobiotics, such as *trans*-stilbene oxide, an epoxide that is not a substrate for the microsomal enzyme. However, the enzyme probably acts primarily on endogenous epoxides, such as the epoxyeicosatrienoic acids. These

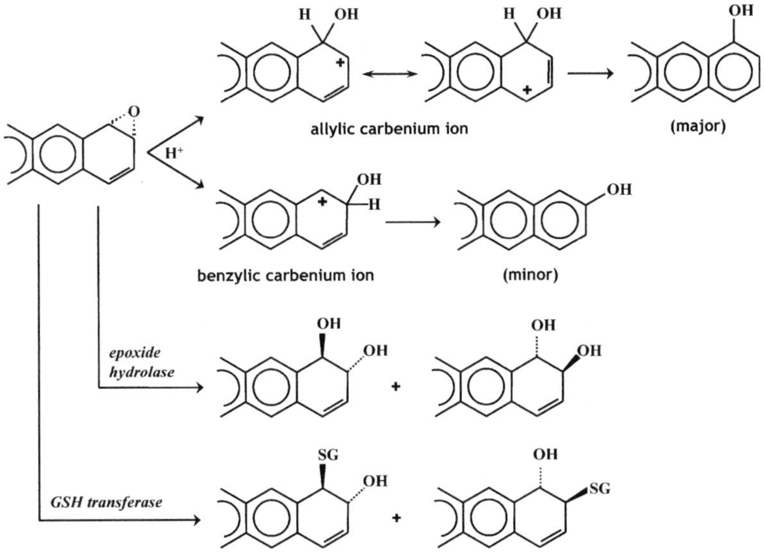

FIGURE 18-12.

Metabolism of an arene oxide. Top row and second row: isomerization to phenols. The reaction also proceeds spontaneously by the "NIH shift" pathway; here, the acid-catalyzed route is illustrated. The direction of opening of the epoxide ring dictates the phenol isomer formed. The allylic intermediate is favored; therefore, for example, naphthalene is metabolized primarily to 1-naphthol, with only a small amount of 2-naphthol formed. Third row: Hydrolysis, catalyzed by epoxide hydrolase, generates *trans*-dihydrodiols, since addition of water (or hydroxide) proceeds with inversion of configuration. Both of the enantiomeric *trans*-dihydrodiols can form, depending on the specificity of the enzyme (see van Bladeren, P. J.; Sayer, J. M.; Ryan, D. E.; Thomas, P. E.; Levin, W.; Jerina, D. M. Differential stereoselectivity of cytochromes P-450b and P-450c in the formation of naphthalene and anthracene 1,2-oxides. The role of epoxide hydrolase in determining the enantiomer composition of the 1,2-dihydrodiols formed. *J. Biol. Chem.* **1985**, *260*, 10226–10235 for further discussion). Bottom row: glutathione conjugation. This reaction is analogous to the reaction with water: the products are *trans* glutathione adducts, with the addition of glutathione occurring at either position, under enzymatic control (see chapter 11). Note that the terminal ring in the products of arene oxide hydrolysis or glutathione addition is a substituted cyclohexene ring: it is not aromatic.

compounds are eicosanoids, oxygenated metabolites of polyunsaturated fatty acids, along with the prostaglandins and leukotrienes.

Additional epoxide hydrolase forms include cholesterol 5,6-oxide hydrolase and leukotriene A_4 hydrolase. The 5,6-double bond of cholesterol (a major component of biological membranes) is oxidized during the process of lipid peroxidation (chapter 1). Cholesterol 5,6-epoxide is cytotoxic and may participate in atherosclerotic disease processes (*33*). Cholesterol 5,6-oxide hydrolase, a microsomal form, metabolizes this compound to cholestane triol (*34*). Leukotriene A_4 is another eicosanoid, an epoxide metabolite of arachidonic acid with potent proinflammatory activity. Leukotriene A_4 hydrolase is a cytosolic enzyme (*35a*) that catalyzes

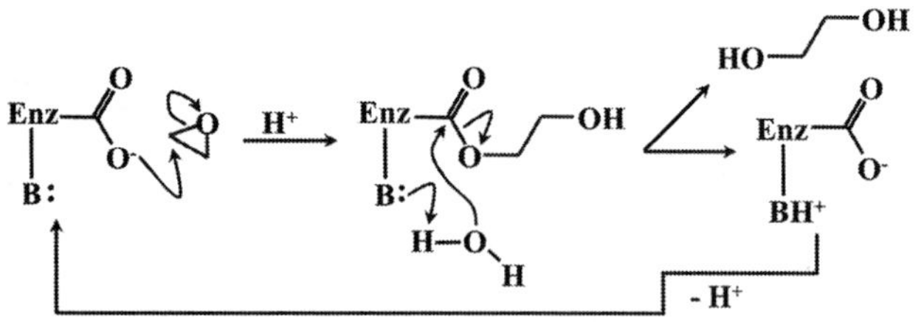

FIGURE 18-13.
Catalytic mechanism of epoxide hydrolase.

the hydrolysis of leukotriene A_4, to produce leukotriene B_4. (As shown in figure 9-21, glutathione conjugation of leukotriene A_4 gives rise to leukotrienes C, D, and E.) Leukotriene A_4 hydrolase is a zinc metalloenzyme that also displays aminopeptidase activity and has structural similarity to thermolysin-like metallopeptidases (35b). Richard Armstrong and co-workers have studied the catalytic mechanism of epoxide hydrolase enzymes (36, 37). An aspartate residue in the catalytic site is essential for activity. Nucleophilic attack by the aspartate side-chain carboxylate group on the epoxide generates a transient covalent (α-hydroxyacyl ester) intermediate, which is then hydrolyzed to form the diol product (figure 18-13).

BAY REGION DIHYDRODIOL EPOXIDES

The discovery that reactive K-region epoxides were metabolic products of PAHs (see above) suggested an explanation for the DNA- and protein-binding activity of these carcinogens. But were the K-region epoxides actually the reactive species responsible for PAH toxicity? Synthetic K-region epoxides were found to cause mutations in bacteria and to react with nucleic acids in vitro; but they were only weak carcinogens in rodents (38) and the chromatographic characteristics of the epoxide-derived adducts proved to be distinct from those of the labeled parent PAHs. However, the K-region (4,5 bond) is not the only site of benzo[a]pyrene epoxidation. Dihydrodiol metabolites are also formed at the terminal ring of benzo[a]pyrene (carbons 7, 8, 9, and 10) (figure 18-14).

When the 4,5- (K-region), 7,8-, and 9,10-dihydrodiol metabolites of benzo[a]pyrene were incubated with DNA and hepatic microsomes, the 7,8-isomer proved to be more than ten times as reactive with DNA as the other dihydrodiol isomers or benzo[a]pyrene itself (39). The 7,8-dihydrodiol was not directly reactive, but required metabolic activation by the microsomal enzymes. What was the activated metabolite of benzo[a]pyrene 7,8-dihydrodiol? Since the dihydrodiol metabolites possess an olefinic double bond, epoxidation was an obvious possibility. In 1974 Peter Sims, Phillip Grover, and colleagues identified 7,8-benzo[a]pyrene dihydrodiol 9,10-epoxide (BPDE) as a potent reactive metabolite of benzo[a]pyrene (40); a historical account of this groundbreaking work has been published recently (41). The key experiments compared the DNA adducts formed from: (a) mammalian cells incubated with benzo[a]pyrene in tissue culture; (b) DNA incubated with synthetic benzo[a]pyrene 4,5-oxide; (c) DNA incubated with liver microsomal preparation and benzo[a]pyrene 7,8-dihydrodiol; and (d) DNA incubated with

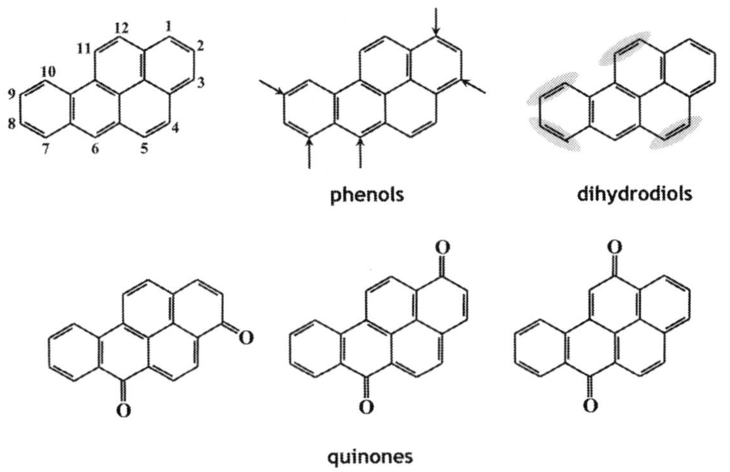

FIGURE 18-14.
Some oxidative metabolites of benzo[a]pyrene (top left). Phenols are formed at the positions indicated by arrows (top row, center). *trans*-Dihydrodiols, formed by epoxide hydrolase-catalyzed hydrolysis of epoxides, are obtained at the 4,5; 7,8; 9,10; and 11,12 regions, as indicated by shading (top row, right). Alternatively, trapping of the epoxides by glutathione yields glutathione adducts. (*Hernandez, O.; Walker, M.; Cox, R. H.; Foureman, G. L.; Smith, B. R.; Bend, J. R. Regiospecificity and stereospecificity in the enzymatic conjugation of glutathione with (+/−)-benzo(a)pyrene 4,5-oxide. Biochem. Biophys. Res. Commun. 1980, 96, 1494–1502.*) Bottom row: isomerization of the epoxides gives rise to phenolic metabolites at the 1, 3, 6, 7, and 9 positions. Further oxidation of the phenols gives 1,6-, 3,6-, and 6,12-quinones. Metabolites bearing hydroxyl groups (such as dihydrodiols and phenols) are conjugated to form glucuronides and sulfates. Epoxidation of the dihydrodiols is the critical pathway for bioactivation. *Note*: A full-color version of this figure appears on the website.

7,8-benzo[a]pyrene dihydrodiol 9,10-epoxide. *The adducts formed from cellular metabolism of benzo[a]pyrene coeluted with the BPDE and benzo[a]-pyrene dihydrodiol-derived adducts, but were distinct from the K-region epoxide-derived adducts.* The critical significance of BPDE was confirmed when BPDE proved to be highly carcinogenic in rodents (*42*) and the DNA adducts formed from benzo[a]pyrene in vivo were also found to coelute with in vitro BPDE-DNA adducts. (Note that BPDE has never been isolated from a metabolic activation system, due to its reactivity; its presence is usually inferred from a study of the DNA adducts formed.)

Formation of BPDE

Let us recapitulate the metabolic pathway leading from benzo[a]pyrene to BPDE (figure 18-15). The first step is P450-catalyzed epoxidation of benzo[a]pyrene to give an arene oxide, benzo[a]pyrene 7,8-epoxide. Epoxidation of an aromatic ring in a PAH such as naphthalene yields a new optically active carbon atom, so there are two enantiomeric naphthalene 1,2-oxides (see chapter 7). Similarly, two enantiomers of benzo[a]pyrene 7,8-epoxide can be formed: (+) (7R,8S)- and (−) (7S,8R)-benzo[a]pyrene 7,8-epoxide. *Trans* hydrolysis of these arene oxides,

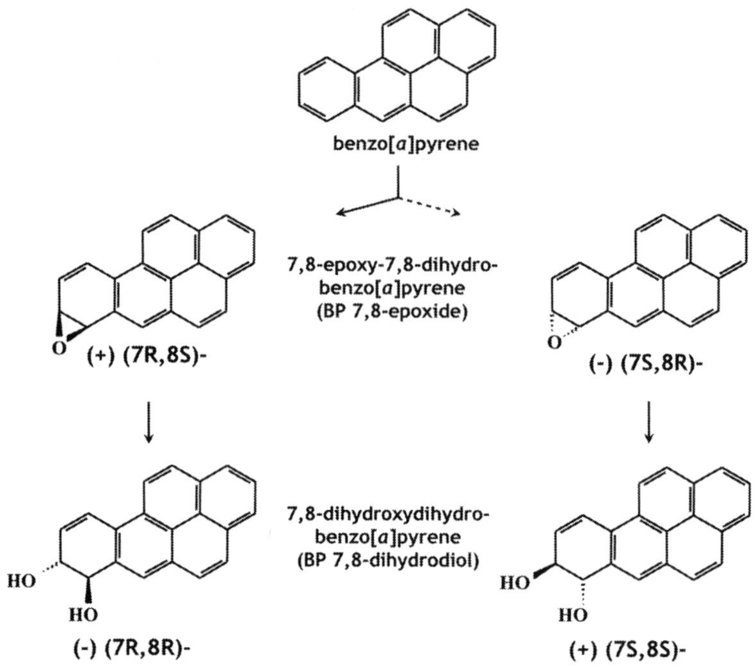

FIGURE 18-15.

Metabolism of benzo[a]pyrene to enantiomeric 7,8-dihydrodiols. Cytochrome P450-catalyzed epoxidation of benzo[a]pyrene is stereospecific. The enantiomeric ratio varies among P450 enzymes. In principle, each enantiomer of the epoxide could be hydrolyzed to both of the dihydrodiols, but microsomal epoxide hydrolase is regiospecific; water attacks at the 8-position only, so that each of the epoxides gives a single dihydrodiol, as indicated. (*Levin, W. et al. An enantiomeric interaction in the metabolism and tumorigenicity of (+)- and (-)-benzo[a]pyrene 7,8-oxide.* J. Biol. Chem. *1980, 255, 9067–9074.*)

catalyzed by epoxide hydrolase, gives 7,8-dihydroxydihydrobenzo[a]pyrene (BP 7,8-dihydrodiol), with each of the enantiomeric forms of the 7,8-epoxide giving a corresponding enantiomer. (Note that the two hydroxyl groups of the dihydrodiol are always *trans*, because of the S_N2 mechanism of enzymatic epoxide hydrolysis.) With the formation of the 7,8-dihydrodiol, the terminal six-membered ring of benzo[a]pyrene is no longer aromatic; it has only one double bond, at the 9,10 position, conjugated to the pyrene moiety. This olefin-like position is now subject to a second P450-catalyzed epoxidation, giving BPDE (figure 18-16). There are four possible BPDE isomers, two from each of the enantiomeric BP 7,8-dihydrodiols. Human P450 forms 1A1, 1A2 (*43, 44*) and 1B1 (*45, 46*) can catalyze the epoxidations of benzo[a]pyrene and 7,8-dihydroxydihydrobenzo[a]pyrene.

THE POTENT CHEMICAL AND BIOLOGICAL ACTIVITIES OF BAY REGION DIHYDRODIOL EPOXIDES

The remarkable activity of bay region dihydrodiol epoxides, compared to any other PAH epoxide metabolites, was first highlighted by Donald Jerina

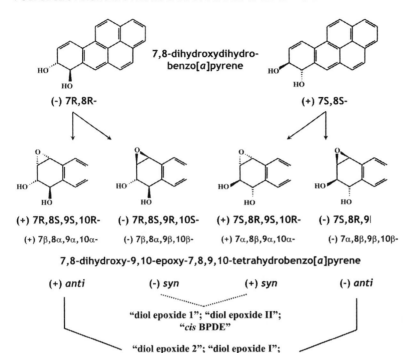

FIGURE 18-16.

Cytochrome P450-catalyzed epoxidation of benzo[*a*]pyrene dihydrodiols yields the "bay region" benzo[*a*]pyrene dihydrodiol epoxides (BPDE). The metabolic conversions show considerable stereospecificity; that is, the ratios of (+) *anti* to (−) *syn*, and of (−) *anti* to (+) *syn*, are not equal to one. The ratios vary with the enzyme systems studied. The BPDE isomers are labeled according to five different conventions; from top: systematic (*R*,*S*) designations; obsolete α,β system used in earlier literature; *syn/anti* designations; bottom rows indicate shorthand designations also used in the literature to distinguish between the *syn* and *anti* diastereomers.

and colleagues (*47*). Studies of the DNA binding, mutagenicity, and carcinogenicity of PAH metabolites have repeatedly confirmed the "bay region theory." It should be borne in mind, as discussed above, that bay region metabolites represent only a small fraction of the total metabolism of the parent hydrocarbon, which occurs at many sites in the molecule (*48*). What makes the bay region unusual? The acid-catalyzed opening of the epoxide ring of bay region dihydrodiol epoxides is particularly favored, because it yields relatively stable benzylic cation intermediates (*49, 50*), as discussed in the sidebar on the reactivity of these epoxides. Also, although epoxides can be detoxified by hydrolysis or glutathione conjugation, bay region dihydrodiol epoxides are relatively resistant to enzymatic hydrolysis or conjugation (*42*), presumably due to the steric inaccessibility of the bay region.

Studies on the biological activities of BPDE analogues have clarified some of the structural features dictating its activity (figure 18-17). Reduction of the 7,8 double bond (which accompanies conversion to the dihydrodiol functionality) is essential but the *hydroxyl groups themselves* are not: synthetic 7,8-dihydrobenzo[*a*]pyrene, which is a precursor to a bay

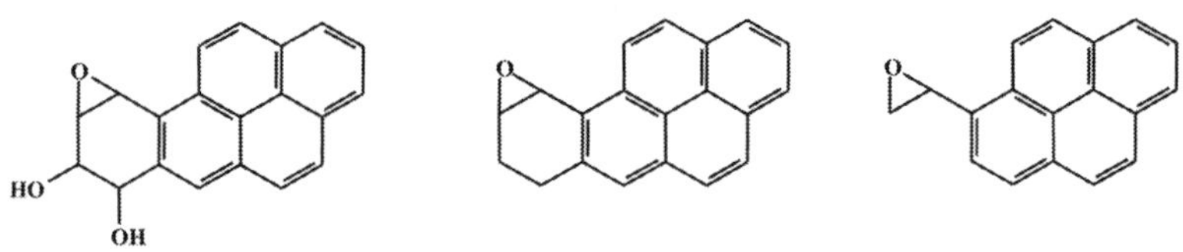

benzo[a]pyrene
7,8-dihydrodiol-9,10-epoxide

tetrahydrobenzo[a]pyrene
9,10-epoxide

1-oxiranylpyrene

FIGURE 18-17.

BPDE analogues.

region epoxide, is a highly potent carcinogen (*51*). Indeed, the bay region epoxide 1-oxiranylpyrene, in which the 7 and 8 carbon atoms of the terminal ring have "disappeared" altogether, is very reactive (*52*). Nevertheless, the presence of the hydroxyl groups in bay region dihydrodiol epoxides probably enhances their reactivity, by hydrogen bonding between the oxygen atom of the closest hydroxyl group and the hydrogen atom of the protonated epoxide, which may facilitate epoxide ring opening (*53*).

▶ **Reactivity of Bay Region Dihydrodiol Epoxides**

Compared to arene oxides, dihydrodiol epoxides are more reactive with nucleophilic targets. Why? This can be explained on the basis of simple aromaticity arguments, which are supported by more sophisticated quantum mechanical calculations (*14, 53*). Consider two competing reactions of an epoxide: ring opening and isomerization to the alcohol versus reaction with a nucleophile (XH$_2$) (figure 18-18). (The toxic processes involve reactions with nucleophiles such as protein and DNA.) In the case of an arene oxide, the isomerization route generates a phenol, whereas reaction with a nucleophile gives a nonaromatic product; isomerization is thermodynamically favored because the product is aromatic. In the case of a dihydrodiol epoxide, the isomerization route generates a triol (or its tautomeric keto/diol form), which, like the product of the reaction with a nucleophile, is nonaromatic. So, in the case of a dihydrodiol epoxide, reaction with nucleophiles competes much more effectively with the alternative detoxication route of rearrangement to an alcohol.

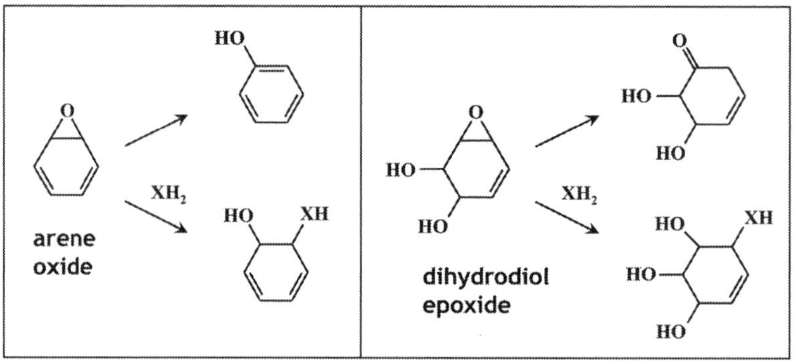

FIGURE 18-18.

The difference in reactivity between arene oxides (left) and dihydrodiol epoxides (right).

The opening of the epoxide ring of a dihydrodiol epoxide could occur in either direction, that is, either of the epoxide C–O bonds could break (figure 18-19). However, the opening will certainly tend to occur in the direction that produces a benzylic cation, rather than in the direction that produces an alkyl cation. In the former case, the positive charge can be delocalized into the aromatic system, whereas in the latter case, it cannot.

Compared to nonbay region PAHs, bay region dihydrodiol epoxides have a greater propensity to undergo epoxide ring opening and form reactive carbonium ions. Why? This can be explained on the basis of the earlier discussion of molecular orbital theory of PAHs. Recall from our previous molecular orbital analysis that we assigned α labels to those positions in the aromatic system that are *nearest neighbors to a ring fusion site* and β labels to those positions that are *next-nearest* neighbors to a ring fusion site. In the case of a bay region dihydrodiol epoxide, the epoxide ring opens to produce a benzylic cation attached to an α position. In the case of a dihydrodiol epoxide metabolite of a PAH that has *no* bay region, the epoxide ring opens to produce a benzylic cation attached to a β position (figure 18-20). Since α sites are better able to stabilize attached charged groups, bay region dihydrodiol epoxides produce more stable benzylic cations. Molecular orbital theory also yields simple rules permitting qualitative predictions of the changes in benzylic cation stability resulting from variations in the parent PAH, including methylation at various positions (53), substitution with a heteroatom, or structure change through ring rearrangement.

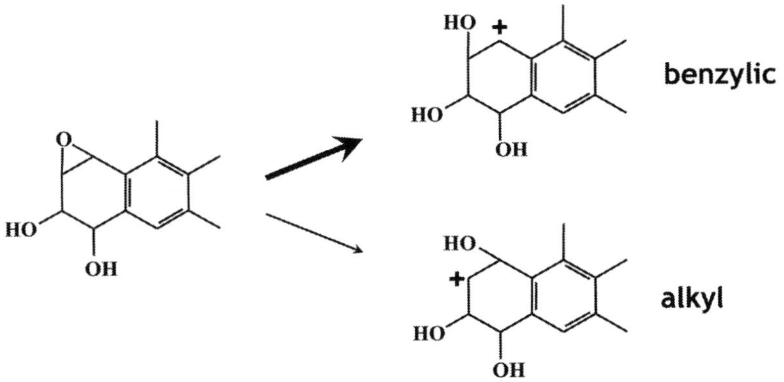

FIGURE 18-19.
Ring opening of the epoxide ring of a dihydrodiol occurs in the direction that produces the more stable benzylic cation.

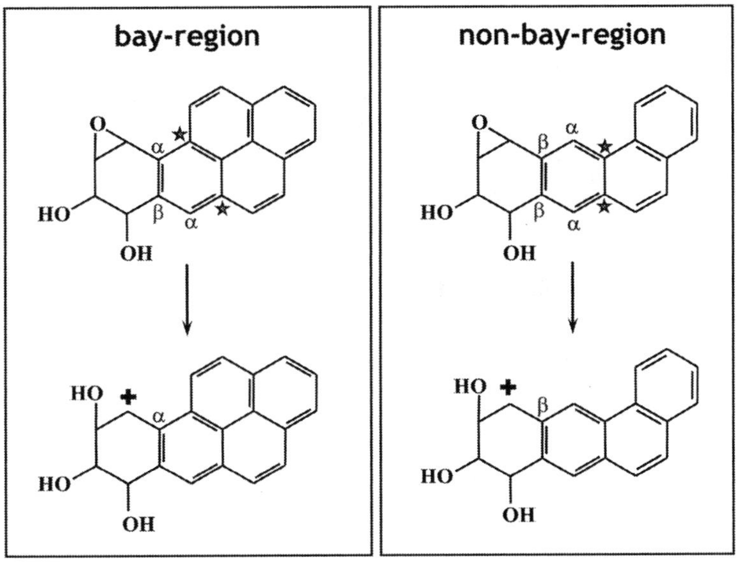

FIGURE 18-20.
Molecular orbital theory analysis of the reactivity of bay region versus nonbay region dihydrodiol epoxides; see text. ◀

DIASTEREOMERIC FORMS OF BPDE

The full name for BPDE is 7,8-dihydroxy-9,10-epoxy-7,8,9,10-tetrahydrobenzo[*a*]pyrene. This cumbersome name is abbreviated to "7,8-dihydroxy-9,10-epoxybenzo[*a*]pyrene"; "7,8-diol 9,10-epoxide" (a potentially misleading abbreviation, since the compounds are dihydrodiols, not catechols); BPDE; and so on. As noted above, four diastereomeric forms of BPDE exist (figure 18-16), comprising two sets of enantiomers.

Two BPDE enantiomers are *anti* (also called *trans*) dihydrodiol epoxides; both terms refer to the relative positions of the 7- and 10-position substituents, which are located on *opposite* faces of the terminal ring. Two BPDE enantiomers are *syn* (also called *cis*) dihydrodiol epoxides, in which the 7- and 10-position substituents are on the *same* face of the ring. The relationship between the *anti* and the *syn* isomers is diastereomeric.

Diastereomers have different chemical properties. We consider the differences in behavior of *syn* and *anti* BPDE below. Enantiomers have identical chemical properties in an optically inactive environment, but will interact differently with optically active biomolecules, such as DNA. Experimentally, enantiomers can be distinguished by *optical polarimetry*: enantiomers have equal and opposite *specific rotatory power*. The enantiomeric forms of BPDE are designated (+) and (−), on this basis. They also have equal and opposite circular dichroism spectra. The absolute stereochemistries of BPDEs have been established, allowing the use of systematic (R,S) designations (*54*).

(Unfortunately, several different BPDE nomenclature systems have been applied. Some authors apply the system used for designation of steroid substituents: α for substituents below the plane of the ring system and β for substituents above the plane; so, for example, the ((+) *anti*) isomer is named as (+) 7β,8α-dihydroxy-9α,10α-epoxy-7,8,9,10-tetrahydrobenzo[*a*]-pyrene. Two other systems are in use, and, frustratingly, they are contradictory. The (±) *anti* and the (±) *syn* diastereomers have been labeled as BPDE 2 and BPDE 1, respectively (Arabic numerals), and also as BPDE I and BPDE II, respectively (Roman numerals).)

BPDEs are highly reactive, forming addition products from the attack of water or other nucleophiles, and binding avidly to macromolecules (*55, 56*). The exceptionally high reactivity of all bay region diol epoxides results from the stabilization of the benzylic cation resulting from the opening of the epoxide ring (see sidebar on reactivity of bay region dihydrodiol epoxides). However, the hydrolytic and electrophilic behaviors of the two classes of diastereomeric diol epoxides are quite different. In tissue culture medium at 37°C, *syn*-BPDE has a half-life of about 30 s whereas *anti*-BPDE has a half-life of about 10 min (*57, 58*). This difference may be due to intramolecular acid catalysis of the opening of the epoxide ring: the 7-hydroxyl proton hydrogen bonds to the epoxide oxygen in *syn*-BPDE. This interaction is geometrically impossible in *anti*-BPDE.

DIHYDRODIOL METABOLITES OF PAHs OTHER THAN BENZO[*a*]PYRENE

The idea that bay region dihydrodiol epoxides are key reactive metabolites of benzo[*a*]pyrene has been successfully extended to many other PAHs, including 5-methylchrysene (*59*), 7,12-dimethylbenz[*a*]anthracene (*60*), benzo[*c*]phenanthrene (*61*), dibenz[*a,j*]acridine (*62*), and so on. Benzo[*c*]-chrysene is a PAH that possesses both a bay region and a fjord region. The biological activities of synthetic dihydrodiol epoxides formed at these two regions have been compared and the fjord region dihydrodiol epoxides

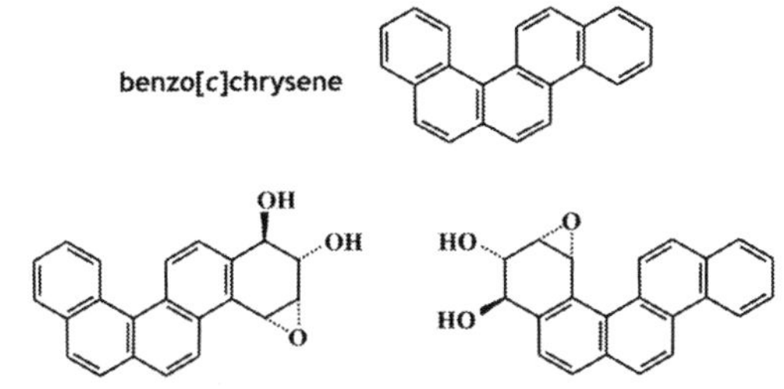

benzo[c]chrysene

anti-1,2,-dihydroxy-3,4-epoxy-
1,2,3,4,-tetrahydrobenzo[c]chrysene
(bay region)

anti-9,10-dihydroxy-11,12-epoxy-
9,10,11,12-tetrahydrobenzo[c]chrysene
(fjord region)

treatment group	number of rats with mammary tumors	number of tumors per rat
bay region diol epoxide	4	0.16 ± 0.3
fjord region diol epoxide	24	3.92 ± 1.7
DMSO (control)	0	0

FIGURE 18-21.
Carcinogenic activity of bay region and fjord region benzo[c]chrysene dihydrodiol epoxides. Four groups of female CD rats (30 days old), 25 rats per group, were used. Rats were given three injections into the mammary tissue of diol epoxide (12.2 μmol total dose) in dimethyl sulfoxide (DMSO), 0.1 mL, or DMSO alone; tumors were scored after 35 weeks. (*Amin, S.; Lin, J. M.; Krzeminski, J.; Boyiri, T.; Desai, D.; El Bayoumy, K. Metabolism of benzo[c]chrysene and comparative mammary gland tumorigenesis of benzo[c]chrysene bay and fjord region diol epoxides in female CD rats.* Chem. Res. Toxicol. **2003**, 16, 227–231.)

proved to be much more carcinogenic than the bay region isomers, based on carcinogenicity assays in young female rats (*63*) (figure 18-21).

BIOLOGICAL ACTIVITIES OF BPDE STEREOISOMERS

The biological activities of the four BPDE stereoisomers are remarkably different. (+)-*anti*-BPDE (i.e., the 7R,8S,9S,10R stereoisomer) is the predominant BPDE isomer formed by benzo[a]pyrene metabolism (*64*) and is also by far the most potent of the BPDE isomers as a skin and pulmonary carcinogen in mice (*65–67*).

BENZO[a]PYRENE-DERIVED DNA ADDUCTS

The general principles of DNA adduct formation, DNA repair, mutagenesis, and carcinogenesis have been presented in earlier chapters. To test the role of a particular reactive carcinogen metabolite, we need to examine the link between this metabolite and specific DNA adducts and mutations occurring in model systems and target tissues. The investigation of the reactivity of benzo[a]pyrene metabolites was accomplished by the synthesis and characterization of metabolites and comparison of the stable end products derived from them with the metabolites produced in biological systems. These stable products include conjugates derived from binding to

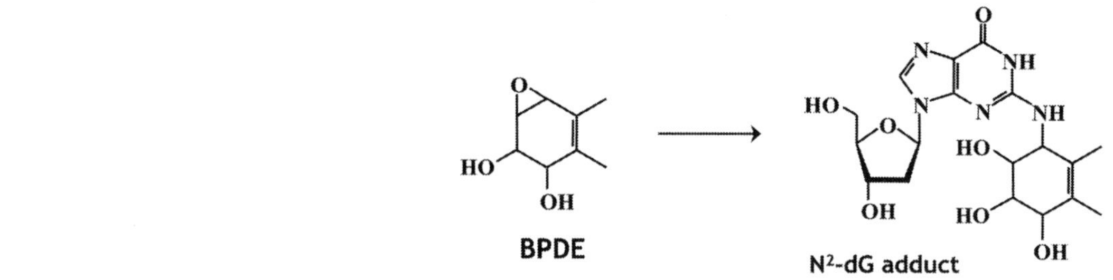

FIGURE 18-22.

Formation of deoxyguanosine adduct.

small molecules, such as GSH, or macromolecules, such as DNA and protein. These studies have shown unequivocally that bay region and fjord region dihydrodiol epoxides of PAH are reactive metabolites that bind covalently to nucleic acids.

Synthetic dihydrodiol epoxides were reacted with homopolyribonucleotides, such as poly(G), which then were hydrolyzed to mononucleosides (68, 69) (see chapter 2). BPDE shows a strong preference for reaction with purine residues, particularly guanosine. The adducted mononucleosides were purified and characterized. With all four benzo[a]pyrene bay region dihydrodiol epoxides, adducts are formed by the attack of the exocyclic nitrogen (N^2) of guanosine on the bay region benzylic carbon (C10) of the PAH (68, 70). The corresponding adduct is formed with deoxyguanosine (figure 18-22) (71). The X-ray crystal structure of a benzo[a]pyrene bay region dihydrodiol epoxide deoxyguanosine N^2 adduct (formed from the 7S,8R,9R,10S stereoisomer) has recently been published (72) (figure 18-23).

Synthetic BPDE adducts were then used as standards for comparison with adducts isolated from biological systems. Application of benzo[a] pyrene to bacteria (73), cultured cells, or animals was followed by the isolation of DNA, enzymatic hydrolysis to mononucleotides or mononucleosides, and characterization of the adducts. The major DNA adduct observed is the *trans* adduct formed between the N^2 atom of deoxyguanosine and (+) *anti*-BPDE, the most highly carcinogenic BPDE stereoisomer (1, 74).

MUTATIONS INDUCED BY BENZO[a]PYRENE

The most common mutation resulting from benzo[a]pyrene treatment of mammalian cells is a G → T transversion (75–77). The predominant *ras* mutations in both skin and lung tumors in benzo[a]pyrene-treated mice are G → T transversions in codon 12 of K-*ras* (78). The same base substitution is commonly seen in p53 mutations in lung cancers from smokers (see chapter 5) (79). How might this G → T transversion mutation arise? One possibility is that, during DNA replication, the N^2-deoxyguanosine adduct mispairs with deoxyadenosine in the daughter strand, and this mechanism is supported by in vitro experiments and molecular dynamics simulations (80, 81). In addition to adduct-induced miscoding, depurination may also contribute to benzo[a]pyrene-induced mutagenesis. The reaction of deoxyguanosine nucleoside with *anti*-BPDE results mainly in the formation of an N^7 adduct (figure 18-24) (82). The presence of an N^7

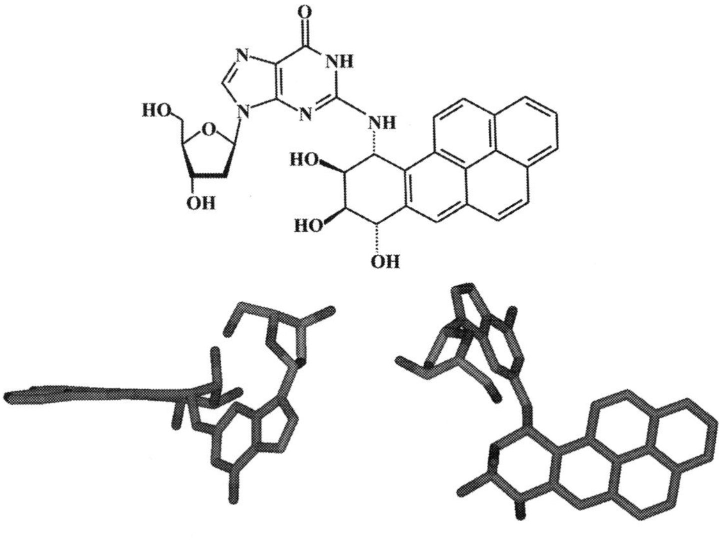

(+)-(7S,8R,9R,10S)-BPDE-derived N²-deoxyguanosine adduct

FIGURE 18-23.

Structure of a deoxyguanosine adduct of benzo[a]pyrene, determined by X-ray crystallography. Top: schematic. Bottom: two views of the structure, in the plane of the pyrene rings (left) and perpendicular to the plane of the pyrene rings (right). The deoxyribose ring carbons are colored orange for clarity. *Note:* A full-color version of this figure appears on the website. (*Karle, I. L.; Yagi, H.; Sayer, J. M.; Jerina, D. M. Crystal and molecular structure of a benzo[a]pyrene 7,8-diol 9,10-epoxide N2-deoxyguanosine adduct: absolute configuration and conformation.* Proc. Natl. Acad. Sci. USA **2004,** 101, 1433–1438.)

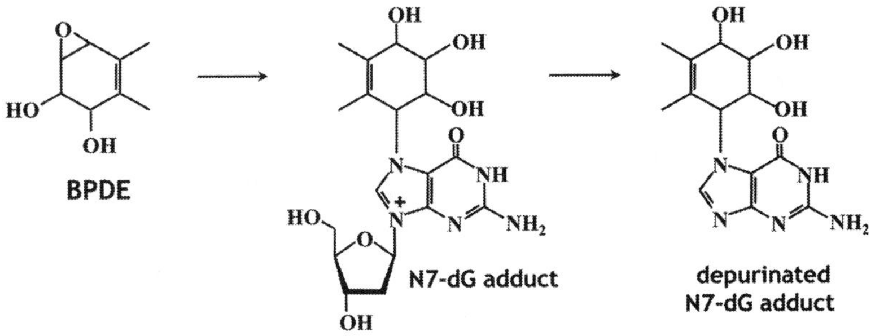

FIGURE 18-24.

Formation of depurinated N^7-deoxyguanosine adduct.

adduct to a purine base destabilizes the glycosylic bond linking the base to the sugar–phosphate backbone of DNA (see chapter 2) and thereby results in apurinic sites. Deoxyadenosine is preferentially inserted opposite apurinic sites by *E. coli* DNA polymerase (*83*), a phenomenon that is referred to as "the A rule." The "A rule" also holds for translesion bypass of apurinic sites by the human Y-family error-prone polymerase (see chapter 4) pol η (*84*). Selective depurination of guanosine residues by formation of BPDE-derived N^7 adducts therefore provides another possible route to G → T transversions: G:C → abasic:C → abasic:A → T:A. Ercole Cavalieri and colleagues have studied the formation of depurinating adducts from PAHs in vivo, and believe that abasic site generation by this route may be a major contributor to PAH-induced mutagenesis and carcinogenesis (85).

CONFORMATIONS OF PAH-ADDUCTED DNA

Alteration of DNA structure due to the presence of a PAH lesion will affect the interaction of the nucleic acid with the DNA replication machinery and may result in a misincorporation event leading to a mutation. Structural studies of PAH–DNA adducts have provided insights into the ways in which PAH adduction alters the structure of DNA and its behavior as a template for replication. Almost all of these studies have been

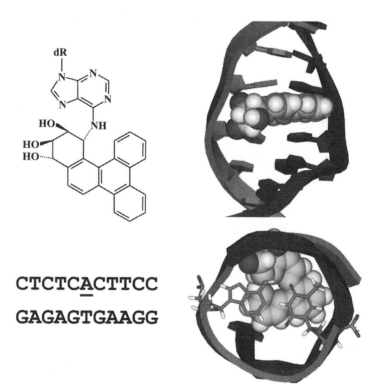

CTCTCACTTCC

GAGAGTGAAGG

FIGURE 18-25.

Structure of a DNA duplex in which a deoxyadenosine base on one strand is modified by benzo[*g*]chrysene adduction. Top left: adduct structure. Bottom left: sequence of duplex; modified base is underlined. Right: two views of the structure. Top: looking into the major groove; the base pairs are shown as rings. The PAH is shown as a space-filling model with the carbon atoms colored green. Bottom: looking along the helix axis. Only the A*:T base pair bearing the adduct is shown, as a stick model. Structure determined by NMR (see chapter 2). *Note*: A full-color version of this figure appears on the website. (*Suri, A. K.; Mao, B.; Amin, S.; Geacintov, N. E.; Patel, D. J. Solution conformation of the* (+)-trans-anti-*benzo[g]chrysene-dA adduct opposite dT in a DNA duplex.* J. Mol. Biol. *1999*, 292, 289–307.)

accomplished by NMR methods (*86*) or molecular dynamics calculations, although X-ray crystallographic analysis of a PAH–DNA adduct has recently been achieved (*87*).

The outcome of an interaction between DNA polymerase and PAH-adducted DNA is influenced by many factors: the covalent structure and the stereochemistry of the adduct; the local sequence context (*88*); whether the modified base is positioned opposite a base or opposite an abasic site; the location of the binding site (e.g., minor groove vs. major groove of the DNA); and the nature of the polymerase enzyme. PAH–DNA adduct structures can be classified into three families, on the basis of adduct location: (a) in the minor groove, without causing significant distortion of the B-DNA duplex (*89*); (b) intercalated into the helix, by displacing the modified base (*90*); and (c) intercalated into the helix, without disrupting the modified base pair (*91*). Figure 18-25 illustrates the third of these cases. The figure shows views of the structure (determined by NMR methods) of a DNA duplex in which one deoxyadenosine base on one strand has been modified by benzo[*g*]chrysene fjord region dihydrodiol epoxide adduction to the exocyclic N6 amino group of the base (*92*). The PAH moiety is positioned in the major groove, intercalated between intact C:G and PAH-modified A:T base-pairs.

Notes

1. Sir John Percivall Pott was a major figure in the transformation of medicine from a craft into a scientifically based discipline. He was a surgeon at St. Bartholomew's Hospital, London, for almost 50 years and wrote influential treatises on the treatment of hernia, head injuries, and other medical subjects. He was appointed to the Royal Society in 1764.

2. Note that the letters in square brackets, which distinguish PAH isomers with different arrangements of fused rings, are italicized English letters, not Greek letters.

References

1. Phillips, D. H. Fifty years of benzo(a)pyrene. *Nature* **1983**, *303*, 468–472.
2. Waller, R. E. 60 years of chemical carcinogens: Sir Ernest Kennaway in retirement. *J. R. Soc. Med.* **1994**, *87*, 96–97.
3. Harvey, R. G. *Polycyclic Aromatic Hydrocarbons*; John Wiley: New York, 1997.
4. Sauvain, J. J.; Vu, D. T.; Guillemin, M. Exposure to carcinogenic polycyclic aromatic compounds and health risk assessment for diesel-exhaust exposed workers. *Int. Arch. Occup. Environ. Health* **2003**, *76*, 443–455.
5. Lin, C. H.; Huang, X.; Kolbanovskii, A.; Hingerty, B. E.; Amin, S.; Broyde, S.; Geacintov, N. E.; Patel, D. J. Molecular topology of polycyclic aromatic carcinogens determines DNA adduct conformation: a link to tumorigenic activity. *J. Mol. Biol.* **2001**, *306*, 1059–1080.
6. Cavalieri, E. L.; Higginbotham, S.; RamaKrishna, N. V.; Devanesan, P. D.; Todorovic, R.; Rogan, E. G.; Salmasi, S. Comparative dose–response tumorigenicity studies of dibenzo[*a,l*]pyrene versus 7,12-dimethylbenz[*a*]anthracene, benzo[*a*]pyrene and two dibenzo[*a,l*]pyrene dihydrodiols in mouse skin and rat mammary gland. *Carcinogenesis* **1991**, *12*, 1939–1944.

7. Sauvain, J. J.; Vu, D. T.; Huynh, C. K. Development of an analytical method for the simultaneous determination of 15 carcinogenic polycyclic aromatic hydrocarbons and polycyclic aromatic nitrogen heterocyclic compounds: application to diesel particulates. *Fresenius J. Anal. Chem.* **2001**, *371*, 966–974.

8. Seidel, A.; Frank, H.; Behnke, A.; Schneider, D.; Jakob, J. Determination of dibenzo[*a,l*]pyrene and other fjord-region PAH isomers with MW 302 in environmental samples. *Polycyclic Aromatic Hydrocarbons* **2004**, *24*, 759–771.

9. Glusker, J. P. X-ray analyses of polycyclic hydrocarbon metabolite structures. In *Polycyclic Hydrocarbons and Carcinogenesis*; Harvey, R. G., Ed.; American Chemical Society: Washington, DC, 1985; pp. 125–185.

10. Glusker, J. P.; Carrell, H. L.; Katz, A. K.; Afshar, C. E. Structural studies of PAHs and their metabolites. *Polycyclic Aromatic Hydrocarbons* **1999**, *14–15*, 87–98.

11. Boyd, D. R.; Jerina, D. M. Arene oxides-oxepins. In *Small Ring Heterocycles, Part 3: Oxiranes, Arene Oxides, Oxaziridines, Dioxetanes, Thietanes, Thietes, Thiazetes*; John Wiley: New York, 1985; pp. 197–282.

12. Lowe, J. P. *Quantum Chemistry*; Academic Press: New York, 1993.

13. Seybold, P. G. Explorations of molecular structure–property relationships. *SAR QSAR. Environ. Res.* **1999**, *10*, 101–115.

14. Lowe, J. P.; Silverman, D. B. Simple molecular orbital explanation for "bay-region" carcinogenic reactivity. *J. Am. Chem. Soc.* **1981**, *103*, 2852–2855.

15. Parke, D. V. Eric Boyland: a pioneer in cancer biochemistry. *Xenobiotica* **1986**, *16*, 887–898.

16. Miller, E. C. Studies on the formation of protein-bound derivatives of 3,4-benzpyrene in epidermal reactions of mouse skin. *Cancer Res.* **1951**, *11*, 100–108.

17. Miller, E. C.; Miller, J. A. Charles Heidelberger: December 23, 1920–January 18, 1983. *Biogr. Mem. Natl. Acad. Sci.* **1989**, *58*, 259–302.

18. Brookes, P.; Lawley, P. D. Evidence for the binding of polynuclear aromatic hydrocarbons to the nucleic acid of mouse skin: relation between carcinogenic power of hydrocarbons and their binding to deoxyribonucleic acid. *Nature* **1964**, *202*, 781–784.

19. Stowers, S. J.; Anderson, M. W. Ubiquitous binding of benzo[a]pyrene metabolites to DNA and protein in tissues of the mouse and rabbit. *Chem. Biol. Interact.* **1984**, *51*, 151–166.

20. Booth, E. D.; Loose, R. W.; Watson, W. P. Effects of solvent on DNA adduct formation in skin and lung of CD1 mice exposed cutaneously to benzo(a)pyrene. *Arch. Toxicol.* **1999**, *73*, 316–322.

21. Keysell, G. R.; Booth, J.; Grover, P. L.; Hewer, A.; Sims, P. The formation of "K-region" epoxides as hepatic microsomal metabolites of 7-methyl-benz(a)anthracene and 7,12-dimethylbenz(a)anthracene and their 7-hydroxymethyl derivatives. *Biochem. Pharmacol.* **1973**, *22*, 2853–2867.

22. Keysell, G. R.; Booth, J.; Sims, P.; Grover, P. L.; Hewer, A. The formation of an epoxide in the microsomal metabolism of 7,12-dimethylbenz(a) anthracene. *Biochem. J.* **1972**, *129*, 41P–42P.

23. Grover, P. L.; Forrester, J. A.; Sims, P. Reactivity of the K-region epoxides of some polycyclic hydrocarbons towards the nucleic acids and proteins of BHK 21 cells. *Biochem. Pharmacol.* **1971**, *20*, 1297–1302.

24. Wolff, T.; Deml, E.; Wanders, H. Aldrin epoxidation, a highly sensitive indicator specific for cytochrome P-450-dependent mono-oxygenase activities. *Drug Metab. Dispos.* **1979**, *7*, 301–305.

25. Csanady, G. A.; Kessler, W.; Hoffmann, H. D.; Filser, J. G. A toxicokinetic model for styrene and its metabolite styrene-7,8-oxide in mouse, rat and human with special emphasis on the lung. *Toxicol. Lett.* **2003,** *138,* 75–102.

26. Omiecinski, C. J.; Hassett, C.; Hosagrahara, V. Epoxide hydrolase: polymorphism and role in toxicology. *Toxicol. Lett.* **2000,** *112–113,* 365–370.

27. Morisseau, C.; Hammock, B. D. Epoxide hydrolases: mechanisms, inhibitor designs, and biological roles. *Ann. Rev. Pharmacol. Toxicol.* **2005,** *45,* 311–333.

28. Fretland, A. J.; Omiecinski, C. J. Epoxide hydrolases: biochemistry and molecular biology. *Chem. Biol. Interact.* **2000,** *129,* 41–59.

29. Argiriadi, M. A.; Morisseau, C.; Hammock, B. D.; Christianson, D. W. Detoxification of environmental mutagens and carcinogens: structure, mechanism, and evolution of liver epoxide hydrolase. *Proc. Natl. Acad. Sci. USA* **1999,** *96,* 10637–10642.

30. Bell, P. A.; Kasper, C. B. Expression of rat microsomal epoxide hydrolase in *Escherichia coli*. Identification of a histidyl residue essential for catalysis. *J. Biol. Chem.* **1993,** *268,* 14011–14017.

31. Beetham, J. K.; Tian, T.; Hammock, B. D. cDNA cloning and expression of a soluble epoxide hydrolase from human liver. *Arch. Biochem. Biophys.* **1993,** *305,* 197–201.

32. Draper, A. J.; Hammock, B. D. Soluble epoxide hydrolase in rat inflammatory cells is indistinguishable from soluble epoxide hydrolase in rat liver. *Toxicol. Sci.* **1999,** *50,* 30–35.

33. Sevanian, A.; Peterson, A. R. The cytotoxic and mutagenic properties of cholesterol oxidation products. *Food Chem. Toxicol.* **1986,** *24,* 1103–1110.

34. Watabe, T.; Ozawa, N.; Ishii, H.; Chiba, K.; Hiratsuka, A. Hepatic microsomal cholesterol epoxide hydrolase: selective inhibition by detergents and separation from xenobiotic epoxide hydrolase. *Biochem. Biophys. Res. Commun.* **1986,** *140,* 632–637.

35. (a) Haeggström, J. Z.; Kull, F.; Rudberg, P. C.; Tholander, F.; Thunnissen, M. M. Leukotriene A$_4$ hydrolase. *Prostaglandins Other Lipid Mediat.* **2002,** *68–69,* 495–510. (b) Thunnissen, M. M.; Andersson, B.; Samuelsson, B.; Wong, C.-H. and Haeggström, J. Z. Crystal structures of leukotriene A$_4$ hydrolase in complex with captopril and two competitive tight-binding inhibitors. *FASEB J.* **2002,** *16,* 1648–1650.

36. Armstrong, R. N.; Cassidy, C. S. New structural and chemical insight into the catalytic mechanism of epoxide hydrolases. *Drug Metab. Rev.* **2000,** *32,* 327–338.

37. Laughlin, L. T.; Tzeng, H. F.; Lin, S.; Armstrong, R. N. Mechanism of microsomal epoxide hydrolase. Semifunctional site-specific mutants affecting the alkylation half-reaction. *Biochemistry* **1998,** *37,* 2897–2904.

38. Levin, W.; Wood, A. W.; Yagi, H.; Dansette, P. M.; Jerina, D. M.; Conney, A. H. Carcinogenicity of benzo[*a*]pyrene 4,5-, 7,8-, and 9,10-oxides on mouse skin. *Proc. Natl. Acad. Sci. USA* **1976,** *73,* 243–247.

39. Borgen, A.; Darvey, H.; Castagnoli, N.; Crocker, T. T.; Rasmussen, R. E.; Wang, I. Y. Metabolic conversion of benzo[*a*]pyrene by Syrian hamster liver microsomes and binding of metabolites to deoxyribonucleic acid. *J. Med. Chem.* **1973,** *16,* 502–506.

40. Sims, P.; Grover, P. L.; Swaisland, A.; Pal, K.; Hewer, A. Metabolic activation of benzo(a)pyrene proceeds by a diol-epoxide. *Nature* **1974,** *252,* 326–328.

41. Baird, W. M.; Mahadevan, B. The uses of carcinogen-DNA adduct measurement in establishing mechanisms of mutagenesis and in chemoprevention. *Mutat. Res.* **2004,** *547*, 1–4.

42. Kouri, R. E.; Wood, A. W.; Levin, W.; Rude, T. H.; Yagi, H.; Mah, H. D.; Jerina, D. M.; Conney, A. H. Carcinogenicity of benzo[*a*]pyrene and thirteen of its derivatives in C3H/fCum mice. *J. Natl. Cancer Inst.* **1980,** *64*, 617–623.

43. Shou, M.; Korzekwa, K. R.; Crespi, C. L.; Gonzalez, F. J.; Gelboin, H. V. The role of 12 cDNA-expressed human, rodent, and rabbit cytochromes P450 in the metabolism of benzo[*a*]pyrene and benzo[*a*]pyrene trans-7,8-dihydrodiol. *Mol. Carcinog.* **1994,** *10*, 159–168.

44. Bauer, E.; Guo, Z.; Ueng, Y. F.; Bell, L. C.; Zeldin, D.; Guengerich, F. P. Oxidation of benzo[*a*]pyrene by recombinant human cytochrome P450 enzymes. *Chem. Res. Toxicol.* **1995,** *8*, 136–142.

45. Shimada, T.; Gillam, E. M.; Oda, Y.; Tsumura, F.; Sutter, T. R.; Guengerich, F. P.; Inoue, K. Metabolism of benzo[*a*]pyrene to trans-7,8-dihydroxy-7,8-dihydrobenzo[*a*]pyrene by recombinant human cytochrome P450 1B1 and purified liver epoxide hydrolase. *Chem. Res. Toxicol.* **1999,** *12*, 623–629.

46. Mammen, J. S.; Pittman, G. S.; Li, Y.; Abou-Zahr, F.; Bejjani, B. A.; Bell, D. A.; Strickland, P. T.; Sutter, T. R. Single amino acid mutations, but not common polymorphisms, decrease the activity of CYP1B1 against (−)benzo[*a*]pyrene-7R-trans-7,8-dihydrodiol. *Carcinogenesis* **2003,** *24*, 1247–1255.

47. Weinshilboum, R.; Wang, L. Pharmacogenomics: bench to bedside. *Nat. Rev. Drug Discov.* **2004,** *3*, 739–748.

48. Conney, A. H.; Chang, R. L.; Jerina, D. M.; Wei, S. J. Studies on the metabolism of benzo[*a*]pyrene and dose-dependent differences in the mutagenic profile of its ultimate carcinogenic metabolite. *Drug Metab. Rev.* **1994,** *26*, 125–163.

49. Lowe, J. P.; Silverman, D. B. Predicting carcinogenicity of polycyclic aromatic hydrocarbons. *Acc. Chem. Res.* **1984,** *17*, 332–338.

50. Lowe, J. P.; Silverman, D. B. Carcinogenicity of polycyclic aromatic hydrocarbons: a dialogue. *J. Mol. Struct.* (*Theochem*) **1988,** *179*, 47–81.

51. Waterfall, J. F.; Sims, P. Epoxy derivatives of aromatic polycyclic hydrocarbons. The preparation and metabolism of epoxides related to benzo(*a*)pyrene and to 7,8- and 9,10-dihydrobenzo(*a*)pyrene. *Biochem. J.* **1972,** *128*, 265–277.

52. Kim, M. H.; Geacintov, N. E.; Pope, M.; Harvey, R. G. Structural effects in reactivity and adduct formation of polycyclic aromatic epoxide and diol epoxide derivatives with DNA: comparison between 1-oxiranylpyrene and benzo[*a*]pyrenediol epoxide. *Biochemistry* **1984,** *23*, 5433–5439.

53. Borosky, G. L. Theoretical study related to the carcinogenic activity of polycyclic aromatic hydrocarbon derivatives. *J. Org. Chem.* **1999,** *64*, 7738–7744.

54. Yagi, H.; Akagi, H.; Thakker, D. R.; Mah, H. D.; Koreeda, M.; Jerina, D. M. Absolute stereochemistry of the highly mutagenic 7,8-diol 9,10-epoxides derived from the potent carcinogen trans-7,8-dihydroxy-7,8-dihydrobenzol[*a*]pyrene. *J. Am. Chem. Soc.* **1977,** *99*, 2358–2359.

55. Harvey, R. G.; Geacintov, N. E. Intercalation and binding of carcinogenic hydrocarbon metabolites to nucleic acids. *Acc. Chem. Res.* **1988,** *21*, 66–73.

56. Szeliga, J.; Dipple, A. DNA adduct formation by polycyclic aromatic hydrocarbon dihydrodiol epoxides. *Chem. Res. Toxicol.* **1998,** *11*, 1–11.

57. Wood, A. W.; Wislocki, P. G.; Chang, R. L.; Levin, W.; Lu, A. Y.; Yagi, J.; Hernandez, O.; Jerina, D. M.; Conney, A. H. Mutagenicity and cytotoxicity of benzo[a]pyrene benzo-ring epoxides. *Cancer Res.* **1976,** *36,* 3358–3366.

58. Doan, L.; Lin, B.; Yagi, H.; Jerina, D. M.; Whalen, D. L. New insights on the mechanisms of the pH-independent reactions of benzo[a]pyrenes 7,8-diol 9,10-epoxides. *J. Am. Chem. Soc.* **2001,** *123,* 6785–6791.

59. Melikian, A. A.; Amin, S.; Hecht, S. S.; Hoffmann, D.; Pataki, J.; Harvey, R. G. Identification of the major adducts formed by reaction of 5-methylchrysene anti-dihydrodiol-epoxides with DNA in vitro. *Cancer Res.* **1984,** *44,* 2524–2529.

60. Cooper, C. S.; Ribeiro, O.; Hewer, A.; Walsh, C.; Grover, P. L.; Sims, P. Additional evidence for the involvement of the 3,4-diol 1,2-oxides in the metabolic activation of 7,12-dimethylbenz[a]anthracene in mouse skin. *Chem. Biol. Interact.* **1980,** *29,* 357–367.

61. Canella, K. A.; Peltonen, K.; Yagi, H.; Jerina, D. M.; Dipple, A. Identification of individual benzo[c]phenanthrene dihydrodiol epoxide-DNA adducts by the ^{32}P-postlabeling assay. *Chem. Res. Toxicol.* **1992,** *5,* 685–690.

62. Xue, W.; Schneider, J.; Mitchell, K.; Jaeger, M.; Nanayakkara, V.; Talaska, G.; Warshawsky, D. *trans*-3,4-Dihydroxy-*anti*-1,2-epoxy-1,2,3,4-tetrahydrodibenz[a,j]acridine involvement in dibenz[a,j]acridine DNA adduct formation in mouse skin consistent with Ha-ras mutation patterns in tumors. *Chem. Res. Toxicol.* **2001,** *14,* 871–878.

63. Amin, S.; Lin, J. M.; Krzeminski, J.; Boyiri, T.; Desai, D.; El Bayoumy, K. Metabolism of benzo[c]chrysene and comparative mammary gland tumorigenesis of benzo[c]chrysene bay and fjord region diol epoxides in female CD rats. *Chem. Res. Toxicol.* **2003,** *16,* 227–231.

64. Thakker, D. R.; Yagi, H.; Akagi, H.; Koreeda, M.; Lu, A. H.; Levin, W.; Wood, A. W.; Conney, A. H.; Jerina, D. M. Metabolism of benzo[a]pyrene. VI. Stereoselective metabolism of benzo[a]pyrene and benzo[a]pyrene 7,8-dihydrodiol to diol epoxides. *Chem. Biol. Interact.* **1977,** *16,* 281–300.

65. Buening, M. K.; Wislocki, P. G.; Levin, W.; Yagi, H.; Thakker, D. R.; Akagi, H.; Koreeda, M.; Jerina, D. M.; Conney, A. H. Tumorigenicity of the optical enantiomers of the diastereomeric benzo[a]pyrene 7,8-diol-9,10-epoxides in newborn mice: exceptional activity of (+)-7β,8α-dihydroxy-9α,10α-epoxy-7,8,9,10-tetrahydrobenzo[a]pyrene. *Proc. Natl. Acad. Sci. USA* **1978,** *75,* 5358–5361.

66. Thakker, D. R.; Yagi, H.; Levin, W.; Wood, A. W.; Conney, A. H.; Jerina, D. M. Polycyclic aromatic hydrocarbons: metabolic activation to ultimate carcinogens. In *Bioactivation of Foreign Compounds*; Anders, M. W., Ed.; Academic Press: Orlando, FL, 1985; pp. 177–242.

67. Kapitulnik, J.; Wislocki, P. G.; Levin, W.; Yagi, H.; Jerina, D. M.; Conney, A. H. Tumorigenicity studies with diol-epoxides of benzo[a]pyrene which indicate that (+/−)-trans-7β,8α-dihydroxy-9α,10α-epoxy-7,8,9,10-tetrahydrobenzo[a]pyrene is an ultimate carcinogen in newborn mice. *Cancer Res.* **1978,** *38,* 354–358.

68. Jeffrey, A. M.; Jennette, K. W.; Blobstein, S. H.; Weinstein, I. B.; Beland, F. A.; Harvey, R. G.; Kasal, H.; Miura, I.; Nakanishi, K. Benzo[a]pyrene-nucleic acid derivative found in vivo: structure of a benzo[a]pyrene-tetrahydrodiol epoxide-guanosine adduct. *J. Am. Chem. Soc.* **1976,** *98,* 5714–5715.

69. Jerina, D. M.; Chadha, A.; Cheh, A. M.; Schurdak, M. E.; Wood, A. W.; Sayer, J. M. Covalent bonding of bay-region diol epoxides to nucleic acids. *Adv. Exp. Med. Biol.* **1991**, *283*, 533–553.

70. Jennette, K. W.; Jeffrey, A. M.; Blobstein, S. H.; Beland, F. A.; Harvey, R. G.; Weinstein, I. B. Nucleoside adducts from the in vitro reaction of benzo[*a*]pyrene-7,8-dihydrodiol 9,10-oxide or benzo[*a*]pyrene 4,5-oxide with nucleic acids. *Biochemistry* **1977**, *16*, 932–938.

71. Straub, K. M.; Meehan, T.; Burlingame, A. L.; Calvin, M. Identification of the major adducts formed by reaction of benzo(a)pyrene diol epoxide with DNA in vitro. *Proc. Natl. Acad. Sci. USA* **1977**, *74*, 5285–5289.

72. Karle, I. L.; Yagi, H.; Sayer, J. M.; Jerina, D. M. Crystal and molecular structure of a benzo[a]pyrene 7,8-diol 9,10-epoxide N2-deoxyguanosine adduct: absolute configuration and conformation. *Proc. Natl. Acad. Sci. USA* **2004**, *101*, 1433–1438.

73. Santella, R. M.; Grunberger, D.; Weinstein, I. B. DNA-benzo[*a*]pyrene adducts formed in a *Salmonella typhimurium* mutagenesis assay system. *Mutat. Res.* **1979**, *61*, 181–189.

74. Koreeda, M.; Moore, P. D.; Wislocki, P. G.; Levin, W.; Yagi, H.; Jerina, D. M. Binding of benzo[*a*]pyrene 7,8-diol-9,10-epoxides to DNA, RNA, and protein of mouse skin occurs with high stereoselectivity. *Science* **1978**, *199*, 778–781.

75. Shibutani, S.; Margulis, L. A.; Geacintov, N. E.; Grollman, A. P. Translesional synthesis on a DNA template containing a single stereoisomer of dG-(+)- or dG-(−)-anti-BPDE (7,8-dihydroxy-anti-9,10-epoxy-7,8,9,10-tetrahydrobenzo[*a*]pyrene). *Biochemistry* **1993**, *32*, 7531–7541.

76. Jernström, B.; Gräslund, A. Covalent binding of benzo[*a*]pyrene 7,8-dihydrodiol 9,10-epoxides to DNA: molecular structures, induced mutations and biological consequences. *Biophys. Chem.* **1994**, *49*, 185–199.

77. Yoon, J. H.; Smith, L. E.; Feng, Z.; Tang, M.; Lee, C. S.; Pfeifer, G. P. Methylated CpG dinucleotides are the preferential targets for G-to-T transversion mutations induced by benzo[*a*]pyrene diol epoxide in mammalian cells: similarities with the p53 mutation spectrum in smoking-associated lung cancers. *Cancer Res.* **2001**, *61*, 7110–7117.

78. Nesnow, S.; Ross, J. A.; Nelson, G.; Wilson, K.; Roop, B. C.; Jeffers, A. J.; Galati, A. J.; Stoner, G. D.; Sangaiah, R.; Gold, A. Cyclopenta[*cd*]pyrene-induced tumorigenicity, *Ki-ras* codon 12 mutations and DNA adducts in strain A/J mouse lung. *Carcinogenesis* **1994**, *15*, 601–606.

79. Pfeifer, G. P.; Denissenko, M. F.; Olivier, M.; Tretyakova, N.; Hecht, S. S.; Hainaut, P. Tobacco smoke carcinogens, DNA damage and p53 mutations in smoking-associated cancers. *Oncogene* **2002**, *21*, 7435–7451.

80. Chary, P.; Lloyd, R. S. In vitro replication by prokaryotic and eukaryotic polymerases on DNA templates containing site-specific and stereospecific benzo[*a*]pyrene-7,8-dihydrodiol-9,10-epoxide adducts. *Nucleic Acids Res.* **1995**, *23*, 1398–1405.

81. Perlow, R. A.; Broyde, S. Toward understanding the mutagenicity of an environmental carcinogen: structural insights into nucleotide incorporation preferences. *J. Mol. Biol.* **2002**, *322*, 291–309.

82. RamaKrishna, N. V.; Gao, F.; Padmavathi, N. S.; Cavalieri, E. L.; Rogan, E. G.; Cerny, R. L.; Gross, M. L. Model adducts of benzo[*a*]pyrene and nucleosides formed from its radical cation and diol epoxide. *Chem. Res. Toxicol.* **1992**, *5*, 293–302.

83. Kunkel, T. A. Mutational specificity of depurination. *Proc. Natl. Acad. Sci. USA* **1984,** *81,* 1494–1498.

84. Kokoska, R. J.; McCulloch, S. D.; Kunkel, T. A. The efficiency and specificity of apurinic/apyrimidinic site bypass by human DNA polymerase η and *Sulfolobus solfataricus* Dpo4. *J. Biol. Chem.* **2003,** *278,* 50537–50545.

85. Casale, G. P.; Singhal, M.; Bhattacharya, S.; RamaNathan, R.; Roberts, K. P.; Barbacci, D. C.; Zhao, J.; Jankowiak, R.; Gross, M. L.; Cavalieri, E. L.; Small, G. J.; Rennard, S. I.; Mumford, J. L.; Shen, M. Detection and quantification of depurinated benzo[*a*]pyrene-adducted DNA bases in the urine of cigarette smokers and women exposed to household coal smoke. *Chem. Res. Toxicol.* **2001,** *14,* 192–201.

86. Geacintov, N. E.; Cosman, M.; Hingerty, B. E.; Amin, S.; Broyde, S.; Patel, D. J. NMR solution structures of stereoisometric covalent polycyclic aromatic carcinogen-DNA adducts: principles, patterns, and diversity. *Chem. Res. Toxicol.* **1997,** *10,* 111–146.

87. Ling, H.; Sayer, J. M.; Plosky, B. S.; Yagi, H.; Boudsocq, F.; Woodgate, R.; Jerina, D. M.; Yang, W. Crystal structure of a benzo[*a*]pyrene diol epoxide adduct in a ternary complex with a DNA polymerase. *Proc. Natl. Acad. Sci. USA* **2004,** *101,* 2265–2269.

88. Yan, S.; Wu, M.; Buterin, T.; Naegeli, H.; Geacintov, N. E.; Broyde, S. Role of base sequence context in conformational equilibria and nucleotide excision repair of benzo[*a*]pyrene diol epoxide-adenine adducts. *Biochemistry* **2003,** *42,* 2339–2354.

89. de los Santos, C.; Cosman, M.; Hingerty, B. E.; Ibanez, V.; Margulis, L. A.; Geacintov, N. E.; Broyde, S.; Patel, D. J. Influence of benzo[*a*]pyrene diol epoxide chirality on solution conformations of DNA covalent adducts: the (–)-trans-anti-[BP]G.C adduct structure and comparison with the (+)-trans-anti-[BP]G.C enantiomer. *Biochemistry* **1992,** *31,* 5245–5252.

90. Cosman, M.; de los Santos, C.; Fiala, R.; Hingerty, B. E.; Ibanez, V.; Luna, E.; Harvey, R.; Geacintov, N. E.; Broyde, S.; Patel, D. J. Solution conformation of the (+)-*cis*-anti-[BP]dG adduct in a DNA duplex: intercalation of the covalently attached benzo[*a*]pyrenyl ring into the helix and displacement of the modified deoxyguanosine. *Biochemistry* **1993,** *32,* 4145–4155.

91. Cosman, M.; Fiala, R.; Hingerty, B. E.; Laryea, A.; Lee, H.; Harvey, R. G.; Amin, S.; Geacintov, N. E.; Broyde, S.; Patel, D. Solution conformation of the (+)-*trans*-anti-[BPh]dA adduct opposite dT in a DNA duplex: intercalation of the covalently attached benzo[*c*]phenanthrene to the 5′-side of the adduct site without disruption of the modified base pair. *Biochemistry* **1993,** *32,* 12488–12497.

92. Suri, A. K.; Mao, B.; Amin, S.; Geacintov, N. E.; Patel, D. J. Solution conformation of the (+)-trans-*anti*-benzo[*g*]chrysene-dA adduct opposite dT in a DNA duplex. *J. Mol. Biol.* **1999,** *292,* 289–307.

THE DISCOVERY OF THE "COAL-TAR ANALGESICS"

The analgesic (painkiller) *acetaminophen* (paracetamol; *p*-acetylamino-phenol; APAP; Tylenol^TM; figure 19-1) is one of the world's most popular nonprescription medications. Its discovery came about through a combination of good science and good luck, and the story spans many decades (*1*). Two antipyretic (fever-reducing) natural products, the extracts of willow bark (salicylic acid) and cinchona bark (quinine; see chapter 16), had been discovered long before the scientific era. However, the former drug had unpleasant side effects and the latter was very expensive. In the late 19th century, an entirely new class of synthetic analgesics and antipyretics was discovered, by chance. The first of these chemicals was acetanilide, *N*-acetylaminobenzene. As recounted by Mann and Plummer:

> In 1886, two Alsatian interns, Drs. Kahn and Hepp, ordered some naphthalene, a treatment for intestinal parasites, from a nearby pharmacist. The substance they received failed to have the expected effect on the parasites but managed instead to reduce the patient's fever. Startled, the two doctors requested more of the same. This time, however, they received a substance that got rid of intestinal parasites but did nothing for fever. Upon further analysis, Kahn and Hepp discovered that they had been the victims of a happy accident; the first material was acetanilide, a coal-tar derivative used in the dye industry, never before given to human beings...The two doctors approached Hepp's brother, a chemist at Kalle & Company of Wiesbaden, the company that had supplied the acetanilide, and told him what had happened.

Kalle & Company began selling acetanilide under the brand name "Antifebrin." At the same time, another German company, Farbenfabriken Bayer, was accumulating tons of unwanted *p*-aminophenol as a byproduct of its synthetic dye production processes (see chapter 17). Chemists at Bayer, under the direction of Carl Duisberg, saw an opportunity to make use of this chemical waste. Acetylation would readily convert the amino group to the acetylamino group, to give *p*-acetylaminophenol. Lacking a commercial route for the removal of the unwanted phenolic hydroxyl group, Bayer's chemists opted to deactivate it by ethylation, giving *p*-ethoxyacetanilide ("phenacetin"). They found this product to be both an antipyretic and an analgesic. Phenacetin was marketed in 1888. As Mann and Plummer observed:

> Duisberg's accomplishment was revolutionary. For the first time, a drug had been conceived, developed, tested, and marketed, all by

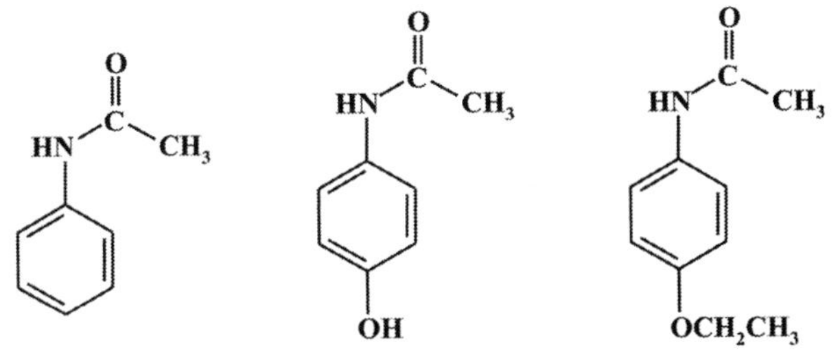

acetanilide | p-hydroxyacetanilide (acetaminophen) | p-ethoxyacetanilide (phenacetin)

FIGURE 19-1.
Acetaminophen and analogues.

> a private company. It marked the creation of the modern drug industry...

Phenacetin was widely used during the influenza epidemic of 1889 and the Bayer company's new pharmaceutical enterprise[1] prospered. Phenacetin remained an important analgesic until concern over its nephrotoxic side effects arose in the 1960s. Heavy use of phenacetin was also associated with increased risk of renal (*2*) and bladder cancers and it was finally withdrawn from sale in 1983.

ACETAMINOPHEN

p-Acetylaminophenol (acetaminophen) had first been synthesized in 1888. Even though it was an intermediate in the synthesis of phenacetin, Bayer chemists did not test this compound as a drug, because phenols were generally regarded as too toxic for medicinal use. In 1889 the Swedish physiological chemist Karl Mörner (later the rector of the Karolinska Institute) discovered that acetaminophen is a urinary metabolite of phenacetin. (We now understand that this biotransformation is a typical P450-catalyzed O-dealkylation reaction; its mechanism was discussed in chapter 7.) In 1893 the German physiologist J.F. von Mering[2] tested acetaminophen and showed that it was also an analgesic and antipyretic. However, phenacetin was already a successful product and acetaminophen was not developed as a commercial drug.

In 1939 a consortium of U.S. proprietary drug manufacturers established the Institute for the Study of Analgesic and Sedative Drugs, with the intention of applying modern pharmacological science to the development and testing of analgesics (*1*, p. 186). The institute organized a symposium to evaluate the evidence about acetaminophen, in 1951. With support from the institute, Bernard Brodie (see chapter 7) and colleagues studied the hepatic metabolism of acetanilide in vitro, and discovered its enzymatic deacetylation (to give aniline) and aromatic hydroxylation (to give acetaminophen). Brodie speculated that acetaminophen might be a useful drug in its own right, as had von Mering, many years earlier. Boréus and Sandberg, at the Karolinska Institute, also obtained encouraging results with acetaminophen (*3*). Several chemical producers began selling the compound over the following years, including Squibb

Pharmaceuticals in New York and McNeil Laboratories in Pennsylvania, which coined the brand name Tylenol[TM]. (In the remainder of this chapter, we refer to this compound generically as acetaminophen.)

NSAIDs

Acetaminophen shares its antipyretic and analgesic properties with a large group of agents known as *nonsteroidal antiinflammatory drugs*[3] (NSAIDs), including acetylsalicylic acid (ASA), ibuprofen, and naproxen (4). However, acetaminophen itself is not an NSAID: it is not strongly antiinflammatory. NSAIDs act (at least, primarily) by inhibiting the enzyme cyclooxygenase (prostaglandin synthase), which catalyzes the first step in the biosynthesis of prostaglandins from arachidonic acid. John Vane shared the 1982 Nobel Prize in Physiology or Medicine for discovering the inhibitory action of ASA on prostaglandin biosynthesis (5). ASA is an irreversible inhibitor: it covalently modifies (by acetylation) a specific serine residue on the cyclooxygenase enzyme (6, p. 333).

Around 1990, molecular cloning revealed the existence of two distinct forms of cyclooxygenase, called COX-1 and COX-2 (7). COX-1 is constitutively expressed in most mammalian tissues. COX-2 is expressed in specific cell types (such as endothelial cells and synoviocytes) and is induced by inflammatory stimuli (8). ASA is a better inhibitor of COX-1 than of COX-2 (9). These advances in the understanding of the pharmacology of NSAIDs provoked the idea of designing specific inhibitors of COX-2. Medicinal chemists hoped that such inhibitors would show analgesic activity against chronic inflammatory conditions while presenting reduced risk of the toxic side effects of earlier NSAIDs (such as the gastrointestinal bleeding sometimes associated with ASA use). COX-2-specific inhibitors (e.g., celecoxib) were developed in the 1990s and, indeed, have been very successful therapeutic agents for arthritis, menstrual cramps, and other painful conditions (10). However, concerns over possible cardiovascular toxicity led to the withdrawal from sale of most COX-2 inhibitors in 2004.

MECHANISM OF THERAPEUTIC ACTION

The coal tar analgesics, such as acetaminophen, were discovered by accident, and their mechanism of action is still not properly understood. There is considerable overlap of activities between acetaminophen and NSAIDs, and they are treated as competitors in the marketplace for over-the-counter analgesics. Nevertheless, in vitro studies show that acetaminophen is not a highly potent inhibitor of COX-1 or COX-2 (although its inhibitory action may be greater under conditions of low ambient peroxide concentration (11)).

In 2002 researchers proposed that a third distinct form of cyclooxygenase, "COX-3," is expressed as a splice variant of the COX-1 gene (12). Canine COX-3, expressed as a protein in insect cells, proved to be highly sensitive to inhibition by acetaminophen, and this inhibition was suggested to account for the drug's analgesic effect. However, further molecular cloning studies (13) failed to confirm the existence of COX-3 in humans and the issue of its possible significance remains unresolved (14).

The search for a convincing mechanistic explanation of acetaminophen's therapeutic activity continues.

ACETAMINOPHEN: HUMAN TOXICITY

Acetaminophen has been used effectively and safely by very large numbers of patients, both children and adults, since its introduction to the consumer market in the 1950s. Despite the drug's safety when used asprescribed, however, acetaminophen toxicity can occur, due to either accidental or deliberate overdose ingestion of the drug (15). Postmortem analysis of fatal acetaminophen poisoning cases showed that death results from liver failure associated with hepatic centrilobular necrosis (16) (figure 19-2). The damaged and dying hepatocytes release, into the serum, characteristic liver enzymes such as aspartate aminotransferase (AST) and alanine aminotransferase (ALT), and measuring the levels of these enzyme activities in the blood provides a reliable clinical measure of hepatotoxicity due to acetaminophen (17) or other agents.

Since acetaminophen pills were often found in household medicine cabinets, children occasionally opened the bottles and swallowed the contents, especially before the introduction of "child-proof" packaging for hazardous products in the 1970s. In 1977 the Analgesic Review Panel of the U.S. Food and Drug Administration (FDA) recommended that all acetaminophen products carry a warning label stating that overdose can cause liver damage (1, p. 205). Unfortunately, acetaminophen continues to be chosen as a poison by suicidal individuals (18). In the U.K., about

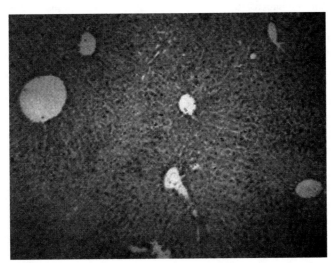

FIGURE 19-2.
Liver section from a mouse treated with acetaminophen (300 mg/kg; 4 hours) and stained with an antibody specific for acetaminophen adducts. The brown stain in the centrilobular regions indicates acetaminophen-protein adducts and the unstained regions are the periportal areas. *Note*: A full-color version of this figure appears on the website. (*Source: Hinson, J. A.; Pike, S. L.; Pumford, N. R.; Mayeux, P. R. Nitrotyrosine-protein adducts in hepatic centrilobular areas following toxic doses of acetaminophen in mice. Chem. Res. Toxicol. **1998**, 11, 604–607. Copyright 1998 American Chemical Society, used by permission.*)

500 deaths occur annually due to acetaminophen overdose, accounting for about 15% of fatal poisonings (*19*).

Because of the high incidence of acetaminophen poisoning cases, there has been ongoing research effort to understand the mechanisms of acetaminophen hepatotoxicity (*20, 21*) and to develop therapeutic interventions that can be administered to victims of acetaminophen overdoses. In discussing these topics, we need to begin by considering the metabolism of acetaminophen.

ACETAMINOPHEN AND ALCOHOL

Alcohol consumption can sensitize individuals to acetaminophen. Jordan Holtzman (*22, 23*) describes how he and his colleagues recognized this hazardous interaction:

> [W]e observed a series of patients who were hospitalized for acute, severe hepatic failure. These individuals had been drinking heavily and had suddenly stopped their alcohol consumption. They had then taken modest doses of acetaminophen for their hangovers and gone into acute hepatic failure. These individuals had aspartate amino-transferases (AST) and alanine aminotransferases (ALT) in the thousands, whereas the usual patient with alcoholic hepatitis has values in the hundreds. This led Dr. Kromhout, the clinical consultant reviewing the cases, to suspect that there was something unusual about these patients. He discovered that all of them had been on a drinking binge, had suddenly stopped drinking, and had taken acetaminophen for their hangovers. All had taken doses that were significantly less than the 16 g per day that is considered to be the minimum toxic dose. In fact, one of the patients who died had consumed only 4 g over 48 h. In light of these clinical observations, we examined the possibility of an interaction between acetaminophen and ethanol consumption in . . . mice. In this study we demonstrated a nearly 50% decrease in the LD_{50} for acetaminophen in mice receiving ethanol in their drinking water for 3 weeks. This report . . . probably represents the only study ever published in the *Journal of the American Medical Association* which included a probit plot for the LD_{50} of a drug in mice.

In 1998 the FDA issued a regulation requiring that acetaminophen products carry the following label: "Alcohol Warning: If you consume 3 or more alcoholic drinks every day, ask your doctor whether you should take acetaminophen. . . . Acetaminophen may cause liver damage."

The mechanism of the alcohol–acetaminophen interaction is still not fully understood. Alcohol induces cytochrome P450 2E1 in humans (see chapter 8) and this enzyme activates acetaminophen to a toxic metabolite, as discussed later in this chapter. Other mechanisms are also believed to contribute, such as ethanol-dependent depletion of hepatic glutathione (*24*).

METABOLISM: CONJUGATION REACTIONS

The phenolic —OH group of acetaminophen is available for metabolic conjugation reactions. At therapeutic doses of the drug, about one-half and

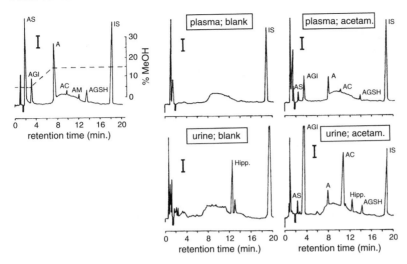

FIGURE 19-3.

Reversed-phase HPLC analysis of acetaminophen metabolites in mice. Top left: mixture of standards. AS = acetaminophen sulfate; AGl = acetaminophen glucuronide; A = acetaminophen; AC = acetaminophen cysteine conjugate; AM = acetaminophen mercapturic acid; AGSH = acetaminophen glutathione conjugate; IS = internal standard (acetanilide). Right: chromatograms of extracts of plasma and urine samples from mice before (left) and after (right) administration of acetaminophen. Hipp = hippuric acid, an endogenous compound found in the urine. (*Source: To, E. C.; Wells, P. G. Repetitive microvolumetric sampling and analysis of acetaminophen and its toxicologically relevant metabolites in murine plasma and urine using high performance liquid chromatography. J. Anal. Toxicol. 1985, 9, 217–221.*)

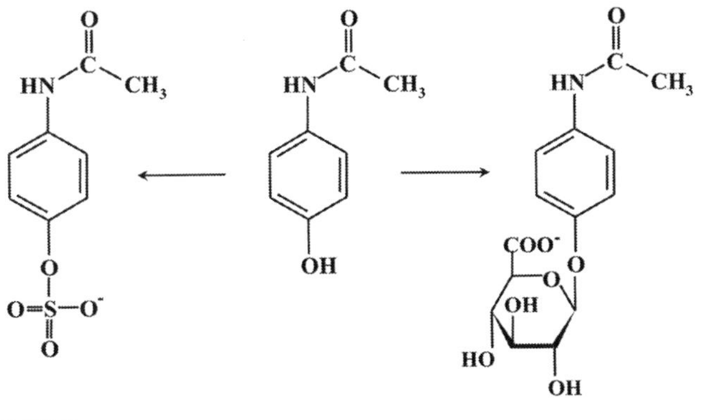

FIGURE 19-4.

Metabolic conjugation of acetaminophen.

one-third of the excreted urinary metabolite is in the forms of acetaminophen *O*-glucuronide and acetaminophen *O*-sulfate, respectively (figures 19-3 and 19-4). These conjugations detoxify acetaminophen. Peter Wells and colleagues have shown, in studies with the UDPGT-deficient Gunn rat and other animal models (*25, 26*), that impairment of glucuronidation results in enhanced acetaminophen toxicity. This increased sensitivity may also obtain in humans with Gilbert's syndrome (27) (see chapter 12). The sulfation pathway becomes saturated at high acetaminophen doses, because of either limited supply of PAPS substrate or limited sulfotransferase enzyme capacity (28). In humans, serum sulfate levels drop after acetaminophen ingestion (29).

OXIDATION OF PHENACETIN AND ACETAMINOPHEN

Quantitatively, only a few percent of an administered dose of acetaminophen undergoes oxidative metabolism, but this process determines the toxicity of the drug.

Before we discuss the oxidation of acetaminophen, it is useful to consider the case of phenacetin and the differences between the oxidation chemistries of these two analgesics. Phenacetin undergoes typical P450-catalyzed oxidation reactions: O-dealkylation to give acetaminophen, as already mentioned; ring hydroxylation to give 2-hydroxyphenacetin and 3-hydroxyphenacetin (30); and N-hydroxylation to give N-hydroxyphenacetin, which accounts for about 0.5% of the urinary excretion of phenacetin in humans (31). N-Hydroxyphenacetin is undoubtedly a more significant primary metabolite than this percentage indicates: most of the metabolite does not reach the urine. N-Hydroxyphenacetin can be bioactivated to reactive mutagenic intermediates (32), such as the nitroso compound p-nitrosophenetole (formed by deacetylation and N-oxidation; figure 19-5, upper panel) and reactive N,O esters formed by sulfation or glucuronidation reactions (33). These processes probably account for phenacetin's carcinogenic activity.

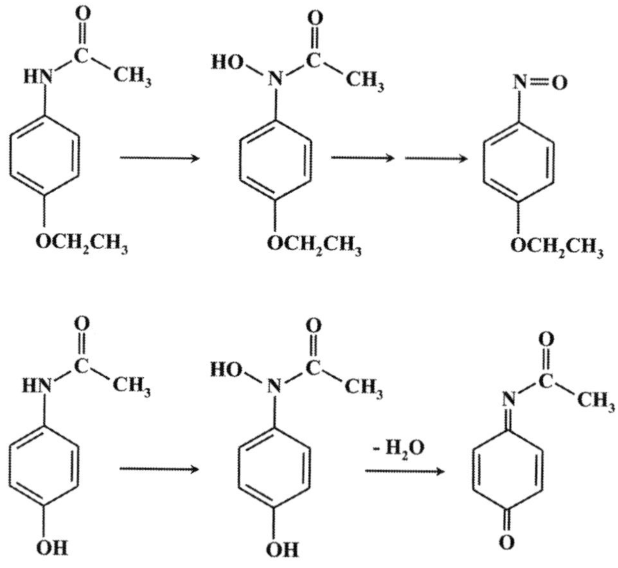

FIGURE 19-5.

Top: production of p-nitrosophenetole from N-hydroxyphenacetin. Bottom: production of N-hydroxyacetaminophen and N-acetyl-p-benzoquinoneimine from acetaminophen.

In the case of acetaminophen, P450-catalyzed N-oxidation might be expected to form *N*-hydroxyacetaminophen. However, the presence of a hydroxy rather than an alkoxy substituent *para* to the amide function makes the chemistry of acetaminophen very different from that of phenacetin. Two distinct two-electron oxidation products of acetaminophen exist: *N*-hydroxyacetaminophen and its dehydration product *N*-acetyl-*p*-benzo-quinoneimine (NAPQI; figure 19-5, lower panel.) In fact, NAPQI, not *N*-hydroxyacetaminophen is observed as a P450-catalyzed metabolite (*34*). Could the *N*-hydroxy derivative be an intermediate in NAPQI formation? Elimination of water from *N*-hydroxyacetaminophen would yield NAPQI (figure 19-6). However, when *N*-hydroxyacetaminophen was synthesized (*35*), its half-life (in aqueous solution at 37°C) was found to be 80 min (*36*), which is much too slow a process to account for P450-dependent formation of the iminoquinone (*34*). A more likely mechanism is one-electron removal from the substrate by P450 to give the cation radical intermediate; deprotonation and transfer of a second electron to the heme group, giving NAPQI, then occurs much more rapidly than oxygen rebound (chapter 7) to give the *N*-hydroxy derivative.

Several human P450 enzymes can oxidize acetaminophen to the iminoquinone, including forms 1A2, 2A6, 2D6, and 2E1 (*37, 38*). The connection between P450-mediated acetaminophen metabolism and toxicity was confirmed by studies with knockout mice. Mice lacking P450 1A2 or P450 2E1 were more resistant to acetaminophen than were wild-type animals (increased LD_{50}). Double knockout mice lacking both P450 1A2 and 2E1 enzymes were very much more resistant to the drug, with almost all of the mice surviving a dose of 1.2 g/kg body weight; half of that dose was already 100% lethal to the wild-type animals (*39, 40*). Knockout mice devoid of the nuclear receptor CAR (see chapter 8) do not

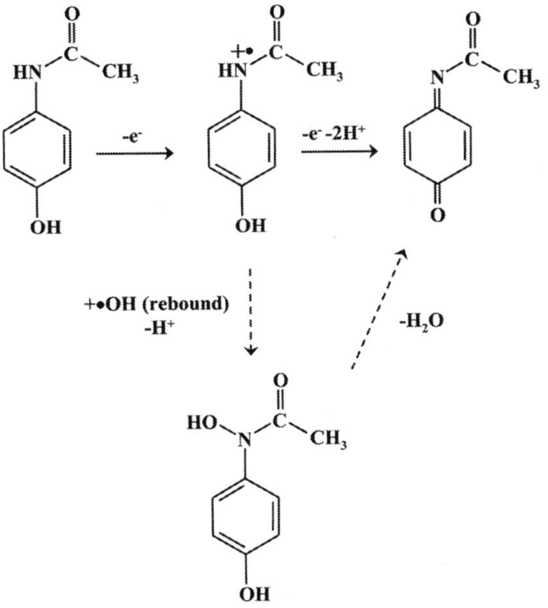

FIGURE 19-6.
Reactions of *N*-hydroxyacetaminophen.

show induction of P450 1A2, P450 3A11 (corresponding to human form 3A4), or glutathione transferase Pi in response to acetaminophen, and are also highly resistant to its hepatotoxicity (*41*).

Peroxidase/hydrogen peroxide systems, which characteristically oxidize organic substrates in one-electron steps, generate the acetaminophen cation radical. The electron paramagnetic resonance (EPR) spectrum of the short-lived radical can be detected in solution, using fast-flow systems (*42, 43*). The radical reacts rapidly with itself to form polymeric products.

REACTIONS OF *N*-ACETYL-*P*-BENZOQUINONE-IMINE; GSH CONJUGATION

The quinoneimine oxidation product of acetaminophen, NAPQI, is a reactive electrophile (*44–46*) (see chapter 10). The spontaneous reaction of NAPQI with GSH is rapid and yields the adduct 3-(glutathion-*S*-yl)acetaminophen via Michael addition; a redox reaction also occurs, giving a lesser amount of acetaminophen plus glutathione disulfide (*47*). Glutathione transferases of several classes can catalyze both reactions. At high acetaminophen doses, liver cells become completely depleted of GSH and the activated acetaminophen binds covalently to cellular proteins (figure 19-7). The major nucleophilic targets in proteins are the thiol groups of cysteine residues (*48*).

The onset of liver damage follows GSH depletion (*49*). Figure 19-8 shows results of a study of acetaminophen toxicity in dogs. Methemoglobinemia occurs with a time-course similar to that of acetaminophen in serum, but this hematological effect is transient and does not cause long-term toxicity. Once hepatic GSH becomes substantially depleted, hepatotoxicity ensues, as indicated by the prolonged rise in liver-derived transaminase and alkaline phosphatase levels in the serum. Also, as mentioned below, intervention to sustain hepatic GSH is an effective treatment for acetaminophen overdose. Most researchers agree that hepatic GSH depletion is the critical trigger for acetaminophen hepatotoxicity (*50*).

COVALENT BINDING TO PROTEINS

James R. Gillette (*51*) was one of the scientists recruited to the Laboratory of Chemical Pharmacology at NIH in the 1950s, by Bernard B. Brodie

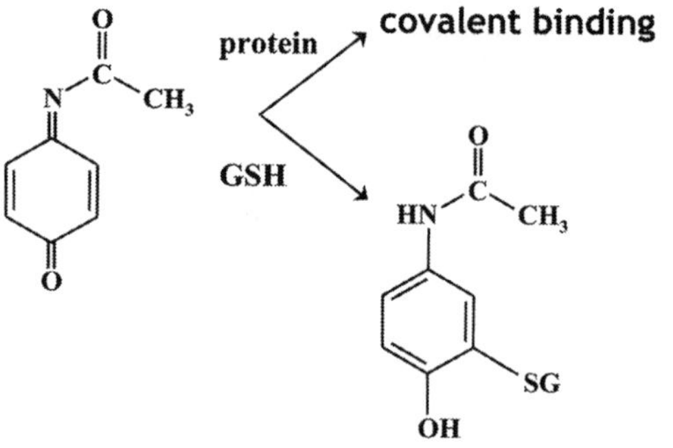

FIGURE 19-7.
Reaction of NAPQI with GSH competing with covalent binding to protein.

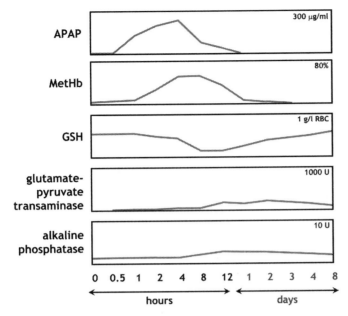

FIGURE 19-8.

Time-course profiles of serum parameters in dogs receiving oral acetaminophen (500 mg/kg). Key: APAP, acetaminophen; MetHB, methemoglobin; GSH, glutathione; the two lower traces show the rise in serum levels of hepatic enzymes, indicating hepatotoxicity. (*Data obtained from Savides, M. C.; Oehme, F. W.; Nash, S. L.; Leipold, H. W. The toxicity and biotransformation of single doses of acetaminophen in dogs and cats.* Toxicol. Appl. Pharmacol. **1984**, 74, 26–34.)

(see chapter 7). In 1973 Gillette, Brodie, and colleagues published a set of four papers delineating the involvement of covalent binding to protein in the mechanism of acetaminophen hepatotoxicity in mice (*52–55*). These influential studies demonstrated that radioactivity of ^{3}H-labeled or ^{14}C-carbonyl-labeled acetaminophen became irreversibly bound to hepatic proteins. Binding was observed in all subcellular compartments examined: nuclear, mitochondrial, endoplasmic reticular, and cytosolic. This binding was far greater in liver than in nontarget tissues (e.g., muscle). Pretreatment of mice with P450 inhibitors decreased both the covalent binding and the hepatotoxicity, whereas pretreatment with P450 inducers increased both parameters. Later studies used immunohistochemistry with antibodies against acetaminophen–protein adducts to show that the histological pattern of covalent adduction matches that of the toxicity, with damage to the centrilobular rather than the periportal regions (*56*). Gillette and colleagues also demonstrated the protective role of glutathione. Understanding the significance of GSH for acetaminophen detoxication led directly to improved clinical therapy for acetaminophen poisoning. Administration of *N-acetyl-L-cysteine*, which replenishes GSH stores (*57*) remains the treatment of choice in human overdose cases (*58*).

PROTEIN BINDING AND HEPATOTOXICITY

Subsequent evidence has supported Gillette's hypothesis that covalent binding to protein following GSH depletion causes hepatocellular necrosis

TABLE 19-1.

Hepatic Proteins Adducted By Acetaminophen (Mouse Liver; Partial List)

ENZYME/PROTEIN	COMPARTMENT
Aldehyde dehydrogenase	Cytosol, mitochondria
ATP synthetase α-subunit	Mitochondria
Glutamine synthetase	ER
Glutathione peroxidase	Cytosol, mitochondria
Glutathione transferase	Cytosol, mitochondria
Glycine N-methyltransferase	Cytosol
3-Hydroxyanthraniliate 3,4-dioxygenase	Cytosol
Tropomyosin 5	Cytoskeleton
Urate oxidase	Peroxisomes

Adapted from James, L. P.; Mayeux, P. R.; Hinson, J. A. Acetaminophen-induced hepatotoxicity. Drug Metab. Dispos. **2003,** 31, *1499–1506.*

and toxicity. As already noted, factors that potentiate or lessen protein binding have corresponding effects on hepatotoxicity. Hinson and colleagues (*59*) used antiserum to the 3-(cystein-S-yl) adduct, formed by reaction of NAPQI with protein cysteine residues, to study acetaminophen toxicity in mice. Patterns of adduct formation correlated with patterns of toxicity, in terms of anatomical distribution within the liver, dose–response, and time-course.

An alternative view is that oxidative stress, rather than protein binding per se, initiates hepatotoxicity. Certainly, many characteristic features of oxidative stress (see chapter 1) are observed in acetaminophen hepatotoxicity, including lipid peroxidation, mitochondrial damage and ATP depletion, and formation of nitrotyrosine adducts in proteins, presumably due to formation of superoxide-derived peroxynitrite (*60*). However, these processes may be consequences of damage mediated by protein adduction, rather than direct causes of hepatotoxicity.

Are there specific proteins that represent critical targets for acetaminophen-mediated hepatotoxicity? Ongoing efforts have been directed to the identification of proteins adducted/inactivated by acetaminophen binding, using radiolabeling, immunological, and proteomic methods, including mass spectrometry (*61*). A sample of acetaminophen target proteins that have been identified is shown in table 19-1.

No single protein or set of proteins, and no specific subcellular compartment, has been found to be a uniquely sensitive target of acetaminophen adduction, although oxidative damage to the mitochondrion may be of particular importance (*62*). For the time being, one concludes that hepatocellular damage results from the aggregated effect of damage to multiple proteins and simultaneous inhibition of many enzymes and cellular functions (*63*).

Notes

1. A few years later, another Bayer chemist, Felix Hoffmann, acetylated salicylic acid to produce acetylsalicylic acid: Bayer "Aspirin."

2. Von Mering is also remembered for his discovery that diabetes can be induced in dogs by removal of the pancreas.

3. The term "nonsteroidal" distinguishes them from the antiinflammatory steroids, such as hydrocortisone.

References

1. Mann, C. C.; Plummer, M. L. *The Aspirin Wars: Money, Medicine, and 100 Years of Rampant Competition;* Knopf: New York, 1991.

2. Gaakeer, H. A.; De Ruiter, H. J. Carcinoma of the renal pelvis following the abuse of phenacetin-containing analgesic drugs. *Br. J. Urol.* **1979,** *51,* 188–192.

3. Boréus, L. O.; Sandberg, F. A comparison of some pharmacological effects of acetophenetidin and N-acetyl-*p*-aminophenol. *Adv. Physiol. Scand.* **1953,** *28,* 261–265.

4. Paulus, H. E.; Whitehouse, M. W. Nonsteroid anti-inflammatory agents. *Annu. Rev. Pharmacol.* **1973,** *13,* 107–125.

5. Vane, J. R. Inhibition of prostaglandin synthesis as a mechanism of action for aspirin-like drugs. *Nat. New Biol.* **1971,** *231,* 232–235.

6. Berg, J. M.; Tymoczko, J. L.; Stryer, L. *Biochemistry;* WH Freeman: New York, 2001.

7. Vane, J. R.; Bakhle, Y. S.; Botting, R. M. Cyclooxygenases 1 and 2. *Annu. Rev. Pharmacol. Toxicol.* **1998,** *38,* 97–120.

8. Crofford, L. J. COX-1 and COX-2 tissue expression: implications and predictions. *J. Rheumatol.* **1997,** *24* (Suppl. 49), 15–19.

9. Mitchell, J. A.; Akarasereenont, P.; Thiemermann, C.; Flower, R. J.; Vane, J. R. Selectivity of nonsteroidal antiinflammatory drugs as inhibitors of constitutive and inducible cyclooxygenase. *Proc. Natl. Acad. Sci. USA* **1993,** *90,* 11693–11697.

10. McMurray, R. W.; Hardy, K. J. Cox-2 inhibitors: today and tomorrow. *Am. J. Med. Sci.* **2002,** *323,* 181–189.

11. Ouellet, M.; Percival, M. D. Mechanism of acetaminophen inhibition of cyclooxygenase isoforms. *Arch. Biochem. Biophys.* **2001,** *387,* 273–280.

12. Chandrasekharan, N. V.; Dai, H.; Roos, K. L.; Evanson, N. K.; Tomsik, J.; Elton, T. S.; Simmons, D. L. COX-3, a cyclooxygenase-1 variant inhibited by acetaminophen and other analgesic/antipyretic drugs: cloning, structure, and expression. *Proc. Natl. Acad. Sci. USA* **2002,** *99,* 13926–13931.

13. Dinchuk, J. E.; Liu, R. Q.; Trzaskos, J. M. COX-3: in the wrong frame in mind. *Immunol. Lett.* **2003,** *86,* 121.

14. Schwab, J. M.; Beiter, T.; Linder, J. U.; Laufer, S.; Schulz, J. E.; Meyermann, R.; Schluesener, H. J. COX-3: a virtual pain target in humans? *FASEB J.* **2003,** *17,* 2174–2175.

15. McClain, C. J.; Price, S.; Barve, S.; Devalarja, R.; Shedlofsky, S. Acetaminophen hepatotoxicity: an update. *Curr. Gastroenterol. Rep.* **1999,** *1,* 42–49.

16. McJunkin, B.; Barwick, K. W.; Little, W. C.; Winfield, J. B. Fatal massive hepatic necrosis following acetaminophen overdose. *JAMA* **1976,** *236,* 1874–1875.

17. Singer, A. J.; Carracio, T. R.; Mofenson, H. C. The temporal profile of increased transaminase levels in patients with acetaminophen-induced liver dysfunction. *Ann. Emerg. Med.* **1995,** *26,* 49–53.

18. Gyamlani, G. G.; Parikh, C. R. Acetaminophen toxicity: suicidal vs. accidental. *Crit. Care* **2002,** *6,* 155–159.

19. Sheen, C. L.; Dillon, J. F.; Bateman, D. N.; Simpson, K. J.; MacDonald, T. M. Paracetamol-related deaths in Scotland, 1994–2000. *Br. J. Clin. Pharmacol.* **2002**, *54*, 430–432.

20. Bromer, M. Q.; Black, M. Acetaminophen hepatotoxicity. *Clin. Liver Dis.* **2003**, *7*, 351–367.

21. Rumack, B. H. Acetaminophen hepatotoxicity: the first 35 years. *J. Toxicol. Clin. Toxicol.* **2002**, *40*, 3–20.

22. Holtzman, J. L. The role of covalent binding to microsomal proteins in the hepatotoxicity of acetaminophen. *Drug Metab. Rev.* **1995**, *27*, 277–297.

23. McClain, C. J.; Kromhout, J. P.; Peterson, F. J.; Holtzman, J. L. Potentiation of acetaminophen hepatotoxicity by alcohol. *JAMA* **1980**, *244*, 251–253.

24. Zhao, P.; Kalhorn, T. F.; Slattery, J. T. Selective mitochondrial glutathione depletion by ethanol enhances acetaminophen toxicity in rat liver. *Hepatology* **2002**, *36*, 326–335.

25. de Morais, S. M.; Chow, S. Y.; Wells, P. G. Biotransformation and toxicity of acetaminophen in congenic RHA rats with or without a hereditary deficiency in bilirubin UDP-glucuronosyltransferase. *Toxicol. Appl. Pharmacol.* **1992**, *117*, 81–87.

26. de Morais, S. M.; Wells, P. G. Enhanced acetaminophen toxicity in rats with bilirubin glucuronyl transferase deficiency. *Hepatology* **1989**, *10*, 163–167.

27. de Morais, S. M.; Uetrecht, J. P.; Wells, P. G. Decreased glucuronidation and increased bioactivation of acetaminophen in Gilbert's syndrome. *Gastroenterology* **1992**, *102*, 577–586.

28. Liu, L.; Klaassen, C. D. Different mechanism of saturation of acetaminophen sulfate conjugation in mice and rats. Toxicol. Appl. Pharmacol. **1996**, *139*, 128–134.

29. Morris, M. E.; Levy, G. Serum concentration and renal excretion by normal adults of inorganic sulfate after acetaminophen, ascorbic acid, or sodium sulfate. *Clin. Pharmacol. Ther.* **1983**, *33*, 529–536.

30. Büch, H.; Pfleger, K.; Rummel, W.; Ullrich, V.; Hey, D.; Staudinger, H. Studies on the oxidative metabolism of phenacetin in rats (in German). *Biochem. Pharmacol.* **1967**, *16*, 2247–2256.

31. Veronese, M. E.; McLean, S.; D'Souza, C. A.; Davies, N. W. Formation of reactive metabolites of phenacetin in humans and rats. *Xenobiotica* **1985**, *15*, 929–940.

32. Nohmi, T.; Mizokami, K.; Kawano, S.; Fukuhara, M.; Ishidate, M. J. Metabolic activation of phenacetin and phenetidine by several forms of cytochrome P-450 purified from liver microsomes of rats and hamsters. *Jpn. J. Cancer Res.* **1987**, *78*, 153–161.

33. Hinson, J. A. Reactive metabolites of phenacetin and acetaminophen: a review. *Environ. Health Perspect.* **1983**, *49*, 71–79.

34. Dahlin, D. C.; Miwa, G. T.; Lu, A. Y.; Nelson, S. D. N-Acetyl-*p*-benzoquinone imine: a cytochrome P-450-mediated oxidation product of acetaminophen. *Proc. Natl. Acad. Sci. USA* **1984**, *81*, 1327–1331.

35. Gemborys, M. W.; Gribble, G. W.; Mudge, G. H. Synthesis of N-hydroxyacetaminophen, a postulated toxic metabolite of acetaminophen, and its phenolic sulfate conjugate. *J. Med. Chem.* **1978**, *21*, 649–652.

36. Calder, I. C.; Hart, S. J.; Healey, K.; Ham, K. N. N-Hydroxyacetaminophen: a postulated toxic metabolite of acetaminophen. *J. Med. Chem.* **1981**, *24*, 988–993.

37. Chen, W.; Koenigs, L. L.; Thompson, S. J.; Peter, R. M.; Rettie, A. E.; Trager, W. F.; Nelson, S. D. Oxidation of acetaminophen to its toxic quinone imine and nontoxic catechol metabolites by baculovirus-expressed and purified human cytochromes P450 2E1 and 2A6. *Chem. Res. Toxicol.* **1998,** *11,* 295–301.

38. Dong, H.; Haining, R. L.; Thummel, K. E.; Rettie, A. E.; Nelson, S. D. Involvement of human cytochrome P450 2D6 in the bioactivation of acetaminophen. *Drug Metab. Dispos.* **2000,** *28,* 1397–1400.

39. Zaher, H.; Buters, J. T. M.; Ward, J. M.; Bruno, M. K.; Lucas, A. M.; Stern, S. T.; Cohen, S. D.; Gonzalez, F. J. Protection against acetaminophen toxicity in CYP1A2 and CYP2E1 double-null mice. *Toxicol. Appl. Pharmacol.* **1998,** *152,* 193–199.

40. Gonzalez, F. J. Role of cytochromes P450 in chemical toxicity and oxidative stress: studies with CYP2E1. *Mutat. Res.* **2005,** *569,* 101–110.

41. Zhang, J.; Huang, W.; Chua, S. S.; Wei, P.; Moore, D. D. Modulation of acetaminophen-induced hepatotoxicity by the xenobiotic receptor CAR. *Science* **2002,** *298,* 422–424.

42. Martin, C. N.; Garner, R. C. The identification and assessment of covalent binding in vitro and in vivo. In *Biochemical Toxicology: A Practical Approach*; Snell, K., Mullock, B., Eds.; IRL Press: Oxford, 1987; pp. 109–128.

43. Mason, R. P.; Fischer, V. Free radicals of acetaminophen: their subsequent reactions and toxicological significance. *Fed. Proc.* **1986,** *45,* 2493–2499.

44. Corcoran, G. B.; Mitchell, J. R.; Vaishnav, Y. N.; Horning, E. C. Evidence that acetaminophen and N-hydroxyacetaminophen form a common arylating intermediate, N-acetyl-p-benzoquinoneimine. *Mol. Pharmacol.* **1980,** *18,* 536–542.

45. Streeter, A. J.; Dahlin, D. C.; Nelson, S. D.; Baillie, T. A. The covalent binding of acetaminophen to protein. Evidence for cysteine residues as major sites of arylation in vitro. *Chem. Biol. Interact.* **1984,** *48,* 349–366.

46. McGirr, L. G.; Subrahmanyam, V. V.; Moore, G. A.; O'Brien, P. J. Peroxidase-catalyzed-3-(glutathion-S-yl)-p,p′-biphenol formation. *Chem. Biol. Interact.* **1986,** *60,* 85–99.

47. Coles, B.; Wilson, I.; Wardman, P.; Hinson, J. A.; Nelson, S. D.; Ketterer, B. The spontaneous and enzymatic reaction of N-acetyl-*p*-benzoquinonimine with glutathione: a stopped-flow kinetic study. *Arch. Biochem. Biophys.* **1988,** *264,* 253–260.

48. Hoffmann, K. J.; Streeter, A. J.; Axworthy, D. B.; Baillie, T. A. Identification of the major covalent adduct formed in vitro and in vivo between acetaminophen and mouse liver proteins. *Mol. Pharmacol.* **1985,** *27,* 566–573.

49. Savides, M. C.; Oehme, F. W.; Nash, S. L.; Leipold, H. W. The toxicity and biotransformation of single doses of acetaminophen in dogs and cats. *Toxicol. Appl. Pharmacol.* **1984,** *74,* 26–34.

50. Bessems, J. G.; Vermeulen, N. P. Paracetamol (acetaminophen)-induced toxicity: molecular and biochemical mechanisms, analogues and protective approaches. *Crit. Rev. Toxicol.* **2001,** *31,* 55–138.

51. Estabrook, R. W. A tribute to James Robert Gillette. *Drug Metab. Dispos.* **2003,** *31,* 1459–1460.

52. Mitchell, J. R.; Jollow, D. J.; Potter, W. Z.; Davis, D. C.; Gillette, J. R.; Brodie, B. B. Acetaminophen-induced hepatic necrosis: I. Role of drug metabolism. *J. Pharmacol. Exp. Ther.* **1973,** *187,* 185–194.

53. Jollow, D. J.; Mitchell, J. R.; Potter, W. Z.; Davis, D. C.; Gillette, J. R.; Brodie, B. B. Acetaminophen-induced hepatic necrosis: II. Role of covalent binding in vivo. *J. Pharmacol. Exp. Ther.* **1973**, *187*, 195–202.

54. Potter, W. Z.; Davis, D. C.; Mitchell, J. R.; Jollow, D. J.; Gillette, J. R.; Brodie, B. B. Acetaminophen-induced hepatic necrosis: III. Cytochrome P-450-mediated covalent binding in vitro. *J. Pharmacol. Exp. Ther.* **1973**, *187*, 203–210.

55. Mitchell, J. R.; Jollow, D. J.; Potter, W. Z.; Gillette, J. R.; Brodie, B. B. Acetaminophen-induced hepatic necrosis: IV. Protective role of glutathione. *J. Pharmacol. Exp. Ther.* **1973**, *187*, 211–217.

56. Hinson, J. A.; Pike, S. L.; Pumford, N. R.; Mayeux, P. R. Nitrotyrosine-protein adducts in hepatic centrilobular areas following toxic doses of acetaminophen in mice. *Chem. Res. Toxicol.* **1998**, *11*, 604–607.

57. Hazelton, G. A.; Hjelle, J. J.; Klaassen, C. D. Effects of cysteine pro-drugs on acetaminophen-induced hepatotoxicity. *J. Pharmacol. Exp. Ther.* **1986**, *237*, 341–349.

58. Smilkstein, M. J.; Bronstein, A. C.; Linden, C.; Augenstein, W. L.; Kulig, K. W.; Rumack, B. H. Acetaminophen overdose: a 48-hour intravenous N-acetylcysteine treatment protocol. *Ann. Emerg. Med.* **1991**, *20*, 1058–1063.

59. Roberts, D. W.; Bucci, T. J.; Benson, R. W.; Warbritton, A. R.; McRae, T. A.; Pumford, N. R.; Hinson, J. A. Immunohistochemical localization and quantification of the 3-(cystein-S-yl)-acetaminophen protein adduct in acetaminophen hepatotoxicity. *Am. J. Pathol.* **1991**, *138*, 359–371.

60. Jaeschke, H.; Knight, T. R.; Bajt, M. L. The role of oxidant stress and reactive nitrogen species in acetaminophen hepatotoxicity. *Toxicol. Lett.* **2003**, *144*, 279–288.

61. Ruepp, S. U.; Tonge, R. P.; Shaw, J.; Wallis, N.; Pognan, F. Genomics and proteomics analysis of acetaminophen toxicity in mouse liver. *Toxicol. Sci.* **2002**, *65*, 135–150.

62. Hinson, J. A.; Reid, A. B.; McCullough, S. S.; James, L. P. Acetaminophen-induced hepatotoxicity: role of metabolic activation, reactive oxygen/nitrogen species, and mitochondrial permeability transition. *Drug Metab. Rev.* **2004**, *36*, 805–822.

63. Coen, M.; Lenz, E. M.; Nicholson, J. K.; Wilson, I. D.; Pognan, F.; Lindon, J. C. An integrated metabonomic investigation of acetaminophen toxicity in the mouse using NMR spectroscopy. *Chem. Res. Toxicol.* **2003**, *16*, 295–303.